Intellectual Disabilities
Toward Inclusion

Intellectual Disabilities
Toward Inclusion

EDITION : 7TH

Editors:
Helen Atherton, BSc (Hons), PhD, RNLD
Lecturer in Nursing
School of Healthcare
University of Leeds, Leeds
United Kingdom

Debbie Crickmore, BSc (Hons), MSc, RNLD
Formerly, Lecturer in Learning Disability
Faculty of Health Sciences
University of Hull, Hull
United Kingdom

ELSEVIER

Notices

Practitioners and researchers must always rely on their own experience and knowledge in evaluating and using any information, methods, compounds or experiments described herein. Because of rapid advances in the medical sciences, in particular, independent verification of diagnoses and drug dosages should be made. To the fullest extent of the law, no responsibility is assumed by Elsevier, authors, editors or contributors for any injury and/or damage to persons or property as a matter of products liability, negligence or otherwise, or from any use or operation of any methods, products, instructions, or ideas contained in the material herein.

ISBN: 978-0-7020-8150-7

Cover image *Jigsaw puzzle of life* by Ria - www.pyramid.org.uk/ria

Content Strategist: Robert Edwards
Content Project Manager: Shivani Pal
Design: Julia Dummitt

Printed in Scotland

Last digit is the print number: 9   8   7   6   5   4   3   2   1

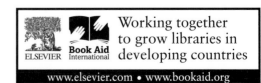

CONTRIBUTORS

Andy Alaszewski, BA, PhD
Emeritus Professor, Centre for Health
Services Studies, University of Kent,
Canterbury, UK

Helen Alaszewski, BA, RGN
Formerly Research Fellow
Centre for Health Services Studies
University of Kent, Canterbury, UK

Salma Ali
Registered & Chartered Forensic
Psychologist
Barnet, Enfield & Haringey NHS Trust
UK

Tom P. Berney, MB, ChB, DPM,
FRCPsych, FRCPCH
The Royal College of Psychiatrists,
UK

Kristin Björnsdóttir, PhD
Professor
Faculty of Education and Diversity,
University of Iceland, Reykjavík
Iceland

Christian Brandt, MD
Head of Department
General Epileptology
Bethel Epilepsy Centre, Bielefeld
Germany

Susan Buell, PhD
Lecturer
School of Nursing and Health Sciences
Dundee University, Dundee
UK

Karen Bunning, PhD
Associate Professor
School of Health Sciences
University of East Anglia, Norwich
UK

Anne-Marie Callus, MEd, PhD
Senior Lecturer
Department of Disability Studies
University of Malta, Msida
Malta

Maria Caples, PGDip TLHE, MSc,
PGDip Ger, RNID, PhD
Lecturer
School of Nursing and Midwifery
University College Cork, Cork
Ireland

Caroline Dalton O'Connor, MSc,
BNS
Lecturer
School of Nursing and Midwifery
University College Cork , Cork
Ireland

Mary Dearing, BSc(Hons), MSc
Formerly Lecturer
Department of Psychological Health &
Wellbeing
The University of Hull, Hull
UK

Mary Doherty, MB BCh, FCARCSI
Consultant Anaesthetist
Our Lady's Hospital, Navan
Ireland

Simon Duffy, MA, PhD
President
Citizen Network
Sheffield, UK

Petri Embregts
Professor
Tilburg University
School of Social and Behavioral Sciences,
Tranzo
Tilburg
Netherlands

Rebecca Fish, BA, MA, PhD
Researcher
Centre for Disability Research
Lancaster University, Lancaster
UK

Ruth Garbutt, BA(Hons), PGDip,
MA, DipSW, PGCLTHE, PhD
Senior Lecturer in Learning Disability
School of Health and Society.
University of Salford.
UK

Susan Hunter
Senior Lecturer in Social Work
(retired)
School of Political and Social Science
University of Edinburgh, UK

Simon Jarrett, BA, MA, PhD
Honorary research fellow
History Classics & Archaeology
Birkbeck, University of London,
London
UK

Joann Kiernan, BSc, MSc, PhD
Consultant Learning Disability Nurse/
Senior Lecturer
Alder Hey Children's Hospital
Liverpool
UK
Faculty of Health Social Care and Medicine
Edge Hill University,
Ormskirk
UK

Peter Langdon, BSc(Hons),
DClinPsy, AFBPsS, CPsychol, PhD
Professor
Centre for Educational Development,
Appraisal and Research, and Centre for
Mental Health and Wellbeing
University of Warwick, Coventry
UK

Jo Lay, MA, BSc(Hons)
Lecturer
School of Healthcare
University of Leeds, Leeds
UK

Susan Ledger, MSc, BA(Hons), PhD
School of Health, Wellbeing and Social Care
The Open University, Milton Keynes
UK

Theresa Lorenzo
Professor
Department of Health and
Rehabilitation Sciences
Faculty of Sciences
University of Cape Town, Cape Town
South Africa

Beth Marks, PhD, RN, FAAN
Research Associate Professor
Department of Disability and Human
Development
University of Illinois at Chicago,
Chicago
Illinois
United States

Lynne Marsh, RNID, BSc (Hons),
MSc, PG Dip, MA TLHE, SFHEA,
Doctor of Nursing (DN),
Senior Lecturer,
School of Nursing and Midwifery,
Queen's University Belfast, Belfast,
Northern Ireland, UK

Anne-Marie Martin, MSc, Grad.
Dip, HDip, PGDip TLHE, BSc, PhD
Lecturer
School of Nursing and Midwifery
University College Cork, Cork
Ireland

Zuzana Matousova, BSc(Hons),
DipResearch, RNLD, PhD
Director, New Beginnings: Intellectual
Disability and Autism Coach,
Cape Town
South Africa

Edward McCann, MSc, PhD, MA,
RN, RPN, RNT, SFHEA, FEANS
Lecturer
Nursing and Midwifery
Trinity College Dublin, Dublin
Ireland

Roy McConkey, BA, PhD
Emeritus Professor
Institute of Nursing and Health
Research
Ulster University, Newtownabbey
Northern Ireland
UK

Ruth Northway, MSc, PhD
Professor of Learning Disability
Nursing
School of Care Sciences
University of South Wales,
Pontypridd
UK

John O'Brien, D Phil
Citizen Network, Lithonia
Georgia
United States

Sharon Paley, PGDip Research
Methodology, PG Cert Intellectual
Disability, RNLD
Head of Quality Risk and Compliance
Quality Risk and Compliance
SEQUAL, Brisbane
Queensland
Australia

Maria Pallisera, PhD
Professor
Department of Pedagogy
University of Girona, Girona
Catalonia
Spain

Linda Diane Parham, PhD, OTR/L,
FAOTA
Professor
Occupational Therapy Graduate
Program, School of Medicine,
University of New Mexico
United States

Jillian Pawlyn, RNLD, SCLD, TCH,
BA Hons, MSc
Lecturer in Nursing, Learning
Disabilities
School of Health, Wellbeing and Social
Care, Faculty of Wellbeing, Education
and Language Studies
The Open University, Milton Keynes
UK

Sue Read, MA, RN, CertEd, PhD
Professor of Learning Disability
Nursing
Nursing & Midwifery
Keele University, Stoke-on-Trent
UK

Stacey Rees, MSc, BN(Hons),
BSc(Hons), PhD
Lecturer
Faculty of Life Sciences & Education
University of South Wales, Pontypridd
UK

Vigdis Reisæter, PhD candidate
Department of Special Need Education
University of Oslo, Oslo
Norway
Department of Welfare and
Participation
Western Norway University of Applied
Science Campus Sogndal
Norway

Pete Richmond, CQSW, MSc
CEO of the Partners for Inclusion
Group
Kilmarnock
Scotland
UK

James Ridley, BSc, Dip Prof Studies,
Dip HE, PGCTLHE, MA
Faculty of Health, Social Care and
Medicine
Edge Hill University, Ormskirk
UK

Julie Ridley, BA(Hons), PhD
Reader in Applied Social Sciences,
School of Social Work, Care and
Community, University of Central
Lancashire, Preston, UK

Kim Scarborough, MSc PMLD and
MSI, Post Grad Certificate Applied
Research, PGCHE, BSc Community
Studies, RNLD, RNT
Senior Lecturer
Health and Social Care
University of Gloucestershire,
Gloucester
UK

Melissa Sebrechts
Assistant Professor
Citizenship and Humanisation of the
Public Sector
University of Humanistic Studies,
Utrecht
Netherlands

Jasmina Sisirak
Research Assistant Professor
Department of Disability and Human
Development
University of Illinois at Chicago, Chicago
Illinois
United States

Alice Squire, BA(Hons), MSc,
DipSW, PGDip
ARC Scotland
Eskbank, Dalkeith
Midlothian, Scotland
UK

David S Stewart, OBE DL BA (Hons)
MA D.Litt.h.c
Oak Field School, Nottingham
UK

Sue Swenson, AM, MBA
President
Inclusion International, Bethesda
Maryland
United States

Laurence Taggart, RNID, BSc,
PGCE, FIASSIDD, PhD
Professor
Institute of Nursing & Health Sciences
Ulster University
Newtownabbey
Northern Ireland
UK

Elizabeth Tilley, BA(Hons), PhD
Senior Lecturer in Health and Social Care
(Learning Disabilities)
School of Health, Wellbeing and Social
Care,
Faculty of Wellbeing, Education and
Languages Studies,
The Open University, Milton Keynes, UK

Elizabeth Walsh, MSc, BSc(Hons),
RN, PhD
Honorary Senior Lecturer in
Psychology and Mental Health
School of Health Sciences
University of Manchester, Manchester
UK

Grete Wangen, BSc, MA
Researcher
Centre for Welfare and Work (SVA) /
Work Research Institute (AFI / WRI)
Oslo Metropolitan University, Oslo
Norway

Angela Wegscheider
Researcher
Institute of Politics and Social Policy
Johannes Kepler University Linz, Linz
Austria

Caroline White, BSc, DipSW, MA
Research Associate
Faculty of Health Sciences
University of Hull, Hull
UK

Michele Wiese, BSc(Hons),
MA(Hons), PhD
Senior Lecturer
School of Social Sciences and
Psychology
Western Sydney University, Kingswood
NSW
Australia

Nathan Wilson, Dip Health Sc
(Nursing), BSocSc, MSc, Grad Cert
Sc (Applied Statistics), PhD
Associate Professor
School of Nursing and Midwifery
Western Sydney University, Richmond
NSW
Australia

In memory of Ivy Angerer and the other victims of the Nazi euthanasia programmes (1939-1945). May their deaths serve as a stark reminder of the capability of human beings.

Inclusion International concerns itself with the human rights of persons with intellectual disabilities and their families. We intervene at a global level because human rights are universal. But we also help people at a personal level because human rights are also plural.

Each of us has different unique or individual needs for supports, services, environments and accommodations to allow us to realise and enjoy our human rights. I suppose a statistical analysis would show us that the needs of people with disabilities and their families are even more plural than those of the general population. Each of us who lives with disability seems to be an 'n of one.' Some of us live our whole lives three standard deviations from what constitutes the norm. We feel this in our bones. We feel the difference, the isolation, the marginalisation, the loneliness. Therefore, individualisation speaks to us. We are hopeful when someone holds out their hand to ask "Are you OK? What do you need?" rather than telling us again the many ways we are not OK and telling us what we need because of some assessment they performed.

Inclusion International's members tell us people with intellectual disabilities and their families want children to be included in school with other children. They want adults with intellectual disabilities to have jobs and be paid fairly. They want the threat of segregation and institutionalisation to be banished from the Earth. They want people with intellectual disabilities to be loved, not in spite of their disability but with their disability. They want the same pride that other disabled communities enjoy. Inclusion International also want the role of families to be honoured and recognised by governments and professionals, and by our brothers and sisters in the disability community, even those whose families have been a source of misery to them.

But here's the thing: we don't want these rights by individual application. We want them to be **universally recognised**. That means designing systems and communities that meet the needs of each disabled person where they are and welcome them in without making them go through assessments and applications and contracts just to have their humanity recognised.

The current global pandemic has underlined how far we are from this ideal. The pandemic has set us back a few decades in that it has thrown more people than ever back on the tender mercies and capabilities of their families even as it has pulled the economic rug out from under those families. Most important, it has highlighted that the progress we hoped we had made was ephemeral because it was not systemic. Education systems have failed to respond to the virtual learning needs of students with disabilities. Health systems have failed to rise above the knee-jerk habit of triage that relies on prejudice, and they have failed to include communication support in patient accommodations. Employment and social supports have moved further out of reach in multiple economies. Many have failed to provide equal access to crucial information in easy read formats. So, despite proclamations of progress, every day, we choose between giving up and moving forward. Which brings me to the purpose of writing this Foreword.

In these chapters, you will find principles, assertions, proposals and ideas to help us move forward to design new solutions and new systems that are better than what we had before. More robust. More real. Designed from the ground up to meet each person's needs. More concerned with supporting the dignity of each person with an intellectual disability and the dignity of the family and the community that (hopefully) surrounds them. Whether you are an advocate, a professional, a policymaker, an academic or whatever your role, these chapters will help you see the best of what we know right now, even as the world is shifting under our feet. These chapters will also help you explore the limits of what we know.

I am old enough (or pessimistic enough) to be certain that the current pandemic will not be the last crisis to affect the world. But I am also optimistic enough to know that if we share ideas with each other in pursuit of the common goal of improving life for people with intellectual disabilities and their families, we cannot fail. Our dream is universal, and our pathways are plural. You can find both here: new ideals, and new ideas to help us make them real.

Sue Swenson
President of Inclusion International

PREFACE

We extend to you a very warm welcome to the seventh edition of this text, titled *Intellectual Disabilities: Toward Inclusion* (more of this name change later). When we commenced revision of the 2011 sixth edition in summer 2019, we could never have predicted we would be concluding it in the shadow of the biggest pandemic to sweep the world since the early part of the 20th century. COVID-19 has impacted the lives of billions of people directly and indirectly. Against this backdrop, it feels little short of a small miracle that we have managed to successfully complete this project, bolstered by the sheer hard work, determination, stamina and health of all our contributors, for which we are eternally grateful. Without their knowledge and expertise, we would not have been able to bring you, the reader, a text we feel is both novel and progressive.

The COVID-19 pandemic has served to accentuate some of the wider health, social and economic problems that have long beset people with intellectual disabilities, on whom this book focuses. Those of you familiar with previous editions of this text will note departure from use of the term *learning disabilities*. Over the thirty-five year life of the book, changes in terminology have been reflected in the titles of its different editions, and the employment of the term 'intellectual disabilities' in this revised text represents the latest step in this evolution. Presently, there is no international agreement on terminology, differing not only between countries but also in the preferences of individuals with intellectual disabilities themselves. Whilst for some the grouping may be an important part of self-identity, for others it represents a description they wish to distance themselves from. Notwithstanding the semantic debate, we felt it important this text used terminology acceptable to an international readership, offering consistency across chapters. People with intellectual disabilities are present in all nations, races and social groups; regardless of nomenclature, it is crucial they are all helped and supported to experience the best quality of life.

COVID-19 may have been largely indiscriminate in its attack, yet because of the health and social vulnerabilities of some groups, including people with intellectual disabilities, its impact has been felt more acutely. People with intellectual disabilities, particularly those with the highest support needs, experience health and living conditions that have made them especially vulnerable to the effects of the pandemic. Indeed, the mortality rate amongst people with intellectual disabilities in the United Kingdom has been reported in the region of 4.1 times (but estimated 6.3 times) higher than in people without. Yet the English actor and playwright, Rory Kinnear, whose sister Karina died from COVID-19 in 2020 wrote that, despite her vulnerability, her life was not disposable. He emphasised that those who 'engaged with her, knew her, loved her … grew to learn, inexorably and unalterably, that *our spirits exist far more tangibly than our abilities*' (our emphasis).

In this new text we take the position that people with intellectual disabilities are people first before any medical label or diagnosis. We have avoided reporting *case studies* in favour of *people's stories*. We have edited using the convention *people (living) with/experiencing … * rather than giving precedence to any condition (for example, the description *epileptic*). Consequently, we have removed content from previous editions that does not reflect this underlying philosophy, an example being the historical chapter on causation and manifestation. We seek not to undermine the usefulness of a diagnosis as for some people this supports both an understanding of their condition and their access to appropriate services. Pragmatically, however, we recognise a textbook is unlikely to be the best source of contemporary information on developments in diagnosing and understanding causes and features of intellectual disabilities, having been surpassed by reputable online sources. Instead, we argue that a clinical label, often imposed by professionals, should not be used to primarily define an individual at the expense of recognising all the additional personal traits that when combined form the 'person'; this includes their unique personal characteristics and lived experiences.

This is paramount as key historical events have taught us that failure to view people with intellectual disabilities as 'people', with the same fundamental human and civil rights enjoyed by others, has resulted in - and in some cases justified - an infringement of rights that includes their abuse or in more extreme cases, destruction. You will note our dedication of this book in memory of Ivy Angerer, a British born victim of Nazi Germany's infamous T4 programme. Ivy, along with more than 70,000 other people, was deemed to have a life unworthy of life. The need to value both the humanity and personhood of people with intellectual disabilities is a central tenet of this book with the *United Nations Convention on the Rights of Persons with*

Disabilities (2006) appearing in many chapters. However, as will be eloquently asserted, such conventions are insufficient unless accompanied by changing social and cultural attitudes. A key aim of this text is to encourage the reader to reflect on the way individuals, services and organisations understand and perceive people with intellectual disabilities and how this can impact on the type and quality of opportunities they provide.

The text is divided into twenty-seven chapters, arranged across three sections. This structure and ordering facilitate reading sequentially or as stand-alone topics. We recognise a range of busy people will want to use the text according to the needs of the individuals they support so we have also linked chapters by providing cross-references. Titles assigned to the three main sections of the text emphasise the individual. These are

- Who am I?
- Maximising my health
- Living my best life.

These have been supplemented by the responses of a number of self-advocates (Alison, Anna, Anna-Marie, Charlotte, Jack, Jez, JoAnne, Josh, and Olivia) to the questions *What do I want from life? How can people best support me to get there?* This represents a further commitment to centralising the voices of people with intellectual disabilities. Additionally, the vibrant cover artwork from Ria represents her considerable creative ability.

Most chapters in the book are the product of a partnership between UK and international contributors with professional backgrounds in many different aspects of intellectual disability. This represents a focused strategy to create a text of utility for anyone for whom people with intellectual disabilities are important, regardless of geographical location. In welcoming back established chapter authors and securing accomplished and new authors we wanted to emphasise that despite material and cultural differences, people with intellectual disabilities across the world share desires to belong, exercise rights and exploit opportunities alongside their non-disabled peers. This is reflected in the passionate Foreword provided by Sue Swenson, president of Inclusion International, who reminds us of the importance of families. Contributors to this book represent Australia, Austria, Germany, Iceland, Ireland, Malta, the Netherlands, Norway, South Africa, Spain, the UK, and the United States of America. Combined, they pay testament to the importance of drawing on international expertise when considering how best to support people with intellectual disabilities in our own countries.

Within the three sections, some new chapters appear. Others have been extended or substantially refreshed. We have been struck, as have some of our contributors, by inconsistent progress in the different areas that comprise the lives of people with intellectual disabilities; some areas have developed markedly, for example sensory integration, whilst others such as employment opportunities may have stalled.

Section 1 opens with two newly developed chapters, *Understanding personhood* and *The importance of the personal narrative,* to set the scene not only for the first third of the text but also the book as a coherent whole. These are bolstered by the foundation chapters encompassing choice, communication, risk, advocacy and safeguarding, with early inclusion of a novel chapter *What's important to me? Using collaborative and creative approaches to shift the power in assessment.* As in the previous edition, additional material in an online resource complements the reader activities found throughout the text.

Section 2 comprises a range of material related to the concept of holistic health and enhancing the experiences of defined groups. A new chapter on *Understanding health* provides the opening for this exploration with reprised chapters operationalising health supporting initiatives across physical and mental wellbeing. We also commissioned a new chapter on *Empowerment through skill development* which we feel sits well here.

Section 3 retains its previous lifespan approach. Popular chapters begin with the family, progress through to childhood and encompass friendships, relationships and milestones including education, employment and *A home of my own.* The section, and the book, closes with positivity and sensitivity in equal measure with *Growing older* and the end of a best life.

We have been acutely aware throughout our editorial task of the responsibility of delivering a text that is not only representative of practice in the second decade of the twenty-first century but also propels it in a more than conservative direction. We hope the gargantuan efforts of our contributors and the care we have taken in editing, and contributing to our own chapters, is matched by your enthusiasm for the seventh edition of *Intellectual Disabilities: Toward Inclusion.* We give our heartfelt thanks to everyone who has supported this endeavour.

Helen Atherton, *Beverley*
Debbie Crickmore, *Kingston-Upon-Hull*

REFERENCES

Atherton H and Schwanninger F (2019) Finding Ivy: a life worthy of life Available at https://www.cl-initiatives.co.uk/finding-ivy-life-worthy-life/ Accessed 5.3.21

Gov.UK 2020 People with learning disabilities had higher death rate from COVID-19 Available online at https://www.gov.uk/government/news/people-with-learning-disabilities-had-higher-death-rate-from-covid-19 Accessed 28.2.2021

Kinnear, R. 2020 My sister died of coronavirus. She needed care but her life was not disposable. Available online at https://www.theguardian.com/commentisfree/2020/may/12/rory-kinnearsister-protect-vulnerable-coronavirus-rory-kinnear Accessed 28.2.2021

United Nations (2006) Convention on the Rights of Persons with Disabilities 2006 Available at: https://www.un.org/development/desa/disabilities/convention-on-the-rights-of-persons-with-disabilities.html Accessed 5.3.21

CONTENTS

Who am I?

I'd like to be an inspiration to other people for other people to look up to me so that I can help them follow their dreams. I'd like to be able to give hope. I need people to care.

Anna-Marie

'I'd like to do more acting, maybe in pantos or in a soap, and also do some dancing. I'd like to be on Britain's Got Talent. I need support with travelling and getting to places on time. I'm happy to still be at home with my family, I'm never bored, there's always something to do.'

Anna

'Most of all I just want people to see me as me; as a person. I'd like to tell people not to be scared – we're not monsters, we're human and we need people to be our friend and we want to be theirs. I'd like to join the Paraorchestra in the future and I'd like to travel and see different countries I've never been to. I'd need support to help me get where I want to be as it's hard to work new routes out.'

Jez

Understanding personhood

Simon Jarrett and Angela Wegscheider

KEY ISSUES

- The idea of personhood tries to define what it means to be a person.
- People with intellectual disabilities, along with other minority groups, have often been regarded as lacking personhood.
- The denial of personhood to some groups of humans can lead to catastrophic events such as the Nazi mass killing of people with intellectual disabilities.

- New models of disability attempt to restore personhood to people with intellectual disabilities, but the denial of personhood continues today.
- Rights are important for people with intellectual disabilities but are only effective if accompanied by inclusion and belonging.

CHAPTER OUTLINE

INTRODUCTION

What is it that makes a person? This can sound like a simple question. It is tempting to give an apparently obvious answer: that to be born human is what makes each one of us a person. If someone is the biological offspring of human parents then they are part of the human species, which distinguishes them from all other animal species, and therefore makes them a person. However, societies across the world for centuries have not been content with such a straightforward answer. Instead they have set all sorts of criteria which dictate whether or not a human can be seen as a person - whether they can be said to have 'personhood'.

The idea of personhood relates to recognition as a person. A human is said to be comprised of a number of characteristics, or traits, that qualify them as a person. These traits, when people try to describe what makes a person, often include having a sense of morality, a sense of reason, an ability to think in an abstract way, and the capacity to form social relations. If a human is seen as lacking these traits, then they are not seen as a full person. Personhood is intimately tied up with ideas of belonging, rights, citizenship, mental capacity and social status. According to the idea of personhood, you can only really belong to a human society if you are seen as a person who has the capacity to understand that you belong, and also to understand the moral responsibilities and reciprocal obligations that go along with belonging. It follows that you can only exercise your rights, and enjoy any form of social status, if you are seen as a person, rather than as a sort of human who lacks personhood for some reason.

Over the centuries people with intellectual disabilities, in particular, have faced, and still face, a struggle to be recognised as full people. From this struggle flows a whole series of other problems, such as lacking rights, the denial of citizenship, outsider status, abuse and discrimination. It is not only people with intellectual disabilities who have suffered the denial of their personhood over time. Women, people of colour, those who experience mental ill health and people with physical disabilities to name just some have all been denied personhood at times, and the legacy of this thinking endures in their lives today. Women have been seen as the property of their husbands, while black slaves were seen as the non-person property of their white owners with, therefore, no rights or social status whatsoever. The feminist movement and civil rights movements have sought to address such discrimination (which is based on denial of personhood) with much success, although severe problems remain and much still needs to be addressed.

For people with intellectual disabilities, however, the denial of personhood has remained a fundamental difficulty that blights their lives. As we will see in subsequent sections, they are a group who, from the nineteenth century, were labelled as 'idiots', unfit to live in society with others. They were therefore cast out into the institutional asylum system. In the late nineteenth century the pseudo-science of eugenics saw them as a threat to the survival of society, the result of 'bad breeding', 'mental defectives' who would contaminate the rest of the population unless they were prevented from producing offspring. Decades of forced institutionalisation, involuntary sterilisation and campaigns for euthanasia ensued. In Britain the Mental Deficiency Act of 1913 condemned 'mental defectives' to life in mental deficiency colonies, or to extensive surveillance and guardianship in the community. There was a terrible culmination of eugenic ideas under the Nazi Regime in Germany. From 1933 the 'mentally unfit' were subject to sterilisation and then to mass killings from 1939–41.

This dark moment in history is explored in detail later in this chapter. All these ideas and actions derived from the fundamental idea that people with intellectual disabilities lack personhood.

While we may feel that things have been improving greatly since the 1980s, when the old long-stay hospitals began to close in some countries, particularly in western Europe, and tens of thousands of people with intellectual disabilities moved back to live within their communities, there are still great threats to their status as people. In the United Kingdom today, for example, there have been a series of scandals involving preventable deaths of people with intellectual disabilities, often due to negligent or misguided approaches by doctors and other medical staff. These have been labelled 'death by indifference' (Mencap, 2012). There have also been examples of young hospital patients with intellectual disabilities being assigned 'Do Not Resuscitate' (DNR) notices, not because they are hospital patients with a painful terminal illness, but simply because they have an intellectual disability (Bass, 2020) (see more on this issue in Chapters 9 and 10). As we discuss later in this chapter, abortion law in Austria, the UK and elsewhere allows for late terminations in cases of fetal abnormality (Statham et al, 2006). New non-invasive antenatal testing for Down syndrome offers prospective parents the option to eliminate not a disease, but a type of human. People regarded as 'challenging' are committed by psychiatrists to 'Assessment and Treatment' units where their stay can turn out to be indefinite, with little recourse to any remedy in law. The idea that a person with an intellectual disability lacks personhood, and cannot make the transition from human to person, endures just as much in contemporary society as it did in the past, it has simply adopted different, more subtle forms and it is these, along with the implications for people with intellectual disabilities, that form the focus of this chapter.

ORIGINS OF PERSONHOOD

How did this idea of personhood, that a human has to develop and meet certain criteria to be recognised as a person, come about? It owes much to the idea of the developing mind, which has been an important mode of thought in psychology since it began. In 1689 John Locke, sometimes known as the father of modern psychology, wrote his *Essay on Human Understanding*. In this he argued that when a human is first born, their mind is effectively empty (this later became known as the 'Blank Slate' theory of the human mind). They are equipped only with senses, such as sight and touch, and through these senses impressions from the outside world gradually form their mind and their capacity to think, speak, reason and imagine. Locke argued that the mind goes through a series of stages of development, from the blank mind of the baby to the fully formed mind of the adult. This gave us the idea of 'developmental milestones' which is so dominant in psychology today. Locke made a distinction between the human and the person. The human is born with an empty mind, and then develops into a person, provided they go through all the developmental stages. Interestingly Locke repeatedly used the examples of what he called 'changelings', 'naturals' or 'idiots' (he used the terms interchangeably) to illustrate what would happen if the mind did not develop in the normal way. Such humans, he argued, could not become a person, because of their lack of mental development. Without personhood, they could not enjoy the rights and privileges allowed by society to the fully developed person.

It was from this way of thinking about the mind that the ideas of Intelligence Quotient (IQ) and mental age developed, based on the level of capacity and competence a child *should* have at any given age. IQ scales and mental age testing were introduced in Paris in the early 20th century by Alfred Binet and fuelled the idea that mental ability could be precisely measured. These measures could then be used to determine who belonged in society and who fell below the cut-off point for personhood (Gould, 1996). An age level was assigned to tasks or questions that were used to assess intelligence. Once a child had reached the last tasks they could perform, this signified their 'mental age'. The gap between the mental age and the true chronological age indicated their general intellectual level. In 1912 the German psychologist W. Stern began dividing mental age by chronological age, giving what became known as the IQ level (Gould, 1996). An adult with an intellectual disability might be assessed as only having the IQ or capacity of a child of six, and for this reason is considered not to have developed into a person. IQ is still widely used, along with the assessment of 'functional' abilities, to assess people with intellectual disabilities and determine their legal status and their capacity to make their own decisions.

Chapter 4 explores limitations of such approaches and offers alternatives.

How do these ideas about personhood play out in the belief systems of modern society, and what are their implications for people with intellectual disabilities today? The struggle for recognition as people still continues. In the United Kingdom the National Association for the Parents of Backward Children was established in 1946, which later became the campaigning organisation known today as Mencap. These parents were effectively put into a position of advocating for the lives, and the human status, of their children. As one activist put it:

> "[We] were trying to get support and recognition as much as anything to try and get people to treat our people as though there was at least a certain amount of normality. They were all human beings … And also to try and get the children, although they weren't children all of them, recognised as people."
>
> Rolph et al, 2005, p. 78

Many modern theories of personhood continue to question whether those who have some form of mental impairment can be seen as fully functioning people, and therefore fully equal citizens. One of the most influential philosophers of the twentieth century, John Rawls, is credited with developing the theoretical justification for equality of justice and equal rights for the citizens of modern democracies. His work is often quoted by judges in American courts of law. Rawls's argument is that human beings count as free and equal persons when they have what he calls the 'moral powers' necessary to engage in social cooperation. The first of these moral powers is that they have the *capacity* for a sense of justice and are therefore able to regard others as equal and treat them accordingly. The second is that they have a concept of what is good and act *rationally* to achieve it. Possessing these so-called powers is known as *moral personhood* (Rawls, 1993, 1999; Wong, 2010, pp. 130–1).

While this theory promotes the idea that the vast majority of people in modern societies can be citizens, with all the rights and benefits that entails, it is clear that this theory excludes people with intellectual disabilities from Rawls's concept of moral personhood. Humans who are seen as unable to act rationally, and unable to understand an abstract concept of justice, are not seen as belonging in a society that requires them to do both of these things. The irony of course is that many people with intellectual disabilities have a strong sense of justice, and of what is good, while many citizens who do not have intellectual disabilities lack a sense of both justice and good. However, in a theory of citizenship that links both of these concepts to having a certain level of intelligence, and an ability to think rationally, it is people with intellectual disabilities who are excluded, while some we might feel to be less worthy citizens are included.

Some thinkers have been even more extreme in their denial of personhood to people with intellectual disabilities. This applies particularly to those who promote animal rights by arguing that higher species of animals have higher capacities than humans with intellectual disabilities. The moral philosopher Peter Singer for example, who wrote the book *Animal Liberation* in 1975, has argued as follows:

> *"Adult chimpanzees, dogs, pigs, and members of many other species far surpass the brain-damaged infant in their ability to relate to others, act independently, be self-aware, and any other capacity that could reasonably be said to give value to life. With the most intensive care possible, some severely retarded infants can never achieve the intelligence level of a dog."*
>
> Singer, 1975, p. 18

Singer has called, and continues to call, for euthanasia for infants with intellectual disabilities (Singer, 1975, pp. 17–22, Singer, 2012, pp. 81–84). To make his position completely clear, he wrote with his co-author Helga Kuhse in 1985 'we think that some infants with severe disabilities should be killed' (Kuhse and Singer, 1985, p. v). The question of the value of the lives of people with intellectual disabilities, and their right to personhood, is still very much alive. Singer, it should be noted, is proud that he has 'for many years … taught intensive bioethics courses for healthcare professionals' (Singer and Winkett, 2020). Singer's colleague Jeff McMahan argues that a 'person' is 'any being with a comparatively highly developed set of psychological capacities' (McMahan, 2002, p. 303), and excludes people with intellectual disabilities as 'nonpersons' from this group. He talks of people with intellectual disabilities as 'human beings who not only lack certain psychological capacities but also, like animals, lack the potential to have them' (McMahan, 2010, p. 346).

The arguments of Singer and McMahan have been attacked by the philosopher Eva Kittay, who is also the mother of a daughter with intellectual disabilities. She argues that although Singer and McMahan claim to know the cognitive capacities of the people they write about, they actually cannot know anything at all about them. She also argues that it is false to set a list of morally significant psychological properties as the only measure of what a human must hold in order to be a person (Kittay, 2010).

Other theorists such as Tim Stainton have fought back against views that deny personhood to people with intellectual disabilities. They have argued for a society based on the formal mechanism of automatic citizenship, with the rights and equality that go with it, and the less formal method of inclusion through participation in everyday life and networks that create belonging (Stainton, 2018). Rather than certain types of human having to achieve personhood by demonstrating that they have certain capacities, personhood simply derives from being born human, and the job of communities is to ensure that everyone belongs. However, as we have seen, the idea first proposed by John Locke in 1689 that a human must pass certain tests before they can be considered a person still endures and has had profound implications for the lives of people with intellectual disabilities through to today. This denial of personhood is not just a theory but is evident in everyday life, in law, social policy, social attitudes, politics and service provision, all of which can serve to isolate people from wider society.

While there have been recent trends towards the recognition of personhood for people with intellectual disabilities in policies and practice, it is still fragile, fragmented and incomplete. However, before turning the spotlight on some current problems, we should consider the historical prelude that involved a total denial of personhood in policy, law and practice in the mid-20th century - the attempt to exterminate people with intellectual disabilities that occurred under the Nazi party in Germany.

PERSONHOOD COMES UNDER THREAT

In this section we will examine what the consequences can be when personhood is denied to people with intellectual disabilities. We will look at the case of Germany and Austria from the late nineteenth century through to the period of Nazi rule from 1933–45 in Germany, and 1938–45 in Austria. We will trace a path which begins with the initial separation of people with intellectual disabilities into a parallel world of institutions and exclusion based on the 'science' of eugenics, and ends with the grotesque policy of deliberate murder that arose from the fatal coming together of eugenic science and the Nazi ideology of racial purity.

Before the nineteenth century intellectual notions about personhood did not unduly affect the daily lives of people with intellectual disabilities, their care and support were accepted as religious or humanist duties. In Austria and Germany, as in many countries, people with intellectual disabilities were generally integrated into their family and the local community and only some were in institutions. It was only after the start of industrialisation towards the end of the nineteenth century that the life situation of people with intellectual disabilities became increasingly precarious. With the changes in family life brought about by industrialisation people with support and care needs could be seen, in some cases, as a financial burden who increased the risk of impoverishment for the whole family. In this way their status as a person, a full member of family and society, was diminished (Schmuhl and Winkler, 2012).

At the same time there was only a rudimentary welfare state and under the law the family remained responsible for all their members, including those with intellectual disabilities. Only very limited local poor relief support was available to those unable to manage. People with intellectual disabilities were increasingly seen as a 'burden', an unwanted form of person, both by the state and the family. This state of affairs continued into the twentieth century (Wegscheider, 2016).

This period saw a parallel structure emerge, of religious and charitable specialised care and educational institutions, federal state-run public hospitals and specialised schools and care facilities which provided shelter for the 'ineducable' or some education for the 'educable'. These facilities had been state of the art at first, but during and after World War I they became overcrowded and poorly resourced, particularly with the emerging economic crisis in the 1930s. The provision of segregating parallel worlds of care and education for those deemed not to have full personhood was costly. Politicians, associations and families were keen

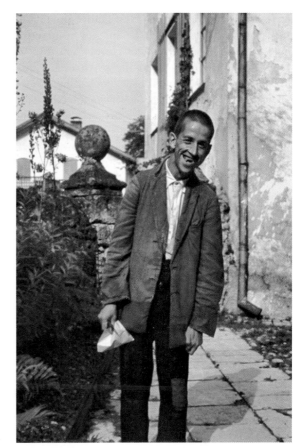

Figure 1.1 Poor house inmate of the small rural municipality, 1939 (Source: Pfarre Maria Ach, Fotosammlung Pfarrer Adolf Theimer)

to get rid of this financial burden (Wegscheider, 2016, 2017, 2020). Segregation and institutionalisation were seen as protecting 'society' from the underprivileged, untalented and in particular, disabled non-persons (Pfahl and Powell, 2011).

A solution was offered by the pseudo-science of eugenics, which emerged in the late-nineteenth century. These new ideas centred around improving the genetic material of humans through the systematic enhancement of the *Volkskörper* (the body of the German people) and the exclusion from reproduction of suspected 'hereditarily inferior' individuals. In eugenic thought the disabled were seen not as people but as 'others' needing to be removed from the breeding stock just like certain animals. Eugenic ideas, in particular the removal of 'undesirables', were discussed and accepted in academia and politics, and in countries across Europe and the rest of the world. They circulated more intensively in Austria and Germany in the aftermath of World War I. In 1920 the lawyer Karl Binding and the psychiatrist Alfred Hoche, both Germans, published a book calling for the 'eradication' of the 'mentally ill', which included people with intellectual disabilities, by euthanasia (Binding and Hoche, 1920).

After the fascist National Socialist Party (or 'Nazis') took power in Germany in 1933, they implemented a radicalised form of eugenics, based exclusively on the superiority of the German race, which they called 'Rassenhygiene' (racial hygiene). It began with the state-mandated sterilisation of the so-called 'hereditarily inferior'. On July 14, 1933, the Nazi dictatorship enacted a 'Law for the Prevention of Genetically Diseased Offspring'. This was followed by the so-called 'Nuremberg Laws' in September 1935, which included a ban on marriage for individuals with disabilities (Schwanninger, 2019). The German Reich was certainly a pioneer of the worldwide eugenic movement but other countries, such as the United States and Sweden, imposed similar provisions to allow sterilisation while an enthusiastic eugenics movement in the United Kingdom brought about the 1913 Mental Deficiency Act to control and isolate the 'mentally defective'. However, decisive differences between Nazi law and other countries could be observed. The sterilisation laws in the United States were not centrally controlled and applied inconsistently (Bock, 1986; Hubbard, 2006). In comparison, approximately 400,000 sterilisations were documented for the German Reich (1933–1945), while the United States registered 65,000 cases over a longer period up to the 1960s (Bock, 1986).

The Nazis enacted their idea of 'eradicating inferior life' to the ultimate end point with their state-controlled euthanasia programme, which was later called Aktion T4. They were able to do this because they created a climate of opinion where personhood was denied to people with disabilities, who were referred to with terms such as 'subhuman organisms.' From 1940, five killing centres were set up in the German Reich. Doctors, employed by an authority in Berlin at the address Tiergartenstrasse 4, (the origin of the name T4 for the killing programme) examined people with intellectual disabilities (and other disabilities) in care facilities or hospitals and decided who should be killed using a criteria sheet. The aim of the programme was to target and eliminate those whose lives were deemed 'life unworthy of living' (Kepplinger, 2009, p. 225). What emerged was a 'differential care' system based on perceived usefulness. While killing those deemed unfit for life, the Nazis intensified education and vocational training for those considered educable and fit to work and therefore allowed to belong to the 'Volksgemeinschaft' (national community). In this way personhood was equated with economic usefulness. This led to an expansion and further professionalisation of specialised education for children with intellectual disabilities through the Gauhilfsschule (Nazi school for children with intellectual disabilities) in the German Reich (Hänsel, 2019).

After Austria merged into the German Reich under Nazism in 1938, Hartheim castle, until then a religious care institution for 'idiots' with 200 patients, was taken over by Nazi authorities and converted into a killing centre. When Aktion T4 started, the first victims to be murdered in May 1940 in Hartheim included at least 63 out of the 191 former inmates of the 'idiot' care institution (Wegscheider, 2017, pp. 44–9).

For their programme of mass-murder the Nazis used their six killing centres across Germany and Austria, which were equipped with gas chambers disguised as shower rooms. They murdered around 70,000 adults with intellectual disabilities, mental health problems or other disabilities with carbon monoxide. 18,000 of them died in Hartheim castle. After gassing, the dead bodies were then cremated on site. The killing stations employed nurses and doctors for medical

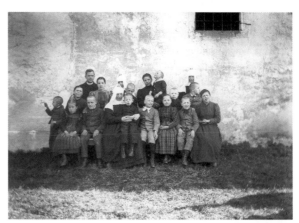

Figure 1.2 Inmates of Schwachsinnigenanstalt, Kretinenanstalt Hartheim castle, 1920 (Source: Dokumentationsstelle Hartheim)

examination and to calm down the incoming victims on the path leading to death. In August 1941, the T4 programme came to a halt. Although the Nazis always tried to hide their murders of people with disabilities, resistance from relatives and the church, and to some extent information relayed to the general public by the German-language programme of the BBC, contributed to Aktion T4 being discontinued (Noack, 2017). Throughout the T4 programme, further killings were carried out by doctors and nurses in the special care facilities and hospitals without a central mandate. Medical staff, willingly and enthusiastically influenced by the cruel Nazi ideology, killed many adults and thousands of children with disabilities by injections, and also through deplorable living conditions.

The death rate in the care institutions and hospitals rose more sharply in the years from 1940 onwards. Until the end of the war in 1945, the gas chambers in Hartheim continued to work, but over this period inmates assessed as unfit to work from the Mauthausen, Gusen or Dachau concentration camps were murdered. In total, there were 30,000 victims in Hartheim and at least 200,000 victims of the Nazi euthanasia policy in the German Reich (Kepplinger, 2009; Schwanninger, 2019).

To change people's views about what or who should be valued as a person, ideas of racial hygiene were propagated to the population through means such as documentaries, feature films, school books and propaganda illustrations (see Figure 1.3). In this way, the ground for the criminal intentions and practices of the Nazi regime was psychologically prepared. The Nazis tried to reframe the mass murdering as 'mercy killing'. In 1941 the propaganda film 'Ich klage an' (I accuse) suggested that 'mercy killings' of severely ill persons were a desirable development. The lives of people with intellectual disabilities were devalued through Nazi terminology such as 'unworthy life', 'hereditarily inferior', 'hereditary sick' or 'ballast existence' with calls for them to be eliminated (Schwanninger, 2019; Kepplinger, 2009; Kammerhofer, 2008). It was not only ideology that drove the Nazi mission, but also cost-benefit calculations. The so-called 'Hartheim statistics', a 39-page report, depressingly demonstrates what had been saved each month through murdering institutionalised people, by calculating the cost savings on food, bread, meat, vegetables, potatoes and butter as well as the costs of medical care and accommodation (Kammerhofer, 2008).

After the war and the defeat of the German Reich, the new authorities aimed to return to the situation before the Nazi area, and silence remained about the atrocities committed against people with disabilities for more than 20 years. There was hardly any discussion or collective memorial. Doctors, nurses and teachers who were involved, or who at least had observed the mass-murder, continued to work. Schools for children with intellectual disabilities, segregated homes, care institutions and soon sheltered workshops were then reopened to meet rising demand from a new population of people with intellectual disabilities. Things continued as if nothing had happened (Wegscheider, 2017), yet the legacy of this period remains today.

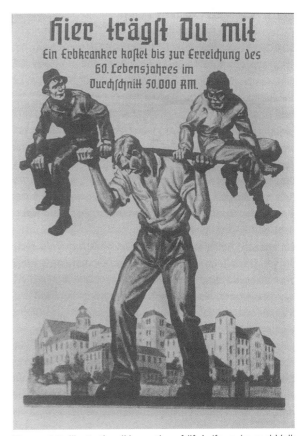

Figure 1.3 Illustration 'Unworthy of life', (from journal Volk and Rasse, 1936 (Source: Dokumentationsstelle Hartheim). *'Here you are also carrying. A hereditary ill patient costs an average of 50,000 Reichsmark until the age of 60.'*

Contemporary threats to personhood

It is important to recognise that the extreme and terrible denial of personhood of the Nazi regime did not end with its defeat. People with intellectual disabilities continue to be deprived of their personhood. We must not make the mistake of looking at the Nazi period as an aberration. Threats to personhood can arise in various different and less obvious ways, often because of ignorance and prejudice. Traditional service provider organisations that claim to be 'values-led', and have an inspiring mission statement, do not always realise the concept of personhood for people with intellectual disabilities (Quinn, 2014, p. 22). The same is true of modern European member states, despite their sophisticated rule of law and welfare systems. The inscription of the cornerstone of the new care institution for people with intellectual disabilities next to Hartheim castle which was set up in the 1960s refers to 'infantibus perpetuis' which means in Latin 'for the eternal children' (see Figure 1.4). People with intellectual disabilities can be seen as retaining 'childhood' status throughout their lives, particularly if they are considered to be unfit to gain their living from work.

In Austria today, there are numerous indications that people with intellectual disabilities are not granted the status of 'full person'. They remain health insured through their parents and receive child benefits as adults. Parents are obliged to provide care for their

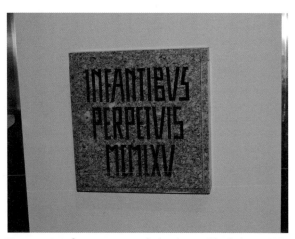

Figure 1.4 Cornerstone of Institute Hartheim, 1965 (Source: Dokumentationsstelle Hartheim)

grown-up child for the rest of their lives. When the parents die, the grown-up child receives an orphan's pension. Though many of them could work within a paid working contract, with personal assistance, they mainly work for pocket money in sheltered workshops. Young people with intellectual disabilities seeking work through Austria's Public Employment Service (PES) have been sent for medical evaluation to prove their economic usefulness. If evaluated as unfit for work they get no further support from PES, and are excluded from nearly all measures to get into the regular labour market (Vianova, 2017). Young people often have too few social insurance contributions to be eligible for a disability pension, and if they have social needs are required to access welfare relief at the federal state level.

In many countries further challenges to the notion of personhood have come in the form of recent developments in the field of non-invasive antenatal tests for Down syndrome and other reproductive technologies that identify, with increasing accuracy, disabled foetuses, giving the option of abortion. Since the 1970s under the Austrian and German criminal codes abortion has been legal for the first three months of pregnancy, but also just before birth if there is suspicion that the child will be mentally or physically severely damaged. UK abortion law (and elsewhere) also allows terminations for fetal abnormality without gestational limit (Statham et al, 2006).

The denial of personhood is also evident in the withholding of specific rights from people with intellectual disabilities. Some countries in Europe, including Poland, Portugal, Bulgaria and Romania, still deny the right to vote to many people with intellectual disabilities. However, in recent years, more countries have granted this right, among them Denmark (2016), France (2018), Spain (2018), and most recently Germany (2019). Limited voting rights persist in Ireland, Belgium, the Netherlands, Estonia, Lithuania, Czech Republic, Hungary, Slovenia, and Greece. In most European countries people who require guardianship will still be automatically deprived or limited in their right to stand for election (Inclusion Europe, 2019). However, on a more positive note, an increasing number of people with intellectual disabilities are presenting themselves as candidates for elections. People with intellectual disabilities have stood for municipal elections (Inclusion Europe, 2020), and a woman with Down syndrome has run for the French municipal elections in Arras (Pailliez and Libert, 2020). In 2015, Gavin Harding became the first UK Mayor with an intellectual disability (Learning Disability Today, 2015).

In this section, we have shown that many of the assumptions that led to the Nazi extermination programmes have not gone away but are being enacted in a more subtle way. Denial of personhood can be observed in contemporary society and policies. This is illustrated in abortion practices after prenatal screening and exclusion from voting. The next section introduces dominant views of disability in society and politics which will be useful when considering full and equal recognition of personhood.

DISABILITY MODELS IN SOCIETY

Disability studies have laid the foundation for new perspectives which regard disability as a social, cultural, relational, human rights and political matter. These perspectives allow greater acknowledgement and understanding of the personhood of people with intellectual disabilities, far more so than traditional perspectives which view intellectual disability as a moral or medical condition.

After a major process of deinstitutionalisation and return to the community began in some European and other Western countries from the 1970s, theorists developed an interest in people with intellectual disabilities that went beyond the old medical and religious understandings. They wanted to know how it was that a certain group of people had come to be understood and perceived as less than human and not fully formed people, and how this could be addressed in order to restore personhood to them. Their interest was in the different ways, or models, that had been used to *construct* certain understandings of people with intellectual disabilities as non- or sub-persons. They also theorised new models which would lead to better understandings of people with intellectual disabilities, and would allow them to be understood as having full personhood. As we will see, whilst the old negative models still persist, these are now being challenged by new, more person-centred models.

Disability as a moral or medical condition

The oldest of all perspectives, which is still current, is based on the idea that disability is related to a divine plan, a moral error, sin, or a test or punishment from God. As recently as 1979 the Tyrolian daily newspaper in Austria reported a conversation of Pope John Paul II with some people with intellectual disabilities:

> *"[The Pope] said to them: 'Your presence is especially precious to us because you are specially connected with Jesus Christ through the cross of your suffering. By humbly accepting and bearing your infirmities as an example and with the power of the suffering Lord, they become a precious source of consolation, purification and strengthening for yourselves and for the Church.'"*

In the moral approach, socio-political or rehabilitative interventions are not necessary since disability is a fate brought by God and equates to suffering, which must be endured patiently and humbly. Motivated by religious virtues, however, the community needs to donate, which helps to alleviate individual suffering. By helping 'the poorest of the poor' the helper and charity-giver also secures personal salvation of the soul (Wegscheider, 2020, p. 177; see also Goodley, 2017, pp. 6–7). In modern secular societies, such donations are related to a patronising, dependency-creating approach, and do nothing to urge the state or society to deal with ensuring personhood through legal capacity, equal rights, and eliminating discrimination and barriers.

This view has had the effect that even today large numbers of people with intellectual disabilities rely on charity and welfare in order to finance their lives and the support they need. Every year in the pre-Christmas period the Austrian Broadcasting Corporation (ORF) carries out the fundraising campaign 'Licht ins Dunkel' (Light in the Dark) and presents people with intellectual disabilities as poor, helpless objects of suffering. By 2017, almost 60,000 people in Austria were under guardianship and lived with substitute decision making in daily life, twice as many as in 2003. The guardianship law is infantilising more than it is useful or desirable and restricts legal recognition as a person (Monitoringausschuss, 2012). Only in 2018 was a new law introduced to foster supported decision-making, with the aim that people with intellectual disabilities become a 'subject' of the law and the political order, and thereby enjoy legal capacity in daily life. Whether this will work in practice depends mainly on the financial resources available for the necessary accompanying professional support.

Medicine, psychology and nursing have tended to conceptualise disability as a pathology, a health threat or a permanent disease. They perceive disability as a personal tragedy and individual problem. Their focus is on defects or faults of physical, mental, and cognitive abilities, which are classified as abnormal and pathological, and sometimes alleged to be caused by individual behaviour. This view treats disability as a medical problem which causes limitations for a disabled individual and casts doubt on their personhood (Goodley, 2017). Interventions in this sense aim at therapeutic, medical or rehabilitative treatments that promise healing, adaptation or compensation. Its strength lies in its ability to justify concrete therapies, treatments, and intervention that are tailored to the needs of the individual (Waldschmidt, 2020). Such interventions are inspired by ideas of medical, therapeutic and technological progress and professional solutions. They are also bolstered by a paternalistic welfare state, which establishes specialised but also segregated living, and a working assumption in Austria until the 1990s that the best and fairest form of integration is seen as the "disabled among disabled people" (Badelt and Österle, 2001, p. 11).

In the medical model, with its questioning of the value of a disabled individual's life and their entitlement to personhood, a disabled baby becomes increasingly undesirable leading to consideration of prenatal termination and euthanasia, which can be either an *active* process e.g. assisted suicide or *a passive* process e.g allowing someone to die. Since Nazism, a paradigm shift has taken place regarding decision making with eugenics-style decision making regarding termination shifting from the state to the individual. With a shrinking welfare state, and without the prospect of receiving adequate practical and financial support, parents are often left alone to make what are essentially challenging and complex ethical decisions.

The possibilities offered through the ongoing development of pre-natal testing procedures are somewhat at odds; on the one hand life-saving medical treatment for a new born could start early, on the other it makes eugenic selection possible and ensures certain kinds of people aren't born. Current and future developments in

READER ACTIVITY 1.2

Read the following blog written by a UK psychiatrist, also carer for her brother with an intellectual disability.
1. Identify the different examples of how people with intellectual disabilities are discriminated against
2. Reflect upon the extent to which a failure to recognise their personhood might perpetuate such actions.

https://blogs.bmj.com/bmj/2020/09/01/covid-19-shows-that-the-lives-of-people-with-a-learning--disability-are-still-not-treated-as-equal/

this area therefore need to be supervised and monitored by the state as well as open to academic, professional and public scrutiny, to allow different perspectives to be debated.

Current developments in society and medicine touch on ground-breaking, existential, moral values about life and death and trigger debates that are sometimes very emotional and heated. Much of this coalesces around the idea of an individual's personhood, and related topics such as value of life, end of life decisions and euthanasia in its passive (allowing someone to die) or active forms. All these issues struggle to find a consensus and agreed legal standards for such difficult ethical questions and dilemmas (Liessmann, 2016).

The Nordic social model and constructionism

The Nordic relational model of disability has developed in the Scandinavian region since the 1960s. This multi-perspective approach originates primarily from non-disabled experts, who formulated disability as an interaction, influenced by contexts and situations, between a person's impairment and their environmental conditions and modes of socio-economic organisation. They called for professional services to help overcome the mismatch between the individual and the environment and thus enable participation in the community and social spaces. Linked to this relational approach are the 'normalisation' concept and the de-institutionalisation movement. Both led to a reorganisation of support for people with intellectual disabilities. It should be noted that this theory has been criticised by left-wing thinkers who argue that it does not address the capitalist mode of production and its mechanisms of exclusion, which they regard as the underlying cause of disability. It has also been criticised on the grounds that it is expert-oriented (rather than emanating from people with disabilities themselves) and ignores the control and disciplining function of social policy (Gustavsson, 2004; Waldschmidt, 2020; Goodley, 2017) Although this approach was developed independently of disability studies and the disability movement, it strengthened the opportunities for personhood through self-determination in people's own life situations, the acquisition of legal capacity and self-representation through self-advocacy. This model ultimately served as an example for many other countries.

First promoted by disability activists in the United Kingdom in the 1970s, constructionism has perceived disability as a product of constructed barriers leading to economic and social disadvantages requiring political action. This approach distinguishes between impairment (which is natural) and disability (which is imposed from the outside). It assumes that barriers, discrimination, social isolation, economic dependence, high unemployment or institutionalisation cause disablement. In the beginning, this idea related to people with physical impairments but it then attracted other groups. The socio-economic perspective points out that certain social practices, structures and institutions are designed in such a way that they exclude people based on specific characteristics and prejudices. In other words, a social denial of personhood leads to exclusion. For example, people with intellectual disabilities enter the workforce at a far lower rate than others. The employment participation rates for those with intellectual disabilities rest at an alarmingly low level. In the United Kingdom, only 5.9 percent of people with intellectual disabilities are in employment (British Association for Supported Employment (BASE), 2020). Many countries now have detailed figures about the employment situation of this group which show a similar picture (see also Chapter 23).

Constructionist theory suggests that the problems of people with disabilities, including the denial of their personhood, are socially caused rather than being a deficit of the individual, and therefore can be solved by society and state interventions. This approach calls for an inclusive economy, with inclusive education and training. It also requires inclusive and flexible social systems with needs-oriented and self-determined support and assistance services through participatory reform processes (Waldschmidt, 2020; Goodley, 2017). Disability policy must therefore enable independent living in the community, active citizenship and self-representation in the sense of 'nothing about us without us', taking into account experiences and interests of people with intellectual disabilities. In order to find adequate solutions for socio-economic disadvantage, it advocates the political participation of those affected by legislation and the design of framework conditions at all levels (Plangger and Schönwiese, 2015).

Cultural model

Since the 1990s, especially in the United States and more recently also in German-speaking countries, humanities scholars began to study disability through analysing literature and so-called 'cultural production'. Cultural production is the process by which shared values, understandings and assumptions are created within a particular culture. The cultural perspective opposes both the medical model view of disability as an individual fate and the social model idea of a socially marginal position. It instead tries to strengthen cultural, historical and cultural-anthropological perspectives on disability (Waldschmidt, 2020). Disability is understood here as a construct of culture and modes of cultural production and questions the distinction between 'normal' and 'not normal'. To deny personhood to a particular individual because a label of 'intellectual disability' is attached to them is simply a product of the normalising assumptions and values of the culture within which the individual lives. Cultural production examines the notion of normalcy and the underlying history of processes of exclusion and stigmatisation.

The cultural perspective assumes that socio-political redistribution and legal recognition (as proposed in the social model) are not enough, but that cultural representations of dis/ablement and ab/normality must be deconstructed to reveal that they are simply representations rather than 'facts' (Goodley, 2017, pp. 13-18). The cultural perspective of disability sees it as both the lived experience of an individual and the cultural context within which their life takes place, and in which assumptions are made about them, including the assumption that they may lack personhood. This approach deconstructs a dominant view and systems of order that devalue and individualise disability and label it as pathological (Plangger and Schönwiese, 2015).

READER ACTIVITY 1.3

You now understand different perspectives of disability.

Identify a movie, television programme or newspaper article in which a person with an intellectual disability appears.

How is this person depicted?

Which model of disability is being promoted there?

People with and without disabilities need to be encouraged to overcome their view of disability as a cause for a stigmatised life situation. By promoting cultural representation and disability pride, the cultural model of disability seeks to strengthen the sense of personhood, belonging and participation in the disability community so that people can claim their rights individually (Waldschmidt, 2020).

The cultural model perspective has been instrumental in sharpening the focus on political, legal, financial, institutional, structural, communicative, social and cognitive barriers, which can weaken recognition as a person with full citizenship rights. It argues that people with intellectual disabilities can live on an equal footing with others and with equal opportunities (Schulze, 2010). Advocates of the cultural model have therefore had a strong influence on a move away from deficit models (such as the moral or medical perspectives) to a focus on human rights, equality and social justice for people with intellectual disabilities as a means of achieving personhood. The issue of rights, and their implications for inclusion, justice and equality, is explored in more detail in the final section of this chapter.

PERSONHOOD, RIGHTS AND JUSTICE

We have seen already how long-standing ideas of personhood can bring into question whether a person with an intellectual disability has the right to full status as a person. This can lead to deep injustices where people are denied status as a citizen or an included member of society, and the rights that are usually accorded with that status. The twentieth century saw the development of universal frameworks of human rights for all people, and in particular rights frameworks for people with disabilities. The *United Nations Universal Declaration of Human Rights*, of 1948 includes rights such as equality before the law, food and shelter, family life, education, and access to healthcare. In 1975, because of enduring systematic discrimination, the United Nations (UN) issued its *Declaration on the Rights of Disabled Persons*, signed or ratified by most countries in the world. The declaration calls for 'reasonable accommodation' (adjustments to ensure equality), accessibility, recognition before the law, access to education and health, and rights of participation and employment. This was followed in 2006 by the *UN Convention on the Rights of Persons with Disabilities* (2006), whose article 12 affirmed that persons with disabilities have the right to recognition everywhere as persons before the law and should enjoy legal capacity on an equal basis with others in all aspects of life.

These frameworks are then adopted regionally, such as the *European Convention on Human Rights* (Council of Europe 1950), and *Convention on the Rights of Persons with Disabilities* which was adopted by the European Union in 2011. Many countries also have their own general human rights or specific disability rights, laws and policies.

This sequence of declarations and conventions indicates that the attachment of rights to people with disabilities, and in particular to people with intellectual disabilities, while highly desirable can also be problematic. After universal declarations of rights for all humans were made by both the United Nations and the European nations, these were followed some years later by specific declarations of rights for people with disabilities. The generalised declarations of human rights were not in themselves sufficient to ensure that people with disabilities were included in their overarching framework. This is often the case for groups that are subject to systematic discrimination, such as women and ethnic minorities, and derives in part from notions of personhood that do not necessarily include all humans. Specific codes and declarations of rights are therefore needed for these groups to ensure that they are encompassed within the wider rights declaration.

We should remember that the famous *Declaration of the Rights of Man and the Citizen* (see Warman, 2016) that marked the French Revolution in 1789 was just what it said it was – a declaration of rights for men, not for women. It also proved problematic for the black citizens of France's colonies and others deemed to lack the capacity to be full citizens. Likewise, the American *Declaration of Independence* of 1776 proclaimed the equality of all 'men' but this did not apply to the enslaved black population who were perceived as lacking personhood (Carson, 2007). Whilst many of the chapters in this book will go on to make reference to human rights policy and legislation, in particular the UN Convention on the Rights of Persons with Disabilities (2006), it is important to remember that even universal human rights, whatever their intention, can in practice be qualified rights, depending on what, or who, is understood as constituting a person.

This problem can be magnified in relation to people with intellectual disabilities whose personhood, and the rights that go with it, are constantly questioned and under threat. For example, in the West African nation of Ghana, although its constitution since independence in 1957 has embedded the rights of people with disabilities as 'citizens of Ghana', the implementation of disability rights has been slow and, in relation to intellectual disability, often non-existent. Ghanaian self-advocates claim that this is the case because society fails to recognise that people with intellectual disabilities are fully human (Abraham and Odoom, 2019). This does not just apply to Ghana. However much it is claimed that rights apply to all persons, enduring transnational practices such as institutional incarceration with little or no legal recourse, denial of the right to family life, education and work, differentiated (and inferior) levels of treatment within health services and abusive treatment even within community-based services demonstrate that universal rights frameworks can be of little value if people are perceived as lacking full personhood.

Some theorists have criticised declarations of rights on the grounds of their efficacy and utility. Is the notion of a 'natural right' that applies to all people no more than moral wishful thinking if there is no viable, concrete, enforcing agency to ensure that the rights are applied? Enforceability, and an effective mechanism for enforcement, are essential for rights to exist at all (Geuss, 2001). Declaring rights without the means to enforce them simply means that they are little more than a morally good idea which we would like to see happen. This can be not just ill-conceived but also harmful, in that such declarations can encourage us to make assumptions that rights are in place for people in the social and political world when in fact they are just an illusion, lacking any

real influence on the lives of people or groups (Geuss, 2001). This illusion can become strongest for those who are most powerless and isolated because it appears to accord them a status in a social sphere they desire, even if the sphere itself is imaginary in the absence of mechanisms for rights enforcement (Geuss, 2001).

It has been argued that the application of a 'one size fits all' set of rights within policy frameworks across all people with intellectual disabilities, from those with the most profound to those with the mildest disabilities, can lead to similar illusions. In England the government's *Valuing People* (2001) policy summed up the civil and legal rights of people with intellectual disabilities as 'a decent education, to grow up to vote, to marry and have a family, to express opinions, with help and support to do so where necessary' (Department of Health, 2001, p. 230). While such aspirations can and should apply to the vast majority of people with intellectual disabilities, their application to people with profound and multiple intellectual disabilities, who have indeterminate levels of cognitive functioning, often accompanied by high levels of sensory impairment, no verbal communication, extremely limited mobility and a need for high levels of care and medical intervention throughout their lives, is problematic. This has been described as the 'as if' application of systems of rights, where an illusion is created 'as if' a person can achieve the aspirations which the rights describe, when in reality the likelihood is that these aspirations will not be achieved (Lyle, 2019). The danger of this form of rights allocation is that when it is stated that 'everybody' can hold and achieve such aspirations this excludes certain people, who cannot achieve these aspirations, from the category of 'everybody'. This can create a dangerous rights vacuum around those who are most profoundly disabled, in much the same way as earlier rights systems excluded some people from notions of personhood.

None of this means, of course, that rights and systems of rights, have no place in the lives of people with intellectual disabilities. Indeed, they are essential as in highly bureaucratised and legalistic modern societies, without the protection of enforceable rights, the risks of discrimination, marginalisation and abuse are extremely high. However, firstly it is important to reflect that while rights are *necessary*, they are not *sufficient* to guarantee people inclusion, protection and equality. Secondly, it is also important that rights should be enforceable and relate to real lives rather than illusory conceptions of people and the social and political world in which they live. Thirdly, past ideas of capacity based on the ability to reason, and the reciprocal responsibilities that are triggered by citizenship rights, act as obstructions to the achievement of rights for people deemed to lack the faculty of reason. Finally, the existence of rights in themselves do not reshape society; they must be accompanied by changing social and cultural attitudes, and a culture of interdependence rather than simple independence, which enable full citizenship and inclusion for groups such as people with intellectual disabilities. These four key points are summarised in Box 1.1.

📄 BOX 1.1   Four points about rights

- They are necessary but not sufficient for inclusion and equality
- They must be enforceable and related to real life
- Past ideas relating rights to capacity must be rejected
- Rights are not enough in themselves – there must also be a change in cultural attitudes

---

The enduring idea that a person's legal status and entitlement to citizenship rest on their mental capacity and autonomy (ability to manage your own life) is now being challenged. Autonomy can be seen instead as 'relational', meaning that a person can be autonomous if they have a level of inter-connectedness with other people that allows them to function within society. Their capacity, seen in this way, is a function of their *interdependence* rather than their *independence*. In this model, citizenship, and the rights and equal status that come with it, can apply to all provided each person has the support necessary to actualise their citizenship through interventions and service programmes.

 READER ACTIVITY 1.4

Can you think of a situation where the rights of a person (or people) with intellectual disabilities have been questioned or ignored?

In what ways has denial of personhood been instrumental in this situation?

How could this be challenged?

Interconnectedness is created around the person to achieve citizenship (Bach, 2017; Leydet, 2017). However, this is no easy task. Many people with intellectual disabilities participate in settings and situations where their low status is assumed, hindering the exercise, or even the recognition, of their rights. Their relationships and relational settings (families, education, support systems etc.) may often actually 'institutionalise social practices and values enforcing their inferior social position' (Carey, 2010, p. 24).

Furthermore, the formal recognition and encouragement of citizenship in law, rights and policy is only part of the story, and on its own is insufficient to ensure that people with intellectual disabilities can live a life with their rights respected. The idea of inclusion is a less formal concept, derived from rights but dependent on attitudes, culture and practice. The starting point for inclusion is that cognitive diversity of any sort is seen not as a justification for exclusion or isolation, because it challenges existing social norms and expectations, but as a trigger for the social environment to adapt so that diversity is embraced (Jordan, 2011). Creating a sense of belonging, leading to inclusion, is essential to enabling citizenship. The concepts of citizenship and inclusion are different but interconnected. One is formal and can be codified in law and statements of rights, while the other derives from an all-embracing understanding and acceptance of human value which is applied across the range of human types. Without legalised citizenship and rights it is difficult, if not impossible, for inclusion to occur. However, without a culture of inclusion and belonging, it is difficult for rights, citizenship and status to have any real meaning (Stainton, 1994, 1998, 2005, 2018; Duffy, 2017; Bach, 2017).

Belonging and the inclusion it entails can appear nebulous concepts, unenforceable by law or codes of rights. However, the desire and the need to belong appear to be a universal human characteristic, given that humans are social beings. It is very possible therefore for communities and societies to understand what is required to create a sense of belonging, given that it is a shared human impulse. Feelings of belonging are built upon places where people feel happy or safe, activities which give them satisfaction and connections between people that are authentic and meaningful. They also derive from environments where people feel respected, noticed and accepted as individuals and thus augments the person-centred approach to care and support that is advocated across the different chapters of this book. As an example, an inclusive hospital environment is one where staff treat a patient with an intellectual disability as a person who needs to be cared for and made well, with medical needs which need to be investigated, identified and treated. An excluding hospital culture sees only the disability, explains all symptoms as a function of the disability, and fails to respond to the presenting person in the same way as they respond to other human types. The person with an intellectual disability may enter the hospital equipped with a full set of rights, but unless an inclusive culture prevails the rights will only become of any interest or use at a subsequent inquiry or inquest. The following chapter in this book builds on this notion by advocating the use of personal narratives as a way of enabling professionals to see beyond the disability to the actual person.

There is finally the matter of 'rights conflict' where the rights of one person or group may clash with the rights of another, or where even simultaneously held rights may conflict within one individual (Geuss, 2001, pp. 148–9). The debate about pre-natal screening for Down syndrome can trigger a conflict between the right of a particular type of human to have life and a woman's right to make decisions and choices about her own body. This can result in complex political interactions where anti-abortion campaigners and intellectual disability activists who are pro-abortion can find themselves unwittingly (and uncomfortably) on the same side. The right to eat what you choose and the right to good health can conflict within an individual and those who support or know them. Each of these examples demonstrates that rights, while necessary and desirable, only take us so far. People live their lives within social contexts where they interact with other people, ideas and events. Beyond a specific right there is a range of situations and interrelationships within which decisions are made and lives are lived. Positive connectedness, and a sense of belonging, enhance the quality of that decision-making, reduce the impact of unwise or wrongful decisions and increase the safety, well-being and self-esteem of the individual. Inclusion is based on, but extends far beyond, a set of rights. Its starting point is the individual, their personhood, their right to belong, and the adjustments and connections that can be made around them to enable belonging to occur.

As we move to conclude this opening chapter, we urge the reader to consider the personal perspectives of self-advocates that appear at the beginning of each of the three Sections of this book. Reader activity 1.5 in the accompanying online resource encourages you to use the insights provided by this chapter to relate them to the concept of personhood.

CONCLUSION

The notion of personhood for people with intellectual disabilities can be discovered in everyday social and political reality and also in the cultural assumptions that underpin societies. It concerns not just people with intellectual disabilities but also communities and ultimately society itself. Personhood is 'about citizenship, mutual support, connectedness to social capital, about independent living, about participation' (Quinn, 2014, p. 39). The recognition of personhood involves a shift away from treating people with intellectual disabilities as 'objects' to be managed or cared for to recognising and respecting them as people. This involves providing pathways for independent living and the restoration of voice, power, authority and choice to each individual (Quinn, 2014).

REFERENCES

Abraham, J., & Odoom, J. O. (2019). Intellectual disability in twentieth-century Ghana. In J. Walmsley & S. Jarrett (Eds.), *Intellectual disability in the twentieth century: transnational perspectives on people, policy and practice.* Bristol: Bristol University Press.

Bach, M. (2017). Inclusive citizenship: refusing the construction of 'cognitive foreigners' in neo-liberal times. *Research and Practice in Intellectual and Developmental Disabilities*, 4(1), 4–25.

Badelt, C., & Österle, A. (2001). *Sozialpolitik in Österreich (Social policy in Austria)* (2nd ed.). Wien: Manz.

BASE (British Association for Supported Employment). (2020). *Employment rates for people with disabilities, 2019–19.* https://www.base-uk.org/employment-rates#:~:text=The%20latest%20figures%20for%20 2018,paid%20employment%20%5BIndicator%20 1E%5D. [Accessed 2 February 2021].

Bass, J. (2020). Learning disabilities should never be a reason for a Do Not Resuscitate order. *Health Service Journal, 25.*

https://www.hsj.co.uk/mental-health/learning-disabilities-should-never-be-a-reason-for-a-do-not-resuscitate-order/7027489.article.

Binding, K., & Hoche, A. (1920). *Die Freigabe der Vernichtung unwerten Lebens (Allowing the destruction of life unworthy of life)*. Leipzig: Felix Meiner.

Bock, G. (1986). *Zwangssterilisation im Nationalsozialismus (Forced sterilisation in Nazi Germany)*. Opladen: Westdt.

Carey, A. (2010). *On the margins of citizenship: intellectual disability and civil rights in twentieth-century America*. Philadelphia: Temple University Press.

Carson, J. (2007). *The measure of merit: talents, intelligence and inequality in the French and American republics, 1750–1940*. Princeton: Princeton University Press.

Council of Europe. (1950) European Convention on Human Rights. Available at: https://www.echr.coe.int/documents/convention_eng.pdf. [Accessed 17 January 2021].

Department of Health. (2001). *Valuing people: a new strategy for learning disability in the 21st century*. London: Department of Health.

Duffy, S. (2017). The value of citizenship. *Research and Practice in Intellectual and Developmental Disabilities, 4*(1), 26–34.

Geuss, R. (2001). *History and illusion in politics*. Cambridge: Cambridge University Press.

Goodley, D. (2017). *Disability studies. An interdisciplinary introduction* (2nd ed.). London: Sage.

Gould, S. J. (1996). *The mismeasure of Man*. New York: Norton.

Gustavsson, A. (2004). The role of theory in disability research – springboard or strait-jacket? *Scandinavian Journal of Disability Research, 6*(1), 55–70.

Hänsel, D. (2019). *Sonderschule im Nationalsozialismus (Special school in Nazi Germany)*. Bad Heilbrunn: Verlag Julius Kinkhardt KG.

Hubbard, R. (2006). Abortion and disability: who should and who should not inhabit the world? In L. J. Davis (Ed.), *The disability studies reader* (2nd ed.) (pp. 93–104). New York: Routledge.

Inclusion Europe. (2020). *Annual report 2019*. Brussels: Inclusion Europe.

Inclusion Europe. (2019). *Right to decide and political life*. Available at: https://www.inclusion-europe.eu/legal-capacity-and-citizenship-briefing/.

Jordan, T. (2011). Moving from diversity to inclusion. *Profiles in Diversity Journal*, March 22.

Kammerhofer, A. (2008). Bis zum 1. September 1941 wurden desinfiziert: Personen: 70.273. Die „Hartheimer Statistik" (Until September 1, 1941, disinfection was carried out: People: 70,273. The 'Hartheim Statistics'). In B. Kepplinger, G. Marckhgott, & H. Reese (Eds.), *Tötungsanstalt Hartheim (Hartheim killing centre)* (pp. 117–130). Linz: Trauner.

Kepplinger, B. (2009). The National Socialist Euthanasia Program in Austria: Aktion T4. In G. Bischof, F. Plasser, & B. Stelzl-Marx (Eds.), *New perspectives on Austrians and World War II* (pp. 224–249). New Brunswick, NJ: Transaction.

Kittay, E. F. (2010). The personal is political: a philosopher and mother of a cognitively disabled person sends notes from the battlefield. In E. F. Kittay, & L. Carlson (Eds.), *Cognitive disability and its challenge to moral philosophy* (pp. 393–413). Chichester: Wiley Blackwell.

Kuhse, H., & Singer, P. (1985). *Should the baby live? The problem of handicapped infants*. Oxford: Oxford University Press.

Learning Disability Today. (2015). *Gavin Harding becomes first UK mayor with learning disabilities*. Available at: https://www.learningdisabilitytoday.co.uk/gavin-harding-becomes-first-uk-mayor-with-learning-disabilities. [Accessed 2 January 2021].

Leydet, D. (2017). Citizenship. In E.N. Zalta (Ed.), *The Stanford encyclopedia of philosophy (Fall 2017 Edition)*.

Liessmann, K. P. (2016). *Neue Menschen! Bilden, optimieren, perfektionieren (New people! Form, optimize, perfect)*. Wien, Zsolnay: Philosophicum Lech (in German).

Locke, J. (1975). In P.H. Nidditch (Ed.), *[1689]. An Essay Concerning Human Understanding*. Oxford: Oxford University Press.

Lyle, D. (2019). *Understanding profound intellectual and multiple disabilities in adults*. Abingdon: Routledge.

McMahan, J. (2002). *The ethics of killing: problems at the margins of life*. Oxford: Oxford University Press.

McMahan, J. (2010). Cognitive disability and cognitive enhancement. In E. F. Kittay, & L. Carlson (Eds.), *Cognitive disability and its challenge to moral philosophy* (pp. 345–367). Chichester: Wiley Blackwell.

Mencap. (2012). *Death by indifference, 74 deaths and counting*. London: Mencap.

Monitoringausschuss (2012). Available at: http://monitoringausschuss.at/sitzungen/wien-17-11-2011-unterstuetzte-entscheidungsfindung-jetzt-entscheide-ich/ (in German). [Accessed 2 January 2021].

Noack, T. (2017). *NS-Euthanasie und internationale Öffentlichkeit (NS euthanasia and the international public)*. Frankfurt am Main: Campus.

Pailliez, C., & Libert, L. (2020). *Down syndrome, so what? One woman's campaign in France's municipal elections*. Available at: https://www.reuters.com/article/us-france-election-candidate-downsyndrom/down-syndrome-so-what-one-womans-campaign-in-frances-municipal-elections-idUSKBN20Q1XR. [Accessed 2 January 2021].

Pfahl, L., & Powell, J. W. (2011). Legitimating school segregation. *Disability & Society, 26*(2), 449–462.

Plangger, S., & Schönwiese, V. (2015). *Behinderung und Gerechtigkeit (Disability and justice)*. Wien: Juridicum.

Quinn, G. (2014). 'Rethinking personhood: new directions in legal capacity law & policy' or how to put the 'shift' back into 'paradigm shift'. In B. Janjic, K. Beker, & M. M. Markovic (Eds.), *Legal capacity and community living: protection of the rights of persons with disabilities. Collection of articles and recommendations* (pp. 17–39). Belgrade: Mental Disability Rights Initiative MDRI-S.

Rawls, J. (1993). *Political liberalism*. New York: Columbia University Press.

Rawls, J. (1999). *A theory of justice*. Cambridge, MA: Harvard University Press.

Rolph, S., Atkinson, D., Nind, M., et al. (2005). *Witnesses to change: families, learning difficulties and history*. Kidderminster: Bild.

Schmuhl, H. W., & Winkler, U. (2012). *Der das Schreien der jungen Raben nicht überhört". Der Wittekindshof – eine Einrichtung für Menschen mit geistiger Behinderung, 1887 bis 2012 (Wittekindshof – an institution for persons with learning disabilities)*. Bielefeld: Verlag für Regionalgeschichte.

Schulze, M. (2010). *Understanding the UN Convention on the Rights of Persons With Disabilities*. New York: Handicap International.

Schwanninger, F. (2019). *The pedagogues of eternal echoes*. Available at: https://www.eternalechoes.org/gb/for-the-classroom/exercises/2-2-racial-hygiene. [Accessed 2 January 2021].

Singer, P. (1975). *Animal liberation*. London: Pimlico.

Singer, P. (2012). *Ethics in the real world: 82 brief essays on things that matter*. Princeton: Princeton University Pres.

Singer, P., & Winkett, L. (2020). The duel: is it more important to save younger lives? *Prospect,* June.

Stainton, T. (2018). *Intellectual disability: towards inclusive citizenship*. Centre for Inclusion and Citizenship, University of British Columbia.

Stainton, T. (2005). Empowerment and the architecture of rights based social policy. *Journal of Intellectual Disabilities*, 9(4), 287–296.

Stainton, T. (1998). Rights and rhetoric in practice: contradictions for practitioners. In A. Symonds & A. Kelly (Eds.), *The social construction of community care* (pp. 135–144). London: Macmillan.

Stainton, T. (1994). *Autonomy and social policy*. Aldershot: Avebury.

Statham, H., Solomou, W., & Green, J. (2006). Late termination of pregnancy: law, policy and decision making in four English fetal medicine units. *British Journal of Obstetrics and Gynaecology*, 113(12), 1402–1411.

United Nations. (1948). *Universal Declaration of Human Rights*.

United Nations. (1975). *Declaration on the Rights of Disabled Persons*.

United Nations. (2006). *Convention on the Rights of Persons with Disabilities*.

Vianova. (2017) Bürgerinitiative betreffend der Diskriminierung von Menschen mit Behinderung durch die österreichische Gesetzgebung (Citizens' initiative concerning the discrimination of people with disabilities by Austrian legislation). Available at: https://vianova-austria.at/buergerinitiative/.

Waldschmidt, A. (2020). Jenseits der Modelle. Theoretische Ansätze in den Disability Studies (Beyond the models. Theoretical approaches in disability studies). In D. Brehme, P. Fuchs, S. Köbsell, & C. Wesselmann (Eds.), *Disability Studies im deutschsprachigen Raum (Disability studies in German speaking countries)* (pp. 56–73). Weinheim: Beltz Juventa.

Warman. (2016). *Tolerance*. Cambridge: The Beacon of Enlightenment Open Book Publishers.

Wegscheider, A. (2020). Dienst an den Ärmsten der Armen' Geschichte und Gegenwart institutioneller Versorgung in Oberösterreich ('Service for the poorest of the poor' History and present of institutional care in Upper Austria). In D. Brehme, P. Fuchs, S. Köbsell, & C. Wesselmann (Eds.), *Disability Studies im deutschsprachigen Raum (Disability studies in German speaking countries)* (pp. 174–181). Weinheim: Beltz Juventa.

Wegscheider, A. (2017). Soziales Engagement im Wandel der Zeit (Social commitment through the ages). In W. Schwaiger (Ed.), *Option Lebensvielfalt (Diversity of lives option)* (pp. 22–84). Linz: Wagner.

Wegscheider, A. (2016). *Differenzierte Hilfe für Menschen mit Behinderungen in Oberösterreich (1918–1938) (Differentiated help for people with disabilities in Upper Austria)*. Available at: http://bidok.uibk.ac.at/library/wegscheider-hilfe.html.

Wong, S. I. (2010). Duties of justice to citizens with cognitive disabilities. In E. F. Kittay & L. Carlson (Eds.), *Cognitive disability and its challenge to moral philosophy* (pp. 127–146). Chichester: Wiley Blackwell.

The importance of the personal narrative in the lives of people with intellectual disabilities

Helen Atherton and Vigdis Reisæter

KEY POINTS

- Pre-conceived ideas and stereotypes exist about what life is like for people with intellectual disabilities and this can hinder the delivery of Person-Centred Practice.
- Personal narratives illustrate the experiences that have shaped people with intellectual disabilities as individuals thus challenging myths, stereotypes and the concept of otherness.
- They can serve to identify what is important to an individual and help others understand how they make sense of the world.

- Personal narratives are central to ensuring that care and support provided to people with intellectual disabilities reflects their individual needs and wishes in different areas of their life
- The generation and use of these personal narratives need to be considered with reference to key ethical principles.

CHAPTER OUTLINE

INTRODUCTION

"Mine is an unexpected journey. When I was young, people were worried that maybe I wouldn't be able to walk. Maybe I wouldn't be able to talk. Many people, often nice people, thought I would have a very limited life."
    Sarah Gordy MBE, University of Nottingham, 2018

The previous chapter has discussed how the notion of personhood has been varyingly understood in terms of people with intellectual disabilities and the consequences this has had for their treatment, care and protection over time. This current chapter will now move this discussion on to consider how understanding someone with an intellectual disability from the perspective of their personal narrative, that is their individual story, can facilitate the development of both personal and professional relationships, ensuring increased life opportunities and care and support that is person centred.

Previous editions of this text included a chapter on causation and manifestation of intellectual disabilities that through necessity drew heavily on the biological/medical aspects of specific conditions. In doing so, it inadvertently aligned itself with the medical model of disability (discussed more fully in Chapter 1), whose primary limitation is the perspective that disability can be solely understood in terms of the presence of (an) impairment(s) [and the effect of this on a person's functional abilities] rather than an acknowledgment of the complex interplay between this and the barriers created by society, whether they be physical or attitudinal. Arguably this preoccupation with impairment stands to inhibit the ability of people interacting with those with intellectual disabilities, either in a personal or professional capacity, to see the person beyond the impairment, or more specifically the key elements that comprise the unique *self*. This is not to say that clinical labels or diagnoses are not important or useful; indeed they can be helpful in providing a preliminary indication of a person's potential needs or prognosis thereby facilitating access to the required treatment and support that Mimmo et al (2018) argue can mitigate against poor outcomes (for interested readers a good resource on specific conditions associated with intellectual disabilities can be found on the website of 'Contact' a UK organisation for families with children with disabilities – see useful addresses in the online resource). However, when a label becomes a stereotype it can result in sweeping assumptions being made about a person including their quality of life or abilities (Aston et al, 2014); as such any interactions, personal or professional, are governed primarily by that label and not by who the person actually is and what is important to them. This carries greater significance when considering that not all children and adults with intellectual disabilities have a definitive diagnosis that could guide the requisite care and support.

A preoccupation with symptoms and treatment can detract from the importance of establishing what it means to be 'me' (Tyreman, 2018). Labels should not become the defining feature of an individual and care should not be based on a set of assumptions or unchallenged perspectives (Rolph and Walmsley, 2006;

Altermark, 2017). Just because someone has Down syndrome does not mean that their life experience will be exactly the same as another with the same diagnosis, nor will be the array of factors that have shaped them as 'people' or what it is that they desire from life. So rather than presuming what it is like to have Down syndrome it is much more important to ask the person *"what makes you, you?"*, *"what do you want?"*, *"how can we help you get there?"*.

The chapter begins by outlining the concept of the personal narrative and considers why an understanding of how people with intellectual disabilities live or have lived their lives is important. It will then move on to look more specifically at the concept of person-centred care or support and how the personal narrative can be best employed to facilitate not only this process but quality interactions with people with intellectual disabilities in general. This provides a basis for subsequent chapters that explore person centred approaches in relation to specific life domains. The chapter concludes by considering the role and responsibilities of the recipient of a person's story, be that a professional or lay person, and some accompanying key ethical issues. Throughout the chapter the voices of people with intellectual disabilities and their significant others will be used to illustrate key points.

WHAT IS THE PERSONAL NARRATIVE?

"I am a great believer in that stories should be told…I just think everything is about stories…I think it has great power telling stories, and it can heal…I think being able to tell your story and to feel that you have been heard …is very important"
Nurse, Brandesburton Hospital 1981–1995

The above quote came from a study undertaken in 2016 to explore the personal experiences of those who lived and worked in a long stay hospital for people with intellectual disabilities in East Yorkshire (Atherton et al, 2017, p. 28). The aim of the study had been to capture personal stories of institutional life that ordinarily would have been lost forever but now exist to help others learn about the past and inform future actions. The concept of the personal narrative or story is as old as time and is an intrinsic part of human life. Ranging from fire side tales to the much more modern medium of digital storytelling, personal stories have allowed us to understand the events that have shaped not only our lives but also the lives of others. They are part of the development of personal, community, societal and national identity and enable connections to be made with others. Dohan et al (2016) define 'narrative' as an account of real life, whether written or spoken by the person who has experienced it. This may range from short anecdotes to longer more complex accounts, and as Edwards (2014) asserts will have meaning and value for the storyteller. Stories emphasise our uniqueness and individuality (Gillman et al, 1997). They also allow us to re-evaluate ourselves and others in light of new information and in some cases alter the way we behave and respond

> *"…I am a pioneer and I can tell my story so others can learn. Finally I get to say what I feel. Someone is listening to me. I've always wanted it that way. Finally everybody can see that I can do things and how I have felt. I can be myself. Then others can learn from me. I have so much to say."*
>
> *Hreinsdóttir et al, 2006, p. 163*

In recent decades, the power of the personal story has been used in a much more focused and deliberate way to improve care, support and treatment for people in different health and social care settings. Varyingly termed life story work, life history, life narrative amongst others, the personal story has been used to encourage behaviour changes, provide better understanding of the self and others, and to change attitudes. For example, in Canada it has been used with people with dementia to improve social connectedness (Hausknecht et al, 2019); in America with people with aphasia to promote a positive sense of self and improve communication skills (Strong et al, 2018); in Norway to support back to work rehabilitation (Brataas and Evensen, 2016) and in Denmark to uncover how people with Borderline Personality Disorder understand themselves and others (Lind et al, 2019).

Historically, little importance has been placed on facilitating people with intellectual disabilities to tell their individual stories and published examples have been few and far between but include *The World of Nigel Hunt* (Hunt, 1967) and *Tongue Tied* by Joey Deacon (Deacon, 1974). More recently have been examples such as David Barron's *A Price to be Born* (Barron, 1996) and *Mabel*

Cooper's Life Story (Cooper, 1997). There also exist written autobiographies of family members of those with intellectual disabilities (for example, Merriman, 2018) and online blogs such as The Future's Rosie (http://www.thefuturesrosie.com/). In addition to these there have been attempts to present the story of people with intellectual disabilities by piecing together their lives using archive research for example *Finding Ivy* (Atherton and Schwanninger, 2019); although useful in challenging people's perspectives on the life course of someone with intellectual disabilities the latter are less useful in presenting the world of that person in their own words.

Atkinson and Walmsley (1999) have referred to the personal stories of people with intellectual disabilities as 'lost voices' and use varying literature to argue that barriers to them telling their story have included a societal perception that they had nothing important to convey about their lives or that they lacked the means or ability to do so. Until recent decades understanding of how they allegedly lived or experienced their lives was largely derived from historical accounts of the impact of changing service philosophies, policy and legislation but individual voices were largely absent leading some to argue that what history they did have did not belong to them but was a history of "…others acting either on their behalf or against them" (Ryan and Thomas, 1987, p. 85). As such there appeared to be little recognition that people with intellectual disabilities themselves may have a perspective that might challenge 'accepted truths' i.e. what people thought they knew about this group and how they experienced the world.

In the past the voice of the person has not been central to the design and delivery of services for people with intellectual disabilities; these have been traditionally driven by 'expert' account (Gillman et al, 1997). Indeed, up until recent years, few developments, either at an individual or societal level, took into consideration the personal stories of people with intellectual disabilities and what they foresaw as being the priorities for their own care and support. This has been disempowering and served to reinforce the notion of their helplessness. Yet gradual changes in societal perceptions about this group coupled with the increasing influence of the self-advocacy movement (as discussed in Chapter 7) and the driver of *'nothing about us without us'* mentioned in Chapter 1 has meant that people with intellectual disabilities have begun to have a voice and a platform from which they can share their personal stories with others. Increasingly, the stories of people with intellectual disabilities have been used to enhance personal wellbeing and facilitate changes in service design and provision at both an individual and societal level as told through a variety of mediums that include the use of life story books (Moya, 2009), rummage boxes (Crook et al, 2015) and digital mediums such as 'Our COVID Voices – a website set up to enable people with intellectual disabilities to share their experiences of the COVID-19 pandemic (https://ourcovidvoices.co.uk/). Chapter 4 contains more detail about the range of media that can be harnessed to support story telling. This chapter focuses specifically on how stories can be employed in the facilitation of person-centred practice.

WHAT IS PERSON-CENTRED PRACTICE?

Person-Centred Practice is strongly connected with the concept of personhood presented in the previous chapter. The history of intellectual disability constructs stories about shifts from institutional to semi-institutionalised systems of care after the closure of long-stay hospitals i.e. group homes, sheltered homes, day services, and so on, towards a new emphasis on normalisation, empowerment, integration and an increasing focus on individualisation and personalisation (Kilbane and McLean, 2008). However, it is important to be aware that these ideas are not new. Individualisation can be traced to Carl Rogers (1965) and empowerment to Paulo Freire (2000), and to activism and the social model of disability. Today, policy documents in many western countries advocate Person-Centred Practice as the preferable way to provide health and social care services (Bigby et al, 2018; Phelan et al, 2020).

There exist a multitude of ways that the main facets of Person-Centred Practice i.e. planning, thinking, care and therapy can be interpreted (Waters and Buchanan, 2017). The approach stems from health care but is now recognised in several other professional fields e.g. education (Phelan et al, 2020). According to McCormack et al (2015, p. 3) person - centredness is defined as:

> *…an approach to practice established through the formation and fostering of healthful relationships between all care providers, service users and others significant to them in their lives. It is underpinned by values of respect for persons, individual right to self-determination, mutual respect and understanding. It is enabled by cultures of empowerment that foster continuous approaches to practice development.*

The aim of Person-Centred Practice is to make sure that the type of service the individual receives is specifically tailored to their own preferences, personal needs and wishes thereby recognising the importance of that unnegotiable value - *human dignity*. All of the activity professionals undertake in Person-Centred Practice - planning, thinking, care-performance and review - must uphold a person's dignity (Thompson et al, 2008). As much as Person-Centred Practice is perceived as a new way of providing care, in opposition to the medical model of disability, it also can be viewed as a part of the ongoing discourse of liberation and the fight for civil rights.

CORNERSTONES OF PERSON-CENTRED PRACTICE

Person-Centred Practice is based on 4 main cornerstones: listening, sharing power, responsive action and citizenship. We now explore each of these key issues in more detail.

Listening

In Person-Centred Practice *listening* is the most fundamental principle; a lack of listening undermines the other core elements that follow. Listening is a fundamental part of communication. In Person-Centred Practice, listening with attention and intention is fundamental. It means *attention* to the wording, either spoken or expressed through an alternative communication system. The wording has to be interpreted in its context, e.g. body language, gesture, clothing, all of which inform the communication. The professional needs to have the *intention* to understand, reveal and act upon what is said. Listening is important at many levels, between individuals, teams, organisations and society in general; it is essential for participation as citizens (Thompson et al, 2008). The ability to engage in multiple ways in searching for solutions requires a high level of interpersonal skills (McCormack and McCance, 2016, p. 44); it also demands creativity.

Sharing power

The principle of *sharing power* is to balance the power between the stakeholders, the service-user and the caregiver (Kilbane et al, 2008). Values, goals and outcome should be developed through a non-dominant and non-hierarchical relationship (McCormack and McCance, 2016, p. 51). Self-determination is an important goal in the attainment of freedom. The concept has gained attention in disability movements and been incorporated within legislation and care. Through this we can see the direct connections between discourses of liberation, self-determination and Person-Centred Practice (Wehmeyer et al, 2017). Phelan and Rickard-Clarke (2020) indicate 'healthy partnerships' as the basis for person-centredness, that include respect for the lived life and the importance of avoiding paternalistic attitudes. However, working with people with intellectual disabilities or people who struggle with ability to make informed choices, there are sometimes instances where we must act in their best interests. This leads us on to the question of autonomy, specifically relational autonomy (Björnsdóttir et al, 2015), where the need for assistance is an accepted part of supporting someone to make the right decisions for themselves although this should not justify doing anything against the person's own will and wishes.

Responsive action

Responsive action obliges the professional to act upon the person's wishes, helping to evolve better or other ways to increase their quality of life. Kilbane et al (2008) hold this to be difficult and complicated, because this may challenge both available resources and the way organisations and care-providers work. They therefore argue that it is important for professionals to be open to new ways of thinking and solving problems. Healthcare professionals need to facilitate active engagement and partnership, regardless of a person's capacity to make decisions or choices:

"For person-centredness to flourish, participants suggested it has to be the norm, with everyone's voice heard and valued. Relationships between all stakeholders within healthcare environments should be characterised by a shared purpose, shared decision making, mutual respect and involvement of all."

Phelan et al, 2020, p. 20

Citizenship

Citizenship is defined as the ultimate destination for Person-Centred Practice (Kilbane et al, 2008). To achieve full citizenship involves formal rights and duties as a citizen, and also the opportunity to make use of the opportunities offered by citizenship, such as participating in local activities in the community, and being engaged socially in political and leisure activities. This is a major issue for people with intellectual disabilities, who often have only limited access to areas of community life which are usually taken for granted. The support needed for individual participation demands effort at both an individual and a political level (Bigby et al, 2018) however, the distribution of resources including finances and staffing may determine the success and feasibility of these.

To conclude this section on the four cornerstones of Person-Centred Practice, the foundation of the approach and support is knowledge and understanding of the person and their wishes and desires. It builds on the notion that everyone is an individual, they are not homogenous; whilst they may share common diagnostic criteria, they have personal identities that have been shaped by a multitude of factors. Care cannot be targeted to individual needs and personal preferences unless professionals explore with the person what is important to them; in essence seeing the person behind the label is essential for tailoring care (Appelgren et al, 2018). The next section of this chapter will consider how the personal narrative can help facilitate this process.

HOW CAN THE PERSONAL NARRATIVE FACILITATE PERSON-CENTRED APPROACHES?

Fundamentally the personal narrative can be employed to challenge what we think we know about a person with an intellectual disability and in doing so can help establish a more realistic picture of their individual wishes and desires that can then form the basis of person-centred care or support. There is a need to challenge the

> "non-disabled assumptions and power relations that govern how people with disabilities are constructed and positioned as objects of professional expertise, rather than subjects of their own lives and decision-making processes."
>
> Fullagar and Darcy, 2004, p. 97

Such assumptions about people with intellectual disabilities exist not only at an individual level but the level of community and societies; they also exist in policy. In such traditional power relationships patients/service users could be construed as having a passive role in the receipt of health care (Naldemirci et al, 2019). Yet, the personal narrative can be an important aid in redressing this imbalance as it encourages professionals to think beyond a diagnosis and to view people with intellectual disabilities as unique individuals with unique stories to tell.

Obtaining the personal narrative has many uses in facilitating person-centred practice. In the following subsections we attempt to discuss four key benefits: identifying what is important, understanding the person and their behaviour, challenging myths, and stereotypes and challenging the concept of otherness.

Identifying what is important

A person's story can illicit important facets of the life of someone with an intellectual disability that can be employed as the basis for person-centred care and support (Roberts et al, 2020). It can offer an alternative to the professional diagnosis, although to be effective, both should be used in conjunction when formulating plans of care. It can facilitate people with intellectual disabilities to bring 'life goals' to the planning process (Naldemirci et al, 2019). Traditional person-centred planning tools such as Essential Lifestyle Planning, Maps and Paths actively employ the personal narrative as a basis for working with an individual to determine their wishes and desires (Lay and Kirk, 2011). Whilst predominantly a feature of social care provision, it is becoming increasingly popular in health care environments to establish individual priorities for care (Socal, 2020).

Where narrative approaches have been employed to connect with the person through their story, this has resulted in increased levels of satisfaction with care delivery (Johnson, 2019). Story tellers derive great benefit from the shift in power that ensues from being able to effectively take control of what is told and how it is told; this is closely connected to the feeling of empowerment that can be emitted from the storytelling experience (Atkinson, 2004). Feeling heard and the chance to release emotions are two further cited benefits, as is the opportunity to revisit and reflect on what has occurred (D'Cruz et al, 2020). This enables individuals to view themselves and their experiences through different lenses to establish new meaning from their story that may also result in a revised perception of the self. People with intellectual disabilities and their carers are often cast in the roles of the 'oppressed' and the 'oppressor' (Barnes, 1996). This is also a narrative which can and should be challenged. If we accept the narrative about the oppressed and the oppressor, then people with intellectual disabilities will be fixed in a position which is difficult to avoid or escape. Story telling has been shown to be effective in allowing people with intellectual disabilities to transition from the role of passive victim to fighter (Stefánsdóttir and Traustadóttir, 2015). We return to the power of storytelling in challenging accepted 'truths' when we consider myths and stereotypes later in this chapter.

Story telling can mean that those supporting people with intellectual disabilities glean a new understanding and perspective of thems as people. Carers in a study exploring the impact of a narrative approach to delivering person centred care in a long-term residential facility for older people talked about 'shining a light' on the person (Buckley et al, 2018, p. 864), enabling them to obtain information that would help build relationships with the person and plan care based on what was important to them. It also increased their awareness of the potential impact of previously unconsidered events such as move to the facility and the accompanying loss of privacy, physical contact and sexuality. In cases where difficulties with communication may hinder a person telling their own story and thus conveying their individual priorities, it has been shown that a personal narrative can be derived through the person's non-verbal communication but interpretation of this depends on working with others who know the person well (Gjermestad, 2017).

In a similar vein, personal stories can be important to facilitating person-centred decision making. Health care decision making that utilises only professional expertise could be considered unidimensional and not particularly person-centred. When people aren't listened to and their own priorities for their life are unacknowledged it can result in behaviour that may be

PERSONAL STORY 2.1

Alice has autism and is in her mid-thirties. She lives in a sheltered home. This story relates to the period of her life when she finished school and moved to a day care centre. At the centre Alice developed severe behavioural difficulties - she screamed, threw chairs and tables and her co-service users were afraid of her. People attributed her behaviour to her autism, particularly her dependency on routines, however her mother was convinced that the behaviour was related to Alice's ideas about having an ordinary job. A lot of effort was needed to convince the staff supporting Alice that this was the case. Despite her own reservations, Alice's mother believed in the importance of giving Alice a chance. Staff eventually took her views seriously and Alice was given the opportunity to change from day-care into work. After a while Alice herself experienced her own difficulties in terms of her ability to undertake work and she returned to the day care centre. However, the behavioural issues vanished. Alice, according to her mother, finally accepted the situation.

Alice's mother laid the groundwork for collaborative decision making. The eventual coming together to try to address Alice's wishes, regardless of the eventual outcome, was an example of good teamwork.

considered challenging (see Personal Story 2.1); however, when personal stories are used in conjunction with medical knowledge it can identify alternative perspectives. Indeed, Dohan et al (2015, p. 724) have concluded that narratives "don't tell patients or clinicians what to do so much as remind them of the pathways and the choices they face." Person-centred and co-created care yields not only positive benefits for people with intellectual disabilities but also those supporting them and in includes increased job satisfaction and mitigation against possible negative aspects such as stress and burnout (Van der Meer et al, 2018).

READER ACTIVITY 2.2

In Personal story 2.1, Alice's mother acted as an advocate for her daughter so her needs and wishes were heard by the people who could effectively respond to these. How might the involvement of the third party, such as parent, relative or significant other impact on the provision of person-centred care?

Whilst the personal narrative, in this case conveyed on Alice's behalf by her mother, can play an important role in finding out more about the person in terms of what is important to them, it can also be employed more widely to determine how people make sense of the world they live in and the experiences that have shaped them as individuals.

Understanding the person and their behaviour

To be able to ascertain what a person wants or needs it may be important to use the personal narrative to understand what has shaped them as individuals. As a qualified intellectual (learning) disability nurse working in a service for people with profound and complex needs the first author supported a gentleman who would regularly lie under chairs. From the stories told by his carers, it emerged that during his time in a long stay institution he would be hit by other residents and would use a chair as a refuge. An account of events that have shaped a person's life might be useful in understanding what causes and maintains individual behaviours (Lovell, 2007) thereby facilitating meaningful forms of support or intervention. In a study exploring nurses' experiences of caring for people with intellectual disabilities and dementia in Ireland Cleary and Doody (2017) demonstrated how a lack of knowledge and understanding of a person's back story can present as a barrier to effective person-centred care:

> "He would run straight to us and call us by their names, clearly these ladies were significant to him but we never found out who they were, and these gaps can be frustrating when they are trying to communicate, we don't have the life story."
>
> *Cleary and Doody, 2017, (p. 626)*

Contrarily when more was known about the person's past life, it was deemed to be helpful and supportive.

> "I knew him as a younger man and there were lots of things I recognised, names of places he had worked and the different individuals he spoke about and I was familiar with him and I was able to reassure him."
>
> *Cleary and Doody, 2017, (p. 626)*

Past experiences play a significant role in shaping our attitudes, beliefs and behaviours and use of personal narrative can aid an understanding of these. Not one person's journey is the same and it is this uniqueness that should drive home the importance of finding out about individuals as people rather than the label or diagnosis they carry. Personal narratives may also serve to counter 'diagnostic overshadowing', a concept that will be frequently revisited in different chapters of this book. Diagnostic overshadowing denotes a phenomenon whereby manifest behaviour is solely attributed to a person's label thus disregarding any other potential factors (Javaid et al, 2019). In terms of people with intellectual disabilities it can be described as the phenomenon of

"symptoms of physical ill health being mistakenly attributed to either a mental health/behavioural problem or as being inherent in the person's learning disabilities."

Emerson and Baines, 2010. p. 9

Without an understanding of a person's life experiences, there is a risk that any behaviour will be wrongly interpreted. This means that the underlying cause of the issue may not be investigated and/or inappropriate treatment and support given. This situation is exemplified in the case of Oliver McGowan in Personal story 2.2.

Evident in both stories of Alice and Oliver are the damaging effects of stereotyping. Stereotyping is inextricably linked to diagnostic overshadowing and therefore can impede the provision of person-centred care or support. Rolph and Walmsley (2006) contend that an important function of personal narratives is to dispel

PERSONAL STORY 2.2

In 2016 18-year-old Oliver McGowan was admitted to a hospital in the UK for treatment relating to his sepilepsy Oliver had a diagnosis of a mild intellectual disability and autism. On admission he began to display distressed behaviour that doctors failed to recognise as being linked to his autism or epilepsy. Without exploring alternatives to support Oliver, they administered Olanzapine, an anti-psychotic medication that Oliver was known to be allergic to. The doctors and nurses did not read his hospital passport which contained vital information about Oliver and his care, they also ignored his pleas when he said *"Please don't give me antipsychotics, I don't like them, they mess with my brain"* (Morris, 2018). Oliver was to die some 17 days later following an allergic response to the medication that caused Neuroleptic Malignant Syndrome, a side effect of the anti-psychotics.

Based on Devine (2018)

prevailing myths, stereotypes or dominant discourses about the lives of people with intellectual disabilities that can overshadow their actual needs and wishes.

Challenging myths and stereotypes

Despite increasing visibility in public life, people with intellectual disabilities continue to be stereotyped as having lower abilities and higher levels of dangerousness than those with other forms of disability (Werner, 2015). A survey of the Dutch population identified commonly occurring stereotypes about people with intellectual disabilities to include being "in need of help" and "unintelligent" all of which, it argued, could potentially lead to restrictions on opportunities to have agency and be self-determining (Pelleboer-Gunnink et al, 2019) Yet stereotypical attitudes and beliefs about people with intellectual disabilities cannot just be confined to the general public but exist amongst the very people delivering professional care and support to this group; these can affect the nature and quality of the working relationship with this group and their families (Lalvani, 2015). A Canadian study conducted by Morin et al (2018), exploring the attitudes of health care professionals and the general population towards people with intellectual disabilities using two vignettes, reported that some health professionals were found to exhibit feelings of pity, sadness or alternatively compassion towards people with intellectual disabilities, and were more likely than the general population to exhibit negative views on interacting with this group in everyday situations. Similarly, Desroches et al (2019) in exploring the attitudes and emotions of nurses in the USA towards people with intellectual disabilities found more negative attitudes towards this group than those exhibited towards people with physical disabilities and a perception that they had lower levels of quality of life.

Stereotypes about people with intellectual disabilities or the way they live or experience their lives can influence the type and quality of care afforded to this group. Altermark (2017) argues that one dominant or widely accepted narrative is that 'citizen inclusion' has been the antithesis to the values of oppression and confinement reflective of the institutional era however this perspective remains largely unchallenged and does not reflect the reality for large numbers of people with intellectual disabilities. Despite the existence of important agreements such as the UN Convention on the Rights of Persons with Disabilities (2006), people with intellectual disabilities still report in their personal narratives having restricted social networks (van Asselt-Goverts et al, 2015) and access to leisure opportunities that remain largely segregated (Hall, 2017). Despite expressing a desire and willingness to work, many do not have meaningful employment or own their homes (McMahon et al, 2019). Some rate the overall quality of their life as lower than those without intellectual disabilities (Simões and Santos, 2016).

Traditional stereotypes of people with intellectual disabilities as eternal children, asexual, childlike or innocent often deny them the opportunity to develop intimate and sexual relationships (Ditchman et al, 2017) despite the fact that personal narratives demonstrate that these are important to this group and when absent can have negative impacts on their lives (Rushbrooke et al, 2014).

> *"I like to touch and kiss. You know, what's wrong with kissing? There's nothing wrong with it. Yeah, we kiss all the time. You know, we just like – we – he comes home from work and I give him a kiss. I say, how was your day?"*
>
> Turner and Crane, 2016, p. 688

Such negative attitudes and presumptions about the capabilities of people also reduce their opportunity to experience parenthood. Whilst some life stories of those growing up with parents with intellectual disabilities have illustrated a range of negative experiences that include lack of basic care and nutrition (Weiber et al, 2019) other studies have shown that it can be a positive experience again emphasising the need to recognise that different personal narratives do exist:

> *"All my childhood, I was stuck at home with my mother. I went out only to school, and then I returned, walked the dog, came back home, cooked, and did the laundry. In the evenings I was so tired of caregiving that I didn't go out anywhere."*
>
> Wołowicz-Ruszowska and McConnell, 2016, p. 488

> *"I grew up with my mother's disability. Disability was part of our relation. But equally important was her nurturance; our deep relation, the fact that we love each other, we argue, and we talk about everything."*
>
> Wołowicz-Ruszowska and McConnell, 2016, p. 488

READER ACTIVITY 2.3

The accompanying online activity 2.3 asks you to consider the story of Sader Issa, a 21 year old dentist from Syria who grew up with a father who has Down syndrome.

Reflect on the different elements of the story and suggest how they challenge particular stereotypes that exist about people with intellectual disabilities.

Negative perspectives amongst health care professionals also extend to the experience of parenting a child with intellectual disabilities. In a study exploring the experience of fathers of children with Down syndrome, the negativity exhibited by health professionals at the point of diagnosis is shown to be in sharp contrast with the very positive aspects of parenting a child with Down syndrome

> *"our experience from what we were told what it was going to be like has been absolutely nothing like what it was really like."*
>
> How et al, 2019, p. 300

Yet the negative stereotypes continue to pervade the information giving process following a diagnosis of an intellectual disability such as Down syndrome (Enoch, 2020) however incorporating personal narratives of parents of children with Down syndrome into the training of professionals can enhance their reported ability to provide more balanced and responsive care (Mugweni et al, 2020).

The stereotypical perceptions of health professionals as to the quality of life enjoyed by people with intellectual disabilities and their families are also at the root of decisions currently being made about the provision of life saving treatment. Over the last few years, there have been increasing concerns raised about the extent to which the label of intellectual disability influences the decisions of doctors to give DNACPR (Do Not Attempt Cardiopulmonary Resuscitation) orders. This situation has been amplified with the COVID-19 pandemic with condemnation of the seemingly blanket application of DNACPRs on the basis of the presence of disability not an objective assessment of individual medical benefits (Chen and McNamara, 2020). It might therefore be assumed that a lack of awareness of how people with intellectual disabilities live their lives can lead to the perception that they lack value; a situation compounded by the fact that many doctors will only meet people when they are unwell (see Personal story 2.3).

Challenging the concept of 'otherness'

Closely linked to the issue of stereotyping is the notion of 'othering' Historically a lack of acceptance of people with intellectual disabilities has stemmed from a perception that they are somehow 'other' from their non-disabled peers. Mengstie (2011, p. 7) defines 'otherness' as the state of not being the same or alike to that experienced or known. Johnson et al (2004) take that definition one step further and consider the

 PERSONAL STORY 2.3   Andrew Waters

In 2011 Andrew Walters, a middle-aged man with Down syndrome and dementia was admitted onto an acute hospital ward in the UK. During his admission he was required to undergo a life enhancing procedure; on discharge his carers found a DNR "Do Not Resuscitate" notice folded up his bag. It stated that in the event of heart or breathing difficulties he should not be resuscitated. The reason given for this course of action was, in part, related to his diagnosis of Down syndrome and intellectual disability.

Neither Andrew's family nor his carers had been consulted about the DNR, nor did it take into consideration Andrew's life outside of his admission that included a love of dancing, swimming and drama.

Adapted from Dreaper (2015)

 READER ACTIVITY 2.4

Use the following link to learn more about Andrew's personal story https://www.bbc.co.uk/news/health-34938832

Think about what might have been your role in supporting Andrew and his family.

How might you have enabled the professionals involved with Andrew's care to find out more about his life outside of the hospital?

How might Andrew have been best supported to tell his personal story?

consequences of othering that include 'marginalization, decreased opportunities and exclusion' (p. 254). People with 'othering' characteristics have often been deemed a curiosity and it is argued that fascination with the idea of otherness still exists today (Ploeger, 2018). The view or belief that people with disabilities are less than human was pervasive in the decision to eliminate tens of thousands of people with intellectual disabilities in Hitler's T4 program (see Chapter 1) yet is still evident in some countries today with Bayat (2015) drawing attention to the murder of the 'spirit' and 'snake' children (those with disabilities) whose existence in West Africa is often ascribed to the work of supernatural forces. Yet, in contrast, this subhuman status, and often mystical quality that accompanies it, has historically given rise to examples where people with intellectual disabilities have been worshipped rather than condemned on the basis of their differences (Miles, 1996).

Yet the concept of 'othering' cannot be confined to developing countries or indeed examples from history as it remains evident in contemporary Western societies and has been linked to the systematic abuse of people with intellectual disabilities (Mathews, 2017). Othering creates and maintains a sense of social distance that can be counterproductive to the development of professional or indeed personal relationships that reflect empathy (Shapiro, 2008). Discomfort may arise from a perception of dissimilar attitudes and abilities as can a lack of awareness and knowledge about this group (Appelgren et al, 2018). In terms of social theories, there is general agreement that interpersonal similarity, defined as the *"level of similarity between the self and another person or persons"*, yields more positive attitudes (Costa-Lopes et al, 2012, p. 34). Where staff deem the people they care for to be 'more like us' whilst simultaneously responding positively to any differences, a more effective working relationship based on the values of 'humanness' ensues (Bigby et al, 2015).

Research has shown that the use of personal narratives can be effective in encouraging people to see the person, beyond the disability and facilitate feelings of empathy (Gona et al, 2018). It can enable disabled and non-disabled people to find common ground that encourages people to see the similarities between them thus reducing the sense of difference leading to a more empathetic response (Shapiro, 2008). Story telling can provide an opportunity for people with intellectual disabilities to connect with others both inside and outside the formal sphere of professional practice (Grove, 2015). In everyday life people exchange personal stories and anecdotes that facilitate a connection, and in some cases this initial connection can be the basis for the development of a friendship or relationship. However, for some people with intellectual disabilities there are limited opportunities to experience a shared identification with another person (Wiesel and Bigby, 2016).

The sharing of stories can promote empathy and understanding of the needs of individuals and others, but they can also lead to more responsive forms of support, not just from professional services but also local communities as illustrated in a study from India (Deepak et al, 2016). They facilitate the forging of connections between professionals and users of services that enable the development of working partnerships required for Person-Centred Practice person-centred planning. In a study exploring the use of personal narratives of people with intellectual disabilities with first year medical students, aspects of these stories were deemed 'relatable'. Having access to these accounts increased self-rated levels of comfort and confidence in providing care to this group (Coret et al, 2018).

WORKING WITHIN AN ETHICAL FRAMEWORK

The earlier sections of this chapter have demonstrated that personal narratives have an important use in facilitating the process of Person-Centred Practice by both challenging stereotypical imagery of people with intellectual disabilities and in doing so encouraging those in both a professional and lay capacity to see beyond a label to the person whose wishes and desires from life can be as individual and unique as those owned and articulated by anyone. Whilst the purpose and medium of choice for the telling or retelling of a story may differ, what is important is that it is both meaningful to the person and facilitates ownership. We all have the right to own our story, similarly we should have the right to be able to decide when, if and to whom a personal story is told. As professionals we are expected to implement evidence-based practice (Kvernbekk, 2017), meaning that best practice should be based on knowledge acquired from research or other sources; ethical guidelines for professionals commit us to reflect upon our use of knowledge

before action, in action and after action (International Council of Nurses, 2012; International Federation of Social Workers, 2018). Much can be learnt from the stories of others, in addition to research evidence, they are an important source of information therefore due consideration also needs to be given to potential ethical issues surrounding their use. To exemplify we ask the reader to reflect on the personal story of Evan (see Personal story 2.4).

As demonstrated in the case of Evan, professionals can play a significant role in the creation, maintenance and sharing of the personal narratives of those for whom they provide care. Evan's narrative was not created or shared by himself but by previous staff working with him; as such it represented their story of Evan, not Evan's story as he himself or those close to him understood or experienced it. This led to a response that was not person-centred, and in many ways reflected historical attitudes and beliefs about the sexuality of people with intellectual disabilities that continue to pervade this group.

Denying a person the right to own and share their personal story undermines the basic ethical principles of

---

👤 PERSONAL STORY 2.4

This a story told by Evan's staff about the planning of his care. Evan has an intellectual disability and has lived in sheltered homes throughout his adult life. Some years ago, he moved to a new group home. Some of the information shared by his old staff with his new staff was a story about a specific incident that Evan had been involved in, and the potential sexual risk they believed he now presented to others. This information was not questioned by the new staff, and no attempt was made to try and establish any alternative perspectives, either by asking Evan to tell his version of events or others who knew him well, e.g. his parents. The information was just accepted as 'fact' and as such served to shape the opinions of the new staff about Evan even before getting to know him as a person and/or reassessing the reality of the risk. These opinions were to significantly influence the care he received that included restrictions on his personal liberties in response to the 'alleged danger' he posed.

autonomy and right to self-determination; an issue that might be more problematic amongst some people with intellectual disabilities, like Evan, where traditional power dynamics mean they lack control over their lives. Stories are often developed and shaped through our interaction with others but for most of us we still retain ownership of them. This might not be so easy for some people with intellectual disabilities, particularly those whose level of intellectual ability and accompanying communication difficulties may mitigate against either the construction or the telling of their own story and thus rely on third party involvement. Gjermestad (2017) argues that such a necessity can increase the risk of a biased narrative emerging that may be countered through discussion and reflection amongst a range of people who know a person well. Related to this is the lack of opportunity to construct a new or revised narrative that would serve to challenge the 'accepted' version (Malacrida, 2006). Naldemirci et al (2019) contend that family members and friends can be an important source of information in the construction of a personal narrative; this said their involvement in adulthood should only be facilitated with the agreement of the individual, or in cases when their consent cannot be obtained, in their best interests.

Another issue concerned Evan's lack of opportunity to consent to the telling of his story - to whom and for what purpose? Most codes of professional conduct uphold the need to maintain patient/service user confidentiality unless there are exceptional grounds such as preventing harm to others; even then attempts must first be made to obtain consent from the person for the sharing of key information (Davies, 2017). The same holds true for personal narratives. People are entitled to privacy and must be supported to make informed choices about how their personal stories might be used. In line with mental capacity guidelines this should involve discussing with the person the pros and cons of sharing their story. This might also include the possibility that sharing their story may evoke strong emotional feelings (Nurser et al, 2018). Whilst the possibility of this should not deter professionals from helping someone tell their story, provision should be made to ensure that they are properly supported and have access to any necessary specialist services.

CONCLUSION

Person-Centred Practice recognises that everyone is an individual with their own wishes and desires however stereotypes and preconceptions as to how people with intellectual disabilities live their lives and what is important to them may mitigate against professionals providing person-centred care and support. Personal narratives, that is the personal stories of individuals with intellectual disabilities, are effective tools for educating people about their lives, what is important to them and what has shaped them as people. They can be used to identify priorities for care, and challenge accepted truths. Where connections can be made through the telling of personal stories, these can be the basis for the forging of greater empathetic relationships between professionals, lay people and those with intellectual disabilities.

REFERENCES

Altermark, N. (2017). The post-institutional era: visions of history in research on intellectual disability. *Disability & Society*, 32(9), 1315–1332.

Appelgren, M., Bahtsevani, C., Persson, K., et al. (2018). Nurses' experiences of caring for patients with intellectual developmental disorders: a systematic review using a meta-ethnographic approach. *BMC Nurse*, 17(51). doi. org/10.1186/s12912-018-0316-9.

Aston, M., Breau, L., & MacLeod, E. (2014). Diagnoses, labels & stereotypes: supporting children with intellectaul disabilities in the hospital. *Journal of Intellectual Disabilities*, 18(4), 291–304.

Atherton, H., Steels, S., & Ackroyd, V. (2017). An exploration of what motivates people to participate in oral history projects. *Learning Disability Practice*, 20(2), 27–31.

Atherton, H., & Schwanninger, F. (2019), Finding Ivy: a life worthy of life, Available at: https://www.cl-initiatives. co.uk/finding-ivy-life-worthy-life/#:~:text=Schloss%20 Hartheim%2C%20an%20old%20castle,programme%20 known%20as%20Aktion%20T4. [Accessed 3 March 2021]

Atkinson, D. (2004). Research and empowerment: involving people with learning difficulties in oral and life history research. *Disability & Society*, 19(7), 691–702.

Atkinson, D., & Walmsley, J. (1999). Using autobiographical approaches with people with learning difficulties. *Disability & Society*, 14(2), 203–216.

Barnes, C. (1996). Disability and the myth of the independent researcher. *Disability & Society*, 11(1), 107–112.

Barron, D. (1996). *A price to be born*. Harrogate: Mencap Northern Division.

Bayat, M. (2015). The stories of 'snake children': killing and abuse of children with developmental disabilities in West Africa. *Journal of Intellectual Disability Research*, 59(Part 1), 1–10.

Bigby, C., Knox, M., Beadle-Brown, J., et al. (2015). We call them people: positive regard as a dimension of culture in group homes for people with severe intellectual disability. *Journal of Applied Research in Intellectual Disabilities, 28*, 283–295.

Bigby, C., Anderson, S., & Cameron, N. (2018). Identifying conceptualizations and theories of change embedded in interventions to facilitate community participation for people with intellectual disability: a scoping review. *Journal of Applied Research in Intellectual Disabilities (JARID), 31*(2), 165–180.

Björnsdóttir, K., Stefánsdóttir, G., & Stefánsdóttir, Á. (2015). 'It's my life': autonomy and people with intellectual disabilities. *Journal of Intellectual Disabilities, 19*(1), 5–21. https://doi.org/10.1177/1744629514564691.

Brataas, H. V., & Evensen, A. E. (2016). Life stories of people on sick leave from work because of mild mental illness, pain and fatigue. *Work, 53*(2), 285–291.

Buckley, C., McCormack, B., Oxon, P., et al. (2018). Working in a storied way – narrative-based approaches to person centred care and practice development in older adult residential care settings. *Journal of Clinical Nursing, 27*(5-6), 858–872.

Chen, B., & McNamara, D. M. (2020). Disability discrimination, medical rationing and COVID 19. *Asian Bioethics Review, 12*, 511–518.

Cleary, J., & Doody, O. (2017). Nurses' experience of caring for people with intellectual disability and dementia. *Journal of Clinical Nursing, 26*(5-6), 620–631.

Cooper, M. (1997). Mabel Cooper's life story. In D. Atkinson, & M. Jackson, & J. Walmsley (Eds.), *Forgotten lives: exploring the history of learning disability*. Kidderminster: BILD.

Coret, A., Boyd, K., Hobbss, K., et al. (2018). Patient narratives as a teaching tool: a pilot study of first-year medical students and patient educators affected by intellectual/developmental disabilities. *Teaching and Learning in Medicine, 30*(3), 317–327.

Costa-Lopes, R., Vala, J., & Judd, C. M. (2012). Similarity and dissimilarity in intergroup relations: different dimensions, different processes. *International Review of Social Psychology, 25*(1), 31–65.

Crook, N., Adams, M., Shorten, N., et al. (2015). Does the well-being of individuals with down syndrome and dementia improve when using life story books and rummage boxes? a randomized single case series experiment. *Journal of Applied Research in Intellectual Disabilities, 29*(1), 1–10.

Davies, M. (2017). Can you breach a patient's confidentiality if you believe they pose a risk to others? *BMJ, 356*, j699.

D'Cruz, K., Douglas, J., Serry, T. (2020). Narrative storytelling as both an advocacy tool and a therapeutic process: perspectives of adult storytellers with acquired brain injury. *Neuropsychological Rehabilitation, 30*(8), 1409–1429.

Deacon, J. J. (1974). *Tongue tied: fifty years of friendship in a subnormality hospital*. London: National Society for Mentally Handicapped Children.

Deepak, S., Kumar, J., Sivarama, C., et al. (2016). Life stories of persons with intellectual disabilities in Mandya District, India. *Knowledge of Management for Development Journal, 11*(1), 8–24.

Desroches, M. L., Sethares, K. A., Curtin, C., et al. (2019). Nurses' attitudes and emotions toward caring for adults with intellecrual disabilities: results of a cross sectional, correlational-predicitive research study. *Journal of Applied Research in Intellectual Disabilities, 32*(6), 1501–1513.

Devine, D. (2018). Interview: 'Oliver McGowan's name should be given to autism and learning disability training'. Available at: https://www.learningdisabilitytoday.co.uk/prevent-avoidable-deaths-by-making-autism-and-learning-disability-training-mandatory. [Accessed 15 March 2021].

Ditchman, N., Easton, A. B., Batchos, E., et al. (2017). The impact of culture on attitudes toward the sexuality of people with intellectual disabilities. *Sexuality and Disability, 35*(2), 245–260.

Dohan, D., Garrett, S. B., Rendle, K. A., et al. (2016). The importance of integrating narrative into health care decision making. *Health Affairs, 35*(4), 720–725.

Dreaper, J. (2015). Hospital sorry for 'do not resuscitate' order on patient with Down's syndrome. Available at: https://www.bbc.co.uk/news/health-34938832. [Accessed 15 March 2021].

Edwards, S. L. (2014). Using personal narrative to deepen emotional awareness of practice. *Nursing Standard, 28*(50), 46–51.

Emerson, E., & Baines, S. (2010). Health inequalities & people with learning disabilities in the UK: 2010. Available at: pureportal.strath.ac.uk/files_asset/7402206/vid_7479_IHaL2010_3HealthInequality2010.pdf. [Accessed 1 March 2021].

Enoch, N. (2020). A life worth living. *British Journal of Midwifery, 28*(1), 9–10.

Freire, P. (2000). *Pedagogy of the oppressed* (30th Anniversary Edition). London: Bloomsberry Academic.

Fullagar, S., & Darcy, S. (2004). Critical points against an Australasian therapeutic recreation association: towards community leisure through enabling justice. *Annals of Leisure Research, 7*(2), 95–103.

Gjermestad, A. (2017). Narrative competence in caring encounters with persons with profound intellectual and multiple disabilities. *International Practice Development Journal*, 7. doi.org/10.19043/ipdj.7SP.007.

Gillman, M., Swain, J., & Heyman (1997). Life history or 'case' history: the objectification of people with learning difficulties through the tyranny of professional discourses. *Disability & Society*, *12*(5), 675–693.

Gona, J. K., Newton, C. R., Hartley, S., et al. (2018). Persons with disabilities as experts-by experience: using personal narratives to affecr community attitudes in Kilifi, Kenya. *BMC International Health and Human Rights*, *18*(18). doi.org/10.1186/s12914-018-0158-2.

Grove, N. (2015). Finding the sparkle: storytelling in the lives of people with learning disabilities. *Tizard Learning Disability Review*, *20*(1), 29–36.

Hall, S. A. (2017). Community involvement of young adults with intellectual disabilities: their experiences and perspectives on inclusion. *Journal of Applied Research in Intellectual Disabilities*, *30*, 859–871.

Hausknecht, S., Vanchu-Orosco, M., & Kaufmann, D. (2019). Digitising the wisdom of our elders: connectedness through digital storytelling. *Ageing and Society*, *39*(12), 2714–2734.

How, B., Smidt, A., Wilson, N. J., et al. (2019). 'We would have missed out so much had we terminated': what fathers of a child with Down syndrome think about current non-invasive prenatal testing for Down syndrome. *Journal of Intellectual Disabilities*, *23*(3), 290–309.

Hreinsdóttir, E. E., Stefándóttir, Lewthwaite A., et al. (2006). Is my story so different from yours? Comparing life stories, experiences of institutionalization and self-advocacy in England and Iceland. *British Journal of Learning Disabilities*, *34*, 157–166.

Hunt, N. (1967). *The world of Nigel Hunt: the diary of a Mongoloid youth*. New York: Garrett Publications.

International Council of Nurses (2012) The ICN Code of Ethics for nurses. Available at: https://ed-areyouprepared.com/wp-content/uploads/2019/01/2012_ICN_Codeofethicsfornurses_-eng.pdf. [Accessed 15 March 2021].

International Federation of Social Workers. (2018). Global social work statement of ethical principles. Available at: https://www.ifsw.org/global-social-work-statement-of-ethical-principles/. [Accessed 15 March 2021].

Javaid, A., Nakata, V., & Michael, D. (2019). Diagnostic overshadowing in learning disability: think beyond the disability. *Progress in Neurology & Psychiatry*, *23*(2), 8–10.

Johnson, J. L., Bottoroft, J. L., Brown, A. J., et al. (2004). Othering and being othered in the conext of health care services. *Health Communication*, *16*(2), 253–271.

Johnson, K. (2019). This is my story: using patient personalization posters to improve nurses' caring.

behaviours Available at: https://sigma.nursingrepository.org/bitstream/handle/10755/17510/Johnson_Kelly_DNP_Paper_May2019.pdf?sequence=3&isAllowed=y. [Accessed 16 October 2020].

Kilbane, J., & McLean, T. (2008). Exploring history and person centred practice. In J. Thompson, J. Kilbane, & H. Sanderson (Eds.), *Person centred practice for professionals*. New York: McGraw Hill Professional.

Kilbane, J., Thompson, J., & Sanderson, H. (2008). Towards person centred practice. In J. Thompson, J. Kilbane, & Sanderson (Eds.), *Person centred practice for professionals*. New York: McGraw Hill Professional.

Kvernbekk, T. (2017). Evidence-based educational practice. *Oxford Research Encyclopedias*. Oxford University Press.

Lalvani, P. (2015). Disability, stigma and otherness: perspectives of parents and teachers. *International Journal of Disability, Development and Education*, *62*(4), 379–393.

Lay, J., & Kirk, L. (2011). Person-centred strategies for planning. In H. L. Atherton, & D. J. Crickmore (Eds.), *Learning disabilities: toward inclusion*. Edinburgh: Churchill Livingstone.

Lind, M., Thomsen, D. K., Bøye, R., et al. (2019). Personal and parents' life stories in patients with borderline personality disorder. *Scandinavian Journal of Psychology*, *60*(3), 231–242.

Lovell, A. (2007). Learning disability aginst itself: the self-injury/self-harm conundrum. *British Journal of Learning Disabilities*, *36*, 109–121.

McCormack, B., Borg, M., Cardiff, S., et al. (2015). Person-centredness – the 'state' of the art. *International Practice Development Journal*, *5*(Suppl), 1–15.

McCormack, B., & McCance, T. (2016). *Person-centred practice in nursing and health care: theory and practice*. Newark: John Wiley & Sons.

McMahon, M., Bowring, D. L., & Hatton, C. (2019). Not such an oridinary life: a comparison of employment, marital status and housing profies oa dults with and without intellectual disabilities. *Tizard Learning Disability Review*, *24*(4), 213–221.

Malacrida, C. (2006). Contested memories: efforts of the powerful to silence former inmates' histories of life in an institution for 'mental defectives'. *Disability & Society*, *21*(5), 397–410.

Mathews, I. (2017). Not like us? Wolfensberger's 'major historic roles' reconsidered. *Disability & Society*, *32*(9), 1351–1365.

Mengstie, S. (2011). Constructions of 'otherness' and the role of education: the case of Ethiopia. *Journal of Education Culture and Society*, *2*, 7–15.

Merriman, A. (2018). *A major adjustment*. London: Down's Syndrome Association.

Miles, M. (1996). Pakistan's microcephalic chuas of Shah Daulah: cursed, clamped or cherished? *History of Psychiatry, 7*, 571–589.

Mimmo, L., Harrison, R., & Hinchcliff, R. (2018). Patient safety vulnerabilities for children with intellectual disability in hospital: a systematic review and narrative synthesis. *BMJ Paediatrics Open*. https://doi.org/10.1136/bmjpo-2017-000201.

Morin, D., Valois, P., Crocker, A. G., et al. (2018). Attitudes of health care professionals toward people with intellectual disability: a comparison with the general population. *Journal of Intellectual Disability Research, 62*(9), 746–758.

Morris, S. (2018). Bristol hospital vows to improve training after death of teenager Available at: https://www.theguardian.com/uk-news/2018/apr/20/bristol-hospital-vows-to-improve-staff-training-over-death-of-teenager-oliver-mcgowan-antipsychotic. [Accessed 4 March 2021].

Moya, H. (2009). Identities on paper: constructing lives for people with intellectual disabilities in life story books. *Narrative Inquiry, 19*(1), 135–153.

Mugweni, E., Lowenhoff, C., Walker, M., et al. (2020). The feasibility of a multi-professional training to improve how heath care professionals deliver different news to families during pregnancy and at birth. *Child: Care, Health and Development*. https://doi.org/10.1111/cch.12758.

Naldemirci, Ö., Britten, N., Lloyd, H., et al. (2019). The potential and pitfalls of narrative elicitation in person-centred care. *Health Expectations, 23*, 238–246.

Nurser, K. P., Rushworth, I., Shakespeare, T., et al. (2018). Personal story telling in mental health recovery. *Mental Health Review Journal, 23*(1), 25–36.

Pelleboer-Gunnink, H. A., van Weeghel, J., & Embregts, P. J. C. M. (2019). Public stigmatisation of people with intellectual disabilities: a mixed method population survey in stereotypes and their relationship with familiarity and discrimination. *Disability and Rehabilitation*. https://doi.org/10.1080/09638288.2019.1630678.

Phelan, A., & Rickard-Clarke, P. (2020). Person-centred approaches in capacity legislation. In A. Phelan (Ed.), *Advances in elder abuse research: practice, legislation and policy* (pp. 23–38). Cham, Switzerland: Springer.

Phelan, A., McCormack, B., Dewing, J., et al. (2020). Review of developments in person-centred healthcare. *International Practice Development Journal, 10*(Suppl 2), 1–29.

Ploeger, E. O. (2018). Otherness as entertainment: the Victorian-era freak show and its legacy in contemporary popular culture. Available at: https://academicarchive.snhu.edu/bitstream/handle/10474/3532/his2018ploeger.pdf?sequence=1&isAllowed=y. [Accessed 6 April 2020].

Roberts, T. J., Ringter, T., Krahn, D., et al. (2020). The 'My Life, My Story' program: sustained impact of veterans personal narratives on healthcare providers 5 years after implementation. *Health Communication*. https://doi.org/10.1080/10410236.2020.1719316.

Rogers, C. R. (1965). *Client-centered therapy: its current practice, implications, and theory*. New York: Houghton Mifflin.

Rolph, S., & Walmsley, J. (2006). Oral history and new orthodoxies: narrative accounts in the history of learning disability. *Oral History, 34*(1), 81–91.

Rushbrooke, E., Murray, C., & Townsend, S. (2014). The experiences of intimate relationships by people with intellectual disabilities: a qualitative study. *Journal of Applied Research in Intellectual Disabilities, 27*, 531–541.

Ryan, J., & Thomas, F. (1987). *The politics of mental handicap* (revised ed). London: Free Association Books.

Shapiro, J. (2008). Walking a mile in their patients' shoes: empathy and othering in medical students' education. *Philsophy, Ethics and Humanitites in Medicine, 3*(10). https://doi.org/10.1186/1747-5341-3-10.

Simões, C., & Santos, S. (2016). Comparing the quality of life of adults with and without intellectual disability. *Journal of Intellectual Disability Research, 60*(4), 378–388.

Socal, M. P. (2020). Patient narratives: a tool for people-centred health systems education. *Medical Science Education, 30*, 1437–1443.

Stefánsdóttir, G. V., & Traustadóttir, R. (2015). Life histories as counter-narratives against dominant and negative stereotypes about people with intellectual disabilities. *Disability & Society, 30*(3), 368–380.

Strong, K. A., Lagerway, M. D., & Shadden, B. B. (2018). More than a story: my life came back to life. *American Journal of Speech Language Pathology, 27*(1S), 464–476.

Thompson, J., Kilbane, J., & Sanderson, H. (Eds.). (2008). *Person centred practice for professionals*. New York: McGraw Hill Professional.

Turner, G. W., & Crane, B. (2016). Pleasure is paramount: adults with intellectual disabilities discuss sensuality and intimacy. *Sexualities, 19*(5-6), 677–697.

Tyreman, S. (2018). Evidence, alternative facts and narrative: a personal reflection on person centred care and the role of stories in healthcare. *International Journal of Osteopathic Medicine, 28*, 1–3.

University of Nottingham. (2018) Honorary doctorate for inspirational actor and campaigner Sarah Gordy. Available at: https://www.nottingham.ac.uk/news/pressreleases/2018/december/honorary-doctorate-for-inspirational-actor-and-campaigner-sarah-gordy.aspx. [Accessed 5 March 2021].

United Nations. (2006). Convention on the Rights of Persons with Disabilities. Available at: https://www.un.org/development/desa/disabilities/convention-on-the-rights-of-persons-with-disabilities.html. [Accessed 5 March 2021].

Van Asselt-Goverts, A. E., Embregts, P. J. C. M., Hendriks, A. H. C., et al. (2015). Do social networks differ? Comparison of the social networks of people with intellectual disabilities, people with autism spectrum disorders and other people living in the community. *Journal of Autism Developmental Disorders, 45,* 1191–1203.

Van der Meer, L., Nieboer, A. P., Finkenflügel, H., et al. (2018). The importance of person-centred care and co-creation of care for the well-being and job satisfaction of professionals working with people with intellectual disabilities. *Scandinavian Journal of Caring Science, 32*(1), 76–81.

Waters, R. A., & Buchanan, A. (2017). An exploration of person-centred concepts in human services: a thematic analysis of the literature. *Health Policy, 121*(10), 1031–1039.

Wehmeyer, M. L., Shogren, K. A., Little, T. D., et al. (Eds.). (2017). *Development of self-determination through the life-course.* Dortdrecht: Springer Natuer.

Weiber, I., Tengland, P. A., Bergland, J. S., et al. (2019). Everyday life when growing up with amother with an intellectual or developmental disability: four retrospective life-stories. *Scandinavian Journal of Occupational Therapy.* https://doi.org/10.1080/11038128.2018.1554087.

Werner, S. (2015). Public stigma and the perception of rights: differences between intellectual and physical disabilities. *Research in Developmental Disabilities, 38,* 262–271.

Wiesel, I., & Bigby, C. (2016). Mainstream, inclusionary, and convivial places: locating encounters between people with and without intellectual disabilities. *Geographical Review, 106*(2), 201–214.

Wołowicz-Ruszowska, A., & McConnell, D. (2016). The experience of adult children of mothers with intellectual disability: a qualitative retrospective study from Poland. *Journal of Applied Intellectual Disability Research, 30,* 482–491.

How can you help me have a choice?

John O'Brien and Simon Duffy

KEY ISSUES

- Many people with intellectual disabilities experience an unacceptable gap between rights established in law and the choices they actually have the freedom to make.
- Closing the gap calls for social invention, the co-creation of new ways of thinking about, organising and delivering the supports a person needs. Social invention reduces the constraints that limit freedom by adapting supports to specific people as they exercise citizenship.
- The ideal of citizenship gives social invention purpose and The Keys to Citizenship provide a practical framework for establishing the conditions that support meaningful choices.
- Successful social inventors – people with intellectual disabilities and their allies – disrupt a culture that takes power-over people with intellectual disabilities for granted. Freedom grows through acting from power-with relationships.
- Increasing the effective control people with intellectual disabilities have over the supports they need and becoming more skilful at supporting choice expands the freedom people with intellectual disabilities have to choose.

CHAPTER OUTLINE

INTRODUCTION

In 2006 the *United Nations (UN) Convention on the Rights of People with Disabilities (CRPD)* proclaimed this general principle in Article 3(1), "Respect for inherent dignity, individual autonomy including the freedom to make one's own choices…". Choice threads through the CRPD in a way that confronts much current reality, especially in residential and day services: Article 19(a), "Persons with disabilities have the opportunity to choose their place of residence and where and with whom they live on an equal basis with others and are not obliged to live in a particular living arrangement". Article 27(1), 'States Parties recognise the right of persons with disabilities to work, on an equal basis with others; this includes the right to the opportunity to gain a living by work freely chosen or accepted in a labour market and work environment that is open, inclusive and accessible to persons with disabilities'. The CRPD calls for deep changes in thinking and practice to establish a meaningful right to make consequential life choices. In particular, Article 12, recognising people with disabilities as persons before the law, disrupts the practice of a Court assuming the right to decide or assigning it to a substitute decision maker. This demands the creation of new ways to support decision making.

As discussed in Chapter 1, established rights do not predict the actual lived experience of having choices. In 2019 Stay Up Late, an English advocacy group that supports access to night life for people with intellectual disabilities, launched the #No Bedtimes Campaign. The campaign aims to abolish staff enforced bedtimes for adults in residential settings (see Box 3.1).

The centrality of choice in the CRPD, the apparent distance between its mandates and the necessity to campaign against enforced bedtimes more than ten years after its ratification all point towards the need for a new way to facilitate choice – that is the use of social invention. Social inventors appreciate and establish the conditions for meaningful choices – from what to eat for breakfast, to where and with whom to live, and how to fulfil the responsibilities of citizenship. Social inventors bring together people with intellectual disabilities and their allies, among which are family members and support providers, to generate new ways to think and act that open the way to greater freedom. Social inventions are necessary in individual circumstances, in organisational structure and culture and in policy. Social inventors take action to discover more liberating ways of thinking and activate co-creative relationships. The result is a growing experience of the benefits and responsibilities of citizenship.

This chapter explores how increasing opportunities for people with intellectual disabilities to have meaningful choices consistent with the rights established by the CRPD can be facilitated. It produces a context for person-specific efforts to inform and support choice and decision making in particular situations. It prioritises pushing back the limits on choice in general over techniques for assisting people with intellectual disabilities to make a specific choice (for ideas about supporting people with intellectual disabilities to choose in a particular situation, see, for example, Minnesota Department of Human Services (MDHS), 2016, which focuses on the choice to work).

We begin the chapter by identifying constraints on choice, including disabling constraints that are attached to differences in body, brain, and mind associated with intellectual disability. Awareness of the ways that current service structures and practices reproduce these constraints is the first step to finding practical ways to reduce their burden.

Next, we establish the ideal of citizenship to orient the search for freedom. Seven Keys to Citizenship offers a practical framework for identifying and developing the conditions that promote community, belonging, mutual responsibility and contribution.

Finally, we frame three challenges that define an agenda for social inventors: shifting a culture that normalises *power-over* people with intellectual disabilities to a culture of *power-with* relationships; increasing the effective control people have over their supports; and decreasing the number of people subjected to substitute decision making.

LIMITS ON CHOICE

The CRPD associates choice with other goods – dignity, autonomy, freedom and independence. Each of these words highlights and amplifies what is desirable about

---

BOX 3.1   The Right to Stay Up Late

The Big Bedtime Audit (Fish, 2018) provides an accessible summary of a study by James, Harvey and Mitchell (2018) that shows the relevance of #No Bedtimes (https://stayuplate.org/our-projects/campaign-resources/). Researchers made two Thursday or Friday evening visits, six months apart, to 263 people resident in supported tenancies, supported living houses, residential care homes and nursing homes to see what they were doing at 8:00pm on a Thursday or Friday. 69% of the residents were in bed or ready for bed. Less than 25% were home and not ready for bed. A small number were out for the evening. Nearly half the staff said that people were in bed because the person chose to be there.

READER ACTIVITY 3.1

In *The Big Bedtime Audit,* about half the staff attribute early bedtimes to people's choice.

Speculate on possible reasons why the staff may explain the situation in this way.

What might be possible consequences for people with intellectual disabilities?

choice and necessary for its exercise. Regardless of disability, every citizen's choices are contingent and constrained; the responsibilities of citizenship, local effects of inequality in the social determinants of health (Marmot, 2015), a community's array of accessible opportunities and assets, a person and family's social status and roles, the breadth, depth and diversity of available relationships, personal capabilities and justified confidence in one's ability to overcome challenges with learning and persistence, and stocks of material resources all interact and shape everyone's degree of autonomy and extent of freedom to choose. However, people with intellectual disabilities experience additional constraints that include:

- dignity and freedom compromised by social devaluation of intellectual disability;
- being perceived as "Other" that generates feelings of fear or disgust or pity or resentment in others, all of which drive social exclusion (see Box 3.2);
- being trapped in restrictive structures and stereotyped social roles;
- a fear of hate crime, shame and trauma following from abuse that encourages social withdrawal and erodes autonomy;
- a history of low expectations and lack of access to relevant learning opportunities that leaves people less capable than they could be and so less free;
- supports that require people's time to be structured according to diagnosis and employ staff to manage them;
- supports that focus heavily on system defined tasks related to physical care, prescribed activity, or family respite;
- services that often mould small, homogeneous relationship networks;
- services designed to assure compliance with prescribed rules and routines claimed as necessary to assure "health and safety" (and avoid liability);
- limited discretionary income; public investment in needed supports is often inadequate, and under regimes of austerity appallingly so.

It's important to honour and support the resilience people with intellectual disabilities display as they encounter a stream of devaluing responses in ordinary life. A growing number of people with intellectual disabilities and their families and allies creatively engage the extra burden of constraint and increase their collective freedom to choose. They free themselves from

BOX 3.2   The Everyday Challenges and Costs of Social Prejudice

The widespread assumption of subordinate status is not confined to intellectual disability or a matter of merely historical interest. Dave Hingsburger, an internationally recognised Canadian action and thought leader in the field of supports to people with intellectual disabilities, writes a blog (*Of battered aspect* http://davehingsburger.blogspot.com) that, among other topics, chronicles what comes to him in life as a wheelchair rider. He describes the toll that accumulates from day to day incidents of degrading comments, indignant responses to his refusals of unwanted and unnecessary help, offence taken at his expectation that public services will live up to their claims to be accessible, and the continual inconveniences and uncertainties of inaccessibility. A strong, articulate voice and a lifetime of advocacy experience can't prevent and do not fully alleviate the effects of the relentless press of devaluation.

restrictions and instead free themselves for the active pursuit of a life of citizenship. Attention to freedom to act matters as much or more than freedom from restriction. Even if a policy makes it clear that people in a group home can choose their own bedtime, people without active support to pursue what has meaning for them can easily fall into filling their time with television or retiring very early.

Over time, the practical meaning of the CRPD principles promoting choice will become clear, not only as policy makers and judges interpret it, but as people with intellectual disabilities live it. The weight of history establishes a sort of generalised power-over people with intellectual disabilities: routine imposition of substitute decision making, professional and bureaucratic surveillance and supervision of daily life, the expectation of deference to service providers, policy that treats access to necessary supports as a bureaucratic gift rather than an entitlement of citizenship. This burden shifts when people with intellectual disabilities join their families and allies to expand their freedom by inventing new ways to live together in power-with relationships. Those who take freedom and choice seriously will organise to invent better answers to questions like these:

- How might we shift the culture that justifies others exercising power-over a person assigned the status of "intellectually disabled" toward a culture that generates power-with relationships that actively support people to pursue the responsibilities of active citizenship?
- How might we increase people's effective control of the supports they need to live a life they and those who love them have good reasons to value?
- How might we support people's decision making in ways that make substitute decision making much less common?

CITIZENSHIP: THE PURPOSE THAT GUIDES SOCIAL INVENTION

Public response to the bundle of impairments currently designated as "intellectual disability" has claimed a variety of purposes since its 19th century inception: containment; shelter; education for usefulness; humane custodial care; protection from a hostile world; protection of society from eugenic threat; medical or psychological treatment to reduce maladaptive behaviour; skill training for independence; active support for engagement in daily life; social integration. Different purposes claim the foreground at different times but even in good times devaluing purposes endure in the background to haunt freedom to choose. Each purpose responds to a perceived lack in what it is presumed necessary to act autonomously and these deficiencies are taken as good reasons to insinuate control into every aspect of the life of someone with an intellectual disability. When a person inhabits services full time, they live under scrutiny and supervision, whether this is justified as for their own good or for the good of society.

Control may be benign: innocents vulnerable to mistreatment deserve shelter that keeps threats outside service walls and offers comfort and pleasure within. Control may be technical: skill development or deceleration of challenging behaviour requires professional control of people's environment and its contingencies. Control may be carceral: meeting the eugenic risk posed by degenerate genes demands segregation and strict discipline if not sterilisation. Control may intend to safeguard: those who serve must steer clear of liability so even ordinary life activities are subject to risk assessment (see also Chapter 6). However gently or harshly control may be imposed, it is taken as

a given that the person must be a client in the oldest sense of the word, "a person under the patronage or protection of another; a dependent" (Oxford English Dictionary, 2020). The risk that professionally certified deficiency will define much of a person's identity is real. So is the risk that people's lives will be wasted in individual efforts to work their way out of deficiency by climbing a professionally defined ladder of goals toward independence.

The differences swept into common understandings of intellectual disability attract unhelpful and risky narratives that encourage people to sacrifice agency and stay passive in the face of social exclusion. While many differences that threaten freedom are constructed from devaluing or confused perceptions, some are real in the sense that they express differences in mind, brain and body that, when insufficiently accommodated, impair a person's capabilities to act as they would choose. Co-creating sufficient accommodations is the work of social inventors, people with intellectual disabilities, their families and support workers who take freedom and choice seriously, as these examples show.

- Brad holds a responsible job and manages his home life. Despite a lot of effort to improve his skills, he still gets tangled up in money matters, so he relies on a trusted supporter to think through money decisions with him. He says his capacity to choose in every area of life has grown better because he has made mistakes and has learned from them with back-up from the direct support workers he has hired (Linnenkamp and Dean, 2019).
- Trusted others sense and turn Rebecca's interests into action. She now occupies valued social roles as a liturgical dancer, an early childhood educator, a museum docent, a volunteer for social justice and a spiritual companion. She disrupts the common sense of choice as the act of a single individual able to unambiguously express and give spoken reasons for their choices. Despite a lifelong search for an effective method of alternative communication, she continues to rely on those she cares about to interpret her limited body movements to discern her will and preferences. Her trust in them activates committed others to join in the continuing process of social invention that supports her good life in community (learn more about Rebecca and her story at https://rebecca-beayni.com/wp/).

Active support to citizenship defines the proper foundation for publicly funded supports to people with intellectual disabilities and guides social invention in terms of ways to increase freedom and inform choice (for more on people with intellectual disabilities and their allies as social inventors, see O'Brien and Mount, 2015).

Although it is possible to confuse the idea of citizenship with national identity and passport-holding, the more fundamental meaning of citizenship is much older and much more important than that. It describes a certain kind of ideal status, not one which is granted from above, but one which is co-created by people who come together in a community of equals. The idea certainly goes back to the world of Ancient Greek democracy, but arguably the same concept can be found in the Bible and in other ancient texts. The resilience of this concept through different times and places is probably due to the way in which it responds to deep human needs.

Firstly, citizens are diverse individuals who come together as members of a community. Citizens value community as an essential condition of their citizenship and membership is vitally important since it responds to the fact that human beings cannot thrive in isolation and need the support, stimulation and opportunities created by living with others, others who are not the same as them.

Secondly citizenship is not just any kind of community membership. Citizenship implies equality, not equality of condition or nature, but equality in dignity and mutual respect. To be in a community of citizens, as opposed to a community that is ordered by hierarchy or some other principle, is to be in a community that makes the equality of all members a first principle.

Thirdly, citizenship implies that people have obligations to each other, and rights that they can expect others to honour. In fact, the ideal of citizenship is possibly more focused on our responsibilities than on our rights, not because rights are not important, but because it asserts the positive value of our commitment to each other, and to the community as a whole. In this sense, focusing on citizenship challenges paternalistic or utilitarian conceptions of social justice. The claim to citizenship is not so much to receive benefits from the community, it is more a challenge to be allowed to make a contribution to the community.

Citizenship thereby reconciles aspects of the human condition where other ideals struggle. Disabled people, and other disadvantaged or marginalised groups, make the claim to citizenship because they recognise that they need to belong, but they also want to be respected as an equal and to make a contribution. Putting citizenship at the heart of public policy is challenging, because the modern world lives within the legacy of many great inequalities and injustices. However, citizenship makes sense as a goal of egalitarian public policy because it creates the conditions to confront the inheritance of injustice and begin to build a more just alternative.

Keys to Citizenship

Citizenship offers a practical framework for supporting others in a spirit of equality. The framework, The Keys to Citizenship, has emerged as a critical but positive response to the theory of normalisation developed by Wolfensberger (1972) and others. Wolfensberger was one of the most important critics of the large-scale institution and his theory drew particular attention to the fact that the wrong kind of support would actually lead to the increased stigmatisation of the person being supported. For instance, forcing people to live in large hospitals, often with high walls around them, sends a message that the people within are a menace to society and that the institution exists to protect citizens from non-citizen people with intellectual disabilities. Good support, on the other hand, needs to help people take up positive and socially valued roles and to avoid or reduce stigma. For example, if someone starts to carry out paid work, as an equal with their non-disabled colleagues, this sends out a message that disabled people belong in the mainstream of life and make a valuable contribution.

Whilst it is worthwhile to minimise stigma, this is an insufficient starting point for helping people build lives of meaning and value. The Keys to Citizenship is a positive framework built around the conditions necessary for the social value inherent in equal citizenship itself. The framework is positive, but it does not treat current social values as an acceptable starting point because many current norms play a role in creating the social injustices that disabled people confront.

The framework has seven elements (see Figure 3.1). The list might start with any Key, the order is not particularly important.

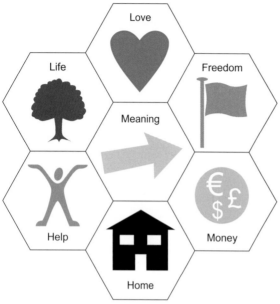

Figure 3.1 Keys to Citizenship

Meaning

The first key to citizenship is **meaning** or purpose. Human beings thrive when what they are doing has meaning for them, and we struggle to respect those who are not doing things they truly value. Living a life of meaning can be hard for everyone, but particularly for people whose lives face severe constraints. A man who loves to be outside and to feel the wind upon his face will always feel something is lacking if he is always made to live and work inside. Without the chance to experiment, try things out, fail or succeed then you will struggle to find a way of life that works for you. Unless you have people in your life who are looking out to support you to engage in the things that have meaning for you then you may always miss out.

Freedom

The second key to citizenship is **freedom**, the ability to make a choice. Freedom has always been one of the benefits of citizenship. Citizens are expected to be free and limitations on our freedom are barriers to our citizenship. Supporting people to make their own decisions is therefore not just a matter of respecting human rights, it is also the means to enable people to be - and be seen as - free agents within the community.

Money

The third key to citizenship is **money** or the resources necessary to enable a reasonable degree of independence. For citizens money is not a goal, but in the modern world a sufficient amount of money may be necessary to be able to live our freedom. Patrick may know that he would like to live a life outside the institution and in a community close to his family, but without the financial resources to adapt his home and provide the extra support he needs he can make no meaningful choice. Ensuring that people get access to the resources they are entitled to, and supporting them to exercise control over their money, become practical issues that supporters must address.

Home

The fourth key to citizenship is to have a **home** and for a citizen home means much more than just a place of shelter. Homes act as foundation stones for citizenship, marking our place within a specific community and enabling us to enter into community life, to retreat into our private life, and to welcome others into our home when we choose. If we are obviously rooted within a community then our opportunities to be welcomed and valued as a member of the community grow. Conversely if we are merely placed within a residential home and are liable to be moved when the services decide, our community status shrinks; so it is important that we explore how to support people to make choices about their own home and explore options like home ownership or secure renting because these are more likely to root the person within the community (see Chapter 24 about living options for people with intellectual disabilities).

Help

The fifth key to citizenship is **help**, more specifically to be someone who needs the help of others. This may seem a rather strange key to citizenship, but it is nevertheless a really important one. For a place where nobody needs anyone else is not a community. The idea of independence - not needing anyone else - actually undermines the idea of citizenship. However, the challenge, which we will discuss in more detail below, is that support is often organised in ways that require that we sacrifice other aspects of our citizenship, particularly our freedom. This is unnecessary and dangerous, and it is the role of supporters to ensure that their assistance strengthens all the other keys to citizenship.

Life

The sixth key to citizenship is **life**, living a life within the community, contributing, playing, growing, caring and working. It is important to note that citizenship is not always about doing worthy or serious activities. If I go to the pub I am not only being present in my community, I am supporting a local business and possibly a local brewer, I can make connections with neighbours and enjoy the love and support of my friends or family. I can also start something new, create a project, form a business, volunteer or get involved in political life. Often the challenge for supporters is that the sense of what citizenship involves has become far too narrow and constrained. It is not just a matter of helping people to choose from some menu of community options, it is much more about creating a life that really builds on what gives meaning to our lives - social invention is critical to supporting citizenship.

Love

Finally, the seventh key - although arguably it could be the first key, is **love**, friendship, sex, marriage and family. Without love we cannot flourish, and when we are seen to lack love our status shrinks. People with intellectual disabilities are as capable of giving and receiving love as anyone else, but to those who do not know them they are often treated as objects of pity or of mild affection. Often families demonstrate the enormous power of love in protecting, supporting and advocating for their relative; but they also fear that when they are gone nobody will be around who can offer the same level of love. For most of us love is the essential ingredient of a good life, but we struggle to talk about love, let alone provide people with the support to find and develop it.

If we start with the assumption that we are all citizens, whether we are someone with an intellectual disability, a family member or a supporter then this changes our approach to the question of how to support choice. Choice stops being a rather empty or consumerist notion - the expression of preference for one product over another. Instead we dignify choice and support for choice becomes an essential part of our shared citizenship, an expression of our freedom and search for meaning. This leads us into deeper listening and more courageous action, as iillustrated in Box 3.3.

 BOX 3.3   Impact of neglecting The Keys to Citizenship

Tom Allen came out of 64 years of institutionalisation with a person centred plan that promised a rich community life. Despite physical impairments and no effective access to augmentative and alternative communication, he recruited help to write a brief but remarkable autobiography (Johnson and Trustadottir, 2005). He describes at p. 161 the cause of a period of deep depression

"Moving into the community did not bring me the freedom I had dreamed about. I was still quite isolated. All the lists I made about all the things I wanted to do seem to have disappeared."

Fortunately, allies among staff took Tom's depression and withdrawal as a signal to listen more deeply and act to rebuild trust. Together they invented and continually revised individualised supports that gave him four years of greater freedom. This allowed him to exercise his citizenship as a vigorous advocate for closing institutions, whether large or small.

 READER ACTIVITY 3.2

Thinking about your own life, review the Seven Keys to Citizenship and describe how each of the Keys shows up for you.

What resources and limitations to freedom does your review identify?

What actions might increase your freedom?

DEVELOPING A CULTURE OF POWER-WITH RATHER THAN POWER-OVER

"Why is there still a question when people with learning disabilities want to do ordinary things for themselves?"

Perez, 2014, cited in Duffy and Perez, 2014, p. 9

The question that hangs over ordinary desires, the question that Wendy Perez brings into focus as an advocate with an intellectual disability, follows on from generations of belief that anyone identified as having intellectual disabilities requires protective supervision from others assumed to be whole in mental functioning. This persistent conviction shapes and justifies a culture of power-over people with intellectual disabilities that constricts their freedom, as described in Box 3.4.

 BOX 3.4   Power-over versus Power-with

Organisation theorist Mary Parker Follett (1940/2013) distinguishes power-over from power-with. Power-over reflects a tradition of hierarchy and competition. It functions transactionally. Those in power employ incentives, influence, and coercion to enforce their will. Power-over presumes certainty about the right way. It asserts and defends its narrative and ignores subordinate voices.

Power-with is collaborative. It functions relationally, creating new possibilities from differences by bringing a variety of perspectives into the open to gain a better understanding of uncertain and unpredictable situations and discovers ways forward that serve and mobilise people's sense of purpose.

Read from an advocate's perspective, the CRPD confronts this belief and calls for correction of its consequences. The work of supporters shifts from taking deficient and inferior others in charge to learning to help and be helped by citizens with equal dignity to their own. The Keys to Citizenship set freedom in the context of the conditions for its exercise and define opportunities for equals to mobilise their differences and co-create good lives as fellow citizens.

Services vary in the amount of freedom people with intellectual disabilities must give up in exchange for assistance. A great deal is at stake when assistance surrounds a person 24 hours every day. Many residential services pass on a legacy of over-generalised interventions and protections that define a person's salient identity in terms of their professionally assessed deficiencies. In contrast, those oriented by the Keys to Citizenship work to individualise support and offer precise assistance to enable a good, ordinary life. This includes personalised supports for decision making and safeguards tailored to a person's particular vulnerabilities in places and activities that matter to them. As a foundation for that assistance they invest in building trust through power-with relationships. They maintain vigilance to detect and correct inevitable slips into imposing power-over on people. Organisations that negotiate person specific assistance to people who live in their own homes, and play active roles in community life, find this work easier than those that package personal assistance with group housing or congregate day services.

Consider the challenges of increasing personal freedom in a six-person group home operated by a respected US organisation to serve people assessed to have moderate to high support needs. In a quality improvement workshop the manager, known for her competency and commitment to residents, identified the following as a positive example of promoting choice: *"We let our individuals take turns choosing the menu for Saturday night dinner."* She sees this as promoting choice because the group home's usual practice is to follow a dietician approved menu sent from the organisation's central office at every meal. Granting this privilege took persistent negotiation. Managers approved an exception to policy. The nurse assigned to the home, and the organisation's dietician, compiled a list of forbidden foods. The team identified a therapeutic possibility and decreed that a person who violates house rules in the week it is their turn to select the menu loses the privilege.

Reflection on the sentence *"We let our individuals take turns choosing the menu…"*– reveals many strands woven in a net of restrictive beliefs and practices that entangles people with intellectual disabilities and the staff who assist them. Its main actors are staff, located on the superior side of a boundary that distances them from, and places them over, those they supervise. From this unequal position they define a privilege and grant it to "our individuals" (a possessive applied to the organisation's practice of calling those they serve "individuals" as an intended form of person centred language). This reflects a culture where power-over people with intellectual disabilities is pervasive and unquestioned. A hierarchy sets direct support workers over people with intellectual disabilities, and management and clinical professionals over direct support workers. It enforces social distance between staff (us, those responsible and capable to supervise and guide) and residents (them, those working to achieve independence under staff tutelage). A staff defined and circumscribed choice is offered as a gift. A parental stance uses a right recast as a privilege as a contingency for appropriate behaviour for "their own good". This culture, taken for granted as "the way we do things here", easily swallows questions that might disrupt it. If a question does come up, there is always a given reason for every limit, either a matter of common sense or clinical necessity. Desire to fit in with the group encourages both staff and people with intellectual disabilities to accept and adapt, at least to the extent of staying quiet and going along.

Culture shapes and is shaped by the group home structure. System case managers place a person in a vacant bed with a group of others the system defines as having similar service needs. If a person has a choice it is between similarly restrictive settings. Staff complements are assigned to manage defined household routines and administer or arrange prescribed services. Detailed rules, policies, reporting requirements and inspections define staff roles and shape staff behaviour. Activities and outings typically involve the whole group. Care managers and staff assume that a person will adapt to the requirements of the place as it is or, if they prove unmanageable, be transferred to another placement. The argument that people have chosen to live in a group, and so must adjust, overlooks the scarcity of available alternatives.

When staff work well within it, a culture that severely limits freedom can support a physically comfortable existence, friendship with other residents, the possibility of caring, even affectionate (if parental), relationships with staff, pleasant at home pursuits like watching favourite videos in one's room or collecting sports memorabilia, enjoyable outings and occasions, and memorable holidays. Those families and people with intellectual disabilities who respond to surveys, such as the US National Core Indicators, usually express satisfaction with their services (Stancliffe et al, 2009). They may defend practices that limit freedom as necessary to assure health, safety and happiness and overlook the costs of limiting freedom.

Not every group home demands as much of people's freedom as the one described in this critique of residential culture. But aspects of power-over compromise the citizenship of enough people with intellectual disabilities to make it worthwhile to learn how to build up power-with people with intellectual disabilities in situations where culture and structure reduces freedom.

Words from authorities are helpful but insufficient. Laws, court decisions, regulations and policies call for greater opportunities to choose. Conferences and training can send expert messages, especially when the voices of people with intellectual disabilities are prominent. Quality measures test for choice. Even when a staff team hear authoritative messages, culture filters their impact. Power-over hides behind a narrative of deficiency, professionally prescribed improvement and protection. This allows imagining that "people here already have as much choice as possible".

At ground level the task is social invention: noticing and owning up to practices that reproduce inequality, surfacing and questioning the beliefs that justify restrictions on choice as necessary, taking responsibility for building power-with relationships that test limiting assumptions, and finding new ways to expand free space, where a person's choice makes a difference. These aspects of social invention happen when people commit to each other and act to cross boundaries. Words from authorities can offer inspiration, insight and ideas. The culture of power-over will absorb any effort that does not engage people with intellectual disabilities, and the people who assist them, in a new form of relationship, in an honest struggle to work as equal citizens who engage their different capabilities to bring purpose into focus and make something meaningful happen.

This is a sign of engaged learning. Looking back on the changes in a person's life over a few months of partnership characterised by intentionally seeking an equal relationship focused on discovering purpose and meaning in community life, a staff person says she is gripped by these questions. "We thought we knew this person inside out. How could we not know that so much more is possible? And how many other people have great possibilities that have been hidden in our routines and stories about them?"

People with intellectual disabilities will have a stronger foundation for choice when the five things in Box 3.5 are (becoming) true.

Support for learning that unmasks inequality and discovers ways to realise the Keys to Citizenship is a worthy investment. These practices have proven useful to organisations with a commitment to change:

BOX 3.5   The Foundations for Choice

- They have experienced a variety of community roles that produce knowledge of their interests and capacities.
- They have confidence, grounded in experience, that in company with others they can take action that makes good things happen, solve problems to overcome obstacles, deal with failures and disappointments, and get help that respects their dignity and competence when they need it.
- They have a hopeful and positive vision of themselves as active and contributing citizens.
- They understand their individual experience of impairment in ways that provide practical knowledge of necessary accommodations, what works and what to avoid in the provision of necessary assistance, and how to cope with risk, including those risks associated with prejudice and discrimination.
- They have a diverse network of personal and family relationships with people who believe they have a positive future as a contributing citizen, will contribute to the thinking and action necessary to establish and sustain good opportunities for them, and include people who can be trusted to support their decision making.

READER ACTIVITY 3.3

What would your first steps be if you wanted to develop more and stronger power-with relationships in your life?

What obstacles would your very first step encounter?

Why would you persist in dealing with these obstacles?

- Investing in learning partnerships between a willing person with intellectual disabilities and a staff member who wants to join them in finding ways to experience more of the Keys to Citizenship. This investment includes a design process for co-creating new opportunities, free time for the learning partners to work together, the ability to negotiate changes in routines, and regular opportunities to meet with other partnerships to share what they are learning. This process not only benefits the people involved, it surfaces practices and assumptions that unnecessarily limit freedom and shapes an agenda for organisational change (O'Brien and Mount, 2005).
- Organising groups of 10–15 organisations committed to developing their capacity to offer individualised supports that significantly increase access to the Keys to Citizenship. Organisational teams follow a process informed by Theory U (Scharmer, 2018) to co-create social innovations with willing people with intellectual disabilities. Over a year or more they alternate work inside their organisations with regular gatherings for shared learning (Meissner, 2020).
- Inviting critical friends from outside the organisation who share commitment to supporting citizenship to visit, inquire and comment on their observations. This can identify opportunities to expand freedom that are hard for insiders to see.
- Developing a distinct organisation committed to co-creating individualised supports within an organisation managing a legacy of group based services (Meissner, 2013).

After diligent effort to increase freedom within group focused structures, some organisations see the need to break out. They choose to close group homes by joining the people who live in them to develop individualised alternatives (Fratangelo and Strully, 2002; Meissner, 2013). Power-with practices have even more possibilities to make a difference in these situations.

SELF-DIRECTED SUPPORTS

In the past many people with intellectual disabilities and their families were faced with a difficult and extreme choice (Ferguson, 2016). Some accepted that their family member would go into institutional care, far from everyone they knew, and into a life which many feared. Others continued to support their family member with little or no additional assistance, and often in the face of many other serious social challenges like poverty and prejudice. Sometimes there was no meaningful choice, and people with intellectual disabilities were forced into institutional care as a form of social control when families were seen as incapable (Wolfensberger, 1975).

Today those choices are less extreme. Many societies offer some support to children and adults to stay with their family and to live in their own communities. Many institutional services have begun to change, there are more choices and people sometimes have greater control over their own support. But these improvements are still quite limited, even in the most progressive societies. There remains a strong bias toward funding institutional services, residential or nursing homes and day centres, placing people there when the need is judged sufficiently acute. Support for individuals and families at home is usually far more limited. There remains a tendency within social care systems to look negatively and distrustfully at people with intellectual disabilities and their families. People and families often find themselves excluded from decision-making and real choices within service systems that tend to be highly constrained.

The social care system sets the scene for the way people with intellectual disabilities are seen and how power and decisions are organised around them. Cultural factors, which reflect long-standing prejudices and assumptions about intelligence, disability and social status, are reinforced by the way money is allocated. What is more, these social care systems are widespread and are integrated with other powerful systems of education, healthcare and welfare. Services for people with intellectual disabilities are not alone in being organised along the lines of the *Professional Gift Model*, where support and services are defined from a position of power-over the person and where the person will be given the service a professional thinks best for them (Duffy, 1996). This top-down approach can seem quite reasonable and even necessary if you assume that the use of resources must be in the hands of the state or its professional agents. However, disabled people and families successfully challenge this assumption by demanding that they should not only be free to make everyday choices for themselves but should also be able to shape the kinds of support that are available to them both individually and collectively. What many people are creating might be called a *Citizenship Model* of support, where the individual is treated as a citizen whose life is located within a community of people and social opportunities (O'Brien et al, 2020). The extra resources that people may need because of their disability are not converted directly into services - in the way that the *Professional Gift Model* assumes - but instead they are treated as entitlements that the citizen can use to help people overcome any barriers to citizenship that have not been removed by wider social change. This is illustrated in Figure 3.2.

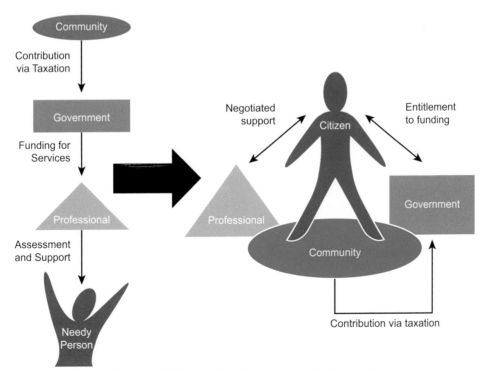

Figure 3.2 Professional gift model and citizenship model

An early instance of implementing this new way of thinking is the emergence of the Independent Living movement led by Ed Roberts which began in Berkeley California in 1965 (Shapiro, 1993).

> "[As a university student] Roberts needed someone to push his wheelchair and help him get dressed and eat. Sometimes a friend helped willingly. But for the most part he hired attendants, including sometimes his brother Ron, also a student at Berkeley. State funding paid for the attendants. California had the nation's first such program."
>
> *Shapiro, 1993, p. 45*

The idea of independent living is often associated primarily with people with physical disabilities, but in fact many people with intellectual disabilities and their families have played critical roles in challenging the old service system to change how it is organised. These ideas have spread around the world, and have been embraced by people with different ages, health conditions or impairments (Duffy, 2018). Increasingly countries are seeking to redesign their whole system of social services around the principle that people themselves should be able to control and direct their own support. For instance, Scotland implemented legislation to make self-directed support a fundamental right in 2013 (Scottish Parliament, 2013).

Even positive legal changes do not guarantee a radical shift in practice or in the relationships that determine how people's lives might change for the better. Just as top-down control of services is ineffective in enabling people to build lives of meaning and citizenship, so is top-down system change in guaranteeing that everyone can benefit from a new approach. Changes in culture and practice seem to depend on a combination of new experiences, stories/examples and support and encouragement in order to take root. Changes in the rules can help, because they create new permissions and provide a powerful signal that the official position of the government has shifted. However, resistance to enabling people to have meaningful choice and control remains, and requires ongoing work.

Reflection on international experience identifies common issues that limit the reach of self-direction and include:

- whilst self-directed support often emerges around one group of people who seek more control, other groups who would benefit are excluded. For instance, people with intellectual disabilities, families, older people, people with mental health problems or people with complex health conditions can be excluded because they are deemed to either not want control over their support, or are seen as in some way incapable of making good decisions for themselves.
- funding for support is often inadequate and while self-directed support is on average more efficient than institutional care (Bogenschutz et al, 2019), systems often resist shifting resources out of older forms of care and avoid fully funding those who have stayed out of institutional care with the support of their families.
- systems typically struggle to give people genuine flexibility in using available resources. There is a tendency to try and regulate what people do with any personal budget for support, and it is often assumed that people should only employ staff or purchase support from a regulated service provider. This means that people are discouraged from seeking the best way of meeting their needs or overcoming any barriers to citizenship. In a sense the system tends to seek to bring the person or family inside its own regulated system and often imposes further controls or restrictions.
- systems also struggle to develop the necessary infrastructure of community supports to make it easier for people to exercise control. Sometimes people need help with getting information, payroll, planning, employment, connecting to community resources or peer support where people can connect to others sharing similar circumstances (Duffy and Fulton, 2010). In particular, only a small number of support organisations seem to have made the shift to change their own ways of working, and to offer people the kind of personalised support that people generally seek (Duffy and Sly, 2017). Box 3.6 identifies some characteristics of these initiatives.

The emergence of self-directed support as a new set of design principles for social services has been slow, but its momentum has continued, largely driven by the persistent desire of disabled people and families to exercise their human rights and take their place as citizens. Such systemic changes are helpful because they both underline the importance of the right to make your own decisions and also give people some practical tools to exercise more authority in

BOX 3.6   Personalised Support

Placing people in large institutions is a common model in the industrialised world, one that began in the nineteenth century and reached its peak in the late twentieth-century. As pressure grew to close these institutions the services which replaced them were often smaller but still highly institutional in character. The combination of care home and day centre could still continue to act as what Goffman calls a Total Institution and exercise control over every aspect of the person's life even away from the old-style institution (Goffman, 1961).

However, some community organisations began to emerge which challenged the institutional model and which aimed to offer support that was liberating and focused on supporting citizenship. Sometimes this support might still be more collective, for example L'Arche communities showed how people with and without disabilities could live together as equals. Other examples were more focused on designing personal support with the person and the family, not expecting the family to do all the work, but creating a mutual partnership of support. Early pioneers of this different approach include Options in Community Living in Wisconsin who developed innovative support solutions to help people who had lived in institutions to live in homes of their own and develop rich and connected community lives (O'Brien et al, 1998). Increasingly, organisations have emerged which assume that a person must shape their own support, select their own supporters, and be enabled to make the best possible use of their budgets (sometimes called an Individual Service Fund). This approach adopts the same principles as self-directed support by assuming the person must be in control but builds a partnership with the person to make this achievable (Fitzpatrick, 2010).

their relationship with services and the community. Money and the right to spend that money in ways which make sense to you are important to the exercise of freedom.

These system changes do not guarantee that the voice of the person will really be heard. Supported decision making, including the art of listening and seeking to support people to exercise choice and control for themselves, will remain a central challenge in its own right.

The reverse is also true, even if the systems around people are imperfect and their rights are limited, it is still possible and important to build power-with the person and to create social inventions that will advance citizenship.

Support for decision making

Article 12 of the CRPD asserts, "persons with disabilities have the right to recognition everywhere as persons before the law" and "persons with disabilities enjoy legal capacity on an equal basis with others in all aspects of life". This creates multiple opportunities for social invention because it confronts common practices that legally remove a person's freedom to choose in all or some situations. These practices rely on the degree to which power-over people with intellectual disabilities is taken for granted.

In many places, courts routinely order people with intellectual disabilities into guardianship or some other form of substitute decision making. These decisions are seldom contested and may be justified by accepting a diagnosis of intellectual disability as sufficient evidence of legal incapacity, or by a professionally endorsed prediction that a person will make bad decisions because of their intellectual disability. Many courts defer to requests to appoint substitute decision makers and don't scrutinise professional or family opinion. While these orders are subject to regular review, and can be challenged, it is unusual for them to be lifted. The court's determination of incapacity puts a substitute decision maker in the person's place before the law and in the exercise of legal capacity. The person themself becomes invisible to the law, a status that has been called "a form of civil death" (Shogren et al, 2018). Within a court's order – which can claim the whole of a person's freedom to decide or only the right to make specified decisions – the substitute decision maker takes over legal capacity to consent to medical treatment, enter into contracts, agree to service plans, manage money, agree to an intimate relationship, and decide in other areas in which life meets the law. A common standard calls on the substitute decision maker to act in the person's "best interests" as the substitute decision maker defines "best interest". In some places, reforms charge substitute decision makers to exercise "substituted judgement", that is to try and imagine the decision the person would make if they had the capacity to do so. Jenny's story (Box 3.7) illustrates the dangers of substitute decision making.

BOX 3.7   The Dangers of Substitute Decision Making

Injured when a driver hit her bicycle with a car, Jenny was referred for guardianship. As she was recovering, a US judge took Down syndrome alone as sufficient reason to order a young woman who held a job, managed life in her own apartment and counted mostly on supportive friends rather than paid services into a guardianship. The guardian sent her to a group home "where she would get the help she needed", made her quit a paying community job and placed her in a sheltered workshop, forbade contact with friends, and even restricted contact with the lawyer who represented her in the two year process of restoring her rights. She has recovered her rights and the life that matters to her and advocates publicly for supported decision making (Shogren et al, 2018).

Article 12 calls for deep change (Centre for Disability Law & Policy, 2012). The presumption of legal capacity in all aspects of life invalidates any approach that presumes generalised incompetence as its starting point. Responsibility shifts from authorising substitute decision makers to creating individualised supports for making specific decisions that build on a person's existing capabilities. The standard for decision making shifts from asserting "best interest" to an active search for ways to understand and respect each person's rights, will and preferences. The role of the court changes from ordering people with intellectual disabilities into legal invisibility to safeguarding people against deprivation of legal capacity, ensuring adequate supports to decision making, and protecting against the abuse of people considered to be impaired in decision making

Social inventors – disabled advocates, family members, support providers, and lawyers – are developing the practical means to replace substituted decision making (see, for example, National Resource Center for Supported Decision-Making, 2020). Because the designation of intellectual disability applies to people with a very wide range of capabilities, supported decision making develops in many different forms. All of these depend on the engagement of others the person trusts who are committed to respect and actively promoting the person's autonomy and rights, to keep learning more about the person's purposes, will and preferences,

and to work with the person to establish the individualised assistance that offers the person freedom. A person might count on family members, friends, advocates who themselves experience intellectual disabilities, and those in past or present helping roles. Their common task is to support the person to form a good understanding of a situation that calls for a decision, consider their purpose and sources of meaning, make and communicate their decision, and if necessary, make and pursue a plan to implement what they have decided. Most people with intellectual disabilities can think with supporters to clarify their will and preferences in a variety of life situations and choose to use (Enduring) Powers of Attorney or Advance Directives to communicate what they want and who represents them. This goes best when people and their supporters are well assisted: sufficient time and privacy in a comfortable place to think together; good communication assistance; necessary personal assistance; opportunities to explore what is possible by learning from other people with intellectual disabilities; access to facilitation if the decision support group gets stuck in conflict.; a capacity for any services the person relies on to assist in implementing their decisions. Practical decision-making aids, such as "When Do I Want Support" can also assist people with intellectual disabilities to develop a Supported-Decision Making agreement (American Civil Liberties Union (ACLU), 2018).

Some jurisdictions overcome uncertainty about legal capacity that poses a barrier to others accepting the person's communication as valid for such matters as consent to medical treatment or entering a contract. The Government of (the Canadian province of) British Columbia (2020), for example, establishes Representation Agreements which allow adults with disabilities to nominate someone to make specified decisions for them, and recognises those decisions as legally valid.

Some people with intellectual disabilities count on others to interpret their will and preferences. The Keys to Citizenship provide a framework for decision supporters' thinking. Building from the reasonable assumption that the question is not whether each Key is important to a person but how it can show up in a way that suits this specific person, supporters can reflect on the experiences they share to identify what they believe a person finds meaningful and what good assistance looks like.

Some people have no obvious members of a supported decision-making network. They may be separated from family and isolated with no others who can bring necessary contributions to good decision making. Until further social inventions consistent with the CRPD emerge, a carefully safeguarded option for substituted decision making needs to be developed to respond to specific, time limited decision situations. The appointed substitute decision maker must make the decision that meets two criteria:

1) it represents their considered understanding of the person's will and preference
2) it encourages development of the person's capacity for decision making.

CONCLUSION

Taking choice seriously disrupts common practices, confronts restrictive service cultures, contests typical structures for offering services, and questions taken for granted assumptions. Social invention, firmly rooted in commitment to citizenship and guided by the Keys to Citizenship, will make progress on closing the gap between legally established rights and available choices. Freedom to choose grows as people learn together how to shift a culture that takes power-over people with intellectual disabilities for granted to a culture consciously committed to building power-with relationships, how to increase the effective control people with intellectual disabilities have over the individualised supports they need in order to act as citizens, and how to better support decision making. This is the work of enabling people to have a choice.

REFERENCES

American Civil Liberties Union (ACLU). (2018). *When Do I Want Support*. Available at: https://www.aclu.org/other/when-do-i-want-support. [Accessed 6 December 2020].

Bogenschutz, M., DeCarlo, J., Hall-Lande, et al. (2019). Fiscal stewardship choice and control. *Intellectual and Developmental Disabilities*, 57(2), 158–171.

Centre for Disability Law & Policy. (2012). *Submission on legal capacity to the Oireachtas Committee on Justice, Defense & Equality*. Available at: https://www.nuigalway.ie/media/centrefordisabilitylawandpolicy/files/archive/Submission-on-Legal-Capacity-to-the-Oireachtas-Committee-on-Justice,-Defence-&-Equality-(August,-2011).pdf. [Accessed 6 December 2020].

Duffy, S. (1996). *Unlocking the imagination*. London: Choice Press.

Duffy, S. (2018). *Self-directed support: if it's so good then why is it so hard*. Sheffield: Centre for Welfare Reform. Available at: https://citizen-network.org/resources/selfdirected-support-resources-english.html. [Accessed 6 December 2020].

Duffy, S., & Fulton, K. (2010). *Architecture for personalisation*. Sheffield: Centre for Welfare Reform.

Duffy, S., & Perez, W. (2014). *Citizenship for all: an accessible guide*. Sheffield: The Centre for Welfare Reform.

Duffy, S., & Sly, S. (2017). *Progress on personalised support – results of an international survey by Citizen Network*. Sheffield: Centre for Welfare Reform.

Ferguson, G. (2016). *Never going back: the Gord Ferguson story*. Toronto: Legacies.

Fish, R. (2018). *Accessible summary: the big bedtime audit*. Available at: https://wp.lancs.ac.uk/cedr/2018/05/16/the-big-bedtime-audit-evening-routines-in-the-community/ [Accessed 9 October 2021].

Fitzpatrick, J. (2010). *Personalised support: how to provide high quality support to people with complex and challenging needs – learning from Partners for Inclusion*. Sheffield: Centre for Welfare Reform.

Follett, M. P. (1940/2013). *Dynamic administration*. Eatstford, CT: Martino.

Fratangelo, P., & Strully, J. (2002). The challenges of person-centered work: how two agencies embraced change. In J. O'Brien & C. Lyle O'Brien (Eds.), *Implementing person-centered planning: voices of experience*. Toronto: Inclusion Press.

Goffman, E. (1961). *Asylums: essays on the social situation of mental patients and other inmates*. New York: Anchor Books.

Government of British Columbia. (2020). *Incapacity planning*. Available at: https://www2.gov.bc.ca/gov/content/health/managing-your-health/incapacity-planning. [Accessed 6 December 2020].

James, E., Harvey, M., & Mitchell, R. (2018). An inquiry by social workers into evening routines in community living settings for adults with learning disabilities. *Practice: Social Work in Action*, 30(1), 19–32.

Johnson, K., & Trustadottir, R. (2005). *Deinstitutionalization and people with intellectual disabilities: in and out of institutions*. London: Jessica Kingsley Publishers.

Linnenkamp, B., & Dean, E. (2019). Supporting decision making: advice and examples from a self-advocate. *Impact*. Available at: https://publications.ici.umn.edu/impact/32-1/supporting-decision-making-advice-and-examples-from-a-self-advocate. [Accessed 6 December 2020].

Marmot, M. (2015). *The health gap: the challenge of an unequal world*. London: Bloomsbury Press.

Minnesota Department of Human Services (MDHS). (2016). *Toolkit to support informed choice in employment.* St Paul: Minnesota Department of Human Services. Available at: *https://mn.db101.org/documents/Informed%20choice%20 toolkit%20v3.pdf.* [Accessed 6 December 2020].

Meissner, H. (2020). *Expanding blue space: the Learning Institute for Social Innovation.* Toronto: Inclusion Press.

Meissner, H. (2013). *Creating blue space: fostering innovative support practices for people with developmental disabilities.* Toronto: Inclusion Press.

National Resource Center for Supported Decision Making. (2020). Available at: *http://www.supporteddecisionmaking. org/.* [Accessed 6 December 2020].

O'Brien, J., Lyle O'Brien, C., & Jacobs, G. (1998). *Celebrating the ordinary: the emergence of Options in Community Living as a thoughtful organisation.* Toronto: Inclusion Press.

O'Brien, J., & Mount, B. (2005). *Make a difference: a guidebook for person-centered support.* Toronto: Inclusion Press.

O'Brien, J., & Mount, B. (2015). *Pathfinders: people with developmental disabilities and their allies building communities that work better for everybody.* Toronto: Inclusion Press.

O'Brien, J., Uditsky, B., & Winter, P. (2020). *Using family managed support to support an inclusive life.* Edmonton, AB: Inclusion Alberta. Available at: *https:// inclusionalberta.org/fms-online-guide/.* [Accessed 6 December 2020].

Oxford English Dictionary. (2020). Client, n. Available at: https://www.oed.com/view/Entry/34279?redirectedFrom= client#eid. [Accessed 6 December 2020].

Shapiro, J. (1993). *No pity: people with disabilities forging a new civil rights movement.* New York: Times Books.

Scharmer, O. (2018). *Essentials of theory U.* San Francisco: Berrett-Koehler.

Scottish Parliament. (2013). *Social care (self-directed support) (Scotland) Act 2013.*

Shogren, K., Wehmeyer, M., Martinis, J., et al. (2018). *Supported decision making: theory, research, and practice to enhance self-determination and quality of life.* New York: Cambridge University Press.

Stancliffe, R., Lakin, K. C., Taub, S., et al. (2009). Satisfaction and sense of well being among Medicaid ICF/MR and HCBS recipients in six states. *Intellectual & Developmental Disabilities, 47*(2), 63–83.

UN Convention on the Rights of Persons With Disabilities. (2006). Available at: https://www.ohchr.org/ EN/HRBodies/CRPD/Pages/ConventionRightsPersons WithDisabilities.aspx. [Accessed 6 December 2020].

Wolfensberger, W. (1972). *The principle of normalization in human services.* Toronto: NIMR.

Wolfensberger, W. (1975). *The origin and nature of our institutional models.* Syracuse, NY: The Center on Human Policy Press.

What's important to me? Using collaborative and creative approaches to shift the power in assessment

Susan June Ledger, Anne-Marie Martin and Elizabeth Tilley

KEY ISSUES

- All people with an intellectual disability have the right to be fully involved in their own assessments and to play an active part in deciding what happens in their lives.
- Historically assessment has been characterised by inequality of power between professionals and people with intellectual disabilities.
- This is beginning to shift – supported by policy and legislation at a national and international level.
- Practitioners must develop and hone skills that will enable them to understand what is most important to the person, how they feel about their life now and what they want to happen in the future.
- This includes skills to work with people who communicate non-verbally and those with complex disabilities.
- Sharing creative and inclusive approaches can help people with intellectual disabilities to take a very active role in the assessment process and so improve outcomes whilst ensuring they continue to benefit from skilled multi-disciplinary support.

CHAPTER OUTLINE

INTRODUCTION

The key features of a collaborative approach to assessment challenge us to leave behind our past, often form-driven, ways of assessing people and to focus instead on listening to their plans, potential and what they want to happen, as opposed to what we, as professionals, believe is best for them. It's a shift in power to co-produced assessments rather than professional-produced assessments (Brown, 2019).

In 1993 the UK self-advocacy group People First published '*Oi It's my assessment: listen to me!*', (People First, 1993) a best practice guide produced by people with intellectual disabilities in response to their own experiences of being assessed by professionals.

"We want things to change. We want assessment to feel more like we're in charge, to be guided by us than being 'done to'. Professionals need to use things like pictures and allow enough time to find out what we want to do

in our lives rather than writing down on a form what we can't do."

Bourlet and Page, 1994

Three decades later, following in the pioneering footsteps of People First, this chapter returns to the subject of assessment and the continued need for creative and inclusive approaches to shift long-standing inequalities of power.

Today, as part of the routine delivery of services, people are formally assessed to determine if they have an intellectual disability (Davidson et al, 2014); to measure academic progress (Standards and Testing Agency, 2018, 2020); to identify the kind and amount of support they might need; to diagnose and treat health issues; to explore possibilities for employment; to secure welfare benefits; to hold their own housing tenancy; to manage risk (Sellars, 2011); and to determine capacity to make decisions (Graham and Cowley, 2015), to give just a few examples.

Accounts from people with intellectual disabilities and their families, combined with research findings, increasingly demonstrate how greater investment of professional time in the assessment process results in better long-term outcomes for the people concerned, often reducing their reliance on traditional and more costly services (Reid et al, 2013; Lemmi et al, 2016; Brown, 2014). Recent studies also show how well conducted screening assessments can enable people with intellectual disabilities to access support with homelessness (McKenzie et al, 2019) and parenting (University of Bristol and Working Together with Parents Network, 2017). However, such progress exists alongside inquiries, investigations and research demonstrating how 'persistent distortions of power and control' (Manthorpe and Martineau, 2015, p. 335) have resulted in people being excluded from society, restricted and abused (Flynn, 2012; Lenehan, 2017). At its worst, the absence of robust, person-centred assessment processes contributed to the premature deaths of some people with intellectual disabilities, as evidenced in England (Heslop et al, 2013).

In the paragraph below Paul Christian shares his reflections on the part assessment has played in his own life and in the lives of his friends, classmates and colleagues:

"Assessment can sometimes feel like you are being probed or tested. Professionals can determine your future through assessment. They have a lot of power. Just because they have the tools and the know how.

But that can't compare to making the time to listen and understand. To find out about people. Today we live in a fast pace society. Often people are in a hurry. It's easier to ask other people their views about us, like today the dentist asked my mum how I was. Give us the time, give us the space, give us the leeway, give us the independence to talk to tell you what life is like even if we don't use words."

Personal correspondence between Paul Christian and Sue Ledger, 2019a

Mirroring Paul Christian's comments, this chapter argues that it remains vital for all practitioners involved in assessment work to critically reflect on their own practice and the steps they can take to improve their own capacity to listen and understand so as to shift power, control and decision-making to those being assessed.

Newman and Wright (cited in Gollins et al, 2016: p. 25) argue that the term assessment is so saturated with notions of professionals as the experts and deciders that it should be abandoned and 'banned'. Promoting models of practice that recognise the person as the leading expert in their own lives, Newman and Wright recommend the use of alternatives such as 'having a conversation'. While this chapter endorses this view, the term 'assessment' has been retained in recognition of its continuing widespread usage in professional training and services and the belief that it is the profoundly enduring and underlying practice and power issues that need to be addressed, regardless of adopted terminology (Oakes, 2012; Manthorpe and Martineau, 2015).

The aim of this chapter is to introduce you to some ideas and approaches that may develop your thinking about assessment. It considers definitions of assessment, with cognisance of the historical context relating to persons with intellectual disability. The chapter reflects upon assessment practice across the life course and the varied contexts in which assessments take place, and shares examples of what we as authors have termed 'collaborative and creative assessment' practice. Throughout, assessment scenarios, individual's stories and illustrations are included to support you to link theory and practice and encourage you to reflect on your experiences.

This chapter is written from a UK/Irish perspective although the principles and illustrations are of relevance to supporting people across international settings.

WHAT IS ASSESSMENT?

Hodgson and Watts (2017) suggest that one of the best definitions of assessment is provided:

> *"Assessment is an ongoing process, in which the client participates, the purpose of which is to understand people in relation to their environment; it is the basis for planning what needs to be done to maintain, improve or bring about change in the person, the environment or both."*

> *Coulshed and Orme (1998)*, p. 21

Hodgson and Watts (2017, pp. 208–9) highlight a number of points from this definition as being particularly useful:

1 The client fully participates
2 That it is an ongoing process
3 That assessment should be a purposeful means of developing understanding about the individual
4 That assessment is a foundation for shared future planning.

A number of writers have suggested that there are different stages to the overall assessment process. Although stages are presented in a chronological order, in reality the practitioner will often move back and forth between these stages as they return to the person, gather more information, check that they have got it right and together re-evaluate the situation and agree the best way forward.

Parker (2013) states that whilst there are many different models and purposes of assessment they all follow a broadly similar pattern and include at least a variation of the following elements:

- preparation, planning, engagement and relationship building
- data collection and creating a view on a given situation
- preliminary analysis and interpretation of information, testing this out with the person
- deeper analysis after testing out data and further interpreting of information with the person
- construction of an action plan or way forward – with the person at the centre.

This reflects a broader paradigm shift over the past thirty years, which has called for the assessment process to be more person-centred and inclusive, shifting greater control to the person being assessed (Symonds et al, 2020). However, definitions of assessment commonly used in health and social care settings demonstrate how concepts of evaluation, judgement and decision-making remain embedded in service descriptions:

> *"The nursing assessment includes gathering information concerning the patient's individual physiological, psychological, sociological, and spiritual needs. It is the first step in the successful evaluation of a patient [..] The assessment identifies current and future care needs of the patient by allowing the formation of a nursing diagnosis."*

> *Toney-Butler and Unison-Pace, 2019*

> *"In adult services for people with learning disabilities in the UK, the support offered to you will be decided through a 'needs assessment', carried out by your local authority. What you need in terms of care and support, healthcare and housing should all be considered as part of this assessment."*

> *Mencap, 2019*

Davidson et al (2014, p. 185) draw attention to the part that cognitive assessment plays in the initial diagnosis of intellectual disability (the authors use the term 'learning disability'):

> *"Central to the diagnosis of learning disability is an IQ score below 70 established by an individually administered cognitive assessment. As the majority of such assessments are conducted by psychologists, this professional group also holds a powerful position."*

These quotations demonstrate the continued reliance on assessment processes to determine eligibility and the amount and type of services to be arranged. Phrases such as 'will be decided' and 'carried out by your local authority' arguably risk communicating the sense that a person with an intellectual disability and their family are the more passive party in an assessment process, being 'done to' by professionals, rather than equal partners and collaborators.

Understanding the historical context

It is important for health and social care professionals to understand and respect that historically many people have endured negative consequences as a result of being assessed and labelled as having an intellectual disability. The outcomes of assessment were in the past often linked to exclusion. In the film No Longer Shut Up: Finding Mabel Cooper's Voice (2015) the late Mabel Cooper, (1944-2013), a leading intellectual disability campaigner, remembers being taken as a child to County Hall in central London for tests 'to see how bad the learning [intellectual] disability was' – a test that concluded she would need care for the rest of her life and resulted in her admission to a long stay institution (Cooper, 1997).

Thousands of people like Mabel Cooper were institutionalised, regarded as a threat to society and separated from their families and communities (Welshman and Walmsley, 2006); others were sterilised and had their children removed (Tilley et al, 2012). Tragically in the 1940s, thousands of children and adults identified as intellectually disabled were murdered in the German Reich as part of the Nazi euthanasia programme known as Aktion T4 programme (Atherton, 2019).

Oakes (2012) argues the importance of professionals appreciating current methods of assessment in their historical context. Following an analysis of intellectual disability care from pre-19th century to present, Oakes concludes that although the roles of professionals have changed, the relationship between those providing and those receiving services has always been, and continues to be, characterised by an inequality of power. Expansion of intellectual disability provision has been accompanied by an increasing range of professionals – including psychiatrists, nurses, social workers and therapists. Oakes argues that professional training and service hierarchies encouraged practitioners to increasingly assume the role of 'experts' (p. 14), arguably leaving people with intellectual disabilities, their families or carers, in the role of the 'amateur' or 'less competent', as opposed to an equal engaged in the process of assessing and planning. Oakes suggests this relational imbalance continues, despite a contemporary international policy landscape that foregrounds principles of rights and citizenship.

Between 2014 and 2018 a group of young people with intellectual disabilities took part in a research project called 'Madhouse: My House?' to explore the history of institutionalisation with the aim of making connections between their own lives today and the experiences of an earlier generation (Ledger and Walmsley with Access All Areas, 2019). The power and consequences of assessment emerged as a key theme, as the young people made links between past and present outcomes of being identified and labelled as intellectually disabled. Despite advances in assessment practice, people from this generation were easily able to identify connections with the experiences of their peers in earlier decades. A visit to the site of a former intellectual disability institution (Access All Areas with Ledger and Walmsley, 2018) triggered contrasts between the outcomes of assessment in the 1950s, 1960s and 1970s, that had led to people being sent away to an institution, and the outcomes of assessment taking place today. One of the young people reflected on how restrictions he had experienced since being assessed as 'ineligible' for social care support had resulted in him feeling cut off from the outside world – a similar consequence to the thousands of adults with intellectual disabilities previously institutionalised following assessment:

> "I don't get help now I've left school as my disability is classed as mild but I still get called names. With no support I can't go out and meet people. In many ways I'm still stuck behind four walls like they were."
> Member of Access All Areas theatre company, Personal Communication, 2015

This reflection reinforces Oakes's conclusion that people with intellectual disabilities remain subject to the decisions of service providers and professionals who assess and decide who is eligible for support and the quality and kind of support that can be given.

> "I think it is really important that professionals know about the history…This is part of why it feels sensitive to be assessed and labelled as a person with learning disabilities today. When you know this happened to people like you, you feel a connection – there is a tension between being assessed and getting good help and being assessed and then your life just getting a lot worse. Now I know this history it helps me to speak up for myself and others. To have confidence to keep speaking up for our right to be listened to and heard."
> Personal communication between Paul Christian and Sue Ledger, 2019b

Policy, legislation: implementing human-rights based approach to assessment

The process of assessment has historically been characterised by an inequality of power between professionals and people with intellectual disabilities (Oakes, 2012; Coalition for Collaborative Care, 2014). However, momentum created by self-advocacy, policy and legislation at national and international levels are demanding changes in practice so all people with intellectual disabilities play a much more active part in their own assessments and in ensuing decision-making, regardless of the complexity of their support. The influence of the social model of disability (Shakespeare, 2014) has been bolstered by international strengthening of policy and legislation to support the rights of people with intellectual disabilities, e.g., the United Nations Convention on the Rights of Persons with Disabilities (2006), Human Rights legislation (see, for example, the UK Human Rights Act, 1998; Joint Committee on Human Rights, 2008) and equalities legislation (see, for example, the UK Equality Act, 2010).

The drive towards co-production

Adoption of co-production is increasingly being advocated across public service delivery in the UK, including the need for co-production to underpin assessment practice (Skills for Care/TLAP, 2018). It refers to active input by the people who use services, as well as – or instead of – those who have traditionally provided them.

> *"Co-production means delivering services in an equal and reciprocal relationship between professionals, people using services, their families and their neighbours Where activities are co-produced in this way, both services and neighbourhoods become far more effective agents of change."*
>
> *Boyle and Harris, 2009*, p. 11

To act as partners, both people with intellectual disabilities and professionals must be empowered. Symonds et al (2020) suggest that in terms of assessment practice in England this may require an extension of policy and practice guidance outlining 'the practitioner should have knowledge and expertise that might be used by people needing support' (p. 14), but that these should be employed in an assessment process which is led by the person, rather than as the basis for organising the assessment meeting. These authors suggest that one possibility could be exploring how the person (or their chosen representative) could set the agenda for, and then chair, the assessment meeting (p. 14). Co-production means involving citizens in collaborative relationships with more empowered frontline staff who are able and confident to share power and accept user

expertise (Cummings and Miller, 2007; Needham and Carr, 2009). Outcomes-based assessment (Miller, 2012) and conversational assessment (Skills for Care/TLAP, 2018) are examples of approaches to assessment that support co-production. Miller argued that an outcome-focused assessment was more likely to treat the person as a citizen with rights, more likely to focus on strengths and capacities, and more likely to draw on the person's family and social network.

Miller (2010, p. 7) identifies a number of key features of an outcomes-based approach to assessment:

- Starting from the person's priorities supports enabling relationships, creates clarity and identifies goals at an early stage. Being listened to, involved and respected supports better outcomes;
- The person's views/preferences are central to decision-making;
- The person is a citizen with rights and responsibilities;
- Semi-structured conversations are undertaken with individuals in assessment, support planning and review;
- Identifying outcomes involves considering a range of solutions/strategies including the role of the person, family supports and community- based resources;
- Analytical skills (as opposed to tick box responses) are involved in assessment;
- Outcomes allow preventive work to take place while services and resources are prioritised for those most in need;
- Outcomes may change in the person's life journey and so should be revisited;
- Involves consideration of difficulties, limitations and aspirations or goals. The priority is to identify what to work towards;
- By focusing on strengths, capacities and goals, while mindful of limitations, the role of the person is maximised. Services do things *with* people.
- Outcomes are what matter to the person, though often consistent with professional and organisational outcomes e.g. being able to get out and about.

The Skills for Care/Think Local Act Personal (2018) in England advocate the use of **conversational assessment**. Drawing on learning from over 150 workforce innovation projects they highlight six key principles that should underpin conversational assessment:

1 It is about people's lives, not just their needs;
2 It recognises that people are expert in their own lives;

3 It is founded on trust, honesty and openness - requiring a relationship of two equals;

4 It starts with a blank sheet;

5 It needs sufficient time and resources;

6 It takes place within the context of the person's whole life and community.

Adopting a mutual model

The social model of disability that was also discussed in Chapters 1 and 2 rejects the idea that disability is a characteristic of an individual person. A person may have an impairment of bodily or mental function, but that only becomes a disability to the extent that society is not structured to cater well for people with that restriction, and other people's interactions exacerbate rather than overcome difficulties. People with intellectual disabilities may find certain skills such as memory and verbal communication more difficult, but equally non-disabled people also lack skills of effective interaction, communication and in building trusted, reciprocal relationships with people with intellectual disabilities. The 'disability' is thus a mutual one, with a need for support and efforts to overcome difficulties on both sides (Williams, 1978, 2009). As practitioners move towards more collaborative ways of undertaking assessment it is critical to reflect on what they can learn from the communications and skills of people with intellectual disabilities and how this can inform and strengthen their assessment practice. The examples in the Getting Creative: responsive and collaborative approaches section below return to the subject of communication and consider how professionals were able to learn directly from people with intellectual disabilities about their earlier lives, health concerns, abilities, networks and local community as part of a more equal and collaborative assessment process.

Person-centred assessment

The concept of a 'person-centred' approach is now well established in health and social care policy in England. The term 'person-centred' can be traced to the work of psychotherapist Carl Rogers (1961). Person-centred planning focuses on organising support so that the right 'environmental conditions' are created for individuals to identify and achieve their own goals (Sanderson et al, 2006). Developed in the 1980s (O'Brien and Lyle, 1988) it originally applied to a model of collaborative life-planning used with people preparing to leave long-stay

institutions and became increasingly widespread in services during the 1990s.

Mansell and Beadle-Brown (2004, pp. 1–2) identify three key features of person-centred planning:

- the focus on the person's own expressed aspirations and capacities;
- the mobilisation of a person's family and social network;
- providing services to support the achievement of goals, rather than limiting goals to fit available services.

In relation to assessment practice these core elements challenge systems of assessment that are deficit-based, bureaucratic and service-led (Symonds et al, 2020, p. 4). In England the government's intellectual disability policy Valuing People (Department of Health, 2001, 2007, 2009) promoted person-centred approaches and some powerful tools were created to support assessment practice. For example, MAPS (Making Action Plans: Forest and Lusthaus, 1989) and PATH (Planning Alternative Tomorrows with Hope: Pearpoint et al, 1993) are frameworks for identifying needs and turning them into a plan of action. These tools depend on a 'circle of support' being organised around the person, consisting of key people interested and willing to assist. This is likely to include family members, friends, neighbours and advocates as well as invited professionals willing to work with the circle - with the person themselves at the core. Symonds et al (2020) highlight how outcomes-based and conversational approaches to assessment, discussed earlier in this chapter, have much in common with elements of person-centred approaches described by Mansell and Beadle-Brown (2004).

Symonds et al (2020) suggest that one attempt to put people in the centre of their assessments was the introduction of provision for disabled people to conduct their own social care self-assessments - also referred to as 'supported self-assessments'. In this form of assessment, the process is led by the individual and not by a professional. A self-assessment can only be offered if the individual is willing and able to carry it out, and they must identify needs and outcomes in line with other assessment formats. Good practice guidance highlights the process as being an iterative one, in which statutory authorities have an obligation to ensure the provision of relevant information to the individual before, during and after the assessment takes place (SCIE, 2015). At the end of the process, statutory authorities must assure themselves that the assessment is a fair reflection of the person's needs. While designed to give disabled people more control over the process, the take up of self-assessments in the UK has remained low and is arguably undermined because of the requirement of local authorities to apply statutory eligibility criteria and standardised budgetary compliance (Slasberg and Beresford, 2017).

Moving from problem-orientated to strengths-based assessment

A key development in the literature on assessment has been the call to shift the focus from 'problem-orientated' (or 'deficits-based') to strengths-based assessment, the key elements of which are illustrated in Figure 4.1. Williams and Evans's work emphasises that the nature and purpose of an assessment is highly related to the values of both the professional and their organisation:

> "although assessment of problems is necessary to allocate resources and seek solutions, we can only capitalise on potential if we perceive some positive value, and for that positive assessment is required."
>
> Williams and Evans, 2013, p. 13

In Table 4.1 Williams and Evans contrast a problem-orientated approach to assessment with that informed by a more positive, strengths-orientated value-base across a number of settings.

Kirst-Ashman (2007) notes the difference between what she refers to as a 'traditional assessment' and strengths-based assessment. In traditional assessments the focus is on identifying and examining problems. In doing so the source or location of these problems is seen as being in the person with a disability. A strengths perspective offers an alternative view. Identification of problems may still be necessary and important as part of the assessment, but a strengths-based approach should be empowering and bring balance by assessing from strengths, opportunities, potentials and resources (Kirst-Ashman, 2007, p. 134, cited in Hodgson and Watts, 2017) It promotes assessment as a collaborative endeavour between practitioner and the person they are working with. This approach is also very mindful of the use of language that may unhelpfully construct deficit assessments-based focus. Labels such as 'challenging behaviour' may become attributed to an inherent or essentialist view of the person's identity (Sly, 2018) (see also Chapter 17). Some labels may work to over-generalise problems, resulting in service-based interventions that are applied to many people with intellectual disabilities as though they all share the same problems and circumstances, when in fact they don't (Brown et al, 2017). Teachers working alongside pupils with complex intellectual disabilities strongly caution against assessment processes that fail to adapt to the child's needs for individualised pacing and physical positioning. Likewise, they highlight the inherent risks associated with practitioners who may 'come to the assessment with their opinions already formed in advance, and then engineer the assessment process to prove their preconceptions correct' (Brown, 2014, pp. 1–2; Hawke, 2019).

Cournoyer (2014, p. 338) explains the best assessment practice brings together the practitioner's knowledge in collaboration with the client's first-hand experience. This is exemplified clearly in Box 4.1 Angela's story.

TABLE 4.1	Problem vs strength-orientated assessment (Williams and Evans, 2013)	
	Problem-orientated assessment involves describing	Strengths-orientated assessment involves describing
Person	What they cannot do	Their interests, achievements, gifts and capacities
Family	The problems the family has	The skills and achievements of the family
Environment	How the environment exacerbates perceived problems	Positive resources in the environment
Service	How the service fails to reach set standards	The pioneer achievements of the service
Community	Rejection and abuse within the community	The wealth and resources available in the community

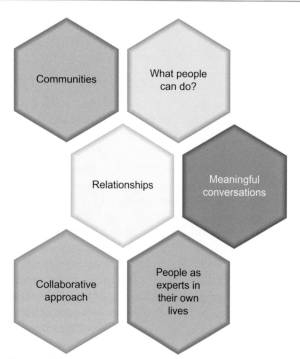

Fig. 4.1 Key elements of strengths-based approach (Colomina and Pereira, 2019)

📋 READER ACTIVITY 4.1

Box 4.1 Angela's story provides a practical example of a problem-orientated approach and a strengths-based approach to assessment.

How does this example demonstrate the difference between these two assessment approaches?

Angela's story provides an example of a professional who adopted a strengths-based approach to assessment; an approach increasingly advocated as good practice. In the next section we turn our attention to the types of assessment that people with intellectual disabilities and their families frequently encounter, considering the shift from traditional to inclusive assessments across the life course.

ASSESSMENT ACROSS THE LIFE COURSE

The experience of assessment recurs across the life course for many people with intellectual disabilities and their families, and continues to feature heavily in training for a wide range of health and social care professionals. A difficulty for people with intellectual disabilities and practitioners

in getting to grips with assessment is the perplexing array of approaches, tools, methodologies, theories and models used by professionals e.g. needs assessments (Painter et al, 2016), dementia screening assessments (Kirk et al, 2006; Dodd, 2017), community mapping (NDTi, 2002); risk assessments (Sellars, 2011; Campbell and McCue, 2013); educational assessments (Standards and Testing Agency, 2018); parenting assessments (Bernard, 2007; McGaw et al, 1998); capacity assessments (Graham and Cowley, 2015); and carers assessments (NHS England/Patient Experience Team, 2016). Different fields of practice utilise different tools and approaches. Depending on the needs of the person, the process of 'assessment' can be undertaken by a range of multi-disciplinary professionals working alongside people with intellectual disabilities, their families and supporters. Some assessment work requires using specific assessment tools (Xenitidis et al, 2000) whereas others require using a blank sheet of paper, good day and bad day headings or relationship circles (Williams and Evans, 2013; Sanderson Associates, 2015).

The predominance of assessment in the lives of some people with intellectual disabilities can be seen in the following extract, in which the mother of Jane, a 45-year old woman with Down syndrome, shares her experiences of assessment over the years.

"Well with Jane she was I suppose first assessed by doctors when they found she had Down's as a baby, and then with me by social services as I was on my own with two children. When she started school there were school assessments before she moved from the local primary to a special school. When she left school there was a school leaving (transition) assessment and then other ones for her health and where she would live. And then about if she could get work, that was with the careers people, or whether she should go to a day centre. At the day centre there was a young man who liked her and followed her and the manager was worried about that so there was a meeting and some tests about that too. Working out how much she could understand and if she liked him. Most recently, since she had her stroke there have been lots of health assessments for her treatment, her depression and more assessments about where she can live next, what she likes to do and who are her friends, boyfriend and family. Mostly it's all been helpful but a lot of paperwork and a lot of different people. Recently, Jane hasn't been involved so much – mainly me."

Interview undertaken for Staying Local Project,
Ledger, 2012

BOX 4.1 Angela's story

Angela, a 43-year old woman, was referred by the family doctor to a multi-disciplinary team for adults with intellectual disabilities in an inner city area. There were concerns regarding her self-care (rapid weight gain and associated health risks), managing of the household and finances. A neighbour had reported that Angela was spending long periods of time in the local café, appeared unwashed and to have put on a lot of weight.

Angela's mother had died nine months previously. The two had been very close, following the death of Angela's father several years earlier. After a period of intensive support from the local intellectual disability team her case had been closed as she was doing well, continuing to live in her family home with her sister.

Angela was visited by a duty social worker. Her initial (and arguably problem-orientated) assessment and recommendations were:

'This person is at risk and struggling to manage in her own home. Seek residential care or supported living placement. Referral to psychiatry for mental health assessment as neighbour feels she may be depressed. Referral to psychology for assessment of ability to manage money'.

The case was then allocated to a community nurse who visited Angela at her house and suggested they visit her local café together. In preparation for the visit the nurse spoke to the speech and language therapist who had previously assessed Angela. On her advice the nurse went prepared with some plain cards, pens, pictures and the knowledge that nine months ago she had a communication book that contained pictures of her family. He called Angela before the visit to arrange a suitable time to meet and ensure she would have sufficient time to be ready. Together they visited the café where she was greeted by a number of her mother's friends and the café owner. At the suggestion of the nurse Angela brought her communication book and the friends were able to refer to this to speak to her and identify members of her family. They explained they had been increasingly worried about Angela since her sister moved away. Angela said she missed her sister. The café owner said that as she seemed lonely he had invited her to stay longer and had taken on providing her with some 'extra meals'.

On the next visit to Angela the nurse took a blank sheet of paper and a relationship map (Mount, 1990). With support and encouragement from the nurse, Angela began to draw what she felt made her happy, what was not so good at present and people she knew in the local area. With Angela's permission the nurse contacted her sister and asked if they could meet up to do some planning together for Angela's future – her sister had been worried about Angela and was only too pleased to join in.

A follow-up meeting was scheduled with Angela, Angela's sister, five of the friends from the cafe and the cafe owner. Together they shared ideas on an equal basis using the mutual model approach. This lively meeting generated a number of ideas and plans, built upon Angela's aspirations for the future. At the meeting it was agreed by all that Angela would benefit from receiving five hours of social care support per week to assist with cooking, cleaning and bills/benefits.

Six months later, Angela was working part-time at the café, enabling her to be active and to maintain contact with family friends. She has made a new friend through the health group and they now go on walks together. Health screening shows a reduction in her weight to within a healthy range. Angela reports feeling much happier.

This account is echoed in findings from research analysing types of referrals received by integrated (health and social care) community teams supporting adults with intellectual disabilities in England (Clare et al, 2019). The purpose of this study was to increase understanding of the support sought by people with intellectual disabilities, their families and staff. The researchers analysed 270 new referrals in relation to 255 people with intellectual disabilities aged from 17 to 78 years. Almost a third of referrals were described as having severe or profound disabilities. Requests for assessment of entitlement to access specialist health care and/or eligibility for specialist social care and/or a review of an existing social care package (including transition to a personal budget) formed the most frequent category. Findings, reported at Figure 4.2, re-affirm the prominence of assessment across the life course with all referrals likely to require some element of assessment work.

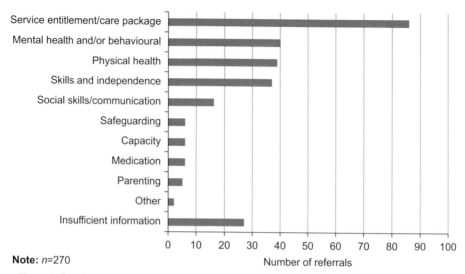

Note: *n*=270

Fig. 4.2 Bar chart summarising the 'primary' reasons for referral (Clare et al, 2019, p. 45)

In the light of the earlier discussion on strengths-based practice, it is interesting to note how this study, and others, indicate a service-centred bias embedded in the description of referral data (Coles and Ellis-Caird, 2019) with 'referral descriptions often locating problems within the bodies of people with intellectual disabilities, whilst constructing the actions of services as appropriate' (Haydon-Laurelut and Nunkoosing, 2016, p. 144). As noted by members of the Supported Loving Network (The Love Project Research Event, 2019; Forrester-Jones, 2019) there are generally very few referrals to services for support going to the cinema, staying up late, taking a holiday or finding a partner - issues which campaigners and researchers consistently identify as key concerns of many people with intellectual disabilities (Forrester-Jones, 2019; Turnpenny and Marriot, 2019).

So why is the process of assessment so predominant across all age groups in the lives of people with intellectual disabilities? In some respects it could be argued that this is no different from those of us who don't live with this label - we will all be assessed in some way if we need medical, dental or social care. Yet in contrast to the general population many people with intellectual disabilities are dependent on a range of services and support (see Department of Health, 2017, for an analysis of the England data). Each of these services and systems often has their own assessment process. In multi-disciplinary settings there may be multiple assessments required to inform the direction of future support. The consequence

is that from birth to old age it is likely that people with intellectual disabilities, their families and supporters will engage with a wide range of assessment processes. Typically, at present, these take place in specific contexts that are typical for people with intellectual disabilities and their families: in family homes, education, employment and care settings, community teams, short breaks services, benefit and finance systems, health care, hospital and crisis intervention services. For some people with more individualised funding, assessments may be completed by the individual, or their advocate and then reviewed by professionals.

> **READER ACTIVITY 4.2**
>
> Risk assessments are a type of assessment that focus primarily on the identification and management of risks. Specifically risk assessments are concerned with gathering information, analysing and weighing up the risks and benefits and using these to inform a plan of action. Using Box 4.2, Billy's story, can you identify sensitive and creative interventions and support you might employ to support Billy in going to the cinema safely?

Although Billy's assessment was focused on risk, you may have identified the potential for practitioners in this situation to adopt a strengths-based and person-centred

BOX 4.2   Billy's story

Going to the cinema: Billy's risk assessment plan

Billy is a 58-year old man of Caribbean origin living in a residential home. He has many friends in the home and area and used to travel independently. He has a particular interest in films from the 1930s–60s. Billy has Down syndrome and 18 months ago was diagnosed with early onset dementia. In recent months he has needed increased support to prepare food and can no longer travel on his own as he finds it hard to remember the route home. He remains a very sociable person and enjoys spending time with his family and friends.

Actions being considered

His sister and keyworker (the residential home worker with named responsibility for Billy's care) have found there are relaxed performances at a local cinema and would like Billy to try it. In England the term 'relaxed performance' refers to performances where adjustments are made so that more people can access community amenities. In a cinema this may include reduction of loud sound effects, arrangements for people to move freely during the screening, increased staffing and welcoming food and drinks. In other countries different terms may

be used, for example in Ireland such sessions are known as 'friendly hours'.

Benefits of the activity

Billy will have the opportunity to watch the type of films he enjoys in a setting tailored for people with dementia. This will provide opportunity to meet new people and make new friends. His sister also enjoys the cinema and will accompany him to the performances when she is not working. Billy really enjoys his sister's company and this could be a shared activity they can enjoy together.

Risks

Since the onset of his dementia Billy has on occasions punched out at other people or at furniture. This is usually if he is frustrated by not being able to achieve something he could previously do or if unable to express something. Risk in general for Billy can be reduced by using suitable visual materials to support communication and repeating activities to build Billy's confidence. The risk is that on visits to the cinema he may hit out and injure staff or other members of the public. Furniture and objects may be damaged and this may place him at risk of police intervention and a conviction.

approach to the situation. Working in a collaborative way like this promotes the opportunity for individuals to be co-designers and co-producers of their future services and support rather than solely passive consumers. Building skills in communicating with people with intellectual disabilities using a range of communication methods and tools is central to the process and will be explored further in the next section.

COMMUNICATION AND ASSESSMENT

Communication is fundamental to any assessment as it provides a means by which people gather or provide information required. However, as discussed in Chapter 5 many people with intellectual disabilities experience difficulties with communication. These communication difficulties negatively impact the extent to which this group are included in assessments. Therefore, it is imperative that each individual is supported to communicate, thus enabling their inclusion in assessments

in the interests of dignity, respect, empowerment, self-determination and autonomy. Such an approach would necessitate the use of a range of communication mediums that are again discussed in Chapter 5.

Ware (1996) in her writing about supporting communication with people with intellectual disabilities uses the term 'responsive communication' and defines it as one in which 'people get responses to their actions, get the opportunity to give responses to the actions of others and have the opportunity to take the lead in interaction', (p.1). In a similar vein, partner sensitivity has been highlighted by several researchers as an important communication facilitator particularly with regard to people with profound and multiple intellectual disabilities (Halle et al, 2004; Coupe O'Kane and Goldbart, 1998). Communication attempts by persons with intellectual disabilities are undetected or not recognised as communicative. Consequently, the person's perspective is not heard or captured. It is particularly problematic for those who communicate idiosyncratically

(Grove et al, 1999; Wilder and Granlund, 2003; Vlaskamp, 2005; Munde and Vlaskamp, 2015). In an assessment situation, this is a missed opportunity to gather valuable information to inform the assessment and subsequent plan. This information is critical to being truly person-centred. Therefore, practitioners must reflect on their own communication skills. Practitioners must develop the self-awareness and sensitivity necessary to communicate successfully and inclusively and respond to people with intellectual disabilities.

Reader Activity 4.3 in the accompanying online resource considers the role of communication in relation to a healthcare scenario.

GETTING CREATIVE: RESPONSIVE AND COLLABORATIVE APPROACHES

In the chapter so far, we have considered how co-production, person-centred, mutual and strengths-based approaches are calling for changes in practice that enable people with intellectual disabilities to lead and shape the assessment process and content. In this section we discuss a number of further, and often inter-related, approaches that have successfully supported people to contribute and be heard in the assessment process. As space is limited, a brief summary is provided with signposting to further reading.

Assessment of Community Resources

A systematic listing of all existing community assets, resources and organisations can make a key contribution to the assessment process – enabling future possibilities to be explored. This could be in the form of a simple list or by using a mapping tool such as the one shown in Figure 4.3 to identify places, volunteering and employment opportunities, and activities of possible interest. Building on their improved understanding of community resources (NDTi, 2002; Salman, 2017; Bown et al, 2017) practitioners have subsequently used community spaces of relevance to the individual as 'talking places or points' leading to improved outcomes for people with intellectual disabilities. Reported improvements include increased self-esteem, improved opportunities for socialising, volunteering and improved fitness.

Self-Building Our Lives (Self Building Our Lives Research Team, 2019), a collaborative social care project, researched how people with intellectual disabilities in England and Scotland are 'self-building' their daily lives when responsibility for daytime social care and support has been given to them to organise. Findings from this research and a resource pack produced by the team emphasise the critical importance of people being able to access information about community resources.

Storytelling

Formal assessment or evaluation, planned in advance, often involves asking people to tell partial stories about aspects of their lives, but the subject-matter of these stories is pre-determined by the assessor or evaluator. Open-ended or informal story-telling leaves control of the story to the storyteller; it is therefore a user-friendly, non-oppressive and empowering method for gaining information.

Storysharing® (Grove, 2014, 2015; Bunning et al, 2016; see also www.openstorytellers.org.uk) is an example of a co-productive approach to telling stories that can be used in assessment. The narrative is co-constructed, with the focus being on what the person with communication disabilities contributes effectively rather than what they fail to do. Grove (2014) provides an assessment protocol; people with intellectual disabilities who have had some training in how to tell stories use a modified version to self-assess when they are working on performance or presentation skills (Grove, 2007).

Life story work

Another way of informing assessment is through life story or life history work. It is often the case that the histories and stories of people with intellectual disabilities are lost in the professional records created in their name (Gillman at al, 1997). Their history may be held in archived childhood records or by staff with whom they no longer have contact (Thompson and Westwood, 2008). These missing records matter as they enable the person to have a voice, to be the expert they are in the life they have lived. If a person doesn't use words to communicate or struggles with remembering or ordering information it can be very hard for them to hold onto their story. Evaluation of life story work, where people are supported to recover and record their stories, is providing clear evidence for the positive effect of investing time in this process (Westerhof et al, 2016).

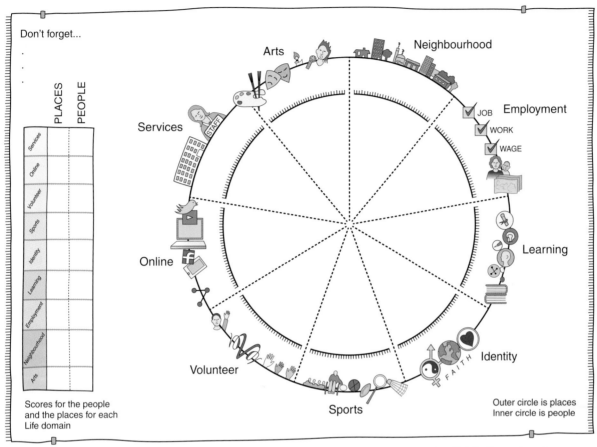

Fig. 4.3 Example of a Community Mapping tool. NDTi (2002). Illustration by Jon Ralph. Reproduced with permission of NDTi.

The aim is not so much to gather and record a complete and detailed history but to build a more informed understanding of the person. The life story can be in whatever form the individual prefers; a sheet of A4 paper, a timeline, some pictures in a scrap book, a memory box, DVD of a memory book. The Wiki website and Life Journey Map (see illustrations in this chapter) are examples of tools that can be used to support people to share aspects of their life stories.

Memory boxes

Memory boxes are a person-centred approach which involves working with an individual to bring together a variety of mementos which represent a time, place, memory, pet or person. These may include, for example, photographs, objects, artwork, music, film and writings. Each item usually has a narrative attached to it which is told and re-told when holding the item. As the approach does not rely heavily on verbal communication, but rather on objects themselves, people with profound intellectual disabilities may find the inclusion of such an approach in assessment beneficial. Memory box work provides a flexible structure for exploring memories and strengthening relationships. They have also been very helpful in supporting bereavement work with people with complex needs (Young and Garrard, 2016).

Photovoice

Photovoice is a visual method that focuses on participant-led photography (Cluley, 2017).

Originally developed by Wang and Burris (1997), the method allows participants the opportunity to voice their perspective visually by giving them a camera to photograph their world independently or with support. For people with intellectual disabilities engaged in assessment this provides a way of concretising issues and concerns that is not reliant on verbal communication. Photovoice provides an accessible method that allows an insight into the lives of people who cannot communicate their experiences via more traditional research methods (Cluley, 2017).

Access to the arts and assessment

Work produced by artists with intellectual disabilities (Ewbank and Mills, 2015; Project Art Works, 2019; Gadiyar, 2019; Eno Amooquaye with Intoart, 2019; City Lit Percussion Orchestra, 2018) demonstrate how access to the arts is providing new mediums and spaces for people to communicate about their lives, feelings and experiences. Bazalgette (2019) and Adams (2019) emphasise the value of art in helping people to understand the life of others – to walk in their shoes. In this respect access to the arts is of value in supporting assessment work. For people who are already working as artists, musicians or performers, access to their work will make a substantial contribution to the assessment process. For individuals who have not had the opportunity to access creative spaces or arts programmes this is an area to explore to support communication and expression.

The illustrations that follow provide examples of responsive and collaborative assessment in practice.

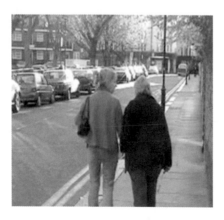

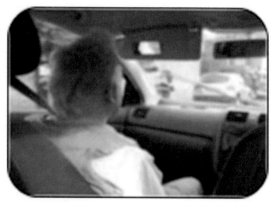

Mobile interviews, on foot and by car, used as part of the assessment process

Using mobile interviews and life journey maps to support collaborative assessment

Between 2008 and 2012 the Staying Local Research Project combined techniques of mobile interviewing, photovoice (Wang and Burris, 1997), and life journey mapping to enable people with complex intellectual disabilities to record and share their life stories and memories (Ledger, 2012, 2019; Department of Health, 2013).

These methods were positively evaluated by people with intellectual disabilities and their support teams (Ledger and Shufflebotham, 2019). This illustration explains how one social worker combined the use of mobile interviews and map-making to support her assessment practice.

Moses is 43 years old and of African-Caribbean heritage. He came to the attention of the Community Learning Disability Team on the sudden death of his father, who lived with him and was his sole carer. This team brings together a range of multi-disciplinary professionals including, for example, nurses, social workers, psychiatrists, speech and language therapists, occupational therapists and physiotherapists to provide community-based support to people with intellectual disabilities.

Father and son had minimal contact with services, although Moses had attended a specialist school for children with severe intellectual disabilities as a child. He has an older sibling who returned to Jamaica 15 years ago but is no longer in contact. He communicates using key words and gestures.

When his father died Moses was admitted on an emergency basis to the local short breaks service. No local residential setting had a vacancy that was felt to be suitable to support him and six months after the death of his father he was still living in the short breaks service whilst the local authority tried to identify a placement.

A Psychiatrist observed that Moses still appeared distressed by his bereavement and the busy environment of the short breaks service was hard for him. He appeared confused and unsettled, and his behaviour was causing increasing concern, necessitating increased staffing to keep him and others safe.

Moses's case was allocated to a new social worker from the Learning Disabilities team, who was tasked with carrying out an assessment in preparation for a move to a specialist placement outside the local area. To inform the assessment and future planning, the social worker felt it was important to identify family and social networks that he may have in the area. Available records revealed a few earlier family addresses but little other useful information.

The social worker met with Moses and established that he enjoys looking at photographs and finds pictures helpful to support his communication. She started the assessment by inviting him to bring photos and objects that he wanted to share. They began to sketch out together all the available autobiographical information on flip chart paper. Utilising graphic facilitation techniques (Mendonca, 2004), Moses and the social worker used drawings and symbols to create an initial accessible record. This resulted in a simple timeline overlaid with photographs, drawings and information from case files (see Figure 4.4).

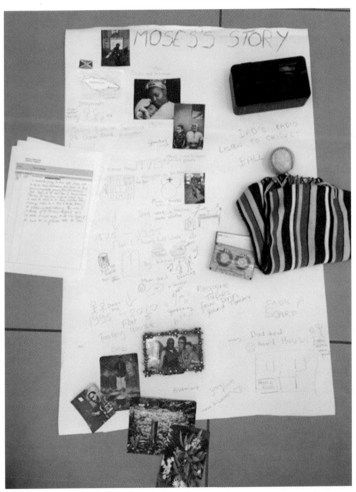

Fig. 4.4 Moses's life story collage following first assessment interview

Moses and the social worker then planned a walk and car journey in the local area, accompanied by a member of the care team. They decided to drive to his former family home and walk around the neighbourhood.

When they arrived at the block where he had previously lived, Moses smiled and seemed really pleased to see his home again. He rang the bell but there was no reply. At this point a neighbour recognised him and came out to greet him. They seemed very pleased to see each other. The neighbour explained that Moses and his father had friends in the area, one of whom ran the local shoe repair shop, which was a place Moses and his father would often visit. The neighbour invited Moses to come back another day for a meal.

Moses, the social worker and her colleague then set off for the shoe repair shop. On the way they passed a church. Moses went into the church and inside handed a candle to the social worker, saying "Mum". In this way Moses was able to communicate that he had previously attended church with his family.

They then walked to the shoe repair shop. Moses was warmly greeted by the owner, who shared some stories about Moses's family, mentioning his father's allotment, which Moses had helped maintain.

Throughout the trip, Moses took photos of the people he met and the places he visited.

During this and subsequent mobile interviews, Moses was able to communicate that he knew his way round the local area and felt comfortable there. It also became clear that he had an existing network of friends and former neighbours.

The social worker then supported Moses to make a life journey map using photos from three sources: those taken during the mobile interviews, existing family photos, and images from the internet. These were superimposed on an image of a street map and Moses's words were added to help him share his story (see Figure 4.5).

Moses used the life journey map to support his communication with people working with him. He appeared much happier and more settled since his trips out with the social worker and the opportunity to communicate his story.

The insights gained by this collaborative assessment process prompted the social worker to contact the housing association which managed the block where Moses had been living. The flat had not yet been re-let as it had been in a poor state of repair. The social worker negotiated with the housing association to re-let the flat to Moses, utilising the second bedroom for staff providing 24-hour support. Several years later Moses remains in his family home. He has maintained links with his former neighbours and family friends and with his faith community.

READER ACTIVITY 4.3

1. Reflecting on Moses's story – how can the methods described support a more collaborative assessment process?
2. Reflecting on your own experiences – can you think of any barriers to the use of these approaches in services?
3. Do you think the outcome might have been different for Moses if the social worker had used a less inclusive approach?

Using multi-media to support inclusive assessment processes

From 2010, RIX Research & Media have been developing RIX Wikis. Rix Wikis are private and easy to use websites that are often used to support person-centred assessment activities and processes:

> "RIX Wikis offer a way to help ensure the needs, wants and aspirations of individuals with learning disabilities are heard by putting them centre-stage. Wikis help people with learning disabilities and all those who live and work with them to communicate better, share information and celebrate achievements."
>
> RIX Research & Media, 2020

The Wiki enables people to upload photos, videos, documents and other content, helping them to share their story. Once a Wiki has been created, other people who are known and trusted can be invited to view or contribute content to it, including family members, friends, colleagues and professionals. Some people with intellectual disabilities will manage their Wikis with very little – or no – support. Other people may benefit from the involvement of someone close to them to help develop their site.

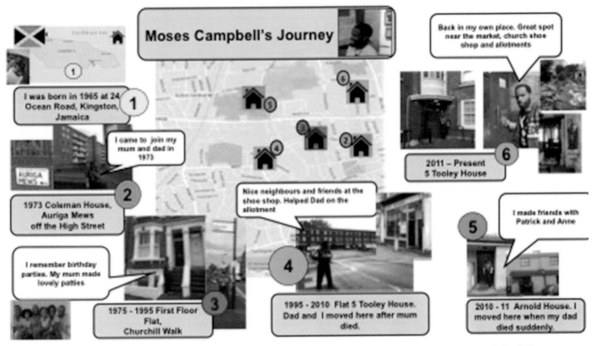

Fig. 4.5 Moses's life journey map. Names and places have been changed to protect confidentiality. Pictures are posed by actor from Access all Areas, a theatre company for people with intellectual disabilities.

Shane and his family were one of the first families to trial RIX Wikis and Shane continues to use his Wiki nearly 10 years later. Shane has intellectual disabilities, cerebral palsy and is registered blind. Commenting in 2011, Shane's mother Sam highlighted how important it was for the whole family to be involved in this process, and that all opportunities were sought to make sure it was as person-centred as possible. This illustration will focus on an early iteration of Shane's Wiki, which highlights how it became an essential tool in assessment and person-centred planning at a key point of transition.

Shane's Wiki contains video and audio reflections from family members that explain how Shane responds in particular situations. The Wiki site also enables practitioners and family members to share learning and information about Shane's progress and achievements, in line with strengths-based assessment. Shane's mother was initially prompted to explore the potential of multi-media to support a more person-centred transitions review process when Shane was 14. Sam explained how prior to this review she felt apprehensive, concerned that the professionals involved in the planning process 'would only be looking at pieces of paper, would only be focusing on Shane's disabilities, on the things he needs help with, and not focusing on Shane as a person'. The Wiki provided an opportunity for Shane and his family to present a more holistic picture of his life and his personality. Sam was hopeful that showing professionals photos and videos of Shane in different contexts would enable a different type of planning process to be undertaken. Most strikingly, the Wiki provided a platform for Shane to attend his annual review meeting in person. Having learned how to operate the website, he was able to show the professionals in attendance about his life, placing Shane firmly in the centre of discussions. Sam said *"prior to this (the Wiki), they (the new professionals in attendance) would not have met him and they would be making decisions purely based on pieces of paper."*

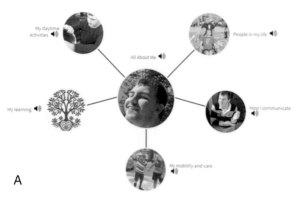

A

Shane's wiki Homepage

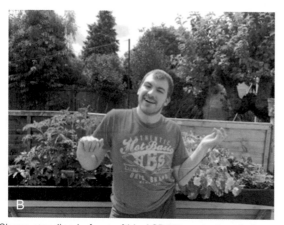

B

Shane standing in front of his ASDAN gardening challenge.

More recently, Shane used his latest Wiki to provide evidence for assessment on ASDAN's Skills for Life. ASDAN is an awarding organisation whose curriculum programmes and qualifications help young people develop knowledge and skills for learning, work and life. The Wiki has also been used in Shane's assessment moving from Children Services to Adult Services (social care), for various Speech and Language and Physiotherapy Assessments, Adult Social Care assessments, and as evidence for personal budgets and support plans. This demonstrates how Shane's Wiki has adapted to reflect wider changes and priorities in his life as he has reached adulthood.

READER ACTIVITY 4.5

Reflecting on Shane's example, in what ways can multi-media support inclusive assessment processes?

Reflecting on your own experiences – personal or professional – can you think of a time when use of a multi-media tool like the RIX Wiki might have led to different outcomes during an assessment process?

Further information about RIX Wikis and a YouTube clip about Shane's wiki can be found in the accompanying online resource.

CONCLUSION

This chapter has introduced you to assessment for people with intellectual disabilities, highlighting that assessment takes many forms and occurs in multiple contexts across the life course. We have argued that assessment must be situated within its historical context, as this is what helps to explain the power imbalances that continue to affect the systems and processes that people with intellectual disabilities and their families experience today. The chapter has highlighted that assessment has been subjected to considerable critiques in recent years, with self-advocates, families, practitioners, policy-makers and academics calling for more person-centred, collaborative and responsive approaches to the process. This chapter has pointed you towards some of the key literature in the field and demonstrated application of new approaches to practice using a number of real-life illustrations. These make plain that approaching assessment with a sense of openness and creativity can make tangible improvements to people's lives. The examples provided here were not dependent on heavy resourcing to achieve the outcomes described. Critically, they were all underpinned by key values of equality and person-centredness, with practitioners taking time to get to know a person and their wider context. Each of these examples highlights the importance of exploring and trying things out, while working collaboratively with people with intellectual disabilities and their families to see what best supports a person to actively participate in – and lead - the assessment process.

However, we do not dismiss the very real barriers facing the implementation of creative, collaborative and responsive assessment practice. Slasberg and Beresford

(2017) highlight the tensions encountered by practitioners when pursuing person-centred approaches within statutory provision based on determining eligibility and funding. In many agencies, recording processes and data systems may not be compatible with highly individualised ways of collecting assessment information (Williams and Evans, 2013). In services providing care, such as residential homes or supported living, research has consistently revealed a lack of life story information to inform assessment and future planning (Gillman et al, 1997; Kaiser and Gaughan, 2012). Hingley-Jones and Ruch (2016) emphasise that repercussions associated with the conflation of risk preoccupied cultures and ideologically driven agendas of financial austerity present additional challenges to practitioners seeking to work in relationship-based ways.

Despite these challenges, this chapter has shown that collaborative, strengths-based assessment can be a positive experience for people with intellectual disabilities and their families. It should be the goal of practitioners to approach assessment critically (understanding the long-standing power dynamics that have shaped the system and people's experience of it), but also with a sense of curiosity and creativity. As Hodgson and Watts (2017, p. 225) write:

> "There are numerous assessment approaches, tools, theories, models and frameworks. The task of the practitioner is to empower people through their approach and at the same time to listen and learn from them in developing their understanding and skills in the art of making good assessments."

REFERENCES

Access All Areas, with Ledger, S., & Walmsley, J. (2018). *Making heritage accessible. The madhouse, my house? history of learning disability project guide.* London: Access All Areas.

Adams, K. (2019). Introduction to awareness raising. Presentation given at Explorers Conference Art, Rights and Representation Conference, Milton Keynes, 20/21 November.

Atherton, H. (2019). Finding Ivy: a life worthy of life. *Community Living*, 33(1), 18–19.

Bazalgette, P. (2019). The empathy instinct. Presentation given at Explorers Conference Art, Rights and Representation Conference. Milton Keynes, 20/21 November.

Bernard, S. (2007). Parents with learning disabilities – the assessment of parenting ability. *Advances in Mental Health and Learning Disabilities*, 1(3), 14–18.

Bown, H., Carrier, J., Hayden, C., et al. (2017). *What works in community led support? First evaluation report.* National Development Team for Inclusion.

Brown, D. (2014). What does 'follow the child' mean? *reSources*, 19(1), 1–8. Available at: http://files.cadbs.org/200002255-952a79623e/reSources%20Brown%202014.pdf. [Accessed 12 January 2020].

Brown, D. (2019). Facilitating strengths-based conversations that support independence and self-agency. Presentation given at Community Care Live 19, London, 16 October.

Brown, M., Janes, E., & Hatton, C. (2017). *A trade in people.* Lancaster: Centre for Disability Studies.

Bourlet, G., & Page, L. (1994). Speaking out on assessment. presentation given at Guidance Launch, London, April.

Boyle, D., & Harris, M. (2009). *The challenge of co-production.* London: NESTA.

Bunning, K., Gooch, L., & Johnson, M. (2016). Developing the personal narratives of children with complex communication needs associated with intellectual disabilities: what is the potential of Storysharing? *Journal of Applied Research in Intellectual Disability*, 30(4), 743–756.

Campbell, M., & McCue, M. (2013). Assessment of interpersonal risk (AIR) in adults with learning disabilities and challenging behaviour – piloting a new risk assessment tool. *British Journal of Learning Disabilities*, 41(2), 141–149.

Christian, P., & Ledger, S. (2019a). *Personal communication, 23 December 2019.*

Christian, P., & Ledger, S. (2019b). *Personal communication, 10 February 2020.*

City Lit Percussion Orchestra in collaboration with the Royal Academy of Music. (2018). Available at: https://www.citylit.ac.uk/percussion-orchestra-royal-academy-music. [Accessed 10 April 2020].

Clare, I., Wade, K., Ranke, N., Whitson, S., Lillywhite, A., Jones, E., Broughton, S., Wagner, A., & Holland, A. (2019), Specialist community teams for adults with learning disabilities: referrals to a countywide service in England. *Tizard Learning Disability Review*, 24(2), 41–49.

Cluley, V. (2017). Using Photovoice to include people with profound and multiple learning disabilities in inclusive research. *British Journal of Learning Disabilities*, 45(1), 39–46.

Coles, S., & Ellis-Caird, H. (2019). Whose story is it anyway? A narrative approach to working with people affected by learning disabilities, their families and networks. In V. Brown & M. Hayden-Laurelut (Eds.), *Working with people with learning disabilities: systemic approaches.* London: Red Globe.

Colomina, C., & Pereira, T. (2019). *Strengths-based approach practice handbook.* London: DHSC.

Coalition for Collaborative Care. (2014). Available at: http://coalitionforcollaborativecare.org.uk/wp-content/uploads/2014/11/C4CC_210x297_final_pages.pdf. [Accessed 21 January 2020].

Cooper, M. (1997). Mabel Cooper's life story. In D. Atkinson, M. Jackson, & J. Walmsley (Eds.), *Forgotten lives: exploring the history of learning disability*. Kidderminster: BILD.

Coulshed, V., & Orme, J. (1998). *Social work practice: an introduction* (3rd ed.). Basingstoke, UK: Macmillan.

Coupe O'Kane, J., & Goldbart, J. (1998). *Communication before speech: development and assessment*. London: David Fulton.

Cournoyer, B. (2014). *The social work skills workbook* (7th ed.). Australia: Brooks/Cole.

Cummins, J., & Miller, C. (2007). *Co-production, social capital and service effectiveness*. London: POM.

Davidson, T., Smith, H., & Burns, J. (2014). The impact of cognitive assessment on the identity of people with learning disabilities. *British Journal of Learning Disabilities*, *42*(3), 185–192.

Department of Health. (2001). *Valuing people: a new strategy for learning disability in the 21st century*. London: The Stationery Office.

Department of Health. (2013). *Learning disabilities good practice project*. London: Crown Copyright.

Department of Health. (2007). *Valuing people now: from progress to transformation*. London: The Stationery Office.

Department of Health. (2009). *Valuing people now: a new three-year strategy for people with learning disabilities*. London: Department of Health.

Department of Health. (2017). *Local support for people with a learning disability*. London: National Audit Office.

Dodd, K. (2017). *The diagnosis and treatment of dementia in people with learning disabilities*. Surrey: Surrey and Borders Partnership.

Eno Amooquaye N., with Intoart. (2019). Artist showcase. Presentation given at Arts, Rights and Representation Conference, Project Artworks, Milton Keynes, 20/21 November.

Equality Act. (2010). United Kingdom. Available at: http://www.legislation.gov.uk/ukpga/2010/15. [Accessed 21 December 2019].

Ewbank, N., & Mills, S. (2015). *Project Art Works: impact analysis an inquiry into cultural engagement for people with complex needs*. Hasting: NEA. https://projectartworks.org/wp-content/uploads/2015/10/PAW-Report Final v2-low-res-spread.pdf. [Accessed 12 January 2020].

Flynn, M. (2012). *Winterbourne View Hospital: a serious case review*. Yate: South Gloucestershire Safeguarding Adults Board.

Forest, M., & Lusthaus, E. (1989). Promoting educational equality for all students: circles and maps. In S. Stainback, W. Stainback, & M. Forest (Eds.), *Educating all students in the mainstream of regular education*. Baltimore: Brookes.

Forrester-Jones, R. (2019). The Love Project. Presentation given at Recent Research from the Tizard Centre, 3 May.

Gadiyar, S. (2019). Artist Showcase – Phoenix Gallery, Brighton. Presentation given at Explorers Conference Art, Rights and Representation Conference, Milton Keynes. 20/21 November.

Gillman, M., Swaine, J., & Heyman, B. (1997). Life history or 'case' history: the objectification of people with learning disabilities through the tyranny of professional discourses. *Disability and Society*, *12*(5), 675–695.

Gollins, T., Fox, A., Walker, B., et al. (2016). *Developing a wellbeing and strengths-based approach to social work practice: changing culture*. TLAP.

Graham, M., & Cowley, J. (2015). *A practical guide to the Mental Capacity Act 2005*. London: Jessica Kingsley.

Grove, N., Bunning, K., Porter, J., et al. (1999). See what I mean: interpreting the meaning of communication by people with severe and profound intellectual disabilities. *Journal of Applied Research in Intellectual Disabilities*, *12*(3), 190–203.

Grove, N. (2007). *Learning to tell: a handbook of inclusive storytelling*. Kidderminster: BILD.

Grove, N. (2014). *The big book of storysharing*. Abingdon: Routledge.

Grove, N. (2015). Finding the sparkle: storytelling in the lives of people with learning disabilities. *Tizard Learning Disability Review*, *20*(1), 29–36.

Hawke, A. (2019). The engagement for learning framework. paper given at Assessment - Readiness to Learn and Evaluating Progress. Medical Needs Professional Learning Network Seminar, London, 11 February.

Halle, J., Brady, N. C., & Drasgow, E. (2004). Enhancing socially adaptive communicative repairs of beginning communicators with disabilities. *American Journal of Speech-Language Pathology*, *13*(1), 43–54.

Haydon-Laurelut, M., & Nunkoosing, K. (2016). Causing trouble: the language of learning disability and challenging behaviour. *Tizard Learning Disability Review*, *21*(3), 144–149.

Heslop, P., Blair, P., Fleming, P., et al. (2013). *Confidential inquiry into premature deaths of people with learning disabilities*. Bristol: Norah Fry Research Centre.

Hodgson, D., & Watts, L. (2017). *Key concepts & theory in social work*. London: Palgrave.

Hingley-Jones, H., & Ruch, G. (2016). 'Stumbling through'? Relationship-based social work practice in austere times. *Journal of Social Work Practice*, *30*(3), 235–248.

Joint Committee on Human Rights. (2008). *A life like any other? Human rights of adults with learning disabilities*.

HL Paper 40 -I HC 73-I. London: The Stationery Office.

Kaiser, P., & Gaughan, A. (2012). *'Your story matters': embedding life stories in practice supporting a human rights based approach*. London: Life Story Network course, Mary Ward Centre, 8 February. Available at: www.lifestorynetwork.org.uk. [Accessed 9 February 2012].

Kirk, L. J., Hick, R., & Laraway, A. (2006). Assessing dementia in people with learning disabilities: the relationship between two screening measures. *Journal of Intellectual Disabilities, 10*(4), 357–364.

Kirst-Ashman, K. K. (2007). *Introduction to social work and social welfare: critical thinking perspectives*. Australia: Thomson Brooks/Cole.

Ledger, S. (2012). *Staying local: support for people with learning difficulties from inner London 1971–2007*. Unpublished PhD Thesis. Milton Keynes: The Open University.

Llewellwyn, N. (Dir.). (2015). *No longer shut up: finding Mabel Cooper's voice* [film]. London: Advocreate and Access All Areas. Available at: https://www.youtube.com/watch?v=BZAgOs4Ngn4. [Accessed 2 January 2020].

Ledger, S. (2019). Stories show the way to stay home. *Community Living, 32*(3), 12–13.

Ledger, S., & Shufflebotham, L. (2019). We were here: sharing stories of local support. *Community Living, 32*(4), 16–17.

Ledger, S., Walmsley, J., & with Access All Areas. (2019). Madhouse: performance artists with learning disabilities sharing the history of institutions. In K. Soldatic & K. Johnson (Eds.), *Global perspectives on disability activism and advocacy*. Abingdon: Routledge.

Lenehan, C. (2017). *These are our children*. London: DH/Council for Disabled Children.

Lemmi, V., Knapp, M., Reid, C., et al. (2016). Positive behavioural support for children and adolescents with learning disabilities and behaviour that challenges: an initial exploration of service use and costs. *Tizard Learning Disability Review, 21*(4), 169–180.

McGaw, S., Beckley, K., Connolly, N., et al. (1998). *The parent assessment manual*. Truro: Trecare NHS Trust.

McKenzie, K., Murray, G., Wilson, H., & Delahunty, L. (2019). A tool to help identify learning disabilities in homeless people. *Nursing Times, 115*(8), 26–28.

Mansell, J., & Beadle-Brown, J. (2004). Person-centred planning or person-centred action? Policy and practice in intellectual disability services. *Journal of Applied Research in Intellectual Disabilities, 17*, 1–9.

Manthorpe, J., & Martineau, S. (2015). What can and cannot be learned from serious case reviews of the care and treatment of adults with learning disabilities in England? Messages for social workers. *British Journal of Social Work, 45*(1), 331–348.

Mencap. (2019) Assessments and eligibility. Available at: https://www.mencap.org.uk/advice-and-support/social-care/assessments-and-eligibility. [Accessed 23 December 2019].

Mendonça, P. (2004). *Rights, independence, choice and inclusion*. London: Learning Disability Task Force.

Miller, E. (2010). Can the shift from needs-led to outcomes-focused assessment in health and social care deliver on policy priorities? *Research, Policy and Planning, 28*(2), 115–127.

Miller, E. (2012). *Measuring outcomes: challenges and strategies*. Glasgow: IRISS.

Mount, B. (1990). *Making futures happen: a manual for facilitators of personal futures planning*. St. Paul, MN: Governor's Council on Developmental Disabilities.

Munde, V., & Vlaskamp, C. (2015). Initiation of activities and alertness in individuals with profound intellectual and multiple disabilities. *Journal of Intellectual Disability Research, 59*(3), 284–292.

National Development Team for Inclusion (NDTi). (2002). *Inclusion web – community mapping tool*. Bath: NDTI.

Needham, C., & Carr, S. (2009). *Co-production: an emerging evidence base for adult social care transformation*. London: SCIE.

NHS England/Patient Experience Team. (2016). *An integrated approach to identifying and assessing carer health and wellbeing*. London: NHSE.

Oakes, P. (2012). Assessment of learning disability: a history. *Learning Disability Practice, 15*(1), 12–16.

O'Brien, J., & Lyle O'Brien, C. (1988). *A little book about person centred planning*. Toronto: Inclusion Press.

Painter, J., et al. (2016). Development and validation of the Learning Disabilities Needs Assessment Tool (LDNAT), a HoNOS-based needs assessment tool for use with people with intellectual disability. *Journal of Intellectual Disability Research, 60*(12), 1178–1188. https://onlinelibrary.wiley.com/doi/abs/10.1111/jir.12340.

Parker, J. (2013). Assessment, intervention and review. In M. Davies (Ed.), *The Blackwell companion to social work* (4th ed.). Chichester: Wiley and Sons.

Pearpoint, J., O'Brien, J., & Forest, M. (1993). *Path: a workbook for planning possible positive futures: planning alternative tomorrows with hope for schools, organizations, businesses, families*. Toronto: Inclusion Press.

People, First. (1993). *Oi it's my assessment*. London: People First.

Project Art Works. (2019). Explorers Conference Art, Rights and Representation Conference, Milton Keynes, 20/21 November.

Reid, C., Scholl, C., & Gore, N. (2013). Seeking to prevent residential care for young people with intellectual disabilities and challenging behaviour: examples and early outcomes from the Ealing ITSBS. *Tizard Learning Disability Review*, 18(4), 171–178.

RIX Research & Media. (2020). Available at: https://rixresearchandmedia.org/software/rix-wikis/. [Accessed 22 April 2020].

Rogers, C. (1961). *On becoming a person: a therapist's view of psychotherapy*. London: Constable and Robinson.

Salman, S. (2017). Community approach to social work delivers more personalised care. *The Guardian*, 11 December. Available at: https://www.theguardian.com/social-care-network/2017/dec/11/community-approach-to-social-work-delivers-more-personalised-care?CMP=ema-1696&CMP=. [Accessed 19 January 2020].

Sanderson, H., Thompson, J., & Kilbane, J. (2006). The emergence of person-centred planning as evidence-based practice. *Journal of Integrated Care*, 14(2), 18–25.

Sanderson Associates. (2015). Good day, bad day. Available at: http://www.helensandersonassociates.co.uk/wp content/uploads/2015/02/gooddaybadday.pdf.

SCIE. (2015). Supported self-assessment. Available at: https://www.scie.org.uk/care-act-2014/assessment-and-eligibility/supported-self-assessment/. [Accessed 2 April 2020].

Self-Building Our Lives Research Team. (2019). Sharing stories about building a life. Presentation given at 'Self-Building Our Lives' National Social Care Research Event, London, 13 November.

Selfbuildingourlives.org. (2019). Resource pack. Available at: http://selfbuildingourlives.org/resources/people_with_learning_disabilities_and_their_supporters/find_out_information/. [Accessed 23 January 2020].

Sellars, C. (2011). *Risk assessment in people with learning disabilities*. Chichester: Blackwell.

Shakespeare, T. (2014). *Disability rights and wrongs revisited*. London: Routledge.

Skills for Care/Think Local Act Personal. (2018). *Using conversations to assess and plan people's care and support*. Leeds: Skills for Care.

Slasberg, C., & Beresford, P. (2017). The need to bring an end to the era of eligibility policies for a person-centred, financially sustainable future. *Disability & Society*, 32(8), 1263–1268.

Sly, S. (2018). I am challenging behaviour. *Community Living*, April.

Standards & Testing Agency. (2018). *Piloting the 7 aspects of engagement for summative assessment: qualitative evaluation*. London: Crown Copyright.

Standards, & Testing Agency. (2020). *The engagement model*. London: Crown Copyright.

www.gov.uk/government/publications.

Symonds, J., Miles, C., Steel, M., et al. (2020). Making person-centred assessments. *Journal of Social Work*, 20(4), 431–447. doi:10.1177/1468017319830593.

The Love Project Research Event. (2019). Audience discussion following 'The Love Project' presentation by McCarthy et al. with My Life My Choice at The Love Project Research Event held at Mary Ward Conference Centre, Bloomsbury, London, 9 April.

Thompson, J., & Westwood, L. (2008). Person centred approaches to educating the learning disability workforce. In J. Thompson, J. Kilbane, & H. Sanderson (Eds.), *Person centred practice for professionals*. Maidenhead: McGraw Hill/Open University Press.

Tilley, E., Earle, S., Walmsley, J., et al. (2012). 'The silence is roaring': sterilization, reproductive rights and women with intellectual disabilities. *Disability and Society*, 27(3), 413–426.

Toney-Butler, T. J., & Unison-Pace, W. J. (2020). *Nursing admission assessment and examination*. Treasure Island, FL: StatPearls Publishing. Available at: https://www.ncbi.nlm.nih.gov/books/NBK493211/.

Turnpenny, A., & Marriot, A. (2019). *The right to a relationship: addressing the barriers that people with learning disabilities face in developing and sustaining intimate and sexual relationships*. Bath: National Development Team for Inclusion.

United Kingdom: Human Rights Act 1998 [United Kingdom of Great Britain and Northern Ireland], 9 November 1998. Available at: https://www.refworld.org/docid/3ae6b5a7a.html. [Accessed 19 January 2020].

University of Bristol. (2017). *Working Together with Parents Network (WTPN) update of the DoH/DfES good practice guidance on working with parents with a learning disability (2007)*.

United Nations. (2006). *United Nations Convention on the Rights of Persons with Disabilities*. New York: UN. Available at: https://www.un.org/disabilities/documents/convention/convention_accessible_pdf.pdf.

Vlaskamp, C. (2005). Interdisciplinary assessment of people with profound intellectual and multiple disabilities. In J. Hogg & A. Langa (Eds.), *Assessing adults with intellectual disabilities: a service provider's guide* (pp. 39–51). Oxford: Blackwell.

Wang, C., & Burris, M. A. (1997). Photovoice: concept, methodology, and use for participatory needs assessment. *Health Education and Behaviour*, 24(3), 369–387.

Ware, J. (1996). *Creating a responsive environment for people with profound and multiple learning disabilities*. London: David Fulton.

Welshman, J., & Walmsley, J. (Eds.). (2006). *Community care in perspective: care, control and citizenship.* Hampshire: Palgrave Macmillan.

Westherhof, G. J., Beernink, J., & Sools, A. (2016). Who am I? A life story intervention for persons with intellectual disability and psychiatric problems. *Intellectual and Developmental Disabilities, 53*(3), 173–186.

Wilder, J., & Granlund, M. (2003). Behavior style and interaction between seven children with multiple disabilities and their caregivers. *Child: Care, Health and Development, 29*(6), 559–567.

Williams, P. (1978). *Our mutual handicap.* London: CMH.

Williams, P. (2009). *Social work with people with learning difficulties.* Exeter: Learning Matters Ltd.

Williams, P., & Evans, M., (2013). *Social work with people with learning disabilities.* London: Sage.

Working Together with Parents Network, Norah Fry Centre for Disability Studies: Bristol. Available at: http://www.bristol.ac.uk/media. [Accessed 18 January 2020].

Xenitidis, K., Thornicroft, G., Leese, M., et al. (2000). Reliability and validity of the CANDID – a needs assessment instrument for adults with learning disabilities and mental health problems. *British Journal of Psychiatry* (176), 473–478.

Young, H., & Garrard, B. (2016). Bereavement and loss: developing a memory box to support a young woman with profound learning disabilities. *British Journal of Learning Disabilities, 44*(1), 78–84.

Inclusive communication

Karen Bunning and Susan Buell

KEY ISSUES

- Communication is not a solitary activity - it takes two to make it happen!
- Communication needs other people - for building meanings together.
- Communication does not happen in a vacuum – the context is integral to the whole process.
- Facilitating communication means building on existing strengths.

- Acceptance of a multi-dimensional view of communication is a good place to start - there are always alternatives to the spoken word!
- Inclusive communication is about an environment that places the least possible restrictions on the people present.

CHAPTER OUTLINE

INTRODUCTION

It is widely acknowledged that communication problems amongst the population with intellectual disabilities are common and multifarious (van der Meer et al, 2017). Since the causes of intellectual disabilities are wide-ranging, so communication difficulties vary (Addebuto et al, 2016). Reported difficulties may affect different aspects of the human communication architecture – an integrated system of: structure (the organisation of sounds in words: speech sounds, and the order of words in sentences: grammar); semantics (vocabulary and meanings); and pragmatics (social use of language covering communicative functions such as requesting information, stating a fact or acknowledging a prior utterance, discourse and conversation). Some individuals may have reasonable language skills but are unable to put their ideas into clear spoken messages due to problems with articulating sounds for speech and/or organising sounds in utterances. For others, the problem may originate in restricted language development resulting in a limited lexicon and/or the ability to process items in sequence, such that understanding and verbal expression are severely challenged. Whatever the particular problem, communication does not happen in isolation. It is part of a complex social process, whereby meanings are created, shared understanding established, views and ideas are exchanged and human connections are forged. This chapter will explore how we can improve social interaction with people with intellectual disabilities by adapting approaches and creating environments where communication can flourish. The reader is encouraged to engage in Activities, reflecting on personal experience, then use chapter content to apply to real-world relationships with people with intellectual disabilities, reflecting the individuality and uniqueness of particular situations.

WHAT IS COMMUNICATION?

There is no doubt about it, communication is a complex business. Take the example of a woman who enters a shoe shop at 5.25 pm. Having ignored the sign on the door that states in bold print – CLOSES AT 5.30pm, she approaches a nearby assistant and asks cheerfully if the shop is still open. The assistant replies quite politely in the affirmative. The woman on hearing the response apologises and leaves the shop rapidly. Now on the face of it, the exchange is all quite straightforward – the woman asks a question and the assistant provides her with an answer. On hearing that the shop is still open, the woman can set about the task in hand – finding a new pair of shoes, except she leaves. So what has gone on here? If we look more closely at the detail of the exchange, we notice the assistant looking fleetingly at her watch whilst answering the woman. Furthermore, we hear the tightness in her voice as she gives her 'yes' response. The 'tut' she utters is barely perceptible as she turns her head to look at her colleague, but if we listen closely, it is there. What are the messages being communicated here? The words suggest that the shop is open because there are 5 minutes to go until closing time. The detail communicates quite a different story. "Yes, the shop is still open, but I am not happy with your request. We are about to close." Suddenly realising her mistake, the woman stumbles her apology and flees in embarrassment vowing never to return to that particular shop. So we see that communication is much, much more than just spoken words as shown in Box 5.1.

So what does this tell us about communication? Firstly, it tells us that it is multi-faceted. It is not just about the exchange of messages through spoken words. For instance, the printed sign on the shop door informed the woman of the closing time. Then of course the tone of voice belies the words spoken by the assistant and conveys, instead, her annoyance at the late request to look at shoes. The way we utter words, the pitch, stress patterns, intonation – all add to the meaning being communicated and are termed para-linguistic phenomena. Non-verbal behaviours are also

 BOX 5.1   The different guises of communication

Here are just some of the different formats we use for communication every day:
- Speech - the strings of words we utter;
- Prosody - our use of intonation and volume, our use of pause, the rate at which we speak, e.g. high pitched and rapid speech denoting excitement, slow, languid delivery with a flat intonation revealing our tiredness;
- Vocal gestures – vocalisations, e.g. gasps to show amazement, screams indicating delight;
- Body gestures - often referred to as body language, e.g. a shake of the fist to convey inner emotional state, leaning forward showing attentiveness to a subject;
- Hand-arm gestures - that hold meaning within a culture, e.g. shaking a fist to convey anger, waving to denote departure;
- Text - the words that we and others write, e.g. in books, on street signs, on websites;
- Images – the pictorial images and symbols that capture a concept or meaning, e.g. the 'female' symbol on the toilet door indicating 'Ladies', the picture on the food packet denoting its contents.

integral to communication (Wharton, 2009). These are behaviours that either contribute to the speaker's overt meaning (the consciously intended message) or to more covert meanings, which may be emitted accidentally. The shop assistant's fleeting look at her watch and her final 'tut' and turn of the head provide evidence of her inner state and signal her displeased state thus we see that the actions and movements used by a person can bear meaning. For example, the person who stamps their foot in expression of anger; the person who grabs hold of a person's sleeve to attract their attention – these all have the potential to convey meaning. Now we see how the communication of the shop assistant is more than just words!

It takes two to communicate!

Communication is something that involves two or more individuals making contributions to a shared construction of meaning. There is usually the coordination of actions so that each person takes turns in the conversation but maintains an active role even when it is not their 'speaking' turn. That is, listening to and interpreting what the other person says and does are as important to the meaning as expressing your own ideas in a communication turn. Consideration of the phenomenon of ambiguity is key. Far from being categorically clear, meanings constructed in interaction are frequently unclear. This is because the intentions behind acts of communication do not map precisely onto the words. The shop assistant's words were probably driven by multiple intentions, not least of which might have been: 1. to perform the role of the courteous shop assistant who perhaps does not want to be reported to her manager; and 2. the shop assistant who does not want to delay getting away from work and therefore wants to let this 'nuisance' of a customer know. Of course, intentions may be conscious and deliberate, but they also may operate at a subconscious level. We just need to be aware that social communication is characterised by multiple intentions and more than one meaning.

All this corresponds very neatly to the inferential model (see Wilson and Sperber, 2012), which simply means that the act of interpreting a message is as important to the resultant meaning as the act of sending a message, therefore communication is achieved through *producing* and *interpreting* the evidence. This means that communication moves beyond two people sending code or words to each other. The meaning behind those words and the accompanying non-verbal behaviour are extracted for sense-making by the individuals taking part in the communication. Related to this is the continuous processing model proposed by Fogel (1993) which describes communication as two or more people working together and co-ordinating their actions in ongoing response to each other and the context (Bunning, 2009; Grove et al, 1999; Olsson, 2004). In this way two people influence the actions of one another: the shop assistant's communication sends the woman out of the shop vowing never to cross its threshold again, and perhaps the stumbling apology and hasty exit of the woman causes the assistant a moment of regret – or maybe not! Fogel's (1993) model offers an important way of thinking about communication with people with intellectual disabilities that implies a shared responsibility for building meanings together (see also Fogel and Garvey, 2007).

The onus for successful exchanges does not rest with just one person, but with the number of people involved in communication at any one time.

READER ACTIVITY 5.1

If communication is multi-faceted, can you think of all the different ways you are able to communicate? Once you have done that, think about a recent conversation you have had with a friend or work colleague, what were the different ways you communicated? What did you do when the other person was talking? How did you let the other person know that you were attending (actively listening) to what they were trying to say?

Making sense

Because for most of us, communication is immediate and spontaneous, we take for granted the way two communicators are able to follow a conversational thread and take their turns as the interaction progresses. The other person says something and we interpret the meaning, which triggers our response. However, many factors influence the way we act in social situations and how meanings are established (see Box 5.2). The person with whom we are communicating will affect our contributions to the conversation. The way we communicate with a close friend is markedly different to the way we communicate with our boss. Our relationship with and experience of the person colours our communicative style. For example, familiarity and closeness with a person enables us to pick up on the little nuances of conversation and shape our responses accordingly. After all, the communication between partners of many years standing will be in marked contrast to the same two people out on a first date! The context in which the communication takes place also plays its part. The degree of informality, the purpose of the context, e.g. workplace, home, classroom; the attributes of the setting, e.g. using a loud voice to make ourselves heard in a noisy environment, using hushed tones in a quiet environment such as a library.

As we have seen, and to repeat our earlier mantra – communication is much more than just words. At this stage it is probably a good idea to put this into some kind of framework. Bronfenbrenner (1979, 2005) proposed a

BOX 5.2   Situational factors affecting communication

- Knowledge and experience each person has of the other.
- Cultural identity and personal values.
- Relationship between the two people whether intimate and highly familiar or else formal and distant.
- Attributes of the physical setting, e.g. ambient noise level, luminescence.
- Purpose of communication, e.g. formal job interview, gossip between two friends.

 READER ACTIVITY 5.2

There are a number of factors that are critical to communication: the individual – the skills and experiences; the other people – your knowledge and experience of them, the relationship you share; the context – the different settings in which you encounter the various people in your life, the purpose of those settings and your role. Now take a blank piece of paper and draw 4 large circles, one inside the other (see Figure 5.1). Write your name inside the circle at the centre. Next reflect on the people with whom you communicate on a daily basis. Write them down in the outer circle. Next, identify the different places or settings where communication happens for you. Finally, tackle the outer circle. What are the key political, social and cultural influences on the communication activities represented in the inner circles? Think about your work, your home life and your leisure outlets. Do the same for someone with an intellectual disability whom you know or have worked with. How do the circles compare?

model to describe human development and functioning in context. Conceived as a series of nested circles which define the different systems in human ecology, the individual is placed at the centre. From here it moves outwards to the immediate and familiar contexts in the person's life, to community settings and finally society. A simplified version of this defines the communication context in three concentric circles around the Individual (1) (source: Bunning, 2004; Bunning and Grove, 2002) – see Figure 5.1. The circle that immediately surrounds the individual is called Communication Partnership (2). It comprises the range of communication partners with whom the individual engages on a daily basis. This may include parents, keyworkers, friends and teachers. The next circle is termed the Communication Environment (3), which represents the various settings in which the individual works, plays and socialises with the communication partners, e.g. the classroom in school, the home, the social club and the local shop. Beyond these inner circles is the Social, Cultural and Political Context (4), where social, political and cultural aspects are represented. This includes government legislation and social policy, which exert influence over the inner two circles.

Finally, what do we find to communicate about? Human beings communicate about a multitude of things and for a variety of reasons. We communicate meanings and exchange information; we make propositions and tell jokes; we share our thoughts and ideas; we express our beliefs and inner emotions; we evince attitudes and report facts (Wilson and Sperber, 2012). We assert our views, make requests, give instructions, accept some things and reject others; access goods and services – the list goes on!

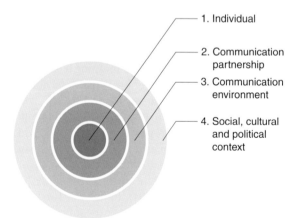

1. Individual
2. Communication partnership
3. Communication environment
4. Social, cultural and political context

Figure 5.1 Communication Ecology

CHALLENGES IN EVERYDAY COMMUNICATION

Having a communication difficulty frequently leads to a breakdown in the ability to exchange information and to engage in social interaction. This may take the form of impaired verbal comprehension (understanding language), difficulties in formulating utterances or speech sounds, or challenges in working out how to use communication skills in different contexts with a range of other people. It also means that opportunities for self-expression and self-determination are likely to be fewer and far between (Bradshaw, 2002; Bunning and Grove, 2002). There are many reasons why this should be the case: person-centred factors interact with factors that are external to the individual – located in the environment (Bunning, 2004). A summary of these factors is provided in Box 5.3.

Communication breakdown

CASE ILLUSTRATION 5.1

Abdullah has a lot to say for himself and shows a great deal of interest in the people around him. He has had a great weekend - he met his sister's new baby for the first time. On Monday morning he greets his tutor at college enthusiastically and starts to tell him about his news. Abdullah's speech is difficult to understand – many of the speech sounds are produced incorrectly. This makes it difficult for the listener to decipher what he is saying. The tutor, who is sorting out the day's work, gives Abdullah only half attention, makes some placatory noises and walks over to some other students. The communication is over and Abdullah's news is unshared and his real competence, i.e. the ability to report an event, remains hidden.

Living with a communication difficulty means that problems with influencing change in your immediate environment and affecting the actions of others happen all too often (Bunning, 2004). Social connections as part of routine interactions are frequently hard-won and misunderstandings crop up frequently. The trouble starts with the unequal share of communication skills in many communication partnerships (Bunning, 2004). Critical differences in the communication skills of the person with an intellectual disability and the people who provide support, e.g.

BOX 5.3   Factors that challenge everyday communication

Person-centred factors
- Compromised or limited communication skills that make it difficult to express ideas and to influence the environment;
- Personal reluctance to challenge those in a position of power because of a fear of failure;
- A lack of confidence in own abilities;
- Individual experience of communication difficulties triggering emotional reactions that protect or sustain self, such as extreme passivity and apathy, defensiveness or aggression.

Factors external to the person:
- A predominantly verbal environment that proves inaccessible to the individual;
- Being placed within a 'carer – being cared for' relationship that nurtures dependence and compromises individual autonomy;
- Limited or inappropriate opportunities to use available skills;
- A lack of sensitivity to the subtle ways an individual may communicate, e.g. eye gaze, vocalisation, facial expression.

carers, teachers, support staff, may lead to an imbalance in what Kagan (1998) refers to as the communication equation. On one side of the equation is the person who is cognitively able and equipped with a full set of linguistic skills for making contributions to the interaction; on the other is the person with an intellectual disability who may have delayed development or restricted cognitive functioning, and impaired communication skills. The chance of something going wrong in an interaction is quite likely. Box 5.4 summarises the chain reaction that occurs when communication breaks down.

For Reader activity 5.3, see online resource.

ADDRESSING COMMUNICATION DIFFICULTIES

So where do we begin to address the problem of living with communication difficulty? The first principle must always be to build on the inherent strengths of the individual. No matter the severity of the

BOX 5.4   Chain reaction of communication breakdown

What happens when communication does not succeed? Using Case Illustration 5.1 of Abdullah we can see a chain reaction where there has been:-

- A struggle to express ideas or to understand what is being communicated, which may lead to.....
- Failure to construct meaning so that communication breaks down, which may lead to.....
- Feelings of disempowerment, where the person with a communication difficulty does not participate, which may lead to......
- Feelings of self-doubt and frustration, which may lead to.......
- Inappropriate ways of responding, withdrawal or problem behaviour, which may result in.....
- Social isolation and exclusion.

(Adapted from Bunning, 2004; Bunning and Grove, 2002)

intellectual disability or the extent of the communication problem, there is always a level at which the individual may connect with the people in the immediate environment, whether it is via fleeting eye gaze, vocalisation, gesture, words or other non-verbal behaviour. We need to respond at whatever level the individual is functioning. It is about optimising communicative potential.

CASE ILLUSTRATION 5.2

Jacqueline is 9 years old with severe to profound and multiple intellectual disabilities. She uses a specialised seating system and is dependent on others for her day to day care. She is able to use her left arm to reach and grab for items. Jacqueline is blind in her right eye but retains some vision in her upper left field of vision. Her hearing is unimpaired. Her teacher has told us that she looks at coloured pictures and objects held in her left field of vision – she smiles, vocalises and jerks her body. She vocalises – using back vowels such as 'ah', mainly making a 'happy' sound and a 'cross' sound. All these things represent starting points with Jacqueline.

Adapting our communication

The art of pitching our communication to the perceived level of the person with an intellectual disability is easier said than done! There are two main types of communication error that may occur in a communication partnership (Bunning, 2004). The first error type involves failure on behalf of the partner to recognise the language and communication skills of the person. This is depicted as a 'cycle of devaluation' in Figure 5.2. In Case Illustration 5.2 this would be paramount to not recognising the discriminating nature of Jacqueline's vocal behaviour and the different meanings they convey. This act of masking the person's competence will limit opportunities for social participation, inclusion and personal development. The second error type is attributing skills and competencies to the person that they do not possess. By inflating an individual's communicative competencies and simultaneously making no adjustments to how communication happens, the partner may literally talk 'over the head' of the person, using vocabulary and linguistic structures that cannot be processed. Similar to error type 1, the person's ability to participate is curtailed by the provision of an inaccessible opportunity for social interaction. The risks associated with these two error-types are defined in two interlocking cycles: (1) 'inflation or over-estimation' of the person's communication skills and (2) the reverse of this, the 'devaluation or under-estimation'. These are illustrated in Figure 5.2 (adapted source: Bunning, 2004, p. 167). The risk of cycle (1) is that the true needs of the person may be overlooked, essential adaptations to communication neglected and expectations of the individual too high, leading to negative or diminished experiences with a corresponding weakening of self-esteem, e.g. the person experiences failure in communication too often. The risk of cycle (2) is that the true competencies of the person may go unnoticed and expectations pitched at too low a level, again leading to a negative or diminished experience that is disempowering to the individual; thus we see the importance of striving for a pitch of communication with which the person can both engage and respond.

Consideration of how to communicate with Jacqueline in Case Illustration 5.2 highlights the risks associated with the two cycles depicted in Figure 5.2. If her communication partners think that she has full understanding of language and make no attempt to adapt their communication to suit Jacqueline's needs,

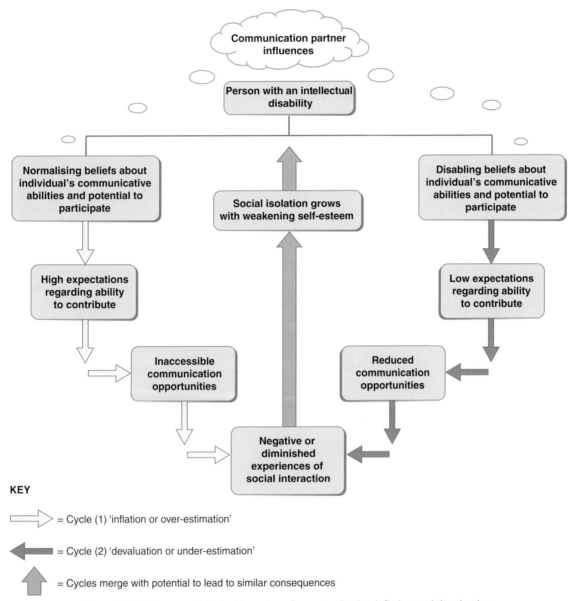

Figure 5.2 Risks associated with cycles of communication inflation and devaluation

there is no opening for Jacqueline to use her skills. The opportunity is inaccessible and her ability to self-determine is overlooked. This is Cycle (1). Conversely, if her communication partners believe that she has no ability to convey her pleasure or disapproval, they will make all decisions without recourse to Jacqueline. There is the failure to tune-in and recognise Jacqueline's own ways of communicating. This is Cycle (2) thus in both cycles Jacqueline is excluded from determining

the things that matter to her and she is prevented from affecting change in her environment.

INCLUSIVE COMMUNICATION

Inclusive communication provides the counterpoint to exclusion due to communication difficulties impacting on expressive and receptive capabilities. If inclusion in education translates as learning in the *least restrictive environment* (Millar, 2003) so inclusive communication must imply an environment free of constraints. This is an interesting proposition as it places the onus on environmental adaptation, which includes the contributions made by the communication partner(s). It is the person with a full set of skills who has the opportunity to promote, or else cast in doubt, the abilities of the person by virtue of their own communicative behaviour (Kagan, 1998); thus an individual's difficulties with communication are not seen as deriving solely from the primary cognitive deficit but rather as by-products of the interactional process (Nind et al, 2001). Far from being static the competencies that each person brings to a partnership are underpinned by 'a relative and dynamic interpersonal construct' (Light, 1989, p. 137) whereby the contributions of one will affect the other and vice versa thus the available skillset of the communication partner needs to be considered.

The skillset of the communication partner is therefore a major consideration for facilitating the communication of people with intellectual disabilities. It would appear that direct support staff are not always prepared sufficiently to provide skilful communication support for the wide range of individual needs they encounter in their work (see Bradshaw, 2002; McConkey et al, 1999). Disparities in the communication process have been observed between staff and individuals with borderline-mild intellectual disabilities, affecting synchrony of verbal and non-verbal aspects (Reuzel et al, 2013a) and turn-taking by staff. Staff tended to use question forms and there was neglect of some spontaneous contributions by service users (Reuzel et al, 2013b). Dalton and Sweeney (2013) found that staff understood the importance of good communicative support to improved quality of life, whilst also recognising deficiencies in their own knowledge and the scarcity of specific resources. Nevertheless, technical knowledge is not sufficient to alter practice (Healey and Noonan Walsh, 2007) and classroom-based learning does not translate automatically into everyday use (Chadwick and Jolliffe 2009). A systematic review of training initiatives delivered to support staff concluded that programmes incorporating opportunities for trying out communication strategies and for receiving feedback on progress were associated with positive outcomes for service users (van der Meer et al, 2017). Thus, it would seem logical that any attempt to improve the social experiences of people with particular communication needs necessitates intervening at the level of the communication partnership in practice.

Augmentative and alternative communication

Human communication is multi-modal. For language reception, this means processing all the available sensory signals that carry meaning, e.g. facial expression, hand gestures, tone of voice. For language expression, this means using a variety of media and behaviours to convey your messages. Where there are significant problems with understanding or expression, a more deliberate approach to language support may be indicated. Augmentative and alternative communication (AAC) offers a wide range of approaches, techniques and tactics for supporting communication (Beukelman and Mirenda, 2013). The main purpose is to bring about tangible benefits to the person's communication through the deliberate use of different ways of representing meaning. AAC is an area of practice whereby 'an individual can supplement or replace spoken communication.' (Royal College of Speech & Language Therapists, 2006, p. 230). Von Tetzchner and Martinsen (2000) identified the different groups of people who may benefit from some form of AAC:

- Augmented group: those who understand and use spoken language but need a system as a back-up.
- Expressive group: those who have good understanding of spoken language but need the system for expression.
- Receptive group: those who need a system to understand as well as to express themselves.

So what are the choices in terms of AAC (see Figure 5.3)? Briefly, the options fall into one or other of two camps: unaided communication and aided communication. Unaided describes typical face to face communication where the interactants or the people who are generating utterances use the characteristics of natural communication, e.g. speech, manual sign, facial expressions and eye gaze. Aided on the other hand includes all types of communication where the linguistic "utterances" (letters, words/graphic symbols, objects) have to be selected from a display e.g. communication boards, books, electronic aids, sets of objects.

Unaided options: signing

Signs have been used with people with communication impairments for around 30 years, beginning in the 1960s in the USA and the UK (Cornforth et al, 1974). Different

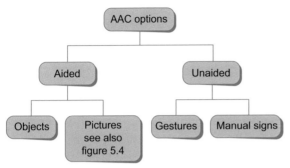

Figure 5.3 Main options for AAC

from the sign languages of Deaf communities, the use of signs with the population with intellectual disabilities provides a compensatory strategy to support deficiencies in communication, e.g. verbal comprehension difficulties, expressive language limitations. The signs themselves are usually taken from sign languages and paired with spoken language thus signing becomes not a replacement for speech but a support. Signing therefore follows the grammatical structure of the spoken language, often known as key word signing where important information carrying words are signed. You can use one sign or several to support the meanings being communicated. Take the sentence 'What do you want for dinner?' There are a number of options for supporting the key meanings being communicated which are based on what we know about the communication needs of the person in front of us. In the Case Illustrations below, the signed supported words are underlined.

 CASE ILLUSTRATION 5.3

Jadine understands one piece of information at a time. Her attention for speech is fleeting but she responds well to facial expression and body language. Her mother asks Jadine: 'What do you want for <u>dinner?</u>' signing <u>dinner</u> in a slow and emphatic way lasting for the length of the spoken utterance.

CASE ILLUSTRATION 5.4

Alexis is able to understand two key pieces of information in an utterance. His carers are trying to get him to use his language to respond to questions asked of him. His carer asks him: '<u>What</u> do you want for <u>dinner?</u>'

CASE ILLUSTRATION 5.5

Nehemiah understands most of what is said to him when key word signing is used. When he attempts to speak himself, it is very difficult for others to understand what he is saying. The main people who communicate with him at school and at home are trying to encourage him to use signing by exposing him to sign support in his environment. They ask him: '<u>What</u> do <u>you want</u> for <u>dinner?</u>'

In the UK two main signing approaches are used:
1. **Makaton** is a vocabulary developed in the early 1970s (see Grove and Walker, 1990). It loosely follows the lines of typical vocabulary acquisition in stages. Used internationally, it draws on the lexicon of the indigenous sign language, e.g. British Sign Language (BSL) in the UK; American Sign Language in the USA. Signs are selected from the range of alternatives available with some consideration given to ease of production e.g. the sign for 'look' is used for both 'look' and 'see'; 'fish' is made with a flat hand in neutral space, rather than being specifically located at chin level with separated fingers as it might be in BSL. There is a core vocabulary of around 350 signs arranged in stages of around 35 signs per stage, starting with those that are highly functional for both the person with an intellectual disability and the teacher. Progression of concepts is evident across the stages as more abstract concepts such as vocabulary associated with time e.g. yesterday, before, next are taught in the later stages. Additional resources are available as a series of topic-based vocabulary sets e.g. sexuality; emotions and relationships; early attainment targets of the National Curriculum; fire and its hazards (The Makaton Charity, 2020).
2. **Signalong** is an extended lexicon which also uses signs from BSL in a broad developmental sequence. Similar to Makaton, it also follows spoken word order. Signalong content is organised according to major topics and themes, 'providing vocabulary for life and learning.' (Signalong – The Communication Charity, 2020).

Use of a manual modality such as sign brings a number of processing advantages. Signing to children can help to disambiguate words and meanings receptively (Loncke et al, 2006). Compared to articulating a string of sounds to represent a spoken word, the physical demands of producing a manual sign are less. Indeed the meaning of the sign appears to be more important to functional usage rather than the distinctive features of the sign itself (Meuris et al, 2014). There are also temporal processing advantages that are helpful to individuals with intellectual disabilities. For example, if we speak a word it disappears almost in the instant that it leaves our lips. Signs and gestures however are produced more slowly allowing for a longer processing time. Furthermore, a sign can be held in space as a model for the other person acquiring a sign. This makes it highly suited to the needs of some individuals with intellectual disabilities. The visuo-spatial structure of signs provides greater opportunity to forge links between the symbol and what it represents. For example, the sign for 'drink' mimics the action of having a drink. There is a correspondence or similarity between the sign and the real life meaning. This is what we call 'iconicity', which is the opposite of arbitrariness where the link between sign and meaning is much more random. Iconicity can make a difference to initial learning – iconic signs are learned more quickly than arbitrary signs by individuals with intellectual disabilities in structured teaching contexts (see Loncke in Grove and Launonen, 2019). Children with Down syndrome quite naturally appear to use more gestural communication than their typically developing peers (Dimitrova et al, 2016).

Regardless of the approach to signing selected, the setting needs to actively support its usage. Various studies have reported a positive association between staff use of signing and the sign usage of people with intellectual disabilities (Grove and McDougall, 1991; Rambouts et al, 2017). Furthermore, staff omitting to use manual signs has been found to have a detrimental effect on the use of signing by service users in prescribed activities (Rambouts et al, 2018). However, the question of how to upskill staff in signing remains. Whilst Chadwick and Jolliffe (2009) reported positive effects of a staff training programme on signing with improved accuracy of signing as one of the outcomes, the transfer of learning from classroom to the natural communication environment was reportedly limited. Box 5.5 provides some brief guidance for creating the optimum sign-friendly environment.

Box 5.6 summarises some key features of positive communication that support social opportunities for optimal communication.

BOX 5.5 Tips for a positive signing environment

- Regular training for all workers who communicate – even after initial training, it is important to maintain your skills!
- Prioritise the use of signs in the environment – make a deliberate effort to use signing with other staff members as well as the people who need it.
- Make sure that the Head of the service is trained as effectively as the frontline staff.
- Enhance the environment so that it reminds people to use signing, e.g. introduce a new, topical sign each week, display line drawings of signs as aide memoires.
- Capitalise on the main events that happen in a setting and make a deliberate effort to include signing, e.g. person-centred planning meetings, school assembly, self-advocacy meetings.
- Train and employ peer tutors who can help to take signing forward in the setting.

BOX 5.6 Principles of a positive communication environment

Van der Gaag (1998) identified a number of core principles considered critical to establishing a positive communication environment:

(a) The communication needs of the individual are at the heart of all practice;

(b) The involvement of significant others in the individual's environment is critical;

(c) The focus is on partnership communication and therefore considers not only communication skills use of service users but also that of significant others;

(d) The remit of speech & language therapists includes assessment of and planning to meet communication needs whilst also encouraging others to have a share in communication;

(e) There is managerial commitment to developments in practice.

Aided communication: objects and images

Aided communication includes those methods where a real-world object is introduced to the person for the purposes of communication. It involves the use of graphic symbols, objects or pictures and written characters set

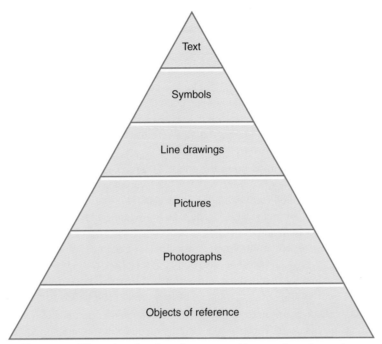

Figure 5.4 Hierarchy of options for representing words and meanings

within a communication board, book or technological device including speech-generating devices (von Tetzchner and Basil, 2011). Context, the attitudes of other people, and the immediate availability of support, are considered to be critical to the functional success of aided communication (Moorcroft et al, 2019). A case series in a rural part of Kenya utilised local resources to ensure cultural meaning and relevance to aided communication (Bunning et al, 2014).

There are many options for graphic representations in aided communication which are dependent on the understanding of the individual user and their preferences. Figure 5.4 summarises the hierarchy of aided communication options. Drawn as a pyramid, the options at the base represent the easiest progressing through to more sophisticated alternatives towards the top.

Objects of Reference

Starting at the base of the pyramid, objects of reference involves the use of 'objects' to stand for categories of events and things. Just as signs are used to represent meanings, so it is with everyday objects. Objects are selected that provide strong associations with

particular events. Unlike spoken or signed communications which do not hang about in the air once they have been delivered, objects are both permanent and open to manipulation presenting lower demands on cognitive abilities, memory and vision. They require only simple motor responses and can be represented at a number of different levels according to the presenting needs of the person (see Park, 1995, 1997, 2002). Table 5.1 provides a summary of the categorisation of the objects of reference by different levels of representation

Graphic symbols

A cornucopia of symbol sets is available in computer software that variously use photographs, pictures, line drawings and symbols and includes Picture Communication Symbols (PCS: Boardmaker, 2020), Makaton Symbols (The Makaton Charity, 2020) and Photosymbols (Photosymbols, 2020). The range of options is reflected in other parts of the world that use advanced learning technologies. As well as being used for communication boards and books, symbols and images from these programmes can be used for creating written work along the lines of a specially adapted word

TABLE 5.1	Objects of reference: different levels of representation
Level	**Examples**
Real objects used in activity – sometimes referred to as 'index' objects.	Fazil is being alerted by his teacher to the fact that it is time to go to the domestic science room at school for the cookery lesson. He has an object box in the classroom that contains a selection of key objects for use in different lessons. The teacher takes out a wooden spoon and gives it to Fazil to represent the shift in activity. He takes the spoon to the lesson and uses it when he is stirring the soup.
Objects not used in activity: Identical objects not used in activity Non-identical objects not used in the activity	Sarah wants to go to the shop to buy a magazine. She gives a small purse containing a few coins to her keyworker who understands that a shopping trip has been requested. He gives Sarah her bag containing the real purse money for her excursion. It is identical to the purse Sarah used to communicate her wish to go shopping. Esme also wants to go shopping. Her object of reference is a green material purse with a zip fastener. The actual purse she uses is a wallet style purse made of red leather that fastens with a popper. Despite these differences, Esme understands that they both symbolise money, which she needs to buy the things she wants.
Associated/partial objects with some corresponding features to real life object	Darren wants to have a bath. He uses a small square of towel to indicate this to his carer. This is a more subtle object of reference, i.e. an item with features (the fabric) relating to the real life object of his bath towel.
Miniature objects providing a smaller and more portable representation of real life object.	Frances is going on a bus trip into town with his parents. He loves going on the bus and will frequently point to the red buses that go down his street. His father shows him a toy double decker bus to let him know what they are going to do.
Abstract objects	The big timetable displayed on the wall of Jason's classroom displays all the different lessons for each week day. Objects are attached by fabric hook and loop fastener (e.g. Velcro) and the teacher directs Jason to pull off the silver whistle, which he loves to blow when he is outside doing gardening. The whistle has nothing to do with the actual activity but there is an association for Jason.

processing package. Change (2016a) have coproduced their own composite line drawings for rendering accessible information, commonly used by self-advocacy organisations.

The question of what to use is dependent on the developmental and cognitive level of the individual, their language ability, sensory issues (for example vision) and any physical issues. Ultimately, it is a question of trying out the different representations with the individual and noting their responses. No matter what type of image used, it is important to check for pre-requisite skills in the areas of:

- attention to pattern (figure-ground discrimination);
- recognition of representational status of pattern;
- recognition of specific meaning.

Questions to ask yourself are: Can this person select a picture when it is named? What about labelling the picture? Can they match object to object and object to picture? What might this mean for day to day communication?

Picture, symbol and photo communication forms are used for a number of purposes including to support language development and literacy skills; to represent meanings in a communication book or board; to facilitate access to information; to support the advocacy process. This can make for a somewhat confusing picture across the lifespan of an individual. For example, PCS tend to be used by speech and language therapists, schools frequently opt for Rebus and adult services, particularly self-advocates use Photosymbols. In low-income settings, access to digitally-generated symbol sets presents challenges. Limited finances and material resources, combined with a lack of power supply in the home affect access. The question of cross-cultural applicability has informed research in South Africa, in particular regarding readability of graphic symbols (Basson and Alant, 2005; Bornman et al, 2009). Some local initiatives have been piloted using photographic images and cultural drawings. For example, Cameron and Markowicz (2013) reported on the development of a communication board for a child in Tanzania, and Crowley and Baigorri (2012) described the development of picture cards for use in the market to support functional communication among young people with intellectual disabilities.

 READER ACTIVITY 5.4

There is an excellent resource entitled *Augmentative Communication in Practice: An Introduction* (Wilson, 1998) available as a free download from the Call Centre at: https://www.callscotland.org.uk/downloads/books/augmentative-communication-in-practice-an-introduction/. Go to pages 19-26.

  What are the key differences among PCS, Rebus, Makaton and Bliss?

  Which symbols are most useful to the people you work with and why?

  Which symbols would present the greatest challenges for people with intellectual disabilities and why?

Communication books and boards

For some people for whom the physical demands of talking are too much, communication through images offers an appropriate alternative. Photographs, pictures and symbols alongside text may be combined to provide the individual with a tailor-made alternative means of communicating their needs, feelings and ideas. The construction of a book or board is achieved through consideration of the layout of images and words (how the display will work in terms of arrangement of pictures on a page and arrangement of pages); the representations to be used (what combination of photographs, symbols, pictures and words); the organisation of content (will it be topic based or linguistic-based?). Various resources are available to support developments in this work, e.g. the Ace Centre, Oxford, UK has produced some practical guidance (Ace Centre, 2020).

Accessible information

Low levels of literacy amongst people with intellectual disabilities means that access to information in text is problematic for many (Morgan et al, 2011). Strategies for circumventing some of the complexities of printed matter have been devised by Mencap (2009). Similar guidelines have also been produced by the European Commission (Freyoff et al, 1998), Inclusion Europe (2020) and Change (2016b). Suggested strategies include covering only one idea per sentence, use of active rather than passive verbs, use of bullet points and avoidance of abstract concepts. The business of producing this kind of material ('easy to read' documentation) is growing steadily and is being used by policy makers and health and social care organisations alike. Inclusion Europe provides a checklist for reviewing Easy Read material and a training programme on how to write accessible texts. Further afield, the South Australian Government (2020) provides an *Online accessibility toolkit*. Countries hosting easy read developments usually display a number of policy documents that have been rendered as 'easy to read' following adherence to published guidelines, e.g. *Willing to Work* (Australian Human Rights Commission, 2016). Accessible information about health is also available in formats that are advertised as eye-catching, use simple words and have photos, symbols and pictures (see Easy Health, 2020) and an 'easy read' version of The World Report on Disability can be accessed on the World Health Organisation website (WHO, 2011). Developments in this area by Mencap and other similar organisations are to be welcomed; however, the best test of accessibility is whether or not it gets a clear response from the person thereby indicating their understanding. It is very often the case that simplifying the linguistic content and altering and enhancing the visual presentation of information is not enough in itself (Buell et al, 2019; Hurtado et al, 2014). Access to meanings in any text need to be supported by significant others who are familiar enough with the reader and the topic to provide relevant explanations contingent on the person's unique literacy and language skillset. There might be occasions when a document with only pictures and no words (for example, Beyond Words®) would be easier for a person with intellectual disabilities to understand. With such books, there is no requirement for reading ability although conveying relevant meaning relies on consistent and reliable explanations from a conversation partner.

Talking Mats

There are occasions where some form of support is needed to enable individuals to express their opinions and make decisions about lifestyle issues. Talking Mats is '…an interactive resource that uses three sets of picture symbols – topics, options and a visual scale' (Murphy and Cameron, 2002, p. 8). It was developed so that people using some form of alternative communication system were able to express their internal judgements and feelings. It involves an ordinary carpet mat, which is typically used on a table top, upon which graphic symbols are placed. On the back of each picture symbol is the hook side of a material fastener (e.g. Velcro®) so that it adheres to the mat when placed. Talking Mats provide support for many different activities, including joint goal planning, planning communication passports, self-perception of intervention outcomes, developing relationships with others and planning activities. The views expressed range from a personal evaluation of activity preferences to feelings about different forms of transport and life course aspirations, e.g. choice of occupation after leaving college, etc. Any one topic explored within a *mat* may be looked at in more detail. These are called *sub mats*. The use of a video camera is recommended to record the views expressed by the individual and to monitor the veracity of the process. A still photographic image provides a permanent record of each completed 'Talking Mat' for feedback to the individual and their significant others. In a scoping review, Stans et al (2019) concluded that Talking Mats provided a useful framework to facilitate conversation between professionals and people with communication difficulties.

Narrative approaches

The ability to share personal narratives and to recount personal experiences with the people that matter in your life is important to the development of social identity and the formation of relationships (Grove and Harwood, 2013; Reese et al, 2010a, b; Soto et al, 2007). By telling our personal stories we invite other people to engage in our experiences and views of the world (Waller, 2006). However, recalling personal experiences is particularly challenging for people with communication difficulties associated with intellectual disabilities. Their narratives tend to lack coherence and are characterised by: restricted use of vocabulary (Scott and Windsor, 2000); limited sequencing and knowledge of how to share a story with others (Soto et al, 2007); absent marking of

relationship between characters with poor ordering of events in time (Grove and Tucker, 2003).

Interest in the development of narrative approaches for individuals with more restricted communication skills has developed over the last decade. Multi-sensory storytelling (MSST) draws on the work of Park (2001; 1998), who developed a multi-sensory approach to drama and Fuller (2013) who created 'Bag Books'. It involves the use of objects and sensory stimuli associated with a focal event or sequence of events thereby diminishing dependence on text and words. The idea is to support social engagement by presenting selected stimuli that may be accessed and appreciated by the individual, although variations in the use of such books have been reported (ten Brug et al, 2012). Young et al (2011) reported improved coping with sensitive issues such as visiting the dentist, understanding epilepsy and masturbation through use of MSST. However, development of staff skills in achieving more attuned interactions with people with intellectual disabilities has been a shared concern. Penne et al (2012) concluded there was a need for specific staff training in how to achieve higher quality interactions during narrative activities. Storysharing® (2020) is an approach to narrative which aims to enable children and adults with severe communication difficulties to recall and share narratives of personal experience. Rather than developing a perfect, well-formed narrative, the emphasis is on developing participation in the act of narrating. The approach employs a range of scaffolding strategies to support narrative development such that even the person with the most complex communication needs may participate in the retelling of his or her own story (see Grove and Harwood, 2013). Positive gains in interactional discourse and in the completeness of the narrative have been found (Bunning et al, 2016), with reports of teachers assimilating the approach into the educational curriculum more broadly (Bunning et al, 2018).

Early stage communication

There are some individuals with severe-profound and multiple intellectual disabilities (S-PMID) whose communication is characterised by subtle or minor body behaviours, e.g. eye gaze, body language, facial expression and vocalisation, which may not be immediately recognisable by others (Grove et al, 1999, 2001); this is in addition to levels of alertness and activity change within short periods of time. Difficulties in signalling affective states and intentions are compounded by idiosyncratic behaviour patterns that lack the salience to convey communicative intentionality.

A number of tools have been produced to help us make sense of communication with people who are functioning at the earliest stages of communication development (see also Goldbart and Caton, 2010).

- *The Affective Communication Assessment* (see Coupe and Goldbart, 1998) provides a structure for exploring the responding behaviours and sensory preferences of individuals. The individual is presented with a range of individualised sensory stimuli which have previously been identified in discussion with significant others. The person's responses are noted on an Observation Recording Sheet together with an interpretation of what they mean.
- *The Early Communication Assessment (ECA)* (Coupe and Goldbart, 1998) utilises 'communicative landmarks' (p. 59) rather than an exhaustive list of communicative behaviours in checklist format. The ECA provides a format for capturing information about an individual against an early communication framework with the joint purpose of keying significant others into the individual's communicative level(s) as indicated by their observed behaviours whilst also highlighting the starting point for establishing communication with the person.
- *The Manchester Pragmatics Profile* (Coupe and Goldbart, 1998) is concerned with the social and functional behaviours that are critical to communication. It is a structured format for recording 'evidence of skills in communicative intentions, social organisation and presupposition' (p. 93). The idea is to reveal information about successes and difficulties, communication partners and contexts, and relevant factors affecting the individual's performance e.g. time of day before developing an intervention that focuses on the individual, communication partners and context.
- *See What I Mean* (Grove et al, 2000) is a set of guidelines designed to help significant others question, check out or validate accuracy of meanings ascribed to an individual's communication. Its starting point is that uncertainty and ambiguity are a part of everyday communication and therefore the intuitive skills that are used by communication partners should form one thread of the assessment. It comprises a series of steps whereby evidence from the individual's

behaviour is gathered to support the different interpretations so that the most likely meaning may be identified.

Mencap conducted a three-year project in partnership with the British Institute for Learning Disabilities (BILD) exploring ways of involving people with S-PMID in decision-making and consultation. They have published practical guidance on using creative strategies to support communication (Mencap, 2011), understand preferences and involve people in everyday events.

Profiling an individual's communication strengths and support needs

Communication passports

A communication passport is a personalised catalogue of information about an individual's communication that is presented in a variety of formats, designed to be accessible and easy to follow. The point of a Communication Passport is to capture the unique and sometimes subtle or idiosyncratic ways an individual communicates and represent this profile to the people who matter to the individual, e.g. carers, teachers, support staff, health practitioner, etc. They can be used to navigate particular junction points in a person's life, e.g. transition from primary to secondary education or just moving from one class to another; or to facilitate communication in a variety of community settings, e.g. a visit to the local medical practice.

Millar (2003) warns that a comprehensive Communication Passport entails a lot of hard work and considered preparation. However, she also points out that the very act of compiling a passport can be an 'enriching process and learning experience' (p. 6) because it brings significant others together around the individual encouraging information pooling and experience sharing. Communication Passports are very often small, portable booklets but can be almost any format that is accessible and meaningful to those involved. They can be wallet-sized cards, wall displays and table mats, videos and other more technical forms of rich and multiple media.

New media

Digital video, still photography, sound, graphics and text have been used to construct multimedia profiles for people with intellectual disabilities. Personal life experiences are stored in the form of video clips, e.g. preferred activities, still life images, e.g. favourite possessions on a computer for access in planning and review meetings (see also Chapter 4). They help to convey the personal agenda of the person with severe-profound intellectual disabilities and complex needs, e.g. physical and sensory impairments. In the UK the Rix Centre has developed Wiki software for use by young people with intellectual disabilities (RIX Research & Media, 2020a). Rich and multiple media are deployed to present information *About Me* in an engaging platform. Video, pictures, sound and words are used in the Wikis enabling the individual to share their stories, communicate their preferences and goals with the key people in their life (see Chapter 4 for further information about the use of Wiki software).

The development of new technologies and applications of rich and multiple media occupy a place in the inclusion debate and in addressing societal marginalisation to which people with intellectual disabilities may be vulnerable. The defining contribution lies in the forging of links between images and meanings, past and present, school and home, so that the need for conventional linguistic exchange is obviated (Bunning et al, 2009). The Rix Centre's mission of 'innovation in learning disability' embraces developments in new media for the enablement and self-advocacy of children and adults with intellectual disabilities (RIX Research & Media, 2020b). They are engaged in action-based research in the development and application of new media technologies with this population.

Total Communication

Total Communication (TC) is just one area that has given rise to service developments across the UK. Total Communication initiatives typically involve multiple agencies and some form of instruction and skills transference to support staff, as well as the development of practical resources to facilitate multi-modal communication (Bradshaw, 2000). Despite the magnitude of service activity in this area, evaluation has been largely restricted to internal audit and interview with service users (see Jones, 2000). Areas of concern include variable compliance rates amongst staff and limited address of individuals who are at the earliest stages of communication development (Jones, 2000). Jones further comments that in spite of the training, staff continued to make errors in the judgement of verbal comprehension. Venditozzi et al (2010) reported on increased knowledge scores of staff participants attending training courses on Total Communication. They state that "referrals are now more specific and the expectations of intervention are more realistic" (p. 24) as an indirect effect of the work. However, such evaluations fall short of any direct measurements of staff-service user communication in the natural environment.

CONCLUSION

So where does all this leave the establishment of a positive and responsive communication environment? The participation of people with intellectual disabilities at every level of society is relevant across the globe (see Imms and Green, 2020), but where does communication come in and what can each of us do to facilitate inclusive communication? We can start by accepting and supporting the diverse ways that people with intellectual disabilities communicate and engage socially. This requires that we place equal value on the different ways people communicate in any given setting. Ware (1996, p. 1) uses the term 'responsive environment' and defines it as one in which '… people get responses to their actions, get the opportunity to give responses to the actions of others, and have the opportunity to take the lead in interaction'. Enough said!

REFERENCES

Ace Centre. (2020). Available at: https://acecentre.org.uk/. [Accessed 28 August 2020].

Addebuto, L., McDuffie, A., Thurman, A. J., et al. (2016). Language development in individuals with intellectual and developmental disabilities: from phenotypes to treatments. *International Review of Research Into Developmental Disabilities*, 50, 71–118.

Australian Human Rights Commission. (2016) Willing to work. Available at: https://www.humanrights.gov.au/sites/default/files/2016_Willing%20to%20Work%20Report%20easy%20read%20summary.pdf. [Accessed 28 August 2020].

Basson, M., & Alant, E. (2005). The iconicity and ease of learning of Picture Communication Symbols: a study with Africaans-speaking children. *The South African Journal of Communication Disorders*, 52, 5–12.

Beukelman, D. R., & Mirenda, P. (2013). *Augmentative and alternative communication: supporting children and adults with complex communication needs* (4th ed.). Paul H. Brookes Publishing Co.

Beyond Words®. Available at: https://booksbeyondwords.co.uk. [Accessed 28 August 2020].

Boardmaker. (2020). Available at: https://goboardmaker.com/pages/picture-communication-symbols.

Bornman, J., Alant, E., & Du Preez, A. (2009). Translucency and learnability of Blissymbols in Setswana-speaking children: an exploration. *Augmentative and Alternative Communication, 25*, 287–298.

Bradshaw, J. (2002). The management of challenging behaviour within a communication framework. In S. Aburdarham & A. Hurd (Eds.), *Management of communication needs in people with a learning disability* (pp. 246–275). London: Whurr.

Bradshaw, J. (2000). A total communication approach: towards meeting the communication needs of people with learning disabilities. *Tizard Learning Disability Review, 5*, 27–30.

Bronfenbrenner, U. (2005). Ecological Systems theory. In U. Bronfenbrenner (Ed.), *Making human beings human – bioecological perspectives on human development.* London: Sage Publications.

Bronfenbrenner, U. (1979). *The ecology of human development: experiments by nature and design.* Cambridge, MA: Harvard University Press.

Buell, S., Langdon, P. E., Pounds, G., et al. (2019). An open randomized controlled trial of the effects of linguistic simplification and mediation on the comprehension of 'easy read' text by people with intellectual disabilities. *Journal of Applied Research in Intellectual Disabilities, 33*(2), 219–231.

Bunning, K., Gona, J. K., Newton, C., et al. (2014). Caregiver perceptions of children who have complex communication needs following a home-based intervention using augmentative and alternative communication in rural Kenya: an intervention note. *Augmentative and Alternative Communication, 30*, 344–356.

Bunning, K., Gooch, L., & Johnson, M. (2016). Developing the personal narratives of children with complex communication needs associated with intellectual disabilities: what is the potential of Storysharing®? *Journal of Applied Research in Intellectual Disabilities, 30*, 743–756.

Bunning, K., Muggeridge, R., & Voke, K. (2018). Teachers and students with severe learning difficulties working together to co-construct personal narratives using Storysharing®: the teacher perspective. *British Journal of Learning Support, 33*, 23–37.

Bunning, K. (2009). Making sense of communication. In J. Pawlyn & S. Carnaby (Eds.), *Profound and multiple intellectual disabilities: nursing complex needs* (pp. 46–51). London: Blackwell Publishing.

Bunning, K. (2004). *Speech and language therapy intervention: framework and processes.* London: Whurr.

Bunning, K., Heath, B., & Minion, A. (2009). Communication and empowerment: a place for rich and multiple media? *Journal of Applied Research in Intellectual Disabilities, 22*, 370–379.

Bunning, K., & Grove, N. (2002). Making connections: understanding and promoting communication. In S. Carnaby (Ed.), *Learning disability today* (pp. 83–94). Brighton: Pavilion Publishing.

Cameron, D., & Markowicz, L. (2013). Augmentative and alternative communication: international perspectives. *Occupational Therapy Now, 11*, 12–14.

Chadwick, D., & Jolliffe, J. (2009). Effectiveness of training caregivers of adults with learning disabilities in how to use twenty signs to communicate. *British Journal of Learning Disabilities, 37*, 34–42.

Change. (2016a). Free easy-read resources. Available at: https://www.changepeople.org/blog/december-2016/free-easy-read-resources. [Accessed 28 August 2020].

Change. (2016b). How to make information accessible. Available at: https://www.changepeople.org/getmedia/923a6399-c13f-418c-bb29-051413f7e3a3/How-to-make-info-accessible-guide-2016-Final. [Accessed 28 August 2020].

Coupe O'Kane, J., & Goldbart, J. (1998). *Communication before speech* (2nd ed.). London: David Fulton Publishers.

Cornforth, T., Johnson, K., & Walker, M. (1974). Teaching sign language to deaf mentally handicapped adults. *Apex, 2*, 23–25.

Crowley, C., & Baigorri, M. (2012). *AAC market cards in Ghana, West Africa for students with autism and intellectual disabilities.* https://www.youtube.com/watch?v=uJG2K0fFBoQ. [Accessed 7 April 2020].

Dalton, C., & Sweeney, J. (2013). Communication supports in residential services for people with an intellectual disability. *British Journal of Learning Disabilities, 41*, 22–30.

Department of Health. (2001). *Valuing people: a new strategy for learning disability in the 21st century.* London: Department of Health Publications.

Department of Health. (2009). *Valuing people now: a new three-year strategy for people with learning disabilities.* London: Department of Health Publications.

Dimitrova, N., Ozcaliskan, S., & Adamson, L. (2016). Parents' translations of child gesture facilitate word learning in children with autism, Down syndrome and typical development. *Journal of Autism and Developmental Disorders, 46*, 221–231.

Easy Health. (2020). Available at: https://www.easyhealth.org.uk/. [Accessed 28 August 2020].

Fogel, A. (1993). Two principles of communication: co-regulation and framing. In J. Nadel, & L. Camaioni (Eds.), *New perspectives in communication development* (pp. 9–22). London: Routledge.

Fogel, A., & Garvey, A. (2007). Alive communication. *Infant Behavior & Development, 30*, 251–257.

Freyhoff, G., Hess, G., Menzel, E., et al. (1998). *Make it simple: European guidelines for the production of easy-to-read information for people with a learning disability*. Brussels: ILSMH European Association.

Fuller, C. (2013). Multi sensory stories in story packs. In N. Grove (Ed.), *Using storytelling to support children and adults with special needs* (pp. 72–77). London: Taylor & Francis.

Gevartera, C., O'Reilly, M. F., Rojeslkia, L., et al. (2013). Comparisons of intervention components within augmentative and alternative communication systems for individuals with developmental disabilities: a review of the literature. *Research in Developmental Disabilities, 34,* 4404–4414.

Goldbart, J., & Caton, S. (2010). *Communication and people with the most complex needs: what works and why this is essential*. London: Mencap. Available at: http://www.mencap.org.uk/page.asp?id=1539. [Accessed 16 January 2020].

Grove, N., Bunning, K., & Porter, J. (2001). Interpreting the meaning of behavior by people with intellectual disabilities: theoretical and methodological issues. In F. Columbus (Ed.), *Advances in psychology research* (Vol. 7) (pp. 87–126). New York: Nova Sciences.

Grove, N., Bunning, K., Porter, J., et al. (2000). *See what I mean: guidelines to aid understanding of communication by people with severe and profound learning disabilities*. Kidderminster: BILD.

Grove, N., Bunning, K., Porter, J., et al. (1999). See what I mean: interpreting the meaning of communication by people with severe and profound intellectual disabilities. *Journal of Applied Research in Intellectual Disabilities, 12,* 190–203.

Grove, N., & Harwood, J. (2013). Storysharing: personal narratives for identity and community. In N. Grove (Ed.), *Using storytelling to support children and adults with special needs* (pp. 102–110). London: Taylor & Francis.

Grove, N., & McDougall, S. (1991). Exploring sign use in two settings. *British Journal of Special Education, 18,* 149–156.

Grove, N., & Tucker, S. (2003). Narratives in manual sign by children with intellectual impairments. In S. von Tetzchner & N. Grove (Eds.), *Augmentative and alternative communication: developmental issues* (pp. 229–255). London: Whurr/Wiley.

Grove, N., & Walker, M. (1990). The Makaton vocabulary: Using manual signs and graphic symbols to develop interpersonal communication. *Augmentative & Alternative Communication, 6,* 15–28.

Healey, D., & Noonan Walsh, P. (2007). Communication among nurses and adults with severe and profound intellectual disabilities: predicted and observed strategies. *Journal of Intellectual Disabilities, 11,* 127–141.

Hurtado, B., Jones, L., & Burniston, F. (2014). Is easy read information really easier to read? *Journal of Intellectual Disability Research, 58*(9), 822–829.

Imms, C., & Green, D. (2020). *Participation: optimising outcomes in childhood-onset neurodisability. Clinics in developmental medicine*. London: Mackeith Press.

Inclusion Europe. (2020). Easy to read. Available at: https://www.inclusion-europe.eu/easy-to-read/. [Accessed 28 August 2020].

Jones, J. (2000). A total communication approach to meeting the communication needs of people with learning disabilities. *Tizard Learning Disability Review, 5,* 20–26.

Kagan, A. (1998). Supported conversation for adults with aphasia: methods and resources for training conversation partners. *Aphasiogy, 12,* 817–830.

Light, J. (1989). Towards a definition of communicative competence for individuals using augmentative and alternative communication systems. *Augmentative and Alternative Communication, 5,* 137–144.

Loncke, F. T., Campbell, J., England, A. M., et al. (2006). Multimodality: a basis for augmentative and alternative communication – psycholinguistic, cognitive, and clinical/educational aspects. *Disability and Rehabilitation, 28,* 169–174.

McConkey, R., Purcell, M., & Morris, I. (1999). Staff perceptions of communication with a partner who is intellectually disabled. *Journal of Applied Research in Intellectual Disabilities, 12,* 204–210.

Meuris, K., Maes, B., De Meyer, A., et al. (2014). Manual signing in adults with intellectual disability: influences of sign characteristics on functional sign vocabulary. *Journal of Policy & Practice in Intellectual Disabilities, 57,* 990–1011.

Mencap. (2009) Am I making myself clear? Mencap's guildelines for accessible writing. Available at: http://www.accessibleinfo.co.uk/pdfs/Making-Myself-Clear.pdf. [Accessed 7 November 2020].

Mencap. (2011). *Involve me practical guide*. Available at: https://www.mencap.org.uk/sites/default/files/2016-06/Involve%20Me%20practical%20guide_full%20version.pdf. [Accessed 28 August 2020].

Millar, S. (2003). *Personal communication passports: guidelines for good practice*. Edinburgh: Call Centre & Scottish Executive Education Department.

Moorcroft, A., Scarinci, N., & Meyer, C. (2019). A systematic review of the barriers and facilitators to the provision and use of low-tech and unaided AAC systems for people with complex communication needs and their families. *Disability and Rehabilitation: Assistive Technology, 14*(7), 710–731.

Morgan, M. F., Cuskelly, M., & Moni, K. B. (2011). Broadening the conceptualization of literacy in the lives of adults with intellectual disability. *Research and Practice for Persons With Severe Disabilities*, 36(3-4), 112–120.

Murphy, J., & Cameron, L. (2002). *Talking mats and learning disability: a low-tech resource to help people to express their views and feelings.* Scotland: University of Stirling.

Nind, M., Kellett, M., & Hopkins, V. (2001). Teachers' talk styles: communicating with learners with severe and complex learning difficulties. *Child Language Teaching & Therapy*, 17, 143–159.

Olsson, C. (2004). Dyadic interaction with a child with multiple disabilities: a systems theory perspective on communication. *Augmentative & Alternative Communication*, 20, 228–242.

Park, K. (1995). Using objects of reference: a review of the literature. *European Journal of Special Needs Education*, 10, 40–46.

Park, K. (1997). How do objects become objects of reference. *British Journal of Special Education*, 24, 108–114.

Park, K. (2002). *Objects of reference: promoting early symbolic communication* (3rd ed.). London: Royal National Institute for the Blind.

Penne, A., ten Brug, A., Munde, V., et al. (2012). Staff interactive style during multisensory storytelling with persons with profound intellectual and multiple disabilities. *Journal of Intellectual Disability Research*, 56, 167–178.

Photosymbols. (2020). Available at: https://www.photosymbols.com. [Accessible 28 August 2020].

Rambouts, E., Maes, B., & Zink, I. (2018). Manual signing throughout the day: influence from staff's sign use and type of activity. *Journal of Intellectual Disability Research*, 62, 737–745.

Rambouts, E., Maes, B., & Zink, I. (2017). Key word signing usage of adults with intellectual disabilities: influence of communication partners' sign usage and responsivity. *American Journal of Speech-Language Pathology*, 26, 853–864.

Reese, E., Suggate, S., Long, J., et al. (2010a). Children's oral narrative and reading skills in the first three years of reading instruction. *Reading and Writing*, 23, 627–644.

Reese, E., Yan, C., Jack, F., et al. (2010b). Emerging identities: narrative and self from early childhood to early adolescence. In K. McLean & M. Pasupathi (Eds.), *Narrative development in early adolescence: creating the storied self* (pp. 23–43). New York: Springer.

Reuzel, E., Embregts, P. J. C. M., Bosma, A. M. T., et al. (2013a). Conversational synchronization in naturally occurring settings: a recurrence-based analysis of gaze directions and speech rhythms of staff and clients with intellectual disability. *Journal of Nonverbal Behavior*, 37, 281–305.

Reuzel, E., Embregts, P. J. C. M., Bosma, A. M. T., et al. (2013b). Interactional patterns between staff and clients with borderline to mild intellectual disabilities. *Journal of Intellectual Disability Research*, 57, 53–66.

RIX Research & Media. (2020a). Available at: https://rixresearchandmedia.org/software/rix-wikis/. [Accessed 28 August 2020].

RIX Research & Media. (2020b). Available at: https://rixresearchandmedia.org. [Accessed 28 August 2020].

Royal College of Speech & Language Therapists. (2006). *Communicating quality 3.* London: RCSLT.

Scott, C., & Windsor, J. (2000). General language performance measures in spoken and written narrative discourse of school age children with language learning disabilities. *Journal of Speech, Language and Hearing Research*, 43, 324–339.

Signalong – The Communication Charity. (2020). Available at: http://www.signalong.org.uk. [Accessed 28 August 2020].

Soto, G., Hartmann, E., & Wilkins, D. P. (2007). Exploring the elements of narrative that emerge in the interactions between an 8-year-old child who uses an AAC device and her teacher. *Augmentative & Alternative Communication*, 22, 231–241.

South Australian Government. (2020). *Online accessibility toolkit.* Available at: https://www.accessibility.sa.gov.au/introduction/welcome. [Accessed 28 August 2020].

Stans, S. E. A., Dalemans, R. J. P., de Witte, L. P., et al. (2019). Using talking mats to support conversations with communication vulnerable people: a scoping review. *Technology and Disability*, 30, 153–176.

Storysharing®. (2020). Available at: https://storysharing.org.uk/. [Accessed 7 November 2020].

Ten Brug, A., can der Putten, A., Penne, A., et al. (2012). Multi-sensory storytelling for persons with profound intellectual and multiple disabilities: an analysis of the development, content and application in practice. *Journal of Applied Research in Intellectual Disabilities*, 25, 350–359.

The Makaton Charity. (2020). Available at: https://www.makaton.org/aboutMakaton. [Accessed 7 November 2020].

van der Meer, L., Matthews, T., Ogilvie, E., et al. (2017). Training direct-care staff to provide communication intervention to adults with intellectual disability: a systematic review. *American Journal of Speech-Language Pathology*, 26, 1279–1295.

von Tetzchner, S., & Basil, C. (2011). Terminology and notation in written representations of conversations with augmentative and alternative communication. *Augmentative and Alternative Communication*, 27, 141–149.

von Tetzchner, S., & Martinsen, H. (2000). *Introduction to augmentative and alternative communication* (2nd ed.). London: Whurr.

Waller, A. (2006). Communication access to conversational narrative. *Topics in Language Disorders, 26*, 221–239.

Ware, J. (1996). *Creating a responsive environment for people with profound and multiple learning difficulties.* London: David Fulton.

Vendetozzi, M., Beltran, H., McMillan, F., et al. (2010). Training others to communicate. *RCSLT Bulletin, 696*, 22–24.

Wharton, T. (2009). *Pragmatics and non-verbal communication.* Cambridge University Press.

Wilson, D., & Sperber, D. (2012). *Meaning and relevance.* Cambridge University Press.

World Health Organisation. (2011). The world report on disability. Available at: https://www.who.int/disabilities/world_report/2011/world_report_disability_easyread.pdf?ua=1. [Accessed 28 August 2020].

Young, H., Fenwick, M., Lambe, L., et al. (2011). Multi-sensory story telling as an aid to assisting people with profound intellectual disabilities to cope with sensitive issues: a multiple research methods analysis of engagement and outcomes. *European Journal of Special Needs Education, 26*, 127–142.

'They won't let me go cycling by myself': challenges of risk taking

Andy Alaszewski, Melissa Sebrechts and Helen Alaszewski

KEY ISSUES

- Individuals take a risk when they undertake an activity that involves possible loss or harm.
- Risk taking provides individuals with opportunities to learn, to develop skills and to experience the pleasure and emotions of having successfully achieved a challenging activity.
- Risk taking is part of everyday life, it can be seen as an intrinsic part of being human and the thrills of successful risk taking and using risk taking for personal learning and development form an important part of most lives.
- Individuals with intellectual disabilities are often defined as vulnerable and needing protection. Safety first regimes often deprive them of the opportunity to take risks.

- Individuals who have severe intellectual disabilities and communication difficulties may have very limited engagement in decision making affecting their lives and depend on significant others to act for and on their behalf. For these individuals risk taking requires trust and effective communication between all those involved in their care.
- Individuals who have mild intellectual disabilities may play a major role in making decisions that affect their lives though significant others may seek to be involved and to influence such decision making as they may be concerned that potential hazards have not been fully factored in.

CHAPTER OUTLINE

INTRODUCTION

In this chapter we explore the nature of risk taking in contemporary society and consider why it is important that individuals with intellectual disabilities have the opportunity to take risks. We explore the issues of risk taking through three contrasted illustrations. We examine ways in which individuals with intellectual disabilities can be supported to take risks.

WHAT IS RISK AND RISK TAKING?

If you search the literature relating to people with intellectual disabilities, using the key word risk, you will identify a substantial number of publications with risk in the title. Most of these articles will use the term 'at risk', in other words they will be about people with intellectual disabilities who are in 'danger of' some form of harm whether this is physical abuse, ill-health, sexual or financial exploitation. You may also find one or two publications that define risk in a different and more positive way, as part of the experience of everyday life enabling people with intellectual disabilities to be active participants in the world around them. In some of these articles, risk taking is defined as a basic human right which individuals with an intellectual disability should have (see for example Greenhill and Whitehead, 2010). In this section we explore the ways in which this tension between risk as something harmful and to be avoided, and risk as an essential part of everyday life and as a way of empowering people, co-exist in everyday discourse drawing on our own and others' research.

As part of our research relating to intellectual disabilities (Alaszewski et al, 2000; Alaszewski and Alaszewski, 2002), we talked to service providers, people with intellectual disabilities and their relatives about risk. There was no consensus over risk. The tension between risk as danger versus risk as empowerment was evident in all groups. Although service providers acknowledged risk was an important part of their practice, they often found it a difficult concept to define. Some practitioners described risk in terms of dangers, often citing specific incidents when things had gone wrong. For example, a student on an intellectual disability training course provided the following negative image:

> "Somewhere I used to work – I took a client to a supermarket and he completely smashed the place up and there were children hanging around. It could have been a risk."

However, other service providers talked about risk as part of everyday life and as a right. As a key worker in a residential facility for people with intellectual disabilities put it:

> "There has to be an element of risk in everybody's lives, walking across the road's a risk … Life is one big risk. Clients have to take risks."

Another service provider working in day care services echoed the same view:

> "If you're going to give people choices and help them to progress, then you've got to take risks, there's no way round it."

A number of service providers did try to reconcile risk as danger with risk as empowerment by balancing the two approaches. An intellectual disability lecturer discussed risk in the following way:

> "Well, risk is a very important area in learning disability [intellectual disability] and anybody working in that area needs to be concerned with it. It is enabling the people you work with to do something, but taking into account the risk that may be involved … for example, you might have somebody who is suffering from epilepsy and you may want them to take part in a certain activity – you need to make a judgement about what the risk to that person is and that's got to be balanced with the experience that they get by taking part."

The relatives of individuals with intellectual disabilities we talked to were aware of the importance of risk and the ways it had to be managed. A minority accepted risk as part of everyday life, for example one family carer observed that: 'Well, I think living life is a risk, so it doesn't really enter into my mind.' However, most relatives we talked to tended to see risk in terms of dangers. They were particularly concerned about the dangers that existed outside the relatively protected environment of their home. One mother discussed the risk her daughter was exposed to outside the home:

> "Well my daughter is at risk if she tries to walk and people expect her to walk because she looks quite normal; but if they expect her to walk then she's likely to fall, so she's at risk whenever she's out of my sight really."

Some parents, while being aware of the dangers, were conscious of the importance of taking risk for personal development and self-esteem. For example, one parent described her strategy for balancing danger and empowerment in the following way:

> "When Brian [her husband] retired and we started going out more, and we had to rush back for Mark coming home from school, well, we thought about giving him a key. So, we put a key on a piece of elastic and it goes in his pocket. The first few weeks, we made sure we were home, just in case, and we hid behind the curtains to see what he'd do… Now it's alright…he just comes in, hangs his keys up… He'll sit quite happy till we come in… That was a risk, but we had to… he's 29-years-old after all."

We also talked to individuals with intellectual disabilities about risk and their views were similar to those of their relatives and service providers. A minority talked about risk taking and the positive feelings they had about successful risk taking:

> "I went to [major seaside landmark] – there was a sand dune – it was hard to get up – we went up. We took pictures. It was risky but worth it. Someone was with us."

Like service providers and relatives, most people with intellectual disabilities talked about risk as a threat. For example, two service users stressed the dangers of living in the community:

> Anthony: *I used to live in an old house and there was a risk of fire because of electrical faults.*

> Brenda: *When it gets dark ... there is the risk of being abused. If you go out at night – people on skate boards – you get abused if you don't get out of the way.*

The tensions between the different definitions of risk are evident in other studies. For example, an innovative project in Scotland (Brookes et al, 2012) brought together University academics, individuals with intellectual disabilities and those supporting them, to jointly explore how risk and other key words could be talked about. They found that key words could be used to convey different meanings depending on the precise context in which they were used. They observed that risk could be given negative connotations, such as threat or control, or more positive ones such as choice, opportunity, fun and daring to do something. One of the participants in the study, Fiona, who helped organise the meeting, explained how her understanding of risk had developed through the project:

> "I had come from a project that was very much about 'adult protection' i.e. how people might best be protected when they are being badly harmed. There was a sense within the Research Planning Group that this was only half a topic, and that the kind of perspective which assumed it was a whole one could be harmful to people using services. I always agreed that some other types of risk can be positive and over–protection can be harmful; but I struggled to see how an approach which constructed risk as a 'good thing' could fit into a coherent project about the types of risk and harm which are definitely bad. But I've come to see that this struggle itself was being pushed into centre stage by the research group."

> *Brookes et al, 2012*, p. 147

The group identified ways in which individuals with intellectual disabilities could be enabled to take risks and identified trust and support as key resources.

Risk taking, therefore, involves a decision to undertake an activity that the risk taker expects to get a benefit from such as pleasure but may, due to unforeseen circumstances, result in undesired, possibly harmful outcomes, affecting not only the risk taker but also other people.

THREE ILLUSTRATIONS

To explore the issues involved in enabling individuals with intellectual disabilities to take risks, we will present and discuss three illustrations which each explore risk taking, albeit in different contexts. The first considers the practical difficulties of making a spontaneous decision by taking very disabled children out tobogganing. The second focuses on the way in which two parents dealt with their son's desire to go cycling by himself in a potentially dangerous urban environment and the third addresses the ways in which young men with mild intellectual disabilities responded to a pseudo-work environment providing care and support.

Illustration 1 'It's snowing in North Wales, let's take the kids tobogganing'
Background
In the early 1990s, Andy Alaszewski and Bie Nio Ong undertook an evaluation of an innovative project based on the principles of normalization (see Wolfensberger, 1972). The project was funded directly by the Department of Health and involved a UK charity, Dr Barnardo's, taking eight very severely disabled children who had been cared for in hospital and providing them with care and support in ordinary houses on a newly built residential estate in Liverpool, Croxteth Park (Alaszewski and Ong, 1990). The unit opened in 1983 when the first four children arrived. All the children had profound intellectual disabilities and additional health problems and were medically fragile. The ideology of the project was:

> "based on the belief that normal patterns of everyday life should be available to [the] children... who used our services."

> *Kendall and Dodson, 2016*

At one of the joint meetings between the researchers and Barnardo's management team, the Project Leader posed the question of how he could enable care staff to take risks for, and on behalf of the children if he was not there. For example, if one Saturday morning it was snowing in North Wales what needed to be in place so that the staff on duty could make a decision to take several of the children tobogganing. Snow falling in North Wales is an unpredictable event and the window of opportunity to make use of it is relatively narrow. Therefore, if this opportunity is to be exploited the staff in the unit need to have the autonomy to assess the potential benefits and hazards and make a decision that was in the best interest of the children.

The nature and distribution of risk

The commitment of the agency and staff was to provide the children in their care with normal patterns of everyday life; outdoor activities such as tobogganing clearly fell within this category.

The children

The children were potential beneficiaries of such risk taking as it would enable them to participate in the thrills and excitement of tobogganing also sharing the physical sensation of the activity. Most of the children could communicate, but often in limited ways, indicating pleasure or pain in the here and now. Thus, they could indicate whether they enjoyed an activity such as tobogganing but only when it was happening. Given the medical fragility of some of the children there was the danger that they might be hurt or experience a health emergency.

When caring for individuals with profound intellectual disabilities, the emphasis is often on assessing and meeting their needs. It is important to be aware that individuals can often communicate their feelings through signs and gestures and such communication can indicate their interest in and consent to activities.

Carers

The children lived in minimally converted bungalows on a newly constructed housing estate. The prime responsibility for their care was undertaken by their care or link worker. The link workers had been selected and trained by Barnardo's and personal status and recognition was inextricably linked to the development and health of the child they were responsible for. The proposed risk taking would enable the link workers to share a normal and valued experience with their child. In preparation for this type of risk taking it would be usual for the link worker or unit leader to do a risk assessment, to identify the potential risks, consider whether they were

reasonable and to make a judgement about the acceptability of the proposed risk taking.

Accountability and blame

Carers are accountable for their actions and given the culture of inquiries, accidents are not seen as chance random events but as preventable injuries for which, with the benefit of hindsight, someone is to blame (Douglas, 1992). In such an environment carers are likely to engage in defensive practice or safety first, and need support if they are to take risks on behalf of those they are caring for. As Robertson and Collinson (2011, p. 161) observed in a study of staff supporting individuals with intellectual disabilities living in the community, anxiety about being blamed meant that 'overcautious, conservative approaches [prevailed] in the lives of some service users'.

Parents and relatives

While the parents and other key relatives such as older siblings were not directly involved in the provision of care or day-to-day decision making, there was a strong ethos within Barnardo's that they should be consulted and involved in all decisions concerning their relative. Barnardo's hoped and anticipated that over time link workers would develop a positive and trusting relationship with parents and other key relatives. However, it was unlikely that care staff would have the time to directly involve parents and other key relations in the decision-making about tobogganing. Parents and other key relatives had to trust care staff although they would clearly expect that if anything went wrong there would be a full investigation identifying and allocating blame and punishment so they could achieve closure.

Values and trust

The parents and relatives depend on and trust Barnardo's and its staff to provide health and social care. Such trust is grounded in a belief that staff are competent and share the parents' values. Risk taking may challenge values that give primacy to safety and protection (for a discussion of trust see Alaszewski, 2003).

The agency

As an organisation, Barnardo's is dependent on its reputation as a competent caring agency to attract support and funds from central and local government and from the public. Even though senior staff in the agency cannot oversee all the activity and actions taking place in each of their care settings, they are vicariously liable; they are ultimately responsible for the actions and decisions of front-line staff. If such actions or decisions cause loss or harm then the agency is liable for the damage, and the publicity linked to any investigation or legal action may damage its reputation which in turn may harm its support and income.

To protect the agency and themselves senior managers need to create systems that minimise risk. These usually involve some form of bureaucratisation, rules and procedures plus documentation of activities and decisions showing adherence to these rules and procedures. The purpose of such systems is to reduce uncertainty and increase predictability but for front-line care staff such systems restrict autonomy and take time and effort. Thus, while front-line care staff might like to take their children tobogganing in North Wales, they may not feel it is worth the extra time and effort to do all the assessments and fill in all the paperwork.

Insurance and risk

Organisations, such as charities, need to protect themselves to ensure their continued existence. One way of doing this is through insurance that provides financial compensation if an accident occurs. An article outlining a legal risk management checklist in Canada noted that not only is a charity liable for the costs of any successful negligence claim but so is each Trustee, and that each charity should ensure that it takes proactive steps to protect against risk, including a 'full written disclosure of all risks to its insurer to avoid denial of coverage' (Carter and Connor, 2005, p. 6).

While the senior manager posed the question of how to facilitate risk taking, in reality facilitating spontaneous risk taking is very difficult. In a normal family setting, parents have the freedom and autonomy to make spontaneous decisions. In residential units, the situation is more complex. The individuals providing the care do not have the autonomy to make decisions as they are embedded in a network of relationships both with their managers and with the children's relatives. Thus, in their decision making they have to consider and engage with this wider network. This can either be done directly through direct communication or indirectly through written documentation. Whichever way it is done will involve some delay and reduced flexibility. There are ways of speeding things up, for example through the use of trust.

Reader Activity 6.1 in the accompanying online resource uses a real-life event – young adults with physical and intellectual disabilities bungee jumping – posted on social media to explore how positive risk taking could be facilitated.

Illustration 2 'Mum and dad go that way and Ian go this way'

Background

This illustration focuses on two parents' decision to allow their son a degree of autonomy and take risks by cycling home without them. It is based on Andy Alaszewski's interview with Ian's mother in 2019 when Ian was 31 years old. In the interview, Ian's mother described him as a gentle giant, who was 6-foot tall and weighed over 14 stone. She felt that as he had got older so Ian's intellectual disability had become more visible and evident which helped those that did not know him understand his situation. His mother described him as very sensitive and as sensible as he could be. He had some developmental delay and some of his behaviour was more appropriate to a young child. He lived most of the time in a shared bungalow with three other young people. They had one-to-one support from 8 in the morning till 10 at night and then a single carer for the night. Every second weekend and most holidays, Ian came back to stay with his parents and he often phoned his mother, sometimes twice a day.

Cycling and risk taking

Ian learnt to cycle when he was 4. His parents were pleased with this as it was one of the few age appropriate skills he had acquired. Everyday his parents would walk to the local shops and Ian would cycle with them. As he got older they taught him basic road safety. They kept it simple, they told him to stop at each road and look for cars, if he could not see any then he could cross. As they acquired trust and confidence in Ian's road skills so they let him cycle further ahead of them until when he was 8 or 9 years old, he cycled off by himself and they lost sight of him. When this first happened they panicked and searched the area looking for him. After a while they gave up and went home and 'there he was'. After this it became part of their daily routine. They trusted Ian and knew he had a good knowledge of the local area so they would all walk to the local shops together; Ian would look at what they had bought and he would then 'bugger off' and would sometimes return home several hours later.

Learning and risk taking

For Ian and his parents, this was a process of mutual learning. As Ian's skills and knowledge developed so did his parent's willingness to 'let him go'. Despite this when he did actually cycle off by himself it was an unexpected surprise. As Näslund and Gardelli (2013) observed in a study in Sweden, individuals with intellectual disabilities need time and support to understand and use technologies, but once they have mastered it they gain a sense of agency and control.

Responding to risk taking: experiencing it as a parent

Ian's mother agreed that Ian's cycling could make her and her husband very anxious especially when he was missing for a long time, 3 hours or more. When this happened, they telephoned the police who were generally very helpful. Although one policewoman did ask if Ian was in a wheelchair and when she replied, no he could walk and cycle, the policewoman said he was not disabled, indicating she did not understand the nature of intellectual disability. When Ian's mother reported him missing, the police officer would take a full description which was then circulated to all patrol cars. After this had happened several times, Ian's parents agreed that the police could have a photo of Ian so that they could identify him more easily if he was reported missing. One of the difficulties was that Ian could not say his address so on one occasion when a police patrol picked him and his bike up, they drove round for an hour and a half looking for his home. There was, however, an on-going problem with the police. Ian's parents were worried about Ian cycling on the road. They would allow him to do so occasionally when they were cycling with him, but they had taught him to cycle on the pavement or sidewalk. As this is illegal in the UK, they had been stopped several times when they were with Ian and they were sure that Ian had been stopped by the police when he was cycling by himself.

Near misses

Ian's mother described one incident that she accepted could be classified as a near miss when Ian sustained some head bruising, had his bike stolen and could have been seriously injured. In the city where Ian and his family live, there were alley ways nearly three metres wide between the back of houses. Ian liked cycling down these as they tended to be traffic free. On one occasion when he was cycling down one of the alleyways he was assaulted by a group of young men who hit him on the head, pushed him off his bike and stole it. His parents were relieved that he was not seriously hurt. They felt that despite the fright Ian had experienced, there was a positive side. Ian's mother said it had been a good learning experience for Ian; he had learnt there were people who might try to hurt him, and it had made him more cautious. Ian's parents had also used it as an opportunity to highlight the benevolent aspect of police. During the night a police helicopter was circling above the area they lived in and Ian's parents told Ian that the police were looking for his bike. In another incident Ian came home wet through even though it was a dry sunny day. Over several days of gentle questioning, his parents found out what had happened. Ian had wanted to wash his bike so when he saw a car in a mechanical car wash, he had taken his bike in for a wash. Give the consequences he was unlikely to do this again.

Dealing with anxiety

The uncertainty associated with risk taking, tends to engender anxiety, especially for carers who often have to act as bystanders as individuals with intellectual disabilities take risks. Learning to cope with such anxiety is an intrinsic part of parenting in the global North but it is not an easy process (see Jenkins, 2006).

The benefits of cycling and risk taking

Ian's cycling was an important skill from which he and his parents (mostly) derived pleasure and enjoyment. Shortly before I interviewed his mother in 2019, the family had been on a cycling holiday in the Netherlands. They had taken an overnight ferry to Rotterdam and then spent two days cycling in the Netherlands before returning home. Ian had coped very well and was only a bit 'dodgy' for the last 20 km. The only times Ian got a bit frightened was when mopeds sped past in the cycle lane. It was a good trip. His mother felt that cycling provided Ian with a way of gaining some independence and control. She commented that when he was in the supported care, it was one-to-one so he was being shadowed all the time and did not have any real independence, so when he came home his parents tried to give him some freedom and independence. The cycling remained important; whenever they went out on a cycle and when they got about half a mile from home and there were two alternative routes, Ian would say to his parents 'Mum and dad go that way and Ian go this way' and they would meet him at home. There was another way in which Ian asserted his independence and took risks. Ian was very keen, almost obsessed, with recycling so at home he had taken responsibility for separating and bagging up all the household recycling. His mother observed that when Ian wanted to be alone and 'needed his own space', he would take some of the bags of recycling and walk by himself through the local streets to the local recycling bins, empty the bags in the bins and then walk back taking his time. He was walking around the local neighbourhood on his own for about half an hour.

Decision making and trust

From Ian's mother's account, it is clear that no explicit decision was taken by them or Ian to take risks. The risk taking associated with Ian's independent cycling evolved over several years and it was very much a case of one thing leading on to another. As Ian's cycling proficiency and road sense developed so his parents were willing to accept his increasing independence and risk taking. However, they had to have ways of managing the anxieties which this risk taking engendered and central to this was trust.

Trust enabled Ian's parents to manage most of the challenges of Ian's risk taking: trust in Ian; trust in those living in the neighbourhood and trust in the police. Ian's parents trust in Ian was based on their direct personal relationship with him and built up over time. It was based on their knowledge that they had taught him how to cycle safely and navigate the hazards of the roads. Occasionally Ian had betrayed this trust, for example not returning home at a reasonable time but these occasional failures did not undermine his parent's overall confidence in him.

Ian's parents also had to trust that those living in the neighbourhood would not be hostile to or hurt Ian. This was a more abstract form of trust as the parents could not personally know everyone who lived in the neighbourhood. However, given their personal experiences of living in and interacting with those living in the neighbourhood, Ian's parents developed a sense that generally their neighbours were good people and there was no reason why they would interfere with and hurt Ian. This trust was only betrayed on one occasion, when the youths attacked Ian in the alleyway and stole his bike. Ian's parent reported the incident to the police, no action was taken as it was not possible to identify the culprits. Ian's parents were able to remind Ian of the potential dangers from other people and Ian's concrete experience has made him more wary of others.

Ian's parents also had to trust the police. If and when Ian did not return home at a reasonable time, then they reported this to the police asking them to look for him. The police force can be seen as an 'abstract system' like the health care system, in that individuals rely on its services often at crucial or fateful moments in their lives, but most people using the system have no real understanding of how it works, what sort of knowledge it uses and have no on-going relationship with it (see Giddens, 1991, pp. 21–23). Ian's parents had to deal with different police officers each time Ian went missing and trust that these officers would take appropriate action to mobilise the relevant sections of the police. Again, Ian's parents' trust in the police was not misplaced. Whenever they telephoned to say he was missing the police took immediate action. Indeed, over time the police service took action to improve their response, for example having a photo so they could give individual police patrols a clearer picture of who they were looking for.

Trust as a way of managing uncertainty

Risk taking creates uncertainty. For most carers, rational ways of managing this uncertainty such as formal risk assessment or insurance are not accessible, so they have to rely on other methods such as trust or hope.

 READER ACTIVITY 6.2 Identifying trust

You can start this exercise by identifying three or four criteria that you use to assess whether a person or organisation is trustworthy. Then complete the following exercises:

- Identify two people and two organisations that you consider trustworthy and write down two or more reasons for your trust in them and at least one occasion in which your trust has been well placed.
- Identify one or more person with an intellectual disability who you know and consider whether they can trust you and why this should be.

This exercise requires reflection on your own circumstances and those of a person with an intellectual disability that you know. It aims to examine the nature of trust, which is a complex concept involving rational (previous knowledge and experience) and non-rational elements (essentially an act of faith). A useful starting point for background reading is Patrick Brown's chapter on Trust and Risk in the *Routledge Handbook of Risk Studies* (Burgess et al, 2016).

Trust combines knowledge built up from previous experiences with an act of faith and is a pragmatic way of managing uncertainty (see Zinn, 2016).

Illustration 3 'It's so boring, let's liven it up'

This illustration draws on research undertaken in the Netherlands by Melissa Sebrechts between 2013 and 2015. In this chapter we use it to examine why a not-for profit (care) organisation funded by central and local government, failed to provide individuals with a mild intellectual disability with opportunities to make positive use of risk taking. The service was used mainly by young men who liked to be referred to as 'co-workers'. To protect their identity, we will refer to the care organisation as 'CareWell'.

The illusion of risk-taking

CareWell provided sheltered employment for individuals with a mild intellectual disability. These facilities were designed for individuals 'who are not (yet) "good enough" for regular employment but too good for occupational activities' (Sebrechts et al, 2018, p. 460). In this chapter, we focus on two sheltered workshops provided by the organisation: a technical workshop, referred to as 'Repair', and a workshop for green maintenance referred to as 'Gardens'.

Both of these sheltered workshops hosted 10 to 20 co-workers. Their publicly stated purpose was to provide those attending them with the opportunity to gain the recognition and benefits that come from work. The aim was to provide co-workers with the opportunity: to become economically self-sustaining; to feel socially and culturally included; and to feel valued for the work done. CareWell stated that individual co-workers should 'experience recognition by participation through sheltered, "meaningful" work' (Sebrechts et al, 2018, p. 462). In addition, the workshops were focused on preparing people with mild intellectual disabilities for employment in regular workplace settings.

The workshops largely failed to achieve the second objective of preparing people with mild intellectual disabilities for work in an open employment setting. In 2015, out of the 671 co-workers in the units, only 15 progressed to open employment and of these 3 were no longer working two years later and the remaining 12 remained on short-term contracts.

The workshops also aimed to provide co-workers with a sense of recognition and valuation for their contribution as workers in the sheltered environment.

Seen from the perspective of risk-taking, they failed to do this as they were unable to replicate the risk reality of the conventional workplace. Co-workers were denied the opportunity to take risks since they were denied the opportunity to carry out work-activities that they considered to be 'meaningful'. They recognised activities as 'meaningful' when they were commissioned by an external party (which could be a department of CareWell) and involved a sense of urgency or time pressure. There did not necessarily have to be additional payments for the work, but the job had to make co-workers feel important, visible to and recognised by people, preferably those outside the sheltered workshop environment.

For co-workers, work in an open employment setting, or in a sheltered setting with 'meaningful' work-activities, can be seen as a form of risk taking in which positive and desired outcomes are balanced against the possibility of negative undesired outcomes. From the perspective of the individual worker, the workplace offers the opportunity to work, which if done diligently and skilfully, should lead to recognition by professionals and colleagues as a skilful worker and, possibly, financial reward in the form of wages. Yet negative outcomes may happen if the worker fails to do the work to the desired standard or fails to come to work; this may result in negative reactions from managers and co-workers, and even financial sanctions culminating in termination of contract.

The sheltered employment settings were intended to replicate the conditions of open employment settings, for example by letting co-workers carry out work tasks that had a sense of urgency to them, but repeatedly failed to do so. Sporadically, the units responded to demands for specific contracts but the work on these was undertaken by paid staff and volunteers plus a small pool of co-workers who had specific skills such as a driving licence or a welding certificate. For the majority, there were few work tasks that had a sense of urgency, and co-workers were repeatedly observed to spend their time sitting around waiting until it was time to go home. In these workshops:

> "Daily life… is characterised by long stretches of sitting and hanging around…in such moments, there is little energy: co-workers stay inside the shed and play with their phones, stare, feel bored, and complain about it."
>
> Sebrechts et al, 2018, p. 463

Most co-workers felt that they were dispensable and that it did not really matter whether they did or did not come to work. For example, one co-worker stated that he did not attend regularly because there was nothing to do (Sebrechts et al, 2018, p. 464).

There were few negative consequences for not coming to work. The professional staff wanted to make the workshops as accessible as possible for co-workers which effectively meant that there were no, or very few, sanctions. Co-workers could easily stay at home and the worst sanction they experienced was getting a telephone call from a professional and/or losing their three-euro attendance allowance. Officially, attendance at the sheltered workshop was a condition for living in CareWell's supported accommodation but staff did not enforce this.

Thus, the opportunity to engage in meaningful work-activities, together with the potential benefits of engaging in such work such as personal recognition and financial rewards, were illusory at the workshops. It is easy to recognise that professional staff were reluctant to use sanctions and were keen to keep providing co-workers with opportunities. However, from the perspective of risk-taking such an approach can be seen as paternalistic; by 'protecting' people with intellectual disabilities from the consequences of their actions, staff are depriving them of the opportunity to learn from their mistakes and to understand that their actions may be harmful to themselves and others.

Creating a false sense of security

Within care agencies there can be a muddled response to risk taking especially when it involves potentially harmful consequences such as sexual abuse. Thompson observed that when men take such risks the initial response is often weak and confused, especially if the victim is another person with intellectual disabilities. Such responses may be unhelpful as these men learn that little will happen if they continue and it does not give them an incentive to change. As a result, they are unprepared for the harsh sanctions that they may face if they carry on taking such risks such as social exclusion or even transfer to secure accommodation. (Thompson, 2000, p. 39)

Risk-taking in the workshops

Given their lack of opportunity to gain recognition through carrying out what they considered to be meaningful work-activities, co-workers had developed alternative ways of obtaining recognition. Sebrechts et al

(2018) identified two alternatives, and while both had features that were problematic, they also involved genuine risk-taking. These are bullying and being street-wise and collaborating on a challenging activity.

Bullying and being street-wise

These are real risk-taking activities that are initiated by the co-workers themselves. In bullying a small group of co-workers, often the more able, pick on one or more of the usually less able co-workers. They may taunt or threaten the less able co-worker. For example, in one incident a group of co-workers flicked a lighter under the nose of a sleeping co-worker threatening to burn him. This bullying can be seen as spontaneous risk taking with immediate benefits for the bullies, but with the possibility that things may go wrong. For the bullies such behaviour marked their social status and could be exciting. It ensured that they were recognised as members of a superior in-group while their victims were categorised as vulnerable outsiders. Bullying was thrilling and pleasurable and it helped pass the time. As Sebrechts et al (2018) observed when discussing the lighter incident, the bullies 'all come to share the excitement that breaks with the earlier atmosphere of boredom' (p. 467). There is some potential danger in bullying. It is an illicit activity that challenges the values of professionals and what they consider acceptable in the workshop. So if things go wrong, for example the victim is injured and the bullies are caught and reported to the professionals, they may be subject to formal investigation and even sanctioned, for example by being suspended from the workshop for a few days or even excluded permanently. A short suspension might not be considered much of a sanction; indeed, it might even be considered 'cool' and enhance the co-worker's social standing.

Collaborating on a challenging activity

An alternative way of gaining recognition was through collaborative work on specific challenging projects. While such collaboration did not often occur, Sebrechts et al (2018) observed an event in which professionals, volunteers and co-workers worked together to demolish an old greenhouse. All participants engaged enthusiastically with the work resulting in the rapid demolition of the greenhouse. The participants appeared to derive pleasure both from engagement with the task and working alongside others and recognition as team members. As

Sebrechts et al (2018) observe in this context 'Recognition arises from inclusion – everybody can participate according to his abilities – and from fulfilling a relatively easy but pressing task' (p. 470). While such recognition was a positive benefit, the demolition work was potentially dangerous. A major accident could happen, if for example one of the heavy pipes at roof top level fell on one of the workers. Indeed, when the unit manager arrived he said that the demolition was too dangerous however his concerns were disregarded by both professionals and co-workers who continued working and he was treated as an outsider and was socially excluded.

Risk taking, personal emotions and group solidarity

As Parker and Stanworth (2005) have observed, risk taking can be a personal challenge in which individuals have to overcome their own sense of fear, but if they do then they can achieve a sense of pleasure and personal achievement and enhance their standing and recognition within a social group. Such risk taking enhances a sense of social solidarity and belonging.

The scenario above has illustrated the complexity of risk and some consequences of not allowing someone to risk take. The situation involving the men who worked at CareWell could have been improved if they had been enabled to take risks by

- *avoidance of illusionary risk taking*
  It is important in risk taking that potential benefits are balanced against possible losses and negative outcomes, and that such benefits and losses are real, not illusionary. While it is tempting to protect individuals with intellectual disabilities from the negative consequences of their choices, this may deprive them of important learning opportunities.
- *channelling of spontaneous risk-taking into socially desirable forms*
  While violence can be seen as an important part of being street wise, there are other ways in which rebelliousness and in-group status can be displayed that are more benign and less harmful, for example through shared cultural symbols such as clothing and music. While any attempt to shape rebelliousness needs to be very subtle if it is not to remove both spontaneity and ownership of the activities, it is not impossible.
- *creating opportunities for collaborative project work*
  In settings such as the CareWell workshops, the emphasis is on the individual co-worker, his skills and

work. In many ways this is similar to the emphasis in other educational establishments such as schools. However, in schools this individual ethos is usually complemented by team activities such as team sports or theatrical productions that provide opportunity for collaborative group work. Such opportunities could and should be provided for individuals with intellectual disabilities.

FACILITATING RISK TAKING: ADVOCACY, TRUST AND COMMUNICATION

Given the challenges of their everyday lives, most people with intellectual disabilities are supported in their decision-making and risk taking by their relatives and/or care agencies. As we have noted, family members can act relatively autonomously, but when faced with risk taking scenarios they still have to be able to manage their own anxieties about possible negative outcomes. Where agencies are involved, things become more complex. Care agencies have systems that are designed to protect both the clients they care for, the staff and the agency itself but such systems are usually not designed to facilitate and support risk taking. The final section of this chapter considers how risk taking can be fostered through advocacy, trust and good communication. It is supported by good practice outlined in Boxes 6.1, 6.2 and 6.3. Box 6.1 gives examples of good practice in identifying aims for positive risk taking and in providing working definitions of risk; Box 6.2 illustrates how a non-profit agency placed the individual at the centre of the subsequent planning process. Good practice in managing inevitable tensions over risk is shown in Box 6.3.

Effective advocacy

In the global North, social relations are based on the assumption that adults have the knowledge and capacity to make decisions and have the capacity to judge whether or not to take risks. However, when individuals have difficulty in accessing or using knowledge then some form of support is needed. As we have already observed, this support can come from relatives or care agencies, but both of these sources of support have limitations. An alternative source of support is advocacy through individuals who are willing to act for and on behalf of, a person. Such relationships depend on the advocate being able to understand the interests and preferences of the

BOX 6. 1   Good practice: aims and definitions

Context

Agency policies should acknowledge the benefits of risk taking and provide a link to, and balance between, issues of safety and those of empowerment. The risk-taking policy should have an explicit definition of risk that recognises the benefits of risk taking. While the potential dangers of risk taking are recognised, these should be set alongside the benefits.

Aims example 1

(NHS trust) "The trust recognises that users of services for learning [intellectual] disabilities, as part of their right to ordinary living opportunities, will be exposed to hazards of daily life. The Directorate acknowledges that if service users are to continue their process of acquiring skills for independence and integration into the local community, they must be allowed to take calculated risks".

Aims example 2

(For-profit agency) "It is our belief that people with a learning [intellectual] disability are entitled to partici-pate in activities and exploit opportunities available to anyone else. We also recognise that our service users are vulnerable to harm and exploitation and need pro-tection. We will strive to achieve an accountable bal-ance between these apparently opposing positions ...

It is our intention to fulfil our duty of care to service users and staffing protecting them from harm, which arises from negligent action, but that is balanced by enabling service users to enjoy freedom, to participate in activities, which involve an element of planned and responsibly managed risk."

Risk definition example 1

(Not-for-profit agency) "A risk situation where benefits can be gained but harms are also possible".

Risk definition example 2

(Local authority Social Services Department) "Risk does not necessarily mean that people are placed in dangerous situations, but that something can go wrong. It may in some situations involve an element of danger".

Risk definition example 3

(NHS trust) "When considering risks, staff are asked to consider the probable outcomes of any activity and whether these outcomes will be beneficial or harm-ful. Staff will also need to consider the likelihood that these outcomes will occur ... Risk can be said to occur when two or more outcomes of an activity are possi-ble but not certain".

 BOX 6.2   Good practice: placing individual's wishes & needs at the centre of planning process

Key issue

It is important that individuals do not get lost in the planning process, therefore, it is important that the individual's wishes are considered before possible risks are considered.

Example 1: Giving priority to an individual's wants and wishes

Before risks can be assessed, an individual's wants and objectives have to be identified. This can be done in a number of ways:

- Where possible talking to the person concerned and to those involved with them.
- Through goal planning.

- Giving people information about resources and opportunities available to enable them to make informed choices.
- Different forums for people to express them-selves, e.g. quality action groups, residents' meetings, community forums.
- Building on and developing individual skills.

Example 2: Developing risk assessment from individual preferences

Exploratory issues:

- What is this person's objective?
- What things have led to this objective being chosen?
- How will achieving this improve the person's life?

BOX 6.3   Good practice: managing tensions over risk

Key issue

Participants in planning and decision making may differ in their assessment of the potential benefits and possible hazards of activities which a person with an intellectual disability would like to undertake. In such circumstances it is important that a process exists for identifying, discussing and resolving these differences.

Example 1: Identifying disagreement

When an individual has identified something they wish to do which involves an element of risk, a full discussion should take place between that individual and a staff member. This discussion should look specifically at what the person wishes to do and what it is likely to entail. It is important to highlight the risks and consequences involved to the individual before continuing. During this meeting a preliminary risk assessment form should be completed with as much information as possible.

Example 2: Assessing the acceptability of risk

The meeting should aim to make a decision on the acceptability of risk that is summarised on a risk-assessment form in the following way:

- Can a decision be taken at this point as to whether this is an acceptable or unacceptable risk?
- If acceptable, please give the reasons why and also the ways in which the person will be enabled to take the risk.
- If unacceptable, please give the reasons why.

Example 3: Planning risk taking

If the risk is considered potentially acceptable then a further meeting may be needed for more detailed planning. This meeting should include the introduction of information contained in the preliminary risk assessment form including the objective, the risks and the other areas highlighted. If individuals are able and wish to do so, they should present this information themselves; if not, it should be presented by somebody of their choice. There should follow a general discussion of the information presented, adding any new points and considerations. The aim should be to reach a joint decision either to go ahead with the risk because it is acceptable or because it is not too great. If all those present are not able to agree then further discussion may need to take place or a majority decision be adhered to.

---

person on whose behalf they are acting and having the skills to make decisions that support these interests and choices. Most people with intellectual disabilities have ready-made advocates – their relatives, especially parents – and this relationship often works well. For example, Christine, who attended a day centre, described the ways in which she made the day-to-day decisions and her mother's role in facilitating this by looking after her money for her:

> "What makes me really happy is playing my music centre – playing my Abba tapes and the Eastenders record I've got. I like to lie on my bed to listen to my music. Sometimes I watch the telly. I bought it myself. I don't know how much money I've got. Mum does it for me."
>
> *Atkinson and Williams, 1990, p. 30*

However, in some circumstances there are difficulties. Parents and their children do not always have the

same interests and perceptions but when they disagree, adolescents often have the resources to resist. In contrast, many people with intellectual disabilities find it difficult to resist well-meaning paternalism. This can cause a tension between paid carers and families as parents can be seen as risk averse or overprotective:

> "The notion of parental 'overprotection'… incorporates a covert value judgement that parents ought to encourage people with learning [intellectual] difficulties to take more risks. The concept of 'letting go'… implies that parents avoid risk for adults with learning [intellectual] difficulties for selfish reasons, because they do not want to give up the parental role."
>
> *Heyman et al, 1998, p. 211*

If agreement cannot be reached over acceptable risk taking, then it may be necessary to identify someone who is able and willing to act on the individual's behalf; with moreover that person should not have a vested interest, that is they should be independent of all the main stakeholders. In the UK a variety of non-profit organisations, such as Mencap. BILD and seAp provide advocacy services for individuals with intellectual disabilities. While these services tend not to foreground risk taking, they do highlight the role of advocacy in enabling individuals to make their own choices and to be independent. For example, seAp (an acronym for Support, Empower, Advocate and Promote) describes advocacy in the following way:

"Advocacy means to speak up for someone. With the help of an advocate people with learning [intellectual] disabilities can gain control over their lives, make their own choices about what happens to them and be as independent as possible."

seAp, n.d.

If independent advocates are to facilitate risk taking then they need the trust of all the key participants and the ability to communicate effectively. The next chapter in this book will encourage you to find out about different advocacy services in your area.

The importance of trust and good communication

Risk-taking involves managing the uncertainties associated with decision making. If an individual lacks the knowledge to assess such risks then they either have to hope for the best or rely on and trust others to assess risks for them. An individual with an intellectual disability who has an advocate must be able to trust that their advocate has the ability to act in and represent their interests (Alaszewski, 2003).

However, where an independent advocate becomes involved, this often indicates that there is some tension between the person with intellectual disability, their parents or relatives and employed carers and/or professionals. The relationship between the person with intellectual disability and their parents or professional carers may have broken down and become one of distrust. Some agencies recognise the possibility of tension with relatives albeit not paid carers. One social service department included the following statement in their specification of who should be involved in decision making:

"There may be some occasions when the person who has a learning [intellectual] disability may express a wish not to involve close relatives in planning and making decisions about their lives. Where this is the case, consideration needs to be given to the importance of their relatives accepting and co-operating with the plans or decisions. Where [a relative is excluded from the] decision making process [this] may lead to conflict, [and] this needs to be explained and discussed with the person with a learning [intellectual] disability."

Alaszewski et al, 1999, p. 40

There is scope for the relationship between parents and professional carers to break down, especially over risk taking. Parents are aware of, and concerned about, the vulnerability of the person with intellectual disability. Parents often have horror stories where their child has been exposed to unacceptable risks (Heyman and Huckle, 1993, p. 1560). In our own study (Alaszewski et al, 2000), we were also told horror stories such as:

"We went to two or three places with Amy ... One of the places was the queerest place I've ever been in my life. We took Amy through the door and the first thing we got was two blokes fighting ... there was one of them on the floor and the other one was kicking the crap out of him ... I didn't want to leave her there ... The other place; well while Amy was there she lost three-quarters of her finger. We don't know how she lost it ... She lost about an inch and half of her finger and they said she must have bitten it off ... it's a great person that could have bitten off like that, never mind a handicapped person ... We think she lost it in a door or something like that."

Alaszewski et al, 2000

However, the participants in our study were not opposed to risk taking per se, indeed they recognised that day care and residential facilities could provide risk taking opportunities that they were unwilling to provide themselves:

"When my sister came here they wanted her to go sailing, now she can't even swim ... she doesn't like water. So I wouldn't have let her go, to be honest, but they were happy to do that."

The parents in our study trusted that the individuals supporting their relative would take reasonable risks. One parent stressed the importance of trust in the following way:

"With most of children not able to speak, you have to have trust, because they couldn't really tell us if there was something wrong; anyway ... we have to believe that what we are told happens to them does happen."

An important element of this trusting relationship was effective communication both with the staff providing the support and also with the service user. Relatives recognised that sometimes things might not work out as planned but they wanted staff to be open and honest when things went wrong. One parent in our study said

"I mean that they have a very good policy of communication with us so if there are any problems they do ring, they don't just sweep anything under the carpet

... you're not thinking, 'Oh, what's going on behind my back?' all the time or anything."

Communication with the person with intellectual disability is more limited but crucial. Relatives want evidence that things are well. Another parent emphasised the importance of non-verbal communication:

"When John was being moved around, trying to find a residential spot for him, we tried three residential homes, and, although he can't talk, he can't tell us, he

---

READER ACTIVITY 6.3   Learning from and avoiding past errors

It is easy to assume that risk is just about the future, about how choices or decisions are likely to play out. However, as Douglas (1992) has observed, risk also plays an important role in making sense of the past, particularly in making sense of poor decisions and bad choices. In the global North, risk plays a key role in making sense of misfortune through the use of hindsight to identify the failure of foresight and the allocation of blame. In this exercise we would like you to consider what lessons can be learnt from disasters. In most democratic countries, disasters, such as the failure to protect individuals with intellectual disabilities are often the subject of open public inquiries, and if this is the case in your country then access and read a report on one such disaster. However, if you are unable to access a report, then you may wish to read the *Independent investigation into the death of CS* (Hussain and Hyde-Bales, 2014). This refers to the investigation into the death of Connor Sparrowhawk. There are a series of reports that explore the wider context of this case as well as newspaper articles, all accessible via an internet search. Once you have read one of the inquiry reports please consider and reflect on the following issues:

- Identify the terms of references of the inquiry and consider how and in what way risk features in them
- Can you identify why the inquiry was set up?
- Briefly summarise the key events and how they resulted in a harmful outcome
- Who was responsible for the care of Connor Sparrowhawk (or the individual(s) in the report you have chosen)?

- Outline what action or inaction contributed to his death (or their harm)
- Who do you think was to blame?

While the past and future seem different—in the past things have happened and cannot be changed while in the future nothing has happened and therefore anything can happen—the concept of risk in the global North, like the concept of sin in religious societies, weaves the past, present and future together. Risk is not just about predicting the future it is also about allocating blame for the past misfortune. In many of the reports on modern disasters there is often a whistle-blower who warned about the poor choices and decisions but whose warnings were ignored. While each disaster is unique, they do tend to share common features. Looking back with the benefit of hindsight, it is clear that the knowledge that would have prevented the disaster did exist at the time but for various reasons, senior managers disregarded information. They did not listen to whistle-blowers, parents and/or front-line staff. Kieran Walsh reviewed Inquiries in the British NHS from 1969 to 2001 and identified five common features of health care disasters:

- The organisational or geographic isolation of the service in which the disaster occurred
- Failure of leadership
- Failure of systems and processes
- Poor communication so early warnings or near misses are ignored
- Lack of a voice for front line staff or patients or clients so problems emerging at the 'coalface' are hidden (Walsh, 2003, pp. 3–4)

walked out of one and he just wouldn't entertain it and the social worker said, 'Well he's voted with his feet, hasn't he!'"

CONCLUSION

Risk taking is a part of every life and people with intellectual disabilities should have a right to their fair share. Identifying what sort of risks a person would like to take is facilitated by communication, and when individuals have limited ability to communicate it can be a challenge to identify their choices and preferences. However, advocates using trust and sensitive communication can play an important role in enabling individuals with intellectual disabilities to take risks.

REFERENCES

Alaszewski, A. (2003). Risk, trust and health. *Health, Risk and Society, 5*(3), 235–239.

Alaszewski, A., & Alaszewski, H. (2002). Towards the creative management of risk: perceptions, practices and policies. *British Journal of Learning Disabilities, 30*(2), 56–62.

Alaszewski, A., & Ong, B. N. (Eds.). (1990). *Normalisation in practice.* London and New York: Routledge.

Alaszewski, A., Alaszewski, A., Ayer, S., et al. (2000). *Managing risk in community practice: nursing, risk and decision making.* Edinburgh: Baillière Tindall.

Alaszewski, H., Parker, A., & Alaszewski, A. (1999). *Empowerment and protection: the development of policies and practices in risk assessment and risk management in services for adults with learning disabilities.* London: The Mental Health Foundation.

Atkinson, D., & Williams, F. (1990). *Know me as I am': an anthology of prose, poetry and art by people with learning difficulties,* London: Hodder and Stoughton.

Brookes, I., Archibald, S., McInnes, K., et al. (2012). Finding the words to work together: developing a research design to explore risk and adult protection in co-produced research. *British Journal of Learning Disabilities, 20*(3), 143–151.

Brown, P. (2016). Trust and risk. In A. Burgess, A. Alemanno, & J. Zinn (Eds.), *2016 Routledge handbook of risk studies.* London: Routledge.

Carter, T. S., & Connor, J. M. (2005). *Legal risk management checklists for charities.* Available at: http://www.krausehouse.ca/krause/Tennis/CCITCRiskManagement.pdf. [Accessed 26 March 2020].

Douglas, M. (1992). *Risk and blame: essays in cultural theory.* London: Routledge.

Giddens, A. (1991). *Modernity and self-identity: self and society in the late modern age.* Cambridge: Polity Press.

Greenhill, B., & Whitehead, R. (2010). Promoting service user inclusion in risk assessment and management: a pilot project developing a human rights–based approach. *British Journal of Learning Disabilities, 39*(4), 277–283.

Heyman, B., & Huckle, S. (1993). Not worth the risk? Attitudes of adults with learning difficulties and their informal carers to the hazards of everyday life. *Social Science & Medicine, 37,* 1557–1564.

Heyman, B., Huckle, S., & Handyside, E. C. (1998). Freedom of the locality for people with learning difficulties. In B. Heyman (Ed.), *Risk, health and health care: a qualitative approach.* London: Arnold.

Hussain, T., & Hyde-Bales, K. (2014). *Independent investigation into the death of CS: a report for Southern Health NHS Foundation Trust.* London: Verita. Available at: http://www.Southernhealth.nhs.uk/EasySiteWeb/GatewayLink.aspx?alid=76277. [Accessed 1 April 2020].

Jenkins, N. E. (2006). 'You can't wrap them up in cotton wool!' Constructing risk in young people's access to outdoor play. *Health, Risk & Society, 8*(4), 379–393.

Kendall, A., & Dodson, G. (2016). Introduction. In A. Alaszewski & B. N. Ong (Eds.), *Normalisation in practice: residential care for children with a profound mental handicap.* London and New York: Routledge.

Näslund, R., & Gardelli, A. (2013). 'I know, I can, I will try': youths and adults with intellectual disabilities in Sweden using information and communication technology in their everyday life. *Disability & Society, 28*(1), 28–40.

Parker, J., & Stanworth, H. (2005). 'Go for it!' Towards a critical realist approach to voluntary risk-taking. *Health, Risk & Society, 7*(4), 319–336.

Robertson, J. P., & Collinson, C. (2011). Positive risk taking: whose risk is it? An exploration in community outreach teams in adult mental health and learning disability services. *Health, Risk & Society, 13*(2), 147–164.

seAp. (n.d.). Advocacy for adults with learning disabilities. Available at: https://www.seap.org.uk/services/learning-disability-advocacy/. [Accessed 5 September 2019].

Sebrechts, M., Tonkens, E., & Bröer, C. (2018). Rituals of recognition: interactions and interaction rules in sheltered workshops in the Netherlands. *European Journal of Cultural and Political Sociology, 5*(4), 455–475.

Thompson, J. D. (2000). Vulnerability, dangerousness and risk: the case of men with learning disabilities who sexually abuse. *Health, Risk & Society, 2*(1), 33–46.

Walshe, K. (2003). Inquiries: learning from failure in the NHS? London: The Nuffield Trust. Available at: https://www.nuffieldtrust.org.uk/files/2017-01/inquiries-learning-from-failure-nhs-web-final.pdf. [Accessed 2 April 2020].

Wolfensberger, W. (1972). *The principle of normalization in human services*. Toronto: National Institute of Mental Retardation.

Zinn, J. O. (2016). 'In-between' and other reasonable ways to deal with risk and uncertainty: a review article. *Health, Risk & Society*, *18*(7-8), 348–366.

7

Self-advocacy and advocacy

Ruth Garbutt and Anne-Marie Callus

KEY ISSUES

- Historically people with intellectual disabilities have not always had choice and control over their lives.
- Self-advocacy is a key way in which people with intellectual disabilities can have a voice and ultimately more choice and control.
- There are different types of advocacy which centre on: an individual speaking up for themselves; an individual speaking up for someone else; and a group of people speaking up together.
- Those who support people with intellectual disabilities should aim to promote self-advocacy in

their practice by supporting people to speak up for themselves.

- Sometimes, it will still be necessary to speak up on behalf of people with intellectual disabilities.
- Policy and legislation support the promotion of self-advocacy.
- The values and attitudes of those who support people with intellectual disabilities are very important in relation to self-advocacy and advocacy.

CHAPTER OUTLINE

INTRODUCTION

The processes of supporting people with intellectual disabilities to speak up for themselves through self-advocacy and by advocating on their behalf both embody the social model of disability (Oliver, 1990, 1996), since they focus on what can be changed in the environment to remove disabling barriers, to uphold disabled people's rights and to ensure that they participate in decision-making processes. As this chapter shows, values and attitudes are very important in self-advocacy and advocacy. We need to start with an attitude of seeing a person with an intellectual disability as

an individual, with their own will and preferences, their own specific goals and aspirations, and with the right to have a voice, make choices and to contribute to their community. Therefore both self-advocacy and advocacy are relevant for those providing support for people with intellectual disabilities. The principles underlying self-advocacy and advocacy emphasise the need to work in a shared and participatory way with people with intellectual disabilities, listening to them and focusing on enabling them to achieve their dreams and goals. They are relevant to those living and working with people with intellectual disabilities across the world, even if they are put into practice in different ways in different sociocultural contexts.

This chapter starts with an overview of the history of self-advocacy from its origins to its developments. Different types of self-advocacy and advocacy are described including a discussion on how a self-advocacy group works. The wider context of substitute and supported decision making is then discussed. The chapter ends with the skills that supporters need to foster when doing work in self-advocacy and advocacy. The chapter also includes activities and an online case study for further exploration of these issues by the reader.

HISTORY OF SELF-ADVOCACY

Self-advocacy can simply mean speaking up for and representing oneself, but for people with intellectual disabilities, it also has additional and more complex meanings. Historically, disabled people have been voiceless, and have been represented from the perspectives of (mostly non-disabled) supporters, family members and benefactors (Driedger, 1989). In fact early on, the disabled people's movement adopted the slogan 'Nothing about us without us' (Charlton, 1998). However, this movement did not include people with intellectual disabilities from its inception, as attested by Campbell and Oliver (1996) and Chappell (1998) among others.

The first people to speak up for the rights of people with intellectual disabilities were their parents and their first campaign was deinstitutionalisation, especially in Scandinavian countries, the UK and North America (Dybwad, 1996). The institutions that had been built in the 19th century in these countries were initially intended to help children with intellectual disabilities to develop and thus be able to return home. However, as Shapland (2019) explains, they evolved into places where these children were effectively abandoned. Mansell and Ericsson (1995) explain how parents in Scandinavia were the first to campaign for community-based residences for their children with intellectual disabilities after the Second World War, followed by parents in the United States. The work of these parents eventually inspired the Campaign for people with Mental Handicaps (CMH) in Britain in the 1970s. Parents have also played key roles in campaigns for the rights of people with intellectual disabilities in many other countries, including Japan (Tsuda, 2006) and Malta (Camilleri and Callus, 2001). In some countries, people with intellectual disabilities themselves who lived in institutions started

to mobilise as a reaction against the horrors of institutionalisation (see for example Hutton et al, 2017, about the campaigning of survivors of institutions in Canada and Mitchell et al, 2006, about their British equivalents).

Another factor that gave momentum to the campaign for the rights of people with intellectual disabilities was normalisation, which originated in Nordic countries (Kebbon, 1997). Normalisation attempted to promote lifestyles for people with intellectual disabilities that were as close as possible to everyday living (Wolfensberger, 1972). O'Brien (1987a) promoted normalisation and the empowerment of people with intellectual disabilities through making sure they had choices, that they were respected and that they were able to participate within their community.

The principles of normalisation are therefore similar to those of self-advocacy, even if the means to putting them into practice vary. It was also around the time when normalisation was being developed that self-advocacy groups started forming. In 1974 the first self-advocacy convention happened in Oregon, USA, when the name 'People First' was adopted (Perske, 1996).

Self-advocacy in the UK developed as a result of a few people with intellectual disabilities from the UK attending a People First conference in the USA in 1984, and on their return, setting up their own People First in London (Hersov, 1996). By the mid-1990s, Dybwad (1996) could write that

> [f]rom its sporadic, tentative beginnings in the 1970s, self-advocacy … has brought forth a well-organized, internationally connected movement that provides an ever-growing voice to what was, until the recent past, a universally rejected minority among a nation's minorities (p. 15).

In the UK, CMH later developed a self-advocacy pack in which they describe the reason for the term 'People First':

> "'People First' is a statement by the members that they are human beings first and that their disabilities are second. People First is a statement that people with disabilities desire to be seen as people who have value and dignity, to be seen as people who can participate and contribute to the community."
>
> CMH, 1986, p. 4

Dybwad and Bersani's (1996) book attests to the development of self-advocacy in Anglophone countries and Scandinavia. Since then, self-advocacy groups have grown in many parts of the world and they are present, to various extents, in, among other countries, Austria, Brazil, Croatia, Germany, India, Italy, Hong Kong, Malaysia, Malta and Romania (Grupp Flimkien Naslu, 2019; Self-advocacy.net, 2019; Soares de Carvalho and Forrester-Jones, 2016; Voices Together, 2019). There are also international networks. The most notable is Inclusion International which also has regional federations in the Middle East and North Africa, Europe, Africa, the Americas and Asia Pacific (Inclusion International, 2020). The model used by Inclusion International and its affiliated organisations is for people with intellectual disabilities and their families to advocate for their rights together.

A number of studies have explored the experience and practice of self-advocacy (e.g. Beart et al, 2004; Dybwad and Bersani, 1996; Gilmartin and Slevin, 2010; Goodley, 2000; Hanna, 1978; Mitchell, 1997; Shoultz, 1997a,b,c; Simons, 1992; Sutcliffe and Simons, 1993; Williams, 1982; Williams and Shoultz, 1982). These studies show how people with intellectual disabilities have developed their own self-advocacy groups and some of the difficulties the self-advocacy movement faces.

The way that self-advocacy has developed in different countries is inevitably influenced by the prevailing culture of each country where it is introduced. One of the best analyses in this regard is that carried out by Tsuda, (2006) about the development of self-advocacy groups in Japan. As both this author and Oka (2013) note, Japanese culture is not homogenous, nor is it untouched by European and American influences. However, both authors also note how these influences have merged with those traditional aspects of Japanese society that have endured. Therefore, the idea of self-determination – which is common to self-advocacy and self-help groups – is inevitably adapted in a culture that favours an emphasis on community and on living 'in a structure of mutual dependence' (Tsuda, 2006 p. 153). In Malta, self-advocacy has developed in a culture that considers parents, or other close family members, as having primary responsibility for decisions concerning the lives of people with intellectual disabilities (Callus, 2013).

Variations in cultures mean that it is difficult to arrive at a comprehensive definition, or even description, of self-advocacy. Ken Simons, who was one of the pioneers in developing self-advocacy in the UK, describes it as:

"a process of individual development through which a person comes to have the confidence and ability to express his or her own feelings and wishes."

Simons, 1992, p. 5

It is therefore envisaged as a process whereby a person speaks up or acts for themselves (Williams and Shoultz, 1982). This can be through peer-advocacy or as an individual, involving such skills as being able to express thoughts and feelings with assertiveness, to make choices and decisions, having clear knowledge of rights and to make changes (Clare, 1990).

Another important aspect of self-advocacy is the role that people, other than those who have intellectual disabilities, play in it. It is worth noting that the self-advocacy of people with intellectual disabilities was partly made possible through the growing realisation of how much they could achieve in a supportive environment. As Dybwad (1996) notes

'people with intellectual impairments have – **in my lifetime** – gone from "feebleminded patients" to empowered agents of social change' (p. 16, author's emphasis).'

Self-advocacy therefore thrives in environments where those who are closely involved in the lives of people with intellectual disabilities see them as capable of representing themselves and provide the necessary support for them to do so. Conversely, in environments where people with intellectual disabilities are considered to be totally dependent on others, even being seen as eternal children, it is very difficult for them to become self-advocates. This is because, in such a context, their lives are likely to be controlled by other adults who do not give them the opportunity to speak up for themselves and who decide, on their behalf, what is best for them. Consequently, an extremely important aspect of self-advocacy is that support is provided – very often by non-disabled people – for people with intellectual disabilities to speak up for themselves.

If one takes self-advocacy as simply meaning speaking up for oneself, the role of the other person may seem to undermine the idea that people with intellectual disabilities can be self-advocates. However, a person can *both* receive support *and* be able to speak up for themselves. Those providing support within a self-advocacy framework do so in a way that enables people with intellectual disabilities to take decisions and act on them.

READER ACTIVITY 7.1

Self-advocacy means speaking up for and represent-ing oneself.

Think about the place where you work or anywhere where you support people with intellectual disabili-ties. To what extent can you demonstrate that the self-advocacy of people with intellectual disabilities is upheld?

READER ACTIVITY 7.2

Think of a self-advocacy group that you know of. Which category would it fit into: the autonomous or ideal model, the divisional model, the coalition model or the service system model?

If you do not know of any self-advocacy groups, think about what kind of group could be set up within the boundaries of your own professional practice.

SELF-ADVOCACY AND OTHER TYPES OF ADVOCACY

Having discussed the history and background of self-advocacy for people with intellectual disabilities, it is important to outline the different types of self-advocacy and to also explore other types of advocacy, namely: citizen-advocacy, collective advocacy, parent advocacy, peer advocacy, short-term/crisis advocacy, legal advo-cacy, systemic advocacy and professional advocacy.

In any given interaction between supporters and peo-ple with intellectual disabilities, advocacy is usually con-sidered when seeking to create change in a person's life. This change can happen through 3 main ways: an individ-ual speaking up for themselves, a person speaking up for someone else and a group of people speaking up together.

People speaking up for themselves
Self-advocacy groups

Apart from referring to a person with an intellectual disability speaking up on an individual basis, the term 'self-advocacy' is also used to refer to groups of peo-ple with intellectual disabilities who work together. In self-advocacy groups, a clear distinction in role is made between the people with intellectual disabilities and their supporters. The former are usually called self-advocates. They are the ones who make decisions. The latter, those who provide support (who tend to be non-disabled people), are there to enable the group members to act on the decisions taken (Chapman, 2005). These groups have various labels including self-advocacy groups, speak-out/up groups, Student Council, trainee committees, working groups and People First.

Crawley (1988) provided an early definition of four key models of self-advocacy groups. In the main, these definitions still hold today and are described below:

i) The 'autonomous' or 'ideal' model

These groups are independent from formal services and will often employ an independent advisor or coor-dinator. They benefit from being independent because they can express their concerns and stand up for their rights without worries about recrimination. The advi-sor/coordinator has no conflicts of interest.

ii) The 'divisional' model

This type is formed as a sub-group of an existing organisation. Examples include Speak Up groups within a Mencap service or a self-advocacy group within an established advocacy agency. These groups can ben-efit from the venues and financial and administrative resources of the organisation. However, there can be a conflict of interest between the self-advocates' requests and the supporters' views. Another disadvantage is that the group can be subservient to the organisation and the organisation would have power in how much priority to give the group amidst its other priorities.

iii) The 'coalition' model

These are usually sub-groups of a wider disability rights organisation, such as the Derbyshire Coalition for Inclusive Living (UK). The advantages here are that people with intellectual disabilities are able to tap into a wider political campaigning process, develop a posi-tive identity as a disabled person and possibly acquire more funding. However, the danger is that people with intellectual disabilities could be overshadowed by more articulate, politically aware members.

iv) The 'service-system' model

These groups are based in a service setting, such as a residents' group within supported accommodation. The advantage of this model is that it has access to trans-port, venues and other resources. It is also easy to access people to make up the group. However, disadvantages include the conflict of interest when members of the self-advocacy group challenge the system or structure of the service. In some cases, this has been known to stop the group (Shearer, 1986).

These four models continue to be used today and are seen as a useful tool to help to identify different types of advocacy groups (see Goodley, 2000). In a recent study by Mallander et al (2018) undertaken in Sweden, they also link these models to 2 theoretical frameworks of Resource-Dependency Perspectives (RDP) and New Institutional Perspectives (NIP) (Johansson, 2006; Fligstein, 2007; Wooten and Hoffman, 2008). In the RDP framework, there is a particular focus on the issues around power and resources, whilst the NIP framework focuses on institutional norms, values and actions. Mallander et al (2018) use the key elements of these theoretical frameworks to compare 2 different types of self-advocacy group in Sweden. In particular, they compare and contrast the groups in relation to organisational field, affinity/membership, expectations of the groups, the role of supporters, power, and control/sanctions.

As a result of being involved in a self-advocacy group, members find that they can influence change and develop skills such as confidence, self-esteem, responsibility, sensitivity, assertiveness, a sense of identity, improved social skills, a greater ability to express themselves and communication (Beart et al, 2004; Gilmartin and Slevin, 2009; Stalker, 1997). They also gain knowledge about the advocacy movement, their own rights and local and wider systems and structures.

How does a self-advocacy group work?

Downer and Ferns (1993) state that a self-advocacy group is defined by the following characteristics:

- Independent of services and workers.
- Has funding without any 'strings' attached.
- Controlled by people with learning difficulties [intellectual disabilities].
- Advised by experienced disabled people and/or non-disabled people skilled in enabling self-advocacy.
- Not shaped by the 'outside' expectations of non-disabled people.
- Given space and time to grow and develop.
- Built on the strength of the group members.
- Taken seriously by services which should not pretend to support self-advocacy when they really do not.
- Has its advice and decisions listened to carefully and acted upon by service workers.
- Has real power and representation in important decisions about services which affect users' lives.
- Becomes a pressure group for positive change in services.
- Empowers group members to change their own lives with the support of other disabled people.

In general, the direction and agenda of most self-advocacy groups is led by the service users. Usually, the group will elect officers to be in the position of chairperson, deputy chairperson, secretary and treasurer. Other people might take on other roles such as helping with refreshments, photocopying the agenda for the meeting, welcoming new people, etc. The minutes and agenda of the meeting would be in an accessible format, such as easy words and pictures. When a group includes people with severe intellectual disabilities, care has to be taken to make sure their views and wishes are expressed. This could happen by an advocate or trusted friend or professional finding out in the previous week what concerns that person has or comments they may want to make. This could be written down for the chairperson of the group to read out at the meeting so that it can be discussed. Communication aids, the use of Makaton or sign language, pictures or photographs might also be appropriate during the meeting so that a person with a severe intellectual disability might be involved (see also Chapters 4 and 5).

In the 'forming' period of the group, emphasis would be on building friendships and trust, developing skills and gaining an understanding of how groups work. Over time, the members of the group would bring their individual and collective concerns to the group and the group would consider their course of action to address the concerns. Examples of issues a group could address include the following:

- Campaigning to the local council for extensions to the hours a disabled person can use their bus pass.
- Better lockers in the day centre.
- Better choice of food in the residential accommodation.
- Investigating hate crime in the area.
- Inviting speakers (such as police, policy makers, researchers, nurses, etc.) to come and talk about a topic of concern.
- Making contact with another self-advocacy group to exchange ideas and meet together.

The role of the advisor of a self-advocacy group

Most self-advocacy groups have an advisor. The advisor can be an independent paid worker, someone working in a voluntary capacity or an existing member of staff of a service or organisation. The advisor should have some knowledge of the local systems, services and structures, and an understanding of the issues involved for people with intellectual disabilities. Most of all, the advisor should uphold the social model of disability and should embody the beliefs, values and principles of self-advocacy.

The advisor's role includes building up the skills of the members of the group and supporting the group in their discussions of possible options and courses of action. The advisor has a responsibility and commitment to the group and is there to be utilised in the way in which the members require. Essentially the advisor can be seen as a resource for the group.

Peer advocacy

'Peer advocacy' is a model where people with intellectual disabilities who have developed confidence, assertiveness and related skills speak up on behalf of their peers, that is other people with intellectual disabilities, who may not yet have developed these skills. For example it could be older people with intellectual disabilities speaking up for younger people with intellectual disabilities (Power et al, 2016; TLAP, 2014). It can also be people with intellectual disabilities joining forces to speak up in solidarity with each other and through mutual empowerment as described by Tideman and Svensson (2015) regarding a Swedish self-advocacy group.

Systemic advocacy

Some self-advocacy groups focus on issues that impact directly on the lives of the members, for example, problems with service-provision or with welfare benefits. Others seek to create change for people with intellectual disabilities more generally. This approach is called systemic advocacy because it aims at bringing about changes to the system. Rich (2015) refers to systemic advocacy in connection with self-advocacy work that is directed at changing laws, public policy and models of service-provision, for example, campaigning for the closure of institutions or for better working conditions for people with intellectual disabilities (a self-advocacy group can of course also fulfil both functions).

A person speaking up for someone with an intellectual disability

Parent/Family advocacy

Parents and families are often required to stand up for their family member with an intellectual disability, especially when the latter is young or if they have additional needs or communication difficulties. Parents and families will often have substantial contact with various supporters and will invariably need to speak up on behalf of their family member on a daily basis. Over time, parents develop wide knowledge about services, systems and structures and find creative ways to try and make their voice heard. As their family member becomes older, with more confidence and skills of their own, tensions can develop between self-advocacy, professional advocacy and family advocacy. For example, in a study by Chadwick et al (2013) which used focus groups to find out about the experiences of family carers of people with intellectual disabilities in Ireland, it was found that key areas of difficulty included:

> "… gaining access to adequate and appropriate supports, services, information and resources for the family, the difficulties in relationships and communication between families and services and professionals; and the need to advocate and fight for services."
>
> *Chadwick et al, 2013*, p. 129

Citizen advocacy

Citizen advocacy was originally conceived by Wolfensberger and Zauha (1973) and supports the notion of attempting to 'import' ordinary aspects of life into services for people with intellectual disabilities. In the citizen advocacy model, a volunteer trained worker (a citizen advocate) is partnered with an individual who finds it difficult to speak up for themselves, with the objective that the advocate will promote and defend the interests of the 'partner'.

A citizen advocate may do many things with the person with an intellectual disability, such as helping that person to deal with personal issues, representing that person at an important meeting such as a case conference, helping to press for changes in a person's living arrangements, or helping a couple get married despite opposition from parents (Pochin, 2002, cited in Gray and Jackson, 2002).

The strength of citizen advocacy is in the appointment of an *independent* person from outside a service who acts on behalf of another person. People with profound and severe intellectual disabilities, who may not be able to express their own will and preferences, can benefit from having an independent citizen advocate appointed to them to help them uphold their rights and represent their views:

> *"Citizen advocacy is needed for people with severe learning disabilities because their access to services and other facilities may depend on their having someone to speak up on their behalf … citizen advocates are needed because others involved in the lives of people with learning disabilities are likely to have pressures on them which prevent them from being independent and objective."*
>
> *Brooke and Harris, 2000.*

Citizen advocacy is well developed in the US (O'Brien, 1987b; Ward, 1986; Wolfensberger and Zauha, 1973), Netherlands and Scandinavia (Cambridge and Ernst, 2006; Health Equality Europe, 2006) but has been slower to develop in the UK and other parts of Europe (Ledger and Tilley, 2006; Traustadottir, 2006).

Short term/crisis advocacy

'Short-term or crisis advocacy' is where an advocate is brought in to stand up for a person who has a particularly pressing or crisis issue, such as having to move house without much warning or a serious medical issue. It is useful if the advocate is someone who has built up a trusting relationship with the service user in the past so that the service user is confident that their views will be represented.

Legal advocacy

'Legal advocacy' is the process of representing clients before courts and tribunals, speaking in court and examining witnesses as part of a professional duty and legal system (Pannick, 1993). Legal advocacy involves debating complex points of law and requires considerable legal training. Legal advocacy is also typically based on a contractual or financial relationship, which does not usually happen in advocacy within health and social care professions or many other settings (Bateman, 2000).

Professional advocacy

Social workers, nurses, care workers, community development workers and other professionals may often be required to play an advocacy role. This can be referred to as 'professional advocacy'. For example, the Professional Standards of Social Work England (2020) include the need for social workers to value each person as an individual, promote the human rights, views, wishes and feelings of individuals, and to enable their access to advocacy as appropriate. From an international perspective, Jugessor and Iles (2009, p. 31) state that:

> *"As a core value in international nursing dominated by western nursing concepts and theories (Davis et al. 2003), advocacy has gained prominence in the Asia-Pacific region, Europe and North America (Leong & Euller-Ziegler 2004), with clients' rights being given prominence in both healthcare reform policies and legislation (Davis et al. 2003)."*
>
> *Jugessor and Iles, 2009, p. 31*

When acting as an advocate within service provision, it is important to be aware of possible conflicts of interest between the service and the needs of people with intellectual disabilities. There is also a specific power relation between the former and the latter. Schwartz (2002), for example, in research looking at the role of health care professionals in patient advocacy in Canada, found that there seemed to be a confusion between a):

> *"advocating for what the patient wants, even if this may not be what the professional thinks is best for the patient and b) doing what the advocate believes is in the patient's best interest, even if this overrides the patient's expressed needs."*
>
> *Schwartz, 2002, p. 38*

The supporter in this case cannot claim to be 'independent'. However, they can provide advocacy that may be appropriate in certain contexts. In situations of abuse, for example, there is a clear expectation within professional standards for a nurse, social worker, or another professional, to advocate on behalf of the person with an intellectual disability (Royal College of Nursing, 2020).

People with intellectual disabilities speaking up together with others

Collective advocacy

'Collective advocacy' is similar to self-advocacy but it is a term used to describe more the way in which groups or user-led organisations raise public awareness, lobby policy makers, become involved in the wider disability movement, have political and economic power and campaign for better treatment and services (CAPS Independent Advocacy, 2020). This approach can bring together people with different types of disabilities, for example as described by Hutchison et al (2007) about user-led disability organisations in Canada. Collective advocacy thus brings people with intellectual disabilities together with other people to have a shared voice in improving rights and working to change the structures of society.

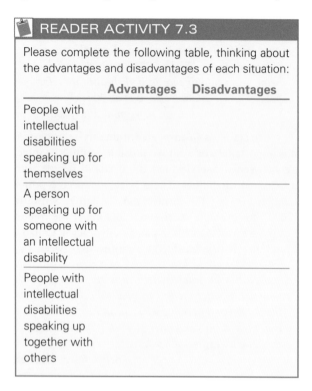

READER ACTIVITY 7.3

Please complete the following table, thinking about the advantages and disadvantages of each situation:

	Advantages	Disadvantages
People with intellectual disabilities speaking up for themselves		
A person speaking up for someone with an intellectual disability		
People with intellectual disabilities speaking up together with others		

This section has indicated the various types of advocacy a supporter might come across in relation to people with intellectual disabilities. Certain types might be more prominent in some countries than others (for instance, citizen advocacy has been more prominent in the USA; parent advocacy is more prominent in countries which have a strong family focus such as Malta (see Azzopardi, 2000). An issue of key importance, regardless of the type of advocacy used, is for people with intellectual disabilities to have a voice and to have their own choices in the way they live their lives. This issue is addressed in the next section.

SUBSTITUTE AND SUPPORTED DECISION MAKING

One of the results of campaigns by the disability rights movement, including by self-advocates with intellectual disabilities, has been an acknowledgement of the importance of establishing the rights of disabled people through legislation. The first disability-related anti-discrimination law was the Americans with Disability Act in 1990. In the following decade, many countries followed suit and enacted their own laws (Breslin and Yee, 2002). In addition, the European Convention of Human Rights (1953) protects human rights and political freedoms in 47 European countries. More recently, in 2006, the United Nations adopted the Convention on the Rights of Persons with Disabilities (UNCRPD) which actively promotes the right of disabled persons to have choice in, and control over, their own lives. This right is upheld most strongly in Article 12 which recognises the capacity of disabled persons to make decisions about their own lives and to act on them (United Nations, 2006). Significantly, Article 12 does not make any distinction regarding type or severity of impairment, thereby asserting that *all* disabled persons have legal capacity.

The implementation of the UNCRPD is monitored by the Committee on the Rights of Persons with Disabilities (henceforth referred to as the Committee). In 2014, this Committee published a General Comment on Article 12, emphasising the need for governments to remove substitute decision-making laws from their statute books and replace it with supported decision-making legislation. Substitute decision-making refers to the practice of removing a disabled person's ability to make decisions and vesting a court-appointed person with the power to make decisions on the disabled person's behalf (Fundamental Rights Agency, 2013). In their General Comment, the Committee (2014) observe that people with intellectual disabilities are among those most disproportionately affected by this type of legislation. There are different types of substitute decision-making laws. These include interdiction and incapacitation, where a person is rendered totally powerless to make any decision, such as signing a housing or employment contract or spending their own money. With other laws, such as guardianship, the level of restriction varies. With plenary guardianship, a person also has their rights taken away from them completely. With partial guardianship, the restriction of rights affects certain aspects of life (for example, in the administration of finances and property). Whether or not a substitute decision-making order covers all or some rights, court-appointed substitute decision-makers are obliged to act in what they deem to be the disabled person's best interest, rather than according to the person's rights, will and preferences, as required by Article 12 of the UNCRPD.

Another problematic aspect of substitute decision-making legislation is that it fails to distinguish between legal and mental capacities. In fact, as the Committee's (2014) General Comment states, these two concepts are often conflated. This conflation comes at a price for those disabled people whose mental capacity to take decisions and act on them may be impaired – including those who have intellectual disabilities. Despite these problems with substitute decision-making, in many jurisdictions this type of legislation is still in force, including the majority of countries that have ratified the UNCRPD.

The Committee (2014) explain that legal capacity is every person's inherent right and refers to 'the ability to hold rights and duties (legal standing) and to exercise those rights and duties (legal agency)' (p. 3). Without legal capacity, a person essentially does not have any rights. For example, a person with an intellectual disability who is under plenary guardianship – and has therefore had all their decision-making rights taken away – cannot enter into an employment contract without the guardian's signature. By law, the guardian has the right to decide whether or not to sign the contract on the basis of what they assume to be in the disabled person's best interest, even if this goes against the will and preference of that person.

As the Committee (2014) continues to explain,

'mental capacity refers to the decision-making skills of a person, which naturally vary from one person to another and may be different for a given person depending on many factors, including environmental and social factors' (p. 3).

Significantly, environmental and social factors are taken into consideration here. A person's decision-making skills are not fixed and can be developed given the right kind of support.

As mentioned above, in their General Comment, the Committee on the Rights of Persons with Disabilities (2014) call for the enactment of supported decision-making legislation, since this addresses all of the concerns associated with substitute decision-making. First of all, it does not take away the disabled person's right to make their own decisions. The person thus retains their legal capacity. Secondly, it makes a distinction between legal and mental capacity. This means that, at the same time as asserting legal capacity as an inherent right, it also acknowledges that some people need support with decision-making. However, since the person's legal capacity is retained, any support provided must be in line with the person's rights, will and preferences. Thus, in the example provided above, a court-appointed supported decision-maker would need to work with the person with an intellectual disability to consider whether the employment they are interested in is the right one for them and whether any support needs to be put in place for the employment to be successful. A third important aspect of supported decision-making is that it is the disabled person who chooses who will provide them with support (Disability Rights Maine, 2019).

One of the objections levelled at supported decision-making is that not all disabled people are in a position to choose who should support them and in what. This is the case, for instance, for people with profound and multiple intellectual disabilities. In such cases, it is the people who live most closely with them who can interpret what the disabled person's will and preferences are (Watson, 2011). This particular process of decision-making can take place within what are known as circles of support, which can comprise family members, friends and staff working with the disabled person. Together, they can help the latter identify their wishes and aspirations and then support them to achieve their goals (Wistow et al, 2016). These circles of support can be informal or they can have legal status (see the discussion by Zhang et al, 2019, about supported decision-making circles in the United States). The fact that there is a group of people working together with the person with an intellectual disability can generate disagreements about the decisions to be taken. When a circle works well, compromises can be found. Although the process of reaching an agreement can be challenging at times, it can help ensure that any decision taken is in line with the preferences of the person concerned (especially in cases where the person cannot directly express their opinion due to profound and multiple intellectual disabilities).

Supported decision-making systems can take many forms. In fact, Lewis (2011) remarks that anything which does not take a disabled person's right to make decisions away from them is supported decision-making. This approach represents a paradigm shift, as attested by Quinn (2010). It perceives people with intellectual disabilities (among others) as having the same rights as everyone else, regardless of their abilities and support needs. It also views the provision of support as a means of ensuring that the person with an intellectual disability can act on their own as much as possible and that in cases where the person does need support, it is provided on the person's own terms. Supported decision-making is therefore very similar to self-advocacy and the two can reinforce each other. After all, supported – as well as substitute – decision-making need not be always formal and carried out through people appointed by a court of law. They can happen informally as well, for example, through circles of support as explained earlier. Family members or staff can take decisions on behalf of a person with an intellectual disability without consulting them. Equally, they can work with the person in those instances where the latter needs support with taking the best decision in line with their rights, will and preferences, and with acting on the decision taken.

READER ACTIVITY 7.4

Consider the country in which you live. Can you identify examples of:

- Supported decision making
- Substitute decision making

  Do you know if attitudes and practices in your country have changed since the implementation of the UN Convention on the Rights of Persons with Disabilities (UN, 2006)?

SKILLS NEEDED TO SUPPORT SELF-ADVOCACY AND ADVOCACY

The focus of this section is the skills that a supporter needs to place a person with an intellectual disability at the centre of the support they provide. The development of these skills is important for all those who live or work with people with intellectual disabilities.

Although, as seen above, there is a crucial difference between advocacy and self-advocacy, the skills presented here are relevant for both when we are supporting people with intellectual disabilities to advocate for themselves and when we are advocating for them. The most basic difference between these two types of advocacy is the amount of intervention by the supporter/advocate and who it is that gets to speak.

Bateman (2000, p. 63) suggests 6 principles when working in an advocacy role (see Box 7.1).

BOX 7.1   Summary of principles needed when working in an advocacy role

1. Act in the client's best interests.
2. Act in accordance with the client's wishes and instructions.
3. Keep the client properly informed.
4. Carry out instructions with diligence and competence.
5. Act impartially and offer frank, independent advice.
6. Maintain rules of confidentiality.

Bateman, (2000, p. 63)

The principles that Bateman (2000) suggests would also apply when we are supporting self-advocates. We also need to keep in mind that the same person can switch between the role of advocate and self-advocacy supporter depending on the person they are supporting and the specific situation they are supporting them in. Therefore, to these we can add the principle that our default position should be that of acting as self-advocacy supporters and only resorting to advocacy where necessary. For this reason, it is important that one of the skills that we foster is that of reflecting on our practice. We need to search for honest answers to these questions and address any issues that we identify in order to ensure that our actions promote choice and control for the people with intellectual disabilities we are working with and are personalised to meet their needs.

The following skills are also important in advocacy and self-advocacy work: communication, providing support to make choices, listening, interviewing, assertiveness, negotiation and recording.

Communication

If people with intellectual disabilities are to participate in a meaningful way, then systems, structures and processes need to be looked at so that participation can really happen. For example, extra time needs to be given, and papers for meetings need preparation in advance so that a person with an intellectual disability has a chance (maybe with assistance from a support worker) to fully understand the agenda and purpose of the meeting. People with intellectual disabilities should be paid fairly for their time. There should be appropriate breaks in meetings so that no-one gets too tired.

People with intellectual disabilities should be appropriately supported or represented so that their voice is heard. Communication tools, such as Makaton, Rebus symbols, smartphones, tablets, accessible information, could be used to help communication in an advocacy situation. Please see Chapter 5 for further information about different communication tools.

 READER ACTIVITY 7.5

Thinking of the suggestions made in the above paragraph around communication, are there any ways in which you could improve your communication with people with intellectual disabilities in your own practice?

Providing support to make choices

One of the supporter's main skills is to provide support to an individual to help them make their own choices. In this way, people with intellectual disabilities are able to express their individuality and personal freedom. An advocate, or a self-advocacy supporter, needs to present information in a clear and concise way, explaining the options without influencing the service user to choose one particular course of action. Here, too, creativity is very important. Again, this involves finding out the best style for the individual. Some people, for example, like to handle objects and have others around them, while others respond more to sounds or other sensory information. The only way to find out is by getting to know the person well (see also Chapter 4).

Once information is gathered, and a clear picture built up, the advocate needs to then provide support to help that person understand the options and give their views and preferences. For people with profound and multiple intellectual disabilities, this may take some time. For some, it may be an unattainable goal, in which case supporters will need to rely on information gathered from the people directly involved in people's lives. Porter et al, (2001) present a case-study involving Peter, a student with profound and multiple intellectual disabilities. Peter does not communicate verbally but through gestures. However, since he does not have control over his body's movements these gestures, for example waving, are subject to interpretation of those around him. The authors describe one incident that happened while Peter's family was in his classroom and he tapped a balloon. Staff interpreted this action as a sign from Peter that he wanted to play, while his family took it to mean that he was pushing the balloon away. If even such a small gesture is open to interpretation, discerning what the will and preferences of Peter are can be very difficult. Through their case study, Porter et al (2001) present an excellent example of how his family and staff at his school can be brought together to build a picture of Peter's abilities and preferences. In this case, it was the researchers who led the process. However, it is a process that can be led by an appropriate practitioner in different settings. In their role of gathering and collating information about Peter, the researchers focused on these areas:

- Physical aspects that affect Peter's communication
- The most important things in Peter's life and how he communicates his likes and dislikes
- How people see their roles in working or living with Peter
- How people communicate with Peter
- What people think about what Peter understands in different situations
- What difficulties people encounter in communicating with Peter
- How Peter's communication is supported
- How people can make sure that they are interpreting Peter's communication correctly.

Using this method enabled Porter et al (2001) to take into account the various perspectives of the people involved in Peter's life over a long period of time and in different contexts. They note that having detailed and updated records about Peter's strengths also played an important role in the process. The authors emphasise that one of the aspects that needs most particular attention is what other people make of Peter's communication. They stress the importance of the people involved in the life of a person with profound and multiple intellectual disabilities to check what they themselves are bringing into the process of interpreting the person's communications. Discussing with others and seeking validation of each other's interpretation plays a crucial role in this regard. Box 7.2 suggests some different ways of discovering a person's identity and working with it.

Listening

Listening is a very important skill in self-advocacy and advocacy, because the supporter or advocate must be clear about the wishes and views of the person with an intellectual disability. The supporter needs to gather facts and show empathy. Active listening involves hearing the information an individual is telling us, reflecting back

BOX 7.2 Different ways you could discover a person's identity and work with it

- Collecting together objects that relate to a person's past, e.g. pebbles from a beach; an object that creates a noise the person likes; a religious symbol.
- Collecting photographs/pictures of significant people/events.
- Visiting places of significance to that person, e.g. a school they went to; a mosque; a street.
- Videoing/recording people/voices/music/scenes.
- Collecting together stories/memories from other people.
- Spending social/leisure/activity time with that person to get to know them.
- 'Dreaming in' about what that person aspires to by talking to significant people in their lives.

to make sure that we have heard them correctly and not being judgemental about the information given. Non-verbal communication is important. It is also important not to rush to advise people with intellectual disabilities or to solve their problems. There needs to be a clear boundary between the listening stage and the discussing of options stage. Nodding and smiling are also useful ways to show that you are actively listening.

Interviewing

Interviewing is a key skill required of supporters doing advocacy and self-advocacy work. An initial interview with the person with an intellectual disability is usually required to find out what the issue is and to work out the best ways of moving forward. It is important to ensure that the means of communication chosen enables the person to express themselves.

The interviewer should carefully explain to the person with an intellectual disability the purpose of the interview. They should be supportive, positive and should offer empathy for the person's situation. Questions should be asked at a level appropriate to the person with an intellectual disability. Leading questions and closed questions should be avoided. The interview should involve active listening, verbal and non-verbal communication, reflecting back, questioning and sensitivity.

Assertiveness

Effective advocates need to be assertive. Their role usually requires them to stand up for other people and to

obtain a satisfactory outcome. Assertiveness when supporting self-advocates is also important – to serve as a role model for the person with an intellectual disability.

Assertiveness involves expressing yourself in a direct, honest, non-manipulative way. To be assertive, a supporter needs to be prepared with all the facts of the case and be clear in their objectives and principles. They also need to believe in their case and to have practised their arguments, thinking through any counter arguments they might come across. They need to have confidence, and to put forward the case without being manipulative or confusing.

Negotiation

Negotiation in an advocacy situation is about getting the best result for the person with an intellectual disability, on their behalf or by supporting them to speak. Sometimes negotiation will be used when there is no other available approach. The goals and interests of the person with an intellectual disability need to be identified. The strengths and weaknesses of the person's position and of the other side's position need to be identified. The options and the possible responses need to be thought through. The following may be a good way forward in the negotiating interview:

1. Obtain information through questioning.
2. Separate the people from the problem:
   - listen to the other side
   - confirm understanding of the other side's problem
   - allow the other party to let off steam.
3. Focus on interests not positions:
   - describe the problem in terms of the impact on the person with an intellectual disability
   - encourage the other side to explain the person's interests and goals
   - explain the interests and goals of the person with an intellectual disability you are working with
   - identify shared interests and goals
   - focus on present and future concerns, not past grievances.
4. Ascertain the scope of the other party's authority.
5. Develop and discuss alternative settlement options.
6. Make offers that are justified by objective criteria.
7. Insist on and probe for objective criteria based on law, precedents, facts or evidence.
8. Be open to reason, closed to threats.
9. Make a note of agreements and concessions as they occur.

(Adapted from Dye 2010, pp. 1–9)

Recording

It is important to record interactions with the person with an intellectual disability. Recording key facts is important for transparency and to have records available if another supporter has to take over, or to provide information for future research. It is important to adhere to the confidentiality arrangements of your profession/organisation. This also means being accountable to other people involved in the life of the person with an intellectual disability. You also need to consider data protection legislation and the right of the person with an intellectual disability to see what is written about them. It is best to write in a concise, factual and non-judgemental way. You may need to keep copies of any letters/e-mails written or any reports that you have written on behalf of the person.

The skills discussed above are also relevant when supporting a self-advocate. The difference is that the focus is on supporting the person with an intellectual disability to be in control of the process. It is important to remember that relationships of advocacy can grow into self-advocacy as both supporters and people with intellectual disabilities become more adept and skilful in speaking up, and in sharing decision-making processes. It is equally important to be aware of limitations and of tokenism, and to be honest about who is giving which input.

These skills will inevitably need to be adapted according to each person's particular situation, which needs to be considered holistically. This means that the person's past needs to be taken into account, as well as their present – including specific familial and/or cultural factors – and their future aims and aspirations. Box 7.3 identifies some of the ways in which relationships of advocacy can turn into self-advocacy.

CONCLUSION

This chapter has discussed various types of self-advocacy – where people with intellectual disabilities speak up for themselves and for others, with support where necessary – and other types of advocacy, where other people speak up on behalf of people with intellectual disabilities. It has been seen that whichever advocacy model is used, it is important to focus on the ability of the person with an intellectual disability to have choice and control in their lives. The chapter has also discussed the difference between substitute and supported decision-making and shown how the latter focuses on acting according to the rights, will and preferences of the person with an

> ### BOX 7.3 Some of the ways in which your relationships of advocacy can turn into self-advocacy
>
> - Skills can be learnt and developed by supporters as well as people with intellectual disabilities. What can only be resolved through advocacy today can turn into self-advocacy in the future
> - Seek opportunities for the person with an intellectual disability to self-advocate. This can start from everyday decisions and grow into an ability to make more important choices in various life domains.
> - Self-advocacy is not an all-or-nothing affair. A person with an intellectual disability may be capable of being a self-advocate in certain aspects of their life, but may need an advocate in others. They may also be more comfortable with someone speaking on their behalf in certain contexts.
> - Keep the person with an intellectual disability informed about what is going on. This will enable them to acquire the information necessary for them to self-advocate.
> - Make incremental changes to enable the person with an intellectual disability to speak up in meetings, and for you as a supporter to develop the skills of supporting the person rather than speaking on their behalf.
> - Be pro-active in seeking different ways in which a person can be supported to self-advocate.
> - Be also ready to take the plunge. It is okay to take a calculated risk – if the person finds self-advocacy difficult, you can always intervene and continue advocating on their behalf.
> - Read about self-advocacy to learn from other people's experiences. The reference list of this chapter and the links to relevant websites on the online resource are a good starting point.

intellectual disability, rather than on what others have determined is in the person's best interest thus emphasising the importance of a person centred approach. The chapter finally presented the skills that are needed to support self-advocacy and to carry out advocacy work especially in a service setting, focusing on the importance of self-reflexivity and striving towards giving people with intellectual disabilities as much control as possible over decisions affecting their lives.

REFERENCES

Azzopardi, A. (2000). A case study of a parents' self-advocacy group in Malta. *Disability & Society*, 15(7), 1065–1072.

Bateman, N. (2000). *Advocacy skills for health and social care professionals* (2nd ed.). London: Jessica Kingsley.

Beart, S., Hardy, G., & Buchan, L. (2004). Changing selves: a grounded theory account of belonging to a self-advocacy group for people with intellectual disabilities. *Journal of Applied Research in Intellectual Disabilities*, 17, 91–100.

Breslin, M. L., & Yee, S. (Eds.). (2002). *Disability rights law and policy: international and national perspectives.* Ardesley, NY: Transnational Publishers.

Brooke , J. & Harris, J. (2000). *Pathways to citizen advocacy.* Kidderminster: British Institute of Learning Disabilities.

Callus, A. M. (2013). *Becoming self-advocates: people with intellectual disability seeking a voice.* Oxford: Peter Lang.

Campbell , J., & Oliver, M. (1996). *Disability politics: understanding our past, changing our future.* London: Routledge.

Cambridge, P., & Ernst, A. (2006). Comparing local and national service systems in social care Europe: framework and findings from the STEPS anti-discrimination learning disability project. *European Journal of Social Work*, 9(3), 279–303.

Camilleri, J., & Callus, A. M. (2001). Out of the cellars. disability, politics and the struggle for change: the Maltese experience. In L. Barton (Ed.), *Disability, politics and the struggle for change* (pp. 79–92). London: David Fulton.

Campaign for People with Mental Handicaps. (1986). *Self-advocacy pack.* London: The Campaign for People with Mental Handicaps.

CAPS Independent Advocacy. (2020). Collective advocacy. Available at: http://capsadvocacy.org/collective-advocacy/.

Chadwick, D. D., Mannan, H., Iriarte, E. G., et al. (2013). Family voices: life for family carers of people with intellectual disabilities in Ireland. *Journal of Applied Research in Intellectual Disabilities*, 26(2), 119–132.

Chapman, R. (2005). *The role of the self-advocacy support-worker in UK People First groups: developing inclusive research.* Ph.D. thesis, Open University. Available at: http://oro.open.ac.uk/59590/1/424812.pdf.

Chappell, A. L. (1998). Still out in the cold: people with learning difficulties and the social model of disability. In T. Shakespeare (Ed.), *The disability reader: social science perspectives.* London: Cassell.

Charlton, J. (1998). *Nothing about us without us: disability oppression and empowerment.* University of California Press.

Clare, M. (1990). *Developing self-advocacy skills.* London: Further Education Unit.

Committee on the Rights of Persons with Disabilities. (2014), General comment No. 1 2014 Article 12: equal recognition before the law. Available at: https://www.ohchr.org/en/hrbodies/crpd/pages/gc.aspx.

Crawley, B. (1988), *The growing voice: a survey of self-advocacy groups in adult training centres and hospitals in Great Britain.* London: Values into Action.

Davis, A. J., Konishi, E., & Tashiro, M. (2003). A pilot study of selected Japanese nurses' ideas on patient advocacy. *Nursing Ethics*, 10, 404–413.

Disability Rights Maine. (2019). Supported decision-making: a user's guide for people with disabilities and their supporters. Available at: http://supportmydecision.org/assets/tools/DRM-SDM-Handbook-Rev.-7.19.19.pdf.

Driedger, D. (1989). *The last civil rights movement.* London: Hurst and Company.

Downer, D., & Ferns, P. (1993). Self-advocacy by Black people with learning difficulties. In L. Ward (Ed.), *Innovations in advocacy and empowerment . Lancashire: Lisieux Hall.*

Dybwad, G. (1996). Setting the stage historically. In G. Dybwad & H. Bersani (Eds.), *New voices: self-advocacy by people with disabilities* (pp. 1–17). Cambridge, MA: Brookline Books.

Dybwad, G., & Bersani, H. (Eds.). (1996). *New voices: self-advocacy by people with disabilities.* Cambridge, MA: Brookline Books.

Dye, T. A. (2010). Winning the settlement – keys to negotiation strategy. ABA Section of Litigation Corporate Counsel CLE Seminar , FL, 11 February.

Fligstein, N. (2007). Organizational field. In M. Bevir (Ed.), *Encyclopedia of governence.* https://doi.org/10.4135/9781412952613.n371.

Fundamental Rights Agency. (2013). Legal capacity of persons with intellectual disabilities and persons with mental health problems. Available at: https://fra.europa.eu/sites/default/files/legal-capacity-intellectual-disabilities-mental-health-problems.pdf.

Gilmartin, A., & Slevin, E. (2010). Being a member of a self-advocacy group: experiences of intellectually disabled people. *British Journal of Learning Disabilities*, 38(3), 152–159.

Goodley, D. (2000). *Self-advocacy in the lives of people with learning difficulties.* Buckingham: Open University Press.

Gray, B., & Jackson, R. (2002). *Advocacy and learning disability.* London: Jessica Kingsley Publishers.

Grupp Flimkien Naslu. (2019). Available at: https://maltacvs.org/voluntary/grupp-flimkien-naslu/.

Hanna, J. (1978). Advisor's roles in self-advocacy groups. *American Rehabilitation*, 4(2), 31–32.

Health Equality Europe. (2006) Challenges facing the health advocacy community – a Europe-wide survey of health campaigners. Health Equality Europe:

Hersov, J. (1996). The rise of self-advocacy in Great Britain. In G. Dybwad & H. Bersani (Eds.), *New* voices: self-advocacy by people with learning disabilities. Cambridge, MA: Brookline Books.

Hutchison, P., Arai, S., Pedlar, A., et al. (2007). Role of Canadian user-led disability organizations in the non-profit sector. *Disability & Society*, 22(7), 701–771.

Hutton, S., Park, P., Levine, M., et al. (2017). Self-advocacy from the ashes of the institution. *Canadian Journal of Disability Studies*, 6(3), 31–59.

Inclusion International. (2020). Who we are. Available at: https://inclusion-international.org/who-we-are/.

Johansson, R. (2006). Nyinstitutionell organisationsteori – från sociologi I USA till socialt arbete i Sverige [New institutional organization theory – from sociology in the US to social work in sweden]. In O. Grape, B. Blom, & R. Johansson (Eds.), *Organisation och omvärld – nyinstitutionell analys av människobehandlande organisationer* (Organization and environment. New institutional analysis of human service organizations). Lund: Studentlitteratur.

Jugessor, T., & Iles, I. K. (2009). Advocacy in mental health nursing: an integrative review of the literature. *Journal of Psychiatric and Mental Health Nursing*, 16, 187–195.

Kebbon, L. (1997). Nordic contributions to disability politics. *Journal of Intellectual Disability Research*, 41(2), 120–125.

Ledger, S., & Tilley, L. (2006). The history of self-advocacy for people with learning difficulties: international comparisons. *British Journal of Learning Disabilities*, 34, 129–130.

Leong, A. L., & Euller-Ziegler, L. (2004). Patient advocacy and arthritis: moving forward. *Bulletin, World Health Organization*, 82, 115–120.

Lewis, O. (2011). Advancing legal capacity jurisprudence. *European Human Rights Law Review*, 6, 700–714.

Mallander, O., Mineur, T., Henderson, D., et al. (2018). Self-advocacy for people with intellectual disability in Sweden – organizational similarities and differences. *Disability Studies Quarterly*, 38(1).

Mansell, J., & Ericsson, K. (1995). *Deinstitutionalisation and community living intellectual disability services in Scandinavia, Britain and the USA*. London: Chapman and Hall http://dx.doi.org/10.18061/dsq.v38i1.

Mitchell, D., Traustadóttir, R., Chapman, R., et al. (2006). *Exploring experiences of advocacy by people with learning disabilities: testimonies of resistance*. London: Jessica Kingsley.

Mitchell, P. (1997). The impact of self-advocacy on families. *Disability and Society*, 12(1), 43–56.

Nursing and Midwifery Council (NMC). (2010). *Standards for pre-registration nursing education*. London: NMC.

O'Brien, J. (1987a). A guide to lifestyle planning: using the activities catalogue to integrate services and natural support systems. In B. W. Wilson & G. T. Bellamy (Eds.), *The activities catalogue: an alternative curriculum for youth and adults with severe disabilities*. Baltimore: Brookes.

O'Brien, J. (1987b). *Learning from citizen advocacy programmes*. Atlanta, GA: Advocacy Office.

Oka, T. (2013). Self-help groups in Japan: historical development and current issues. *International Journal of Self-help & Self-Care*, 7(2), 217–232.

Oliver, M. (1990). *The politics of disablement*. Basingstoke: Macmillan.

Oliver, M. (1996). *Understanding disability: from theory to practice*. Basingstoke: Macmillan.

Pannick, D. (1993). *Advocacy*. UK: Oxford Paperbacks.

Perske, R. (1996). Self-advocates on the move: a journalist's view. In G. Dybwad & H. Bersani (Eds.), *New voices: self-advocacy by people with disabilities* (pp. 18–34). Cambridge, MA: Brookline Books.

Pochin, M. (2002). Thoughts from a UK citizen advocacy scheme. In B. Gray & R. Jackson (Eds.), *Advocacy and learning disability*. London: Jessica Kingsley Publishers.

Porter, J., Ouvry, C., Morgan, M., et al. (2001). Interpreting the communication of people with profound and multiple learning difficulties. *British Journal of Learning Disabilities*, 29(1), 12–16.

Power, A., Bartlett, R., & Hall, R. (2016). Peer advocacy in a personalised landscape: the role of peer support in a context of individualized support and austerity. *Journal of Intellectual Disability*, 20(2), 183–193.

Quinn, G. (2010). *Personhood & legal capacity: perspectives on the paradigm shift of Article 12 CRPD. Conference on Disability and Legal Capacity Under the CRPD*. Boston: Harvard Law School (20), 3–5.

Rich, a (2015), Standing *together and finding a voice apart:* advocating for intellectual disability rights. Washington DC: AAIDD.

Royal College of Nursing. Available at: https://www.rcn.org.uk/clinical-topics/safeguarding.

Schwartz, L. (2002). Is there an advocate in the house? The role of health care professionals in patient advocacy. *Journal of Medical Ethics*, 28(1), 37–40.

Self-advocacy.net. (2019). Welcome to self-advocacy.net. Available at: https://www.selfadvocacy.net.

Shapland, S. (2019). A source of affection then shame. *Community Living*, 32(4), 30.

Shoultz, B. (1997a). More thoughts on self-advocacy: the movement, the group and the individual. Available at: http://soeweb.syr.edu/.

Shoultz, B. (1997b). The self-advocacy movement. Available at: http://soeweb.syr.edu/.

Shoultz, B. (1997c). The self-advocacy movement. Ppportunities for everyone. Available at: http://soeweb.syr.edu/. http://soeweb.syr.edu/.

Shearer, A. (1986). *Building community with people with mental handicaps, their families and friends.* London: CMH/King's Fund.

Simons, K. (1992). 'Sticking up for yourself': self-advocacy and people with learning difficulties. Community Care publication in association with the Joseph Rowntree Foundation.

Soares de Carvalho, E. N., & Forrester-Jones, R. (2016). Country profile: intellectual disability in Brazil. *Tizard Learning Disability Review, 21*(2), 65–74.

Social Work England. (2020). Professional standards. Available at: https://www.socialworkengland.org.uk/media/1640/1227_socialworkengland_standards_prof_standards_final-aw. [Accessed 29 March 2020].

Stalker, K. (1997). Choices and voices: a case study of a self-advocacy group. *Health and Social Care in the Community, 5,* 246–254.

Sutcliffe, J., & Simons, K. (1993). *Self-advocacy and adults with learning difficulties: contexts and debates.* Leicester: National Institute of Adult Continuing Education.

Tideman, M., & Svensson, O. (2015). Young people with intellectual disability: the role of self-advocacy in a transformed Swedish welfare system. *International Journal of Qualitative Studies on Health and Well-being, 10*(1).

TLAP (Think Local, Act Personal). (2014). *Social care jargon buster.* London: TLAP.

Traustadottir, R. (2006). Learning about self-advocacy from life history: a case study from the United States. *British Journal of Learning Disabilities, 34,* 175–180.

Tsuda, E. (2006). Japanese culture and the philosophy of self-advocacy: the importance of interdependence in community living. *British Journal of Learning Disabilities, 34*(3), 151–156.

United Nations. (2006). United Nations Convention on the Rights of Persons with Disabilities. Available at: https://www.un.org/development/desa/disabilities/convention-on-the-rights-of-persons-with-disabilities/convention-on-the-rights-of-persons-with-disabilities-2.html.

Voices Together. (2019). Self-advocacy around the world. Available at: https://www.voicestogether.com.au/

wp-content/uploads/2019/01/Self-Advocacy-Around-the-World.pdf.

Ward, J. (1986). A point of view: citizen advocacy: its legal context. *Journal of Intellectual and Developmental Disability, 12*(2), 91–96.

Watson, J. (2011). Supported decision-making for people with severe or profound intellectual disability: 'we're all in this together aren't we?' In C. Bigby and C. Fyffe (Eds.), *Services and families working together to support adults with intellectual disability. Proceedings of the Sixth Annual Roundtable on Intellectual Disability Policy*(pp. 38–48). Available at: https://www.researchgate.net/publication/258997307_Watson_J_2012_Supported_decision_making_for_people_with_severe_or_profound_intellectual_disability_'We're_all_in_this_together_aren't_we'_Paper_presented_at_the_6th_Roundtable_on_Intellectual_Disabili.

Williams, P. (1982). Participation and self-advocacy. *CMH Newsletter, 20*(Spring), 3–4.

Williams, P., & Shoultz, B. (1982). *We can speak for ourselves.* London: Souvenir Press.

Wistow, G., Perkins, M., Knapp, M., et al. (2016). Circles of support and personalization: exploring the economic case. *Journal of Intellectual Disabilities, 20*(2), 194–207.

Wolfensberger, W. (1972). *Normalisation: the principle of normalisation in human services.* Toronto: Leonard Crainford.

Wolfensberger, W., & Zauha, H. (1973). *Citizen advocacy and protective services for the impaired and handicapped.* Toronto: National Institute on Mental Retardation.

Wooten, M., & Hoffman, A. J. (2008). Organizational fields: past, present and future. In R. Greenwood, C. Oliver, R. Suddaby, & K. Sahlin (Eds.), *The SAGE handbook of organizational institutionalism.* London: Sage. Publications. https://doi.org/10.4135/9781849200387.n5.

Zhang, D., Walker, J. M., Leal, D. R., et al. (2019). A call to society for supported decision-making: theoretical and legal reasoning. *Journal of Child and Family Studies, 28,* 1803–1814.

8

Safeguarding against abuse and harm

Caroline White

KEY ISSUES

- People with intellectual disabilities are at risk of abuse, neglect and harm in a variety of settings and circumstances.
- While individuals may demonstrate resilience and coping strategies, the emotional impact of abuse for people with intellectual disabilities and their families may be significant.
- Practitioners should have an understanding of abuse and take steps to prevent the onset of abuse;

respond to abuse which occurs; and provide support to those who have been abused.
- People with intellectual disabilities have the potential to play an active role in their own protection; this should be recognised, while ensuring that individuals are not isolated from the support of practitioners and others.

CHAPTER OUTLINE

INTRODUCTION

The United Nations Convention on the Rights of Persons with Disabilities (2006) highlights the rights of disabled people to live lives that are free from exploitation, violence and abuse. Further, in many countries, current policy, values and thinking stress the importance of rights, personalisation, inclusion, choice, control, participation and independence in the lives of people with intellectual disabilities (Department of Health (DH), 2001; Scottish Government, 2013, 2019). However, in

contrast to these important aims, inquiries and research have demonstrated that people with intellectual disabilities face risks of abuse, neglect and harm. Establishing the prevalence of abuse is difficult due to varying definitions and methodologies, and because not all abuse is reported (Northway et al, 2013a,b; Hewitt, 2014); however studies indicate that abuse appears more prevalent among people with intellectual disabilities than among non-disabled people (Hollomotz, 2009; Beadle-Brown et al, 2010; McCarthy, 2014). Abuse and harm may have a profound impact on individuals' lives. Those who support people with intellectual disabilities need to be aware of the risks they face from abuse; however awareness of such risks should not prevent individuals from exercising their rights to make informed choices, choose to take risks, and develop friendships and relationships. As Fyson (2009) has observed:

> *"What value does freedom from abuse have if it comes at the cost of losing all independence? ... What value does independence have if it comes at the cost of being abused?"*
>
> *Fyson, 2009, pp. 23–24*

This chapter will give examples of how people with intellectual disabilities have been abused in a range of settings and circumstances. It considers definitions of abuse and explores the different kinds of recognised abuse. Some of the underlying reasons why people with intellectual disabilities appear to be at risk of abuse will be explored, as well as some of the potential consequences and impacts. Practice responses to prevent the onset of abuse, and to support people with intellectual disabilities who have been abused, will be outlined. Finally, the importance of supporting people with intellectual disabilities to play active roles in their own protection will be highlighted. Although both children and adults with intellectual disabilities experience abuse and harm in a range of settings, this chapter focuses specifically on the abuse of adults.

 READER ACTIVITY 8.1

The term 'abuse' could be considered a subjective concept.

What does the term mean to you?

How would you define it?

What are some of the different ways people can be abused and harmed?

Compare your responses to the ideas presented in this chapter.

BACKGROUND AND HISTORICAL OVERVIEW

Our awareness of the abuse of people with intellectual disabilities has developed over time. An early scandal was reported by the Ely Hospital Inquiry in 1968/1969, which investigated the treatment of people with intellectual disabilities in a long-stay hospital in Wales (UK), typical of service provision for people with intellectual disabilities

at that time. The abuses reported included examples of cruel and threatening treatment (such as beatings, hosing patients down with cold water), theft of items belonging to the hospital and patients, a lack of care, and indifference by senior staff to complaints (Butler and Drakeford, 2005). Further examples of abuses within intellectual disability services in the UK were revealed by inquiries during the 1960s and 70s (Martin, 1984) leading to some recognition of the failings within institutional care at that time. However, any assumptions that such abuses were due to outmoded practice and service delivery have been challenged by more recent examples of abuse within contemporary services; Marsland et al (2015a, p. 135) have observed that

> *'perhaps the greatest and most enduring challenge faced by modern services is the abuse of people who receive those services'.*

In 2006, an inquiry into services for people with intellectual disabilities in Cornwall (UK) found examples of abuse and ill treatment. These included hitting, mocking, withholding food, giving cold showers, inappropriate use of residents' money, and violence between residents. It was reported that "one person spent 16 hours a day tied to their bed or wheelchair, for what staff wrongly believed was for that person's own protection" (Commission for Social Care Inspection/Healthcare, Commission 2006, p. 5). In 2011 the UK documentary programme Panorama undertook covert filming in a private hospital (Winterbourne View) for people with intellectual disabilities and/or autism. The broadcast showed:

> *"Patients wrestled to the floor with support workers lying on them and/or they were immobilised with furniture. Patients were slapped, punched, subjected to unequal games of strength and kicked. They had their hair pulled, their fingers, wrists and arms bent back, they were teased and soaked in water. Their distress was deliberately induced."*
>
> *Flynn and Citrella, 2013, p. 174*

More recently, further undercover filming was undertaken by the Panorama programme which revealed similar abusive practices at Whorlton Hall, a private hospital for people with intellectual disabilities (Murphy, 2019; Plomin, 2019).

The above examples have highlighted the abuses experienced by people with intellectual disabilities in settings which should have provided support and care, and promoted their safety and wellbeing. They have focused on abuses within large scale services which have attracted considerable attention, however people with intellectual disabilities also experience abuse in smaller community settings and care homes, as well as other forms of care delivery such as home care (Hanley and Marsland, 2014).

Abuse also occurs within family relationships, although this may receive less public attention in contrast to more high profile cases (such as those in service settings) involving greater numbers of people (Manthorpe and Martineau, 2015). People with intellectual disabilities have reported examples of physical, emotional, financial and sexual abuses within their families (Gravell, 2012; Hollomotz, 2012). For example, one woman with intellectual disabilities spoke of her experiences when living with a family member:

"Many times I was locked in a room all day and all night. [...] I had a bucket [to go to the toilet]. And [...] he's taken all the money [benefits] off me. He wouldn't let me have any money, unless I asked him for it and he'd be watching over while I had that."

Hollomotz, 2012, p. 124

A report from Australia (Ombudsman New South Wales, 2018) found examples of physical abuse and assault, over-medication to control behaviours, sexual abuse and neglect by family members. They cautioned that within family contexts:

"There is an inclination to look the other way, not interfere, and to see the conduct as part of the family dynamic. Instances of physical abuse are viewed as harsh or tough behaviour rather than domestic violence and criminal conduct."

Ombudsman New South Wales, 2018, p. 25

People with intellectual disabilities may also experience abuse from people they meet within their communities. Some may appear to befriend them, although such friendships may be abusive and exploitative, sometimes referred to as 'mate crimes' (McCarthy, 2014). A participant in research shared such an experience:

"They made out they were friends, came back here, had food and that, slept here sometimes, watched TV here, did their drugs here. I thought they was friends but ... they would only turn up here when I had my benefits, you know my money."

Gravell, 2012, p. 23

Taken together the examples above demonstrate that people with intellectual disabilities can be at risk of abuse and neglect in a variety of settings and relationships (though it should not be forgotten that many enjoy positive and supportive relationships in addition to high quality care and support). The above cases illustrate the need for practitioners to recognise signs of abuse and to act appropriately and effectively to prevent and respond to abuse and harm across a range of settings.

The examples given above are primarily from the UK however, the abuse of people with intellectual disabilities is an international issue. For example, at the time of writing, the Australian Government has set up a Royal Commission into Violence, Abuse, Neglect and Exploitation of People with Disability, to explore and respond to the abuse of disabled people, including those with intellectual disabilities (Australian Government, 2019). The abuse of people with intellectual disabilities and other groups have led, in some countries, to the development of policy and legislation which seek to prevent and inform responses to the occurrence of abuse and neglect. As these vary between nations these are not explored within this chapter, however, it is recommended that readers explore and familiarise themselves with their local policy and legislative framework.

DEFINITIONS AND CATEGORIES OF ABUSE

Definitions of abuse have been much debated. Early policy in England defined abuse as:

"A violation of an individual's human and civil rights by any other person or persons."

DH, 2000, p. 9

Many different types of abuse are recognised. In England current guidance (Department of Health and Social Care (DHSC), 2018) recognises ten forms of abuse which may be experienced by adults. These are:

- Sexual abuse
- Physical abuse
- Psychological abuse
- Financial or material abuse
- Neglect
- Self-neglect
- Organisational abuse
- Domestic violence
- Discriminatory abuse
- Modern slavery

Previous policy (DH, 2000) recognised six categories of abuse, suggesting that our understanding of the multiple ways in which people can be hurt and harmed is growing.

Sexual abuse

A wide range of acts are encompassed within the category of sexual abuse. Brown and Turk (1992) observed that sexual abuse may involve contact or non-contact acts. Contact abuse includes acts such as rape, penetration, masturbation and sexual touch. Non-contact abuse includes acts which do not involve touch such as harassment, indecent exposure, involvement in pornography, all of which can be distressing and harmful.

A key issue in respect of sexual abuse is whether or not an individual has consented to sexual acts. The British Psychological Society (Herbert et al, 2019) cautions that the law in respect of sexual crimes differs between areas, and there are different definitions of consent, underscoring the importance of practitioners understanding how these are defined within local legislation. They report that within legislation in England, Wales and Northern Ireland consent to sexual acts is determined by whether the person agrees to a sexual act by choice, and whether they have the freedom and capacity to make that choice. Thus, important questions in respect of consent to sexual acts are:

- Does the person consent to the act?
- Do they have the capacity to consent; for example do they understand the act and possible consequences (such as pregnancy)? In some cases their capacity and understanding may be developed, for example, through sex education (Herbert et al, 2019).
- Are they free to consent? The ability to consent may be undermined if the person is pressurised, threatened, or if the person carrying out the sexual act is in a position of power or authority such as a member of staff, a practitioner, a family member (Brown and Turk, 1992).

Working to establish whether consent has been given or withheld can be complex, especially perhaps when both individuals have an intellectual disability. However, it is an issue which requires clear and careful consideration. In the absence of such consideration there are risks that either safe, consenting and mutually satisfying relationships are prohibited, or that relationships in which one individual is frightened, hurt and exploited are supported or condoned. People are placed at risk both when their rights to a consenting sexual life are ignored, and when a desire to support choice and adult lifestyles mean that indicators of fear, distress and a lack of meaningful consent are ignored.

Physical abuse

Physical abuse includes assault, hitting, slapping, rough handling, pushing (NHS England, 2019; Social Care Institute for Excellence (SCIE), 2018; DHSC, 2018). It also includes the misuse of medication, such as over-sedating people (SCIE, 2018). People may also receive inappropriate sanctions or punishments, and restraint may be used illegally or inappropriately (NHS England, 2019; SCIE, 2018; DHSC, 2018); for example, in Winterbourne View restraint was used dangerously, illegally and on a very frequent basis (DH, 2012; Flynn and Citrella, 2013). It was reported that:

> "One family provided evidence that their son was restrained 45 times in 5 months, and on one occasion was restrained 'on and off' all day. It is very difficult to see how such high numbers of interventions could possibly be seen as normal."

> DH, 2012, p. 14

Psychological abuse

NHS England, (2019, p. 21) has described psychological abuse as

> 'behaviour that causes mental distress or has a harmful effect on an individual's emotional health and development';

it includes making threats, frightening or humiliating people, verbal abuse and intimidation (Robinson and Chenoweth, 2012; SCIE, 2018; DHSC, 2018; NHS England, 2019). It may also include ignoring people, isolating them (for example from family, friends and advocates), preventing people from meeting their cultural or religious needs, and from making choices (Robinson and Chenoweth, 2012; SCIE, 2018).

Financial and material abuse

Financial abuse of people with intellectual disabilities appears to have received little research attention

(McCarthy, 2014). Such abuse involves the theft or misuse of individuals' money, benefits and property, putting people under undue pressure in respect of their money or financial affairs, and fraud (SCIE, 2018; DHSC, 2018; NHS England, 2019). Scams conducted online or by post are also examples of financial abuse (DHSC, 2018). Careful consideration is required by services to enable people with intellectual disabilities to manage their own money and make financial choices, while at the same time protecting them from abuse and exploitation (Livingstone, 2006).

Neglect and Self-neglect

The types of abuse defined above involve acting or doing something *to* another person. In contrast, neglect involves a failure or omission to do something *for* another. This includes ignoring or failing to meet physical, emotional, social and health care needs, such as the provision of medication, nutrition, heating, personal care, and access to health, care and educational services (SCIE, 2018; DHSC, 2018; NHS England, 2019). In addition to neglect carried out by others, individuals may neglect themselves. This may involve neglecting their care needs (including neglect in respect of their health, nutrition and/or personal hygiene) and their environment (Braye et al, 2015).

Organisational abuse

Organisational abuses include neglect and poor care in settings such as care homes, hospitals and by home care services; such abuses arise as a result of poor care practices, policies and cultures (Robinson and Chenoweth, 2012; DHSC, 2018). Brown (2007) has observed that organisational abuse is not a 'type' of abuse, but instead consists of a range of factors which interact to promote poor or abusive practice and include:

- Poor quality environments
- Rigid and oppressive routines
- Neglecting the needs and wishes of residents
- Practice which does not reflect accepted professional behaviours
- Acts of cruelty from individuals or staff groups
- Negligent practice and exposing residents to risks.

Domestic abuse and violence

The UK Government defines domestic violence and abuse as:

"Any incident or pattern of incidents of controlling, coercive or threatening behaviour, violence or abuse between those aged 16 or over who are, or have been, intimate partners or family members regardless of gender or sexuality."

DHSC, 2018.

While the terms domestic violence and domestic abuse are both used, the latter is viewed as 'wider-ranging' (Dixon and Robb, 2016, p. 775), emphasising the range of abuse experienced within intimate and familial relationships.

Although men also experience domestic abuse, research has mainly studied experiences of domestic abuse and violence among women with intellectual disabilities. This research has uncovered accounts of relationships in which women have experienced psychological, physical, sexual and financial abuses from partners, as well as curtailment of their freedom and isolation from family and friends (Walter-Brice et al, 2012; McCarthy et al, 2017). Their experiences of domestic abuse have had profound consequences, which include injury (often serious), debt, impacts on their self-esteem and mental health, and anxiety about the wellbeing of their children, who in some instances were removed from their care. Reporting domestic abuse did not always lead to helpful responses, however being listened to and believed did help the women, who valued the opportunity to access sources of support such as counselling and women's groups, thus highlighting the importance of professionals being aware of domestic violence and offering appropriate support.

Discriminatory abuse

This is abuse which is grounded in discrimination based on an individual's disability, ethnic origin, gender or gender identity, sexual orientation, age or religion (DH, 2018; NHS England, 2019). A refusal to respect an individual's religious or cultural needs, for example, by failing to provide an appropriate diet (Brown, 2003), refusing to provide supports required by a disabled person such as a communication aid (SCIE, 2018), or belittling an individual on the grounds of their disability, all constitute discriminatory abuse.

Modern slavery

Modern slavery includes human trafficking, slavery, forced labour and domestic servitude, and may operate across international borders (Home Office, 2014). Although not extensively documented to date, people with intellectual disabilities are among those who have been coerced or forced into slavery ('UK family found guilty', 2017).

Although this section has explored distinct forms of abuse, research indicates that many people with intellectual disabilities experience multiple forms of abuse, sometimes from the same person, or in different episodes of abuse over time (Beadle-Brown et al, 2010; Rowsell et al, 2013; Hewitt, 2014; McCarthy et al, 2017; DHSC, 2018). It is also important to remember that some acts of abuse are also crimes, for example, rape, theft, fraud (DHSC, 2018), and therefore legal responses and reporting to law enforcement agencies may be required.

SETTINGS OF ABUSE

The examples of abuse outlined above indicate that people with intellectual disabilities can be abused in a range of settings. These include individuals' own or family homes, care homes and hospitals; in addition to these locations, individuals may also experience abuse in day centres, and when out in public places (Beadle-Brown et al, 2010). People with intellectual disabilities may also be at risk of abuse and exploitation in virtual spaces.

The internet can offer many positive opportunities to people with intellectual disabilities, however, they have also reported being subject to insults, bullying, sexual and financial exploitation, and unwanted experiences such as being sent sexual photographs when online (Holmes and O'Loughlin, 2014; Chiner et al, 2017). Therefore awareness of, and support to navigate online risks, are required.

When taken together the above research highlights that individuals may be at risk of abuse in settings such as their homes, where there is – or should be – an expectation of safety, as well as in more public spaces, including the online world.

PERPETRATORS OF ABUSE

Abuse may be carried out by a range of different perpetrators. This includes
- Family members
- Members of staff/managers
- Other people with intellectual disabilities
- Partners
- Friends (and people who pose as friends)
- Strangers.

(Beadle-Brown et al, 2010; Hewitt, 2014):

While concern often surrounds the risks posed by strangers, abuse is frequently carried out by people known to the person and with whom there should be an expectation of trust and of positive, caring relationships.

The previous section has given examples of abuses perpetrated by care staff, managers, family members and friends. Additionally, people with intellectual disabilities may experience abusive or unwanted behaviours from other people with intellectual disabilities with whom they share a service setting such as a care home or day centre. However, it appears that this issue is often overlooked within services and people with intellectual disabilities may be encouraged by staff to tolerate or ignore these behaviours (Hollomotz, 2012). The label of 'challenging behaviour' is often used within services. This may reduce the stigma attached to such behaviours but can also distort and soften perceptions of the behaviours, so that the impact upon others may not be recognised and abusive behaviours remain unreported and unchallenged (Brown, 1999, 2003; Joyce, 2003). In such circumstances:

> "Many people with intellectual disabilities are encouraged by staff to tolerate behaviours from their peers that few other people would want to put up with from their friends, flatmates or colleagues."
>
> *McCarthy and Thompson, 1996*, pp. 213–214

There is a need to consider clearly the impact of challenging behaviours on other service users, and to respond effectively and in ways which recognise and respect their feelings and needs for safety and security. A clear acknowledgement of abuse among people with intellectual disabilities helps ensure that those at risk of being abused are protected, and that those at risk of abusing receive appropriate support to manage their behaviour.

THE IMPACT OF ABUSE

Understanding, recognising and responding to the abuse of people with intellectual disabilities is a vital area of work, because of the potential costs and consequences to those who are abused. McCarthy (1999), who carried out research into the sexual experiences of women with intellectual disabilities, found high levels of sexual abuse among those she interviewed. Her work also highlighted the resilience of the women and she observed that, although some experienced difficulties:

> "Generally speaking ... the personal strength and resilience shown by the women in coming to terms with what had happened to them and in some cases was continuing to happen, was to their great credit."

> *McCarthy, 1999, p. 217*

McCarthy's work offers an important reminder that people with intellectual disabilities who have experienced abuse should not be perceived simply as 'victims', but also as survivors with personal coping skills and resources.

However, there is also evidence that the experience of abuse can be traumatic, severe and enduring. People with intellectual disabilities have spoken about some of the ways they can be affected, illustrating the emotional impact of abuse (Northway et al, 2013a, p. 369):

> "Like a headache, you just can't get it out of your head."

> "I feel like I had been turned inside out and gone through the mangle."

> "You can get nightmares when people abuse you. Nightmares about it. I always have nightmares when people abuse me and take advantage."

Studies by O'Callaghan et al (2003) and Sequeira et al (2003) explored the impact of abuse on people with intellectual disabilities, the majority of whom had been sexually abused. O'Callaghan et al (2003) identified that the experience of abuse had had a devastating, profound and long-lasting impact upon survivors. Both studies identified symptoms of post-traumatic stress disorder and a range of behavioural and mental health problems among the survivors (see also Rowsell et al, 2013). O'Callaghan et al (2003) reported the following effects of abuse:

1. Behavioural changes including:
   - self-harming
   - challenging behaviours
   - stopping communicating
   - avoiding places associated with the abuse
   - re-enacting the abuse, including demonstrating sexualised behaviours.

2. Emotional changes including:
   - appearing depressed
   - showing signs of fear
   - becoming tearful and withdrawn
   - experiencing flashbacks and nightmares.

3. Physical changes, including weight loss.

They also found that abuse could lead to other consequences for survivors. For example, the majority (89%) experienced changes to their services, either moving to different residential placements or stopping using respite services, following the abuse. While these changes may have been intended to protect individuals from repeated abuse and further harm, this also suggests that survivors of abuse are at risk of experiencing change, discontinuity and disruption, at a time when they are especially vulnerable (O'Callaghan et al, 2003). While O'Callaghan et al observed that the individuals in their study had experienced very severe, multiple abuses, and that their experiences may not have been typical of all abuse survivors, their study does provide a powerful indication of the extent and impact of the harm that may be caused by abuse.

O'Callaghan et al's (2003) study also highlighted the profound consequences for the families of those who had been abused. These included feelings of distrust of other people and services, feelings of guilt and anger, developing mental health problems (such as depression) and personal problems (such as alcohol abuse, problems in their relationship with their partner). While the provision of therapeutic support to survivors of abuse was identified as 'patchy', they found that although family members were experiencing trauma, they were offered little support.

In summary, while people with intellectual disabilities may demonstrate resilience in the aftermath of abusive experiences, for many abuse has a lasting impact, both for individuals and their families. This therefore underscores the importance of acting to prevent abuse from occurring, and of providing effective support to those who have been abused and their families.

WHY ARE PEOPLE WITH INTELLECTUAL DISABILITIES ABUSED?

People with intellectual disabilities not only experience abuse and neglect, they also appear to experience

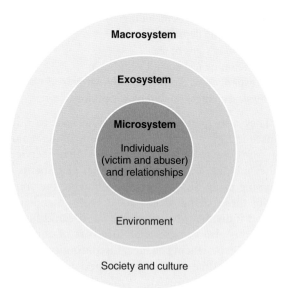

Figure 8.1 An ecological model of abuse (Adapted from Sobsey (1994); Hollomotz, 2009)

these to a greater extent than non-disabled people (Hollomotz, 2009; Beadle-Brown et al, 2010; McCarthy, 2014). This therefore raises the question of why abuse is so prevalent among this group; this section will explore some of the underlying reasons such abuses may occur.

A key message with regard to the causes of abuse is that there are no easy or simple explanations; there are instead a wide range of factors which may account for the risks faced by people with intellectual disabilities. Sobsey (1994) and Hollomotz (2009) have both outlined an 'ecological model' of abuse (see Figure 8.1). This clearly illustrates that the occurrence of abuse cannot simply be attributed to individual 'vulnerability' arising as a result of having an intellectual disability; instead a range of factors associated with other people's behaviours, relationships, the way people with intellectual disabilities are treated, and societal influences all contribute to abuse (Hollomotz, 2009; Hough, 2012). These ecological models group risk factors within three systems:

1. **The microsystem** – which is concerned with individuals and the social networks around them; this therefore focuses on those who are abused, those who carry out abuse, and the relationships between them.
2. **The exosystem** – which is concerned with the environments in which people with intellectual disabilities live, as well as their neighbourhoods and the places they spend their social, leisure and working time.

3. **The macrosystem** – which is concerned with wider cultural, political and societal factors.

The Microsystem

This section will consider the characteristics and behaviours of individuals.

People who are abused

Several aspects of living with an intellectual disability have been associated with risk of abuse, these include:

A lack of opportunities to make choices

Some people with intellectual disabilities live in situations where others tend to make decisions for them; this can make it difficult for people to feel able and empowered to make their own decisions, to say no to others who may also be in positions of greater authority and power, or to speak out about abusive experiences (Hollomotz, 2009; Fraser Barbour, 2018). Furthermore, where people with intellectual disabilities are reliant on others to deliver support, they and their families may lack the power to readily leave these relationships and access alternative sources of support (Hanley and Marsland, 2014).

Limited understanding of rights in respect of abuse

People with intellectual disabilities may not have had opportunities to learn about abuse and their right to be safe. The implications of this were highlighted by Northway et al (2013a,b):

> "If you are unsure as to what is acceptable and unacceptable, the unacceptable may come to be accepted as the norm. This could lead to people with intellectual disabilities accepting abuse as part of their lives; or as one [person] noted, it is 'just how things are'."
>
> *Northway et al, 2013b*, p. 242

Similarly, research in Australia with disabled people (including people with intellectual disabilities) noted that

> 'silences around violence were an ongoing problem'
> (*Robinson et al, 2020*, p. 11).

These limited opportunities for discussion and learning mean that people with intellectual disabilities may lack information which helps them avoid risky situations, or report and address abuse which occurs.

Communication difficulties

Some people with intellectual disabilities may experience communication difficulties which make reporting abuse difficult; this may place them at risk of ongoing abuse. Sobsey (1994) has noted that communication may also be impaired by factors external to individuals such as being isolated from support, not being listened to, or believed.

Lack of sex and relationship education and information about sexual rights

Sex education, while important in its own right, may also have a potentially protective role. Where people with intellectual disabilities have not had opportunities for formal sex education, their only opportunities to learn about sex and sexual relationships may come through personal experience, including experiences of abuse (McCarthy, 1999; Sobsey, 1994). Studies by McCarthy (1999) and Fitzgerald and Withers (2013) have explored the sexual lives of women with intellectual disabilities. The women in their studies appeared to have little understanding of their sexual rights, and limited recognition or expectation of sexual pleasure, although this was perceived as something that men could expect. Some women have also been found to be unaware of their right to reject unwanted sexual experiences (Olsen and Carter, 2016). Opportunities for sex education and to discuss relationships may help men and women with intellectual disabilities to better understand their sexual rights, how they should expect to be treated, and to treat others. Some people with intellectual disabilities may lack the vocabulary to name intimate body parts (Tinney et al, 2014), which can better enable them to report unwanted or abusive experiences; sex education may help provide individuals with such a vocabulary.

Confusion about the boundaries of friendship

Tinney et al (2014) found that some people with intellectual disabilities were unclear about different kinds of friendship (for example, close friends, acquaintances, strangers who are friendly); accordingly they found it difficult to recognise appropriate behaviours with and from different kinds of friends. Confusion about the term 'online friend' has also been noted (Holmes and O'Loughlin, 2014), which may contribute to risk. For example, Holmes and O'Loughlin (2014) highlight the story of Sarah, who:

"Accepted anyone who posted a friend request, and as a result had 600 'friends' she had never met. Initially, Sarah suffered cyber bullying, with messages heavily laden with personal remarks about her appearance and activities on Facebook. Sarah, although admittedly hurt by the remarks, did not want to 'block' these people as she believed they were her 'friends'."

Holmes and O'Loughlin, 2014, p. 5

Subsequently, she was also targeted by 'friends' for sexual exploitation and received unwanted and upsetting sexually explicit messages. This highlights how the language of online spaces may confuse, and a need to enable people to understand the potential risks from online friends.

A focus on people with intellectual disabilities can be useful in highlighting areas in which change and development are required; for example through highlighting the need for awareness raising and the provision of information or education. However, this is also a focus which has been criticised, since focusing on the risks associated with individuals may lead to 'victim blaming', in which the reasons for abuse are perceived to be the fault of the person experiencing the abuse (Brown, 2003; Sobsey, 1994; Wishart, 2003). The ecological model moves beyond a focus on people with intellectual disabilities by highlighting the importance of additional factors, such as wider environmental and cultural factors; Sobsey (1994) has observed that 'society's response to disability may be more important than the disability itself' (p. 103).

Individual abusers

Abuse may arise for many reasons and includes abuses which are carried out unintentionally as well as deliberate acts (DHSC, 2018). For example, abuse may arise unintentionally as a result of a carer, such as a family carer, lacking information about the best ways to provide support or struggling to manage (DHSC, 2018); in such cases they may need support to ensure both that their own needs and the needs of the person receiving support are met. However, our ideas about the causes of abuse frequently attribute abusive behaviours to the psychopathology of the individual abuser, in which abuse is perceived as arising from individual malice or deviance (White et al, 2003). While this may account for some of the underlying reasons for abuse, especially with regard to sexual abuse (Brown, 2007), there is a strong consensus that individuals' behaviours are also shaped or influenced by external factors (for example, Brown, 2007; Manthorpe and Stanley, 1999; Martin, 1984), the significance of which will be explored below.

Additionally, abuse may also be understood as arising in a context of power inequalities and misuse which enable abuse and exploitation to occur (Hanley and Marsland, 2014).

The Exosystem

Our ideas about abuse often locate the causes of such abuse with individuals and their behaviours, however there are also wider explanatory factors. The environments in which people with intellectual disabilities live can expose them to significant risk. This has been most clearly documented with regard to residential services, and it has been argued that such services may develop cultures and practices which increase the likelihood of abuse occurring (White et al, 2003; Marsland et al, 2007; Robinson and Chenoweth, 2012). Culture can be defined as

> 'the predominating attitudes and behaviours that characterise the functioning of a group or organisation'
> Francis, 2010, p. 152.

Cultures and attitudes can be passed on within services, from staff member to staff member (Marsland et al, 2015b). They may

> 'encourage the practices of well-intentioned staff to deteriorate; they may also allow the actions of intentional abusers to remain hidden and unreported'
> Marsland et al, 2007, p. 8.

Important factors underpinning and shaping care cultures include the following:

The quality of management

Research and inquiries into abusive services have highlighted the significance of management. Where leadership in services or organisations is weak and supervision of staff is infrequent, managers lack opportunities to challenge poor or abusive practice and to set positive standards for the provision of care (Cambridge, 1999; Marsland et al, 2007). Managers may set the tone for a service, for example, at Winterbourne View management were judged to have 'allowed a culture of abuse to flourish' (DH, 2012, p. 8).

Staff skills and competence

A staff group which is skilled, knowledgeable and well trained will be aware of accepted practice and able to recognise poor or abusive practice (White et al, 2003).

Where staff lack such skills and awareness, people with intellectual disabilities may be at risk of abuse, and this abuse may remain unrecognised and unchallenged. Without adequate training staff may lack the skills to provide effective care and support; for example, if they lack training in safe responses to behaviours which challenge services there is a risk that they may respond inappropriately due to a lack of awareness of the most appropriate, safe and dignified responses.

Staff attitudes and behaviours

How staff perceive the people with intellectual disabilities they support is important and can influence the way they treat individuals. Wardhaugh and Wilding (1993) introduced the term 'neutralisation of normal moral concerns' to describe the process by which people receiving care may become dehumanised or perceived as fundamentally different. Where people with intellectual disabilities are perceived as of lesser value than staff or other members of society, there is a risk that poor or abusive treatment, which would normally be viewed as unacceptable, can be justified.

Isolation

Although in many countries residential homes are now typically placed within the community (in contrast with historically segregated services), services for people with intellectual disabilities can still be isolated from the support and vigilance of external professionals, family and friends. Isolation may allow abuse to occur (because ideas about good practice are not being brought into the service) and enables abuse to remain concealed (because there are few external people to observe and report poor practice) (Sobsey, 1994, in White et al, 2003). People with intellectual disabilities may be especially isolated when they are placed 'out of area' and at a distance from families and support networks; this may place people at a particular risk of abuse, and the use of such placements has been criticised (Beadle-Brown et al, 2010; DH, 2012). Winterbourne View provides an illustration of the different ways in which services can isolate people; it was located within a business park, away from the wider community; families were only able to visit their relatives in designated areas, not on the wards; many patients were placed out of area, creating further difficulties for visiting families (DH, 2012; Flynn and Citrella, 2013; Hanley and Marsland, 2014).

This exploration of the exosystem, or the environments in which support is provided, helps to illustrate how, while individual attributes and characteristics are important (and individual responsibility for behaviour should not be ignored), the services, settings and cultures in which people with intellectual disabilities live are also significant. For example, where services are poorly managed, isolated from external support, and staff are given little training, abusive practice may develop and become entrenched. Such settings may provide a safe haven for those whose individual characteristics predispose them to abuse others, as well as creating the conditions in which well-intentioned staff commit acts of abuse or fail to challenge the abuses of others (Marsland et al, 2007).

While abuse may be associated with poor service cultures, a lack of provision and support may leave some individuals isolated and effectively hidden from view (Ombudsman New South Wales, 2018), in such contexts they may be both vulnerable to abuse, and to signs of such abuse being rendered invisible.

The Macrosystem

Wider cultural, societal and political factors may also contribute towards the vulnerability of people with intellectual disabilities. Robinson and Chenoweth (2011) have noted that:

"The constructions of people with intellectual disability as 'other', as damaged, as less than human, and as needing to be 'kept in their place' are powerful and dominant modes of social and cultural operation, and they have informed the development of the structures, including the disability services systems, within which people live today."

Robinson and Chenoweth, 2011, p. 64

These factors influence the ways in which people with intellectual disabilities are treated and services are planned, designed and commissioned. For example, people with intellectual disabilities and their families may explicitly be left out of, or marginalised, within discussions and initiatives to improve services (Marsland et al, 2015a) so that their experiences and perspectives do not inform future planning and safety initiatives, the success of which may therefore be compromised. Service design and commissioning may fail to reflect knowledge about factors which help to create or militate against safety, therefore placing people in situations of risk.

The attitudes held within our societies can also place people at risk of abuse. Early consideration of the abuse of people with intellectual disabilities outlined the importance of 'cultural myths' in shaping societal and individual beliefs about the value of people with

intellectual disabilities, and which can be used to justify abusive behaviours and minimise the impact of abuse; these myths are summarised in Table 8.1 (Sobsey and Mansell, 1990).

Overall, the ecological model highlights the diverse factors which underpin the abuse of people with intellectual disabilities; it also highlights that the actions required to reduce risks are diverse, and reflect all levels of the model, not simply those targeted at people with intellectual disabilities (Hough, 2012).

RESPONDING TO ABUSE AND HARM

The findings with regard to the impact of abuse demonstrate the importance of taking steps to prevent people with intellectual disabilities from being abused, and of responding wisely and appropriately when abuse does take place. Brown (2003) and May-Chahal et al (2006) outlined useful models for considering the prevention of abuse, which will be used within this section. These models define three levels of prevention:

1. Primary prevention, which includes strategies to reduce risk and prevent the onset of abuse.
2. Secondary prevention, which is concerned with ensuring the prompt identification of abuse and responding effectively to prevent its reoccurrence.
3. Tertiary prevention, which focuses on the need to support individuals who have been abused, seeking to reduce the impact of the harm and trauma that may follow on from abusive experiences.

Primary Prevention

As has already been seen, the experience of abuse can lead to individuals being hurt, harmed and distressed. Therefore, a critical element of adult safeguarding work concerns actions to prevent abuse from happening at all. However, it has been argued that

'we are better able to respond to abuse which has already occurred than to protect people before they are abused'

(White et al, 2003, p. 2).

In England the importance of prevention has been highlighted in guidance:

Agencies should stress the need for preventing abuse and neglect wherever possible. Observant professionals and other staff making early, positive interventions with individuals and families can make a huge

TABLE 8.1	**Sobsey and Mansell's Cultural Myths**
Dehumanisation myth	People with intellectual disabilities are perceived as less than fully human; this enables abuse to be more readily justified.
Damaged merchandise myth	People with intellectual disabilities are perceived as having a poor quality of life. Such beliefs can help justify carrying out abuse and alleviate guilt
Feeling no pain myth	People with intellectual disabilities are wrongly perceived as not experiencing pain or distress; this permits the belief that they do not understand and are not hurt by abuse
Disabled menace myth	This positions people with intellectual disabilities as in some way dangerous or deviant, allowing the cause of the abuse to be located in their behaviour, and not that of the person carrying out the abuse.
Helplessness myth	Where people with intellectual disabilities are believed to be helpless, they may be perceived as 'ideal victims' who will be unable to stand up for themselves.

difference to their lives, preventing the deterioration of a situation or breakdown of a support network.

DHSC, 2018

This highlights the importance of ensuring that individuals and their families have the support they need as an important element of abuse prevention, as well as contributing to individual and family wellbeing.

This section will consider two further forms of primary prevention:

- Actions to identify unsuitable or inappropriate staff and support workers.
- The recognition of 'early indicators' of abuse.

Actions to identify unsuitable or inappropriate staff

There is a particular irony that people with intellectual disabilities may be abused by those who are paid to offer support, care and protection. Consideration has been given to ways of ensuring the suitability of staff whose roles involve providing care and support. In some countries or states there are systems for conducting pre-employment checks of potential candidates for roles supporting people with intellectual disabilities (and others), ensuring, for example, that they do not have a history of convictions for certain crimes (Robinson and Chenoweth, 2011; Manthorpe and Lipman, 2015). However, such checks are only effective if criminal (and other relevant) activity has been detected, and therefore should not be considered the sole means by which suitable staff can be identified and abuse prevented.

Good staff recruitment can help ensure that people with positive values, attitudes and practices are employed. Involving people with intellectual disabilities is an important way of ensuring that they have a voice in the selection of new staff, choosing people with whom they feel comfortable. People with intellectual disabilities can be involved in staff selection through activities such as identifying the qualities they wish to see in staff; choosing interview questions; taking part in interviews; being involved in decision making – this could include having a right of veto over any applicants (Hurtado et al, 2012). Interviewing can be a demanding process, so it is important that people with intellectual disabilities receive support to enable their participation; it is also important that they have a real choice and say in recruitment decisions, and that payment for the work undertaken is considered (Hurtado et al, 2012).

While efforts to screen out unsuitable individuals can play an important role in preventing abuse, this approach has been criticised as focusing energy and resources on individuals who are perceived as causing risk, with less emphasis placed on other factors which promote abuse (Manthorpe and Stanley, 1999).

The recognition of 'early indicators of abuse'

Although abuse has often been considered the result of individual failings, there are other factors that contribute to abuse, meaning that it is important to think beyond individuals. As already highlighted, the cultures and organisation of care services may place people at risk and contribute to abuse and neglect. Recognising aspects of service cultures which may place people at risk can therefore contribute to the prevention of abuse. Marsland et al, (2007) carried research out to identify 'early indicators of abuse'. Early indicators are visible signs or warnings that service cultures and conditions are such that residents are being placed at significant risk of abuse and neglect in the places they live; they do not provide evidence that abuse is occurring, but of worrying levels of risk.

Recognising, reporting and responding to the presence of early indicators in a service can enable practitioners to take steps at an early stage to protect residents and prevent the onset of abuse, or prevent abuse from becoming ongoing. Examples of the early indicators identified are presented in Box 8.1.

Secondary Prevention: Responding Effectively

Actions to prevent abuse from occurring at all should be a priority. However, it is also vital to know how to recognise signs that abuse may have taken place, and how to respond effectively when abuse does occur. This section will consider both how abuse is recognised and responses to abuse.

Recognising abuse

Abuse may come to light in different ways. In some instances, the person who has been abused will tell another person – sometimes termed making a disclosure. An early publication developed guidance on responding to disclosures of abuse (ARC/NAPSAC, 1996), this continues to provide useful information, summarised in Table 8.2.

READER ACTIVITY 8.2

Read Leo's story in the online resource and consider whether there are any circumstances which give you cause for concern.

 BOX 8.1   Early indicators of abuse in residential services (adapted from Marsland et al, 2007)

The decisions, attitudes and actions of managers.
- The managers can't or don't want to make decisions or take responsibility for things
- The managers don't make sure staff meetings and supervision take place
- The manager has relatively little experience of working with people with intellectual disabilities and/or little understanding of the care needs of people with intellectual disabilities

The behaviours and attitudes of staff.
- Members of staff do not manage behaviours in a safe, professional or dignified way
- Restraint is used frequently and as a first option before other approaches are tried
- The members of staff do not appear to value people with intellectual disabilities and treat them as different from themselves and other people
- There is denial or a lack of concern where the possibility of abuse is raised.

The behaviours of people with intellectual disabilities.
- Residents are expressing emotional changes – for example becoming withdrawn, weepy or anxious
- There are residents who control, bully or harm other residents

Isolation.
- There is little input from outsiders and external professionals
- Members of staff try to manage very complex situations (such as aggression, severe distress) without or against the advice of external professionals
- Important meetings are arranged at very short notice

Service design, placement planning and commissioning.
- Agreed programmes or plans are not being carried out
- The residents are incompatible
- Residents with a history of abusing are placed alongside other vulnerable people

Fundamental care and the quality of the environment
- There is poor or inadequate support for residents with health problems who become ill or have special needs (e.g. sensory impairments)
- Residents are not given support to change inappropriate or harmful behaviours
- There are no or few activities for residents

TABLE 8.2   Guidance on responding to disclosures of abuse (ARC/NAPSAC, 1996)

Do	• Believe the person and listen to them • Stay calm • Offer reassurance that they are doing the right thing • Follow agency guidelines • Write a factual account of what the person said, using their own words as far as possible • Show sympathy and concern • Explain what you are going to do
Do not	• Ask the person for details • Make judgements or appear shocked or angry • Promise to keep what they have said a secret • Make promises that they will never be abused again • Confront the person they said abused them

 READER ACTIVITY 8.3

You are the social worker for Rachel, a young woman with an intellectual disability. Rachel lives at home with her mum Barbara; her dad Ian died almost a year ago. Several times a year Rachel goes away for the weekend for respite and enjoys spending time away from home with other young people her age.

Barbara phones to talk to you about Rachel. She tells you that in the last few weeks Rachel has 'not been herself at all'. She has taken to spending a lot of time shut in her room and is reluctant to leave the house. She is eating very little and often says she feels sick. Rachel seems in 'very low spirits' but will not speak to Barbara about what is upsetting her. Rachel is due to go to the respite unit next weekend but cried and said she didn't want to go when Barbara reminded her.

What are possible explanations for Rachel's behaviour and distress?

What initial steps might you take to understand better what is happening for Rachel?

Disclosing abuse may be a stressful experience (Joyce, 2003) and people with intellectual disabilities may need encouragement to express and discuss negative feelings and experiences, and to trust that others are willing to listen if they raise difficult and painful issues. However, disclosures are not always made. Feelings of embarrassment; fear of what will happen or of reprisals; blaming themselves for the abuse; communication difficulties and lack of specific language to articulate abusive experiences may prevent people with intellectual disabilities from speaking out (Northway et al, 2013a,b; Tinney et al, 2014; Fraser Barbour, 2018; McGilloway et al, 2018; SCIE, 2018). Taken together these factors mean that it cannot be assumed that people with intellectual disabilities will always speak up when abuse has occurred. People with intellectual disabilities have stressed the importance of having a trusted person to whom they can talk (Northway et al, 2013a,b); this highlights the importance of ensuring that people with intellectual disabilities have a network of safe and trusting relationships with people such as family, friends and advocates, to whom they can report abuse and who will listen and believe them when they experience abuse or feel at risk (Bruder and Stenfert Kroese, 2005; Northway et al, 2013a,b). Bruder and Stenfert Kroese (2005) highlight the importance of regularly making time to ask people with intellectual disabilities how they are and whether anything or anyone has upset them. Taking such steps can help create a culture in which people with intellectual disabilities feel able and permitted to disclose difficult, abusive or hurtful experiences.

When disclosures are made it is also vital that people are believed, taken seriously and actions taken, however there is evidence that people are not always believed and may be told to ignore other people's behaviours (Hollomotz 2012; Northway et al, 2013a,b). Moreover, Hollomotz (2012) found that they may be labelled as 'challenging' or 'drama queens' which may mask the importance of their complaints.

There are therefore many barriers to disclosure. It is important that people with intellectual disabilities are provided with the resources and support to facilitate disclosure, and also that others, such as families, friends and professionals, are able to recognise signs that people have been abused, so that identification of abuse is not solely dependent on individuals speaking out. This includes attending to the ways in which they communicate experiences and feelings through behaviour, observable behavioural changes, the behaviours of others, as well as other circumstances. Table 8.3 details signs that may indicate that abuse is occurring.

TABLE 8.3 Indicators of abuse (McCarthy et al, 2017; SCIE, 2018)	
Type of abuse	**Examples of possible indicators**
Physical	Injuries such as bruising, welts, hair loss in clumps Frequent injuries, or injuries which are unexplained or for which there are inconsistent explanations Changed behaviour in the presence of certain person/people
Sexual	Physical signs – including sexually transmitted infections, bruising – especially to the thighs, buttocks, upper arms Fear of personal care or being alone with specific people Changes in behaviour, including uncharacteristically sexually explicit language Poor concentration, withdrawal, sleep disturbance
Psychological	Signs of distress Low self-esteem Changed appetite, weight loss or gain Insomnia
Financial	Missing money or possessions Unexplained lack of money or withdrawal from accounts Other people showing an unusual interest in the person's money or assets Evasiveness or a lack of cooperation by people responsible for managing finances
Neglect	Lack of hygiene or appropriate clothing Build-up of medications Malnutrition, unexplained weight loss Untreated injuries or medical problems, reluctance for contact with health or social care professionals
Domestic violence	Becoming isolated and having less contact with family, friends, professionals Having less money than before they met their partner Physical injuries Fear of outside intervention Damage to the home
Modern slavery	Being isolated from others Appearing to be controlled by others Lack of personal possessions and documents Fear of talking to others Signs of being malnourished, being unkempt or withdrawn

Recognising signs of abuse may be complex and problematic. Many indicators have multiple potential causes, so are not clear and unambiguous, and their presence does not necessarily indicate that abuse has occurred (SCIE, 2018). For example, depression is associated with abuse, however, it may also be a response to bereavement, change or other factors. Despite these limitations, the signs listed in Table 8.3 highlight that something is very wrong for individuals, that a supportive response is required, and that the possibility that abuse is occurring should be considered as one of a range of possible causes.

Responding to abuse

The recognition of abuse, or the possibility of abuse, is an important step. Once abuse has been disclosed, witnessed or suspected, it is essential that this is reported, so that actions can be taken to support the person who has been abused and ensure their future safety (and the safety of others). Furthermore, actions may need to be taken in respect of the person(s) who has carried out the abuse.

Ignoring abuse, or concerns, is not an option. Different countries, areas and agencies have different laws and policies which stipulate how professionals should respond if they have evidence or are concerned that someone has been abused. It is outside the scope of this book to outline these; instead it is essential for all practitioners to be aware of the policies and legislation in effect in their own area and agency, and to ensure that they know how to respond to and report abuse. In England guidance (DHSC, 2018) states clearly that:

> *"No professional should assume that someone else will pass on information which they think may be critical to the safety and wellbeing of the adult. If a professional has concerns about the adult's welfare and believes they are suffering or likely to suffer abuse or neglect, then they should share the information with the local authority and, or, the police if they believe or suspect that a crime has been committed."*

There have been many examples where inquiries have recognised that different professional groups had not shared their concerns or information which could have led to an earlier or preventative response; therefore it is important that practitioners share concerns (even where these fall short of clear evidence of abuse), enabling a clear picture of individuals' circumstances to be developed (DH, 2012; DHSC, 2018).

READER ACTIVITY 8.4

An important element of adult safeguarding is for practitioners to be sure that they know what to do when they have concerns or evidence of abuse.

Find out what policies and legislation govern responses to adult abuse in your country, area and agency.

Although there is a professional duty to report concerns, this is not always easy. In some situations or settings, people may lack faith that their concerns will be taken seriously and fear the possible consequences of reporting such as intimidation or harassment by colleagues; in such circumstances, reporting can be a courageous act (Calcraft, 2005). Where managers are involved in abusive or poor practice, or fail to respond to reports of abuse, workers may take their concerns outside the usual management structures and report to external agencies; such action is referred to as 'whistleblowing' (Calcraft, 2005; Gaylard, 2008). In some areas there is legislation in place to protect those who whistle-blow in good faith; local whistleblowing policy and legislation is an important area for practitioners to explore.

When abuse has occurred there are a range of actions which may be taken with the aim of stopping further abuse and ensuring that the person and others are safe in the future. Potential responses to abuse may include considering whether additional or different forms of care and support are required; providing support to a family carer to enable them to provide safer support (for example, this might include information, training, provision of services such as respite, paid carers); disciplining or dismissal of staff; reporting to professional registration bodies if relevant; criminal investigations where a crime may have been committed (DHSC, 2018).

In addition to responses directed at those who have carried out abuse (whether deliberately or unintentionally) it is important to ensure that the welfare and wellbeing of the person who has been abused is considered (DHSC, 2018). This may include the provision of emotional or therapeutic support which is considered below.

Tertiary Prevention: Emotional Support and Aftercare

As has been seen, the experience of abuse can be traumatic and distressing. Therefore, in addition to taking practical action to ensure the safety of individuals and reduce the risk of future abuse, it is also important to consider the emotional needs of those who have been abused.

Post-abuse support has been described, primarily with regard to sexual abuses and domestic violence. However, accessing support may be difficult; for example, the availability of appropriate therapeutic support may be limited (Rowsell et al, 2013). Women with intellectual disabilities leaving abusive relationships may have limited access to services such as refuges and may have to leave their local area to access support or move to services which do not meet their needs (Olsen and Carter, 2016; McCarthy et al, 2019).

Supports available following sexual abuse include counselling, group work and therapy. Such approaches may be beneficial, although working through such difficult experiences can also be a challenging and painful process (O'Malley et al, 2019). For example, Peckham et al (2007) described the work of a support group for women survivors of sexual abuse. They concluded that the participants appeared to develop increased sexual knowledge, and that symptoms of depression and trauma decreased; however, they also identified that 'challenging behaviour appeared to get worse before it got better' (Peckham et al, 2007, p. 243), illustrating the emotional demands which such work asks of participants. Additional benefits of support groups have also been identified; for example, women attending a group for survivors of domestic abuse were able to form friendships and meet women who had undergone similar experiences, which helped to combat the isolation they had previously experienced (Walter-Brice et al, 2012).

Accounts of providing individual or group support to people with intellectual disabilities indicate that such work is complex and may require significant time (and therefore resources). Further, the provision of such support is a skilled role, requiring training, support and supervision. However, while the provision of therapeutic support may be a specialist role, this is not to suggest that other practitioners should not be willing to hear and acknowledge painful experiences and to take a supportive and empathetic approach. O'Malley et al (2019) found that staff members could be an important 'bridge' between individuals and those providing skilled support (such as psychologists and counsellors), enabling them to explore worries and feelings of distress, and implement practical strategies. The importance of all staff and professionals being willing to offer support to people who have been abused is illustrated by Olsen and Carter (2016) who found that:

> "All services… from hospital accident and emergency nurses to intellectual disability outreach services, thought that supporting a person with an intellectual disability after rape was someone else's problem. Without exception all workers present said that their most likely course of action would be to take some details then refer the person on to what they believed would be a more appropriate service."
>
> *Olsen and Carter, 2016*, p. 36

Given the identified difficulties in accessing support for people with intellectual disabilities who have been abused, research has been conducted in respect of mainstream, post-abuse services. Olsen and Carter (2016) explored the support available to women with intellectual disabilities who had experienced rape (while recognising that rape is also experienced by men). They found that women with intellectual disabilities were seldom referred to generic rape services and were not always aware of sources of support and where to go for help. Furthermore, staff within such services identified communication issues as a barrier to working with people with intellectual disabilities, and lacked understanding of their lives and circumstances, which impacted on the appropriateness of the support offered. They concluded that there was a need both for information for those who have experienced abuse and for training for workers in generic services to enable them to better support people with intellectual disabilities.

This section suggests that finding appropriate and skilled sources of emotional support to reduce the impact of abuse may be difficult. However, where the experience of abuse appears to have been traumatic, steps should be taken to attempt to identify – or develop – appropriate and compassionate sources of support.

SAFEGUARDING – TOWARD INCLUSION

Work to safeguard people with intellectual disabilities, which often uses the language of 'vulnerability' and 'protection', is open to charges of paternalism, and that it is something that is done 'for' or 'to' people, and not 'with' them (Collins and Walford, 2008). In a book that considers the journey of people with intellectual disabilities toward inclusion, it is important to reflect upon how the focus of safeguarding work could move towards greater partnership working with people with intellectual disabilities, and how individuals can play a part in their own protection.

Hollomotz (2009) noted that people with intellectual disabilities can and do have strategies to protect themselves and should not be considered passive in the face of risk. However, studies reviewed in this chapter have also indicated that some people with intellectual disabilities lack important information, education and knowledge, which could help them to better recognise and take actions to avoid risk, and to report abusive or harmful experiences, enabling them to access support. A range of actions have been suggested to support people with intellectual disabilities. These include supporting individuals to:

- Be aware of their rights, ensuring they know how to recognise and report abuse and access support
- Recognise appropriate (and inappropriate) behaviours across a range of different relationships
- Recognise acceptable touch (and develop language to report inappropriate touch and name intimate body parts)
- Develop an understanding of sex and their sexual rights, including an expectation that sex should be mutually pleasurable
- Be aware of online risks and safety strategies
- Access information about individuals and organisations that can offer help and support

(Holmes and O'Loughlin, 2014; Tinney et al, 2014; Chiner et al, 2017; McCarthy et al, 2017; Fraser Barbour, 2018).

Ensuring that information and education is delivered in accessible formats and including people with intellectual disabilities in their design and delivery have also been identified as important (Northway et al, 2013a,b; see also Chapter 5).

While it is important to enable people with intellectual disabilities to gain information, knowledge and skills to help them to protect themselves, this work should never be perceived as a substitute for good support and detection of abuse by practitioners and others. People with intellectual disabilities may learn to recognise, respond to and avoid abusive or risky situations, however, they may not always be able to use these skills in practice (Bruder and Stenfert Kroese, 2005; Hollomotz, 2012). Where people are frightened, intimidated or are being abused by someone in a powerful or trusted position, it may be very difficult for them to resist or report abuse. McCarthy and Thompson (1996) have cautioned that an emphasis on education risks 'victim blaming' when people with intellectual disabilities 'fail' to avoid abuse, offering a reminder that steps to empower people with intellectual disabilities must take place alongside attempts to change the behaviours of others, as well as the environmental and societal factors that place individuals at risk (Hollomotz, 2009). However, despite the importance of ensuring that the full weight of responsibility is not placed upon people with intellectual disabilities, it remains important to identify ways of ensuring that they have opportunities to become active participants in their own protection.

CONCLUSION

This chapter has highlighted the risks faced by people with intellectual disabilities in their lives. Such abuse can be distressing and traumatic, although the resilience and coping skills of this group should not be overlooked. The risks of abuse for people with intellectual disabilities means that practitioners have a professional duty to take steps to prevent the onset of abuse, to recognise and respond to the abuse of individuals, as well as to work alongside them, ensuring they have the necessary skills, strategies and knowledge to enable them to address their own protection.

REFERENCES

ARC/NAPSAC. (1996). *It could never happen here! The prevention and treatment of sexual abuse of adults with learning disabilities in residential settings.* Nottingham: ARC/NAPSAC.

Australian Government. (2019). *Royal Commission into Violence, Abuse, Neglect and Exploitation of People with Disability.* Available at: https://disability.royalcommission.gov.au/Documents/fact-sheet.pdf.

Beadle-Brown, J., Mansell, J., Cambridge, P., et al. (2010). Adult protection of people with intellectual disabilities: incidence, nature and responses. *Journal of Applied Research in Intellectual Disabilities, 23,* 573–584.

Braye, S., Orr, D., & Preston-Shoot, M. (2015). Learning lessons about self-neglect? An analysis of serious case reviews. *Journal of Adult Protection, 17*(1), 3–18.

Brown, H. (1999). Abuse of people with learning disabilities – layers of concern and analysis. In N. Stanley, J. Manthorpe, & B. Penhale (Eds.), *Institutional abuse: perspectives across the lifecourse* (pp. 89–109) London: Routledge.

Brown, H. (2003). *Safeguarding adults and children with disabilities against abuse.* Strasbourg: Council of Europe Publishing.

Brown, H. (2007). Editorial. *The Journal of Adult Protection, 9,* 2–5.

Brown, H., & Turk, V. (1992). Defining sexual abuse as it affects adults with learning disabilities. *Mental Handicap, 20,* 44–55.

Bruder, C., & Stenfert Kroese, B. (2005). The efficacy of interventions designed to prevent and protect people with intellectual disabilities from sexual abuse: a review of the literature. *The Journal of Adult Protection, 7,* 13–27.

Butler, I., & Drakeford, M. (2005). *Scandal, social policy and social welfare* (2nd ed). Bristol: ASW/Policy Press.

Calcraft, R. (2005). *Blowing the whistle on the abuse of adults with learning disabilities*. Nottingham: Ann Craft Trust.

Cambridge, P. (1999). The first hit: a case study of the physical abuse of people with learning disabilities and challenging behaviours in a residential service. *Disability and Society, 14*, 285–308.

Chiner, E., Gomez-Puerta, M., & Cardona-Molto, M. C. (2017). Internet use, risks and online behaviour: the view of internet users with intellectual disabilities and their caregivers. *British Journal of Learning Disabilities, 45*, 190–197.

Collins, M., & Walford, M. (2008). Helping vulnerable adults keep safe. *The Journal of Adult Protection, 10*, 7–12.

Commission for Social Care Inspection/Healthcare Commission. (2006). *Joint investigation into the provision of services for people with learning disabilities at Cornwall Partnership NHS Trust Commission for Healthcare*. London: Audit and Inspection.

Department of Health. (2000). *No secrets. Guidance on developing and implementing multi-agency policies and procedures to protect vulnerable adults from abuse*. London: Department of Health.

Department of Health. (2001). *Valuing people: a new strategy for learning disability for the*. London: Century Department of Health.

Department of Health. (2012). *Transforming care: a national response to Winterbourne View Hospital*. London: Department of Health.

Department of Health and Social Care. (2018). *Care and support statutory guidance*. Available at: https://www.gov.uk/government/publications/care-act-statutory-guidance/care-and-support-statutory-guidance.

Dixon, J., & Robb, M. (2016). Working with women with a learning disability experiencing domestic abuse: how social workers can negotiate competing definitions of risk. *British Journal of Social Work, 46*, 773–788.

Fitzgerald, C., & Withers, P. (2013). 'I don't know what a proper woman means': what women with intellectual disabilities think about sex, sexuality and themselves. *British Journal of Learning Disabilities, 41*, 5–12.

Flynn, M., & Citrella, V. (2013). Winterbourne View Hospital: a glimpse of the legacy. *The Journal of Adult Protection, 15*, 173–181.

Francis, R. (2010). *Independent inquiry into care provided by Mid Staffordshire NHS Foundation Trust January 2005–March 2009*. London: Stationery Office.

Fraser Barbour, E. F. (2018). On the ground insights from disability professionals supporting people with intellectual disability who have experienced sexual violence. *The Journal of Adult Protection, 20*, 207–220.

Fyson, R. (2009). Independence and learning disabilities: why we must also recognise vulnerability. *The Journal of Adult Protection, 11*, 18–25.

Gaylard, D. (2008). Policy and practice. In A. Mantell & T. Scragg (Eds.), *Safeguarding adults in social work* (pp. 9–30). Exeter: Learning Matters.

Gravell, C. (2012). *Loneliness and cruelty. People with learning disabilities and their experiences of harassment, abuse and related crime in the community*. London: Lemos and Crane.

UK family found guilty of enslaving homeless and disabled people. (2017). *Guardian*. Available at: https://www.theguardian.com/uk-news/2017/aug/11/uk-family-found-guilty-of-enslaving-homeless-and-disabled-people.

Hanley, J., & Marsland, D. (2014). Unhappy anniversary? *The Journal of Adult Protection, 16*, 104–112.

Herbert, C., Joyce, T., Gray, G., et al. (2019). *Capacity to consent to sexual relations*. Leicester: British Psychological Society.

Hewitt, O. (2014). A survey of experiences of abuse. *Tizard Learning Disability Review, 19*, 122–129.

Hollomotz, A. (2009). Beyond 'vulnerability': an ecological model approach to conceptualizing risk of sexual violence against people with learning difficulties. *British Journal of Social Work, 39*, 99–112.

Hollomotz, A. (2012). 'A lad tried to get hold of my boobs, so I kicked him': an examination of attempts by adults with learning difficulties to initiate their own safeguarding. *Disability and Society, 27*, 117–129.

Holmes, K. M., & O'Loughlin, N. (2014). The experiences of people with learning disabilities on social networking sites. *British Journal of Learning Disabilities, 42*, 3–7.

Home Office. (2014). *Modern slavery: how the UK is leading the fight*. Available at: https://assets.publishing.service.gov.uk/government/uploads/system/uploads/attachment_data/file/328096/Modern_slavery_booklet_v12_WEB__2_.pdf.

Hough, R. E. (2012). Adult protection and 'intimate citizenship' for people with learning difficulties: empowering and protecting in light of the No Secrets review. *Disability and Society, 27*, 131–144.

Hurtado, B., Timmins, S., & Seward, C. (2012). The importance of being earnest: our experience of involving service users with complex needs in staff recruitment. *British Journal of Learning Disabilities, 42*, 38–44.

Joyce, T. (2003). An audit of investigations into allegations of abuse involving adults with intellectual disability. *Journal of Intellectual Disability Research, 47*, 606–616.

Livingstone, J. (2006). *My money matters. Guidance on the best practice in handling the money of people with learning disabilities*. Chesterfield: ARC.

McCarthy, M. (1999). *Sexuality and women with learning disabilities*. London: Jessica Kingsley.

McCarthy, M., & Thompson, D. (1996). Sexual abuse by design: an examination of the issues in learning disability services. *Disability and Society, 11*, 205–218.

McCarthy, M. (2014). Brick by brick: building up our knowledge base on the abuse of adults with learning disabilities. *Tizard Learning Disability Review, 19,* 130–133.

McCarthy, M., Hunt, S., & Skillman, K. (2017). 'I know it was every week, but I can't be sure if it was every day': domestic violence and women with learning disabilities. *Journal of Applied Research in Intellectual Disabilities, 30,* 269–282.

McCarthy, M., Hunt, S., Triantafyllopoulou, P., et al. (2019). 'Put bluntly, they are targeted by the worst creeps society has to offer': police and professionals' views and actions relating to domestic violence and women with intellectual disabilities. *Journal of Applied Research in Intellectual Disabilities, 32,* 71–81.

McGilloway, C., Smith, D., & Galvin, R. (2020). Barriers faced by adults with intellectual disabilities who experience sexual assault: a systematic review and meta-synthesis. *Journal of Applied Research in Intellectual Disabilities, 33,* 51–66.

Manthorpe, J., & Lipman, V. (2015). Preventing abuse through pre-employment checks: an international review. *The Journal of Adult Protection, 17,* 341–350.

Manthorpe, J., & Stanley, N. (1999). Conclusion. Shifting the focus from 'bad apples' to users' rights. In N. Stanley, J. Manthorpe, & B. Penhale (Eds.), *Institutional abuse: perspectives across the lifecourse* (pp. 223–240). London: Routledge.

Manthorpe, J., & Martineau, S. (2015). What can and cannot be learned from serious case reviews of the care and treatment of adults with learning disabilities in England? Messages for social workers. *British Journal of Social Work, 45,* 331–348.

Marsland, D., Oakes, P., & White, C. (2007). Abuse in care? The identification of early indicators of the abuse of people with learning disabilities in residential settings. *The Journal of Adult Protection, 9,* 6–20.

Marsland, D., Oakes, P., & Bright, N. (2015a). It can still happen here: systemic risk factors that may contribute to the continued abuse of people with intellectual disabilities. *Tizard Learning Disability Review, 20,* 134–146.

Marsland, D., Oakes, P., & White, C. (2015b). Abuse in care? A research project to identify early indicators of concern in residential and nursing homes for older people. *The Journal of Adult Protection, 17,* 111–125.

Martin, J. (1984). *Hospitals in trouble.* Oxford: Basil Blackwell.

May-Chahal, C., Bertotti, T., Blasio, P., et al. (2006). Child maltreatment in the family: a European perspective. *European Journal of Social Work, 9,* 3–20.

Murphy, G. (2019). Whorlton Hall: a predictable tragedy? *British Medical Journal, 366,* l4705.

NHS England. (2019). *Safeguarding policy.* Available at: https://www.england.nhs.uk/wp-content/uploads/2019/09/safeguarding-policy.pdf.

Northway, R., Melsome, M., Flood, S., et al. (2013a). How do people with intellectual disabilities view abuse and abusers? *Journal of Intellectual Disabilities, 17,* 361–375.

Northway, R., Bennett, D., Melsome, M., et al. (2013b). Keeping safe and providing support: a participatory survey about abuse and people with intellectual disabilities. *Journal of Policy and Practice in Intellectual Disabilities, 10,* 236–244.e.

O'Callaghan, A. C., Murphy, G., & Clare, I. C. H. (2003). *Symptoms of abuse in adults with severe learning disabilities Final report to the Department of Health.* Canterbury: Tizard Centre, University of Kent.

O'Malley, G., Irwin, L., Syed, A. A., et al. (2019). The clinical approach used in supporting individuals with intellectual disability who have been sexually abused. *British Journal of Learning Disabilities, 47,* 105–115.

Olsen, A., & Carter, C. (2016). Responding to the needs of people with learning disabilities who have been raped: co-production in action. *Tizard Learning Disability Review, 21,* 30–38.

Ombudsman New South Wales. (2018). *Abuse and neglect of vulnerable adults in New South Wales – the need for action.* Sydney, Australia: NSW Ombudsman. Available at: https://www.ombo.nsw.gov.au/__data/assets/pdf_file/0003/62139/Abuse-and-neglect-of-vulnerable-adults-in-NSW-November-2018.pdf.

Peckham, N. G., Corbett, A., Howlett, S., et al. (2007). The delivery of a survivors group for learning disabled women who have been abused. *British Journal of Learning Disabilities, 35,* 236–244.

Plomin, J. (2019). *Whorlton Hall hospital abuse and how it was uncovered.* BBC News. Available at: https://www.bbc.co.uk/news/health-48369500.

Robinson, S., & Chenoweth, L. (2011). Preventing abuse in accommodation services: from procedural response to protective cultures. *Journal of Intellectual Disabilities, 15,* 63–74.

Robinson, S., & Chenoweth, L. (2012). Understanding emotional and psychological harm of people with intellectual disability: an evolving framework. *The Journal of Adult Protection, 14,* 110–121.

Robinson, S., Frawley, P., & Dyson, S. (2020). Access and accessibility in domestic and family violence services for women with disabilities: widening the lens. *Violence Against Women, 0,* 1–19.

Rowsell, A. C., Clare, I. C. H., & Murphy, G. H. (2013). The psychological impact of abuse on men and women with severe intellectual disabilities. *Journal of Applied Research in Intellectual Disabilities, 26,* 257–270.

Sequeira, H., Howlin, P., & Hollins, S. (2003). Psychological symptoms associated with sexual abuse in people with learning disabilities: case control study. *Br J Psychiatry*, *183*, 451–456.

SCIE. (2018). *Types and indicators of abuse.* Available at: https://www.scie.org.uk/safeguarding/adults/introduction/types-and-indicators-of-abuse.

Scottish Government. (2013). *The keys to life. Improving the quality of life for people with learning disabilities.* Edinburgh: The Scottish Government. Available at: https://keystolife.info/wp-content/uploads/2019/03/the-keys-to-life-full-version.pdf.

Scottish Government. (2019). *The keys to life. Unlocking Futures for People with Learning Disabilities implementation framework and priorities 2019–2021.* Available at: https://keystolife.info/wp-content/uploads/2019/03/Keys-To-Life-Implementation-Framework.pdf.

Sobsey, D. (1994). Sexual abuse of individuals with intellectual disability. In A. Craft (Ed.), *Practice issues in sexuality and learning disabilities.* London: Routledge.

Sobsey, D., & Mansell, S. (1990). The prevention of sexual abuse of people with developmental disabilities. *Developmental Disabilities Bulletin*, *18*, 51–66.

Tinney, G., Forde, J., Hone, L., et al. (2014). Safe and social: what does it mean anyway?? *British Journal of Learning Disabilities*, *43*, 55–61.

Walter-Brice, A., Cox, R., Priest, H., et al. (2012). What do women with learning disabilities say about their experiences of domestic abuse within the context of their intimate partner relationships? *Disability and Society*, *27*, 503–517.

Wardhaugh, J., & Wilding, P. (1993). Towards an explanation of the corruption of care. *Critical Social Policy*, *37*, 4–31.

White, C., Holland, E., Marsland, D., et al. (2003). The identification of environments and cultures that promote the abuse of people with intellectual disabilities: a review of the literature. *Journal of Applied Research in Intellectual Disabilities*, *16*, 1–9.

Wishart, G. (2003). The sexual abuse of people with learning difficulties: do we need a social model approach to vulnerability? *The Journal of Adult Protection*, *5*, 14–27.

Maximising my health

'I want to live independently. At the moment I still rely on my mum to cook my tea, but I want to be in a flat, not too far away. I feel confident being on my own. I'll need support to learn how to use a cooker, and I need help finding places.'

JoAnne

'As a general rule, getting a paid job is what I'd like. It's hard to get the benefits you deserve. The people asking have made the system more cruel as they make it out that you can do more than you can. Even the form is inaccessible and I often don't really know what they're asking. Because I try to go for jobs I think I can do, I need support with travel, which can be a big problem, particularly on buses. I panic and get off too soon or too late. I once got on a bus that went somewhere I didn't recognise so I got off and had to ask where I was. I ended up being late. Thankfully, I'm now used to buses in Leeds, but if I go somewhere new, I don't really know what I'm look-ing for.'

Alison

'I'd like a job – maybe in a supermarket. My family will need to help me get that job.'

Jack

Understanding health

Beth Marks, Jasmina Sisirak and Joann Kiernan

KEY ISSUES

- Understanding health conceptualisations and health challenges for people with intellectual disabilities is critical for ensuring that health is an everyday resource for people to live, learn, work, recreate, and thrive in their communities.
- Addressing social determinants of health and illness for people with intellectual disabilities can improve health outcomes.
- Incorporating the Ottawa Charter strategies of "advocate, enable, and mediate," can shift the view of health not as a single amorphous condition, but a complex state comprised of multiple levels of wellness.
- Using an ecological framework can optimise health outcomes by engaging people with intellectual disabilities, building capacity among their supports, and promoting health- and disability-friendly communities.

CHAPTER OUTLINE

INTRODUCTION

Understanding health and health challenges for people with intellectual disabilities is critical for ensuring that health is an everyday, equitable resource for this group to live, learn, work, recreate, and thrive in communities. This chapter will explore the concept of health among people with intellectual disabilities and their unique vulnerabilities to health and illness as compared to their non-intellectually disabled peers. Specifically, we will delineate conceptualisations of health, social determinants of health and illness, and an ecological framework to optimise health outcomes by engaging people with intellectual disabilities. Aligned to this are the structures. that may hinder or facilitate access to relevant health care and opportunities for health promotion within the context of individual disabilities. We consider how capacity can be built among people's supports, promoting health- and disability-friendly communities. We begin, however, by exploring the three core strategies of the Ottawa Charter- "advocate, enable, and mediate" (World Health Organization (WHO), 1986). This will serve to demonstrate how the conceptualisation of health among people with intellectual disabilities has shifted beyond the dichotomous and negative perspective (e.g., freedom from disease) to a view of health, not as a single amorphous condition, but as a complex state comprised of multiple levels of health and wellbeing. The roles of multisectoral stakeholders in optimising social, economic, and environmental factors to improve health outcomes for individuals with intellectual disabilities will also be discussed.

UNDERSTANDING THE CONCEPT OF HEALTH

The Ottawa Charter for Health Promotion definition of health as a resource for everyday life and a positive concept emphasising social and personal resources (WHO, 1986) provides a framework for broadening our understanding of health for people with intellectual disabilities and the challenges they face. Traditionally, health promotion for people with intellectual disabilities was situated in the health sector. However, a widening responsibility for promoting health across the different settings where people with intellectual disabilities live, learn, work, and access recreation provides opportunities to further consider the range of social determinants that impact on health outcomes for this group. The WHO defines a setting as a "place or social context in which people engage in daily activities in which environmental, organizational, and personal factors interact to affect health and wellbeing" (World Health Organization, 1998a). This may include schools, worksites, municipalities, community centres, recreational facilities, or hospitals.

Sundsvall Statement

Building on the Ottawa Charter (WHO, 1986), the Sundsvall Statement of 1991 connects health with our physical environments and calls for the creation of supportive environments that encourage everyone, including people with intellectual disabilities, to be engaged in maintaining optimal health ('Supportive environments for health: The Sundsvall Statement', 1991). In 1997, the Jakarta Declaration on health promotion further emphasised the value and role of community settings to implement public policy, create supportive environments, promote community action, while developing personal skills and reorienting health services ('The Jakarta Declaration on health promotion in the 21st century', 1998). Promoting health and addressing health challenges among people with intellectual disabilities, who are often an underserved and marginalised group worldwide, requires the development of new partnerships for health across all community sectors and levels of society and government.

Broad multisectoral alliances increase the capacity for social, economic, and environmental supports for people with intellectual disabilities to enable access to health promoting options and the achievement of optimal health outcomes. Addressing the broad determinants of health that may range from home and neighbourhood, education, work, transport, food and nutrition, social support, and care can achieve the goal of health for all people with intellectual disabilities (World Health Organization (WHO), 1998b). Because people with intellectual disabilities often have little input into the way their health and health concerns are perceived and addressed, considering health as a resource and addressing the wider determinants of health can provide better supports for this group to function in their communities.

By virtue of variations in stages of social, cognitive and emotional development, health challenges among people with intellectual disabilities must be considered within the context of person-centeredness. People with intellectual disabilities often have little to no control over decisions made regarding their lives, have limited choices and lack the opportunity to input or consent (Debenham, 2020). Figure 9.1 illustrates the journey that many individuals with intellectual disabilities experience in their attempts to access health services.

Social determinants of health

Article 25 and the other articles within the 2006 United Nations Convention on the Rights of Persons with Disabilities (UNCRPD) provide a global impetus to secure community-integrated, sustainable health promotion initiatives so people with intellectual disabilities can enjoy optimal health without discrimination. Health risks and health outcomes for people with intellectual disabilities are affected by conditions known as social determinants of health in the places where they live, learn, work, and access recreation opportunities (Centers for Disease Control and Prevention (CDC), 2018). Strategies to reduce health disparities must include attention to the multiple social determinants that influence health

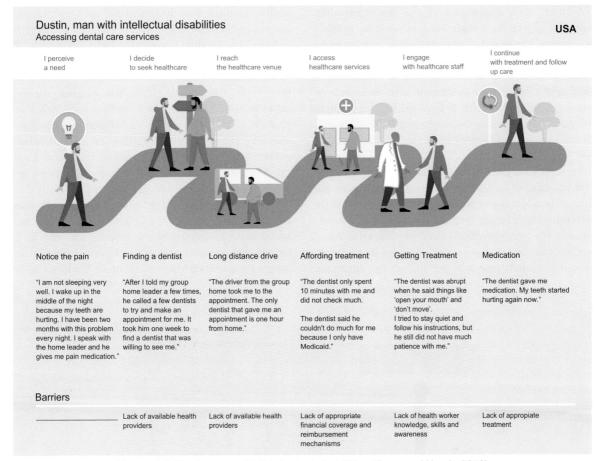

Figure 9.1 Dustin, man with intellectual disabilities (Kuper and Heydt, 2019)

outcomes (Krahn and Fox, 2014). Integrating a multi-level, social determinants approach to improve health outcomes for people with intellectual disabilities focuses available resources on social and economic factors, social support networks, physical and social environments, access to health services, and social and health policies (Koh et al, 2010). Addressing the myriad of challenges to the health of people with intellectual disabilities requires understanding environmental and structural barriers along with social determinants (Bodde and Seo, 2009).

Triple burden of disease

Today's global health concerns for people with intellectual disabilities reflect a 'triple burden of diseases' from communicable diseases, newly emerging and re-emerging diseases, as well as the unprecedented rise of non-communicable chronic conditions (Kumar and Preetha, 2012). The COVID-19 pandemic highlights a "narrow margin of health" for many people with intellectual disabilities as the interaction between non-communicable chronic conditions and a highly contagious communicable disease is resulting in new diseases that have potential for long term illnesses among this group. Additionally, COVID-19 has exposed structural weaknesses of social care systems for people with intellectual disabilities around the world that were ill-prepared to support healthy lifestyles. With poorly managed multiple chronic conditions such as high cholesterol, hypertension, cardiovascular disease, and obesity, many people with intellectual disabilities found that their congregate care settings were "hotspots" for COVID-19 infections and that they were more likely to die from COVID-19 than their non-intellectually disabled peers (Turk and McDermott, 2020).

A variety of the ongoing threats that challenge public health initiatives for people with intellectual disabilities around the world, including lack of resources to take care of the most vulnerable, become immediately apparent with any crisis. Whilst people with intellectual disabilities continue to struggle with issues related to hunger, food insecurity, sedentary lifestyles, climate changes, and increasing frequency of natural disasters, financial crises, and security risks, the implied value of their lives is "less worthy."

As seen with the COVID-19 pandemic, an urgent need was created across many communities worldwide to actively address the social determinants of health. Determinants of health including economic and political stability, neighbourhood environment, education, food, community and social networks, are increasingly associated with having a bigger impact on improved health outcomes than the health care sector which often focuses solely on biomedical care (Kumar and Preetha, 2012). The Health Rankings Model in Figure 9.2 (University of Wisconsin Population Health Institute (UWPHI), 2014) uses a model of population health that emphasises various factors that can help communities become healthier places to live, learn, work and play for people with intellectual disabilities by understanding the factors that influence an individual's overall quality of life and life expectancy. This model can be used in communities as a framework to identify how various factors influence the health of individuals (health factors) and in the future (health outcomes). For example, the physical environment, along with social and economic factors, account for 50% of the factors that impact a person's health outcomes by limiting or supporting options to make healthy choices,

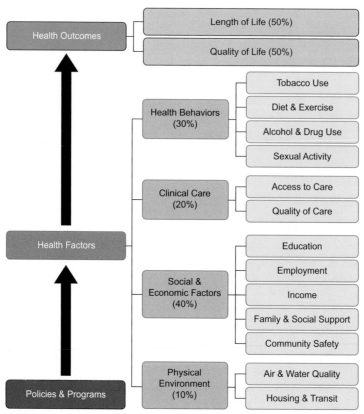

Figure 9.2 Health Rankings Model (University of Wisconsin Population Health Institute (UWPHI), 2014)

have social support, obtain quality health care, enjoy safe, clean housing and communities, manage stress, access transportation to work, school and recreation.

As shown in Figure 9.2, a population's health is shaped 10% by the physical environment, 20% by clinical health care (access and quality), 30% by health behaviours (largely determined by social and physical environments), and 40% by social and economic factors. In using this model to improve health outcomes for adults with intellectual disabilities living in the community, the social and economic factors are a major predictor of health outcomes and strongly impact health behaviours. With safe communities and sufficient economic, social, and environmental support, people are more likely to engage in, and sustain, health promoting activities. For people with intellectual disabilities, addressing the social determinants of health is *even more* imperative today given global public health issues and the inherent vulnerability this group experience within their communities. Research documents the long-lasting biological effects on health from social determinants and adverse life events (National Academies of Sciences, Engineering and Medicine, 2019).

In the United States of America, communities were galvanised to advocate with and for people with intellectual disabilities to obtain access to quality healthcare, social and family support, and health promoting and disease prevention programmes during the COVID-19 pandemic. For example, Disability Rights Pennsylvania (2020) successfully advocated for an exception to its COVID-19 visitation policies to permit access to support persons for people with intellectual disabilities to be able to understand and participate in their treatment as required by federal anti-discrimination laws.

 READER ACTIVITY 9.1

Identify difficulties encountered by people with intellectual disabilities, and those supporting them, in relation to the COVID-19 pandemic in your country or region.

Consider if and how they were overcome.

Based upon this, reflect on whether you would feel better equipped should a similar situation (re-) occur.

HEALTH CHALLENGES

Unfortunately, people with intellectual disabilities are experiencing more complex health conditions, earlier onset of age-related conditions, and premature age-related changes in their health compared to their peers without disabilities (Bowers et al, 2014; Carmeli and Imam, 2014; Esbensen, 2010; Krahn and Fox, 2014). In comparison to people without disabilities, people with intellectual disabilities are often the most underserved with regard to health services, and in consequence often experience premature deaths (University of Bristol, 2013; Scott and Havercamp, 2014). Additionally, because people with intellectual disabilities frequently live in settings devoid of inclusive and accessible health promoting environments and communities, they experience a number of issues related to negative determinants of health (e.g., environmental exposures, social circumstances, poor healthcare access, unhealthy behaviours) (Scheepers et al, 2005; Sisirak et al, 2016). For example, in the United States the prevalence of being overweight and obese is documented as equal or higher amongst people with intellectual disabilities than found in the general population (Segal et al, 2016; Rimmer et al, 2011).

Many people with intellectual disabilities experience a number of co-existing chronic conditions which are often poorly managed. (Reichard et al, 2011; Rimmer et al, 2010). There is reportedly an increased risk of mental health concerns amongst this group in addition to a range of undetected vision and oral health problems (Krahn et al, 2015). A higher prevalence of sleep difficulties, including less stable and more fragmented sleep, is also more prevalent in this group (Shanahan et al, 2019).

People with intellectual disabilities have 2.5 times more health problems related to epilepsy, dental disease, osteoporosis, and Alzheimer's disease and related dementias as compared to the general population (O'Dwyer et al, 2016). Similar to older adults in the general population, they may also experience negative consequences related to polypharmacy/overmedication with potentially inappropriate medications (O'Dwyer et al, 2016, 2017; NHS England, 2017), and limited physical and mental stimulation at earlier ages compared to their non-disabled peers (Flood, 2018).

People with intellectual disabilities also experience a higher prevalence of comorbid circulatory, respiratory, and endocrine diseases across all age groups. Potential negative health outcomes are compounded by reduced uptake of health screenings, for example cancer screenings, and preventive services. Overall limited access to health care services leads to generally poorer health outcomes amongst this group including lowered life expectancy.

Life expectancy

Tailored health care services and health promotion programming is urgently needed for people with intellectual disabilities to be able to live, work, learn, and benefit from recreation opportunities in communities and settings of their choice. With improved access to health care, increased availability of diagnostic technology, medication and surgical interventions, many people with intellectual disabilities in developed countries are experiencing improved health outcomes and decreased mortality rates (Bittles and Glasson, 2004). However, 80% of all people living with a disability worldwide (which will include people with intellectual disabilities) reside in developing countries where these benefits may not be seen. Additionally, 90% of children with a disability do not attend school, increasing the likelihood of living in poverty as an adult with poor health outcomes (Marchildon, 2018).

Yet despite people with intellectual disabilities in developed countries experiencing decreased mortality, their overall mortality rates remain higher than those found in the general population. In 2019 the Learning Disability Mortality Review (LeDeR) Programme reported significant differences in life expectancy of people with intellectual disabilities compared to the general population in England with men with intellectual disabilities dying on average 23 years earlier than men without intellectual disabilities and women on average 27 years earlier than their non-intellectually disabled peers (NHS England and NHS Improvement, 2019). With life expectancy of people with intellectual disabilities predicted to rise over the next two to three decades, with many living into their 70s and 80s, primary health care is a significant worldwide need for this group.

Globally, primary health care is basic health care that is universally accessible and acceptable to people with intellectual disabilities and their supports, located in their communities at an affordable cost (World Health Organization, 1978). As an approach to health policy and service provision it includes services ranging from individual care from a primary care provider (primary care services) to population-level "public health-type" functions (Awofeso, 2004; Muldoon et al, 2006). While primary care is person-focused, with an ideal of a sustained partnership between people with intellectual disabilities and their health care provider over time (Institute of Medicine (IOM), 1996; Muldoon et al, 2006; Starfield, 1998), it also includes core components of universal access to care; commitment to health equity oriented to social justice; community participation in developing and implementing health goals; and intersectoral approaches to health (Muldoon et al, 2006; Scott and Havercamp, 2016; World Health Organization (WHO), 2003).

Facilitating primary health care

On an individual level, it is imperative in primary care that people with intellectual disabilities receive accessible services around health promotion, disease prevention, health maintenance, counselling, patient education, diagnosis and treatment of acute and chronic illnesses. While access to linguistic and culturally relevant care is a global challenge across all community sectors, it can be particularly problematic for people with intellectual disabilities. To date very few professional health care training programmes address disability issues in their curricula (Havercamp and Scott, 2015; Holder et al, 2009; Minihan et al, 2011; Phillips et al 2004; Thierer and Meyerowitz, 2005). Even within countries where there exists field specific training for nurses, for example the UK and Eire, a shortage of intellectual (learning) disability nurses remains an issue (Royal College of Nursing, 2018).

Nurses report knowledge gaps concerning the health care needs of people with intellectual disabilities with minimal if any training into how to effectively communicate with this group (Melville et al, 2005). Studies among health professionals document stress, lack of confidence, fear and anxiety, and poorer treatment interventions for people with intellectual disabilities (Oulton et al, 2018; Pelleboer-Gunnink et al, 2017). There is agreement that accreditation bodies should stipulate standardised disability content across different health professions' educational programmes in a bid to increase confidence and skills in working with people

BOX 9.1 Main practitioner training needs to improve health of people with intellectual disabilities

General communication
Knowledge/information
Profession-specific needs to reduce the high prevalence of poor physical and psychiatric health among people with intellectual disabilities
(Hemm et al, 2015)

who have various disabilities (Ong et al, 2017; Roll et al, 2017). Box 9.1 lists the main training needs related to this group

With the lack of disability content across health professions' education, people with intellectual disabilities continue to experience a cascade of disparities (Krahn et al, 2006). Treatment plans and risks may not be communicated in an accessible way; health care providers may be unable to complete physical examinations, diagnostic procedures, and screening and preventive care due to economic and structural policies that do not accommodate people with intellectual disabilities who may require access to adjusted health care environments. This may include physical accessibility (e.g. wheelchair accessible waiting rooms); longer appointment times, accessible examination tables and diagnostic equipment amongst others (Minihan et al, 2011). Attitudinal biases may also still prevail among many health care providers, and present unnecessary barriers which may negatively affect the quality of care. This includes 'diagnostic overshadowing', which is an assumption made by a health professional that a health concern reported by or on behalf of someone with intellectual disabilities is related to their disability rather than an emerging physiological or psychological condition (Javaid et al, 2019; Lewis and Stenfert-Kroese, 2010).

Health systems can reduce inequities and improve health outcomes through clinical care by incorporating local and national legal mandates such as the Equality Act 2010 in the UK and the Americans with Disabilities Act (ADA) of 1990, both of which aim to prevent discrimination against people with disabilities (ADA, 1990; UK Equality Act, 2010). Additionally, health and social systems can attend to the following strategies to improve access among people with intellectual disabilities: accessible formats for health information to accommodate various learning and language needs;

wayfinding signage design, and sign language interpreters for people who are deaf or hard of hearing; large print formats for people with low vision; and readers for people who are blind or visually impaired (Marks and Sisirak, 2013). Methods of promoting access to healthcare are discussed in more detail in the following chapter.

In summary, people with intellectual disabilities will likely experience improved health outcomes when health care becomes equitable and inclusive at the primary care level (Lennox et al, 2015). Moreover, to address many of the issues related to ineffective or absent health care delivery (Ali et al, 2013), the provision of evidence-based didactic and clinical preparation for health care professionals can increase their knowledge and confidence in providing health care to this group (Holder et al, 2009). To address health inequities and have access to necessary resources to control health determinants, such as culturally and linguistically relevant care, the Ottawa Charter of 1986 clearly states the need for political action (WHO, 1986) to ensure "health care for all" through primary health care.

KEY DETERMINANTS OF HEALTH

The next section of this chapter considers in more detail some of the reasons why people with intellectual disabilities may experience poorer health than their non-intellectually disabled peers. These are considered in relation to three key areas – disability, health behaviours including access to health education and health promotion and social, economic and environmental factors.

Disability

An etiological cause of disability may be associated with medical conditions in 40-60% of adults with intellectual disabilities (Battaglia et al, 1991; Lennox, 2002; Majnemer and Shevell, 1995). The more significant the intellectual disability, the more likely the etiology is identifiable, along with greater multi-morbidity burden, which occurs at a much earlier age (Cooper et al, 2015; Gustavson et al, 1977; Lennox, 2002). In addition, many people with intellectual disabilities who have specific syndrome-related conditions (e.g., Down, Fragile X, Prader-Willi, Williams, Rett, Angelman syndromes, tuberous sclerosis, cerebral palsy) may also be predisposed to specific health conditions related to their disability. People with intellectual disabilities may also have higher rates of epilepsy, psychiatric conditions, gastrointestinal concerns, and sensory and mobility disabilities compared to their non-disabled peers (Robertson et al, 2015; Traci et al, 2002).

Disability etiology, syndromes, and associated health conditions can be supported by tailored development of accessible health care services and health promotion interventions that can maximise a person's quality of life (Lennox, 2002). For example, syndrome-related conditions may predispose a person with intellectual disability to having issues such as difficulty eating or swallowing, dental problems, reduced mobility, bone demineralisation, gastroesophageal reflux, arthritis, decreased muscle tone, and progressive cervical spine degeneration (Marks and Sisirak, 2013; White-Scott, 2007).

Health behaviours

Similar to people without disabilities, health behaviours of people with intellectual disabilities can directly influence health status. Researchers in Portugal found numerous and diverse unmet needs that could impact on the health of this group (see Box 9.2).

Key behavioural factors of health include physical activity, diet, hand washing, alcohol, tobacco, and other drug use (Office of Disease Prevention and Health Promotion, 2020). Studies continue to report low levels of physical activity, poor fitness, poor nutrition, and a

higher risk of falls among people with intellectual disabilities. For many adults with intellectual disabilities, the combination of sedentary lifestyles, high fat and low fruit and vegetable diets is a major factor for the increased risk for acquiring chronic health conditions.

Many people with intellectual disabilities are frequently prescribed psychotropic and anti-seizure medications on a long-term basis for behavioural issues which can often be more easily managed with complementary care approaches, such as acupuncture, spinal manipulation, and massage therapy (Bowring et al, 2017; Perry et al, 2018). Medications prescribed for people with intellectual disabilities can contribute to a higher risk of falling (Hsieh et al, 2012) and for osteoporosis (brittle bone disease), which may be compounded by the lack of physical activity and a diet limited in calcium and vitamin D (Bolton et al, 2017). Proactive healthcare management and elimination or modification of behavioural risk factors associated with either the onset or the management of a chronic condition can mitigate more serious health issues related to multiple chronic conditions (Roll, 2018).

Many people with intellectual disabilities receive limited or no health education during their primary education. Moreover, if they were taught health information, they may not have received disability-specific health education or health education that was accessible for their particular learning needs. Consequently, people with intellectual disabilities often have low health literacy impacting their self-care and management of their own health, resulting in high use of treatment services, increased hospitalisation rates and use of emergency services, low utilisation of preventive services, and high health care costs (Baur, 2007; National Center for Education Statistics, 2003). Additionally, many may have had early negative experiences with healthcare, which creates challenges and barriers to their ability to interact with health care providers and use of health care facilities (Ali et al, 2013).

Health promotion is a continuous process affected by daily circumstances, context, and life stages and must begin in infancy so that people with intellectual disabilities, who may have a higher risk of various health conditions across their lifespan, can achieve positive health outcomes. Cardell (2015) argues that factors associated with individual lifestyles, preferences, motivation for health behaviours, disabilities, mental health

 BOX 9.2   Unmet needs impacting on health of people with intellectual disabilities

1. Literacy
2. Handling of money
3. Information on rights
4. Self-care
5. Information on services
6. Communication
7. Occupation at holidays and weekends
8. General physical health
9. Cognitive rehabilitation
10. Daytime activities
    (Albuquerque and Carvalho, 2020)

and interdependence of individuals on others may all affect access and implementation of health promotion activities; as such, tailoring health promotion programmes to enable people with intellectual disabilities to live healthy lives is recommended.

Social, economic and environmental factors

People with intellectual disabilities often live in homes and communities that are devoid of inclusive and accessible health promoting environments (Scheepers et al, 2005; Sisirak et al, 2016a). They are also more likely to be unemployed, under-educated, have lower incomes, and greater disparities in health care (Krahn et al, 2015; Ward et al, 2010). As health begins in our homes, schools, workplaces, neighbourhoods, and communities, creating social and physical environments that promote good health for all is critical for people with intellectual disabilities (Office of Disease Prevention and Health Promotion (ODPHP), 2016).

Socioeconomic and environmental factors which affect health status, include "rapid and often adverse social, economic and demographic changes that affect working conditions, learning environments, family patterns, and the culture and social fabric of communities" (World Health Organization (WHO), 2005). However, the vulnerability and exclusion of people with intellectual disabilities across the lifespan who are isolated and marginalised in many communities remains a challenge (Cummins and Lau, 2003; Wilson et al, 2017). Where people with intellectual disabilities live, work, and access recreation matters. Financial stability and money also matter, as poverty is one of the most prevalent risk factors of poor health (Emerson and Hatton, 2007). For example, in a study with a nationally representative cross-sectional sample of 7070 British families supporting children aged 0–16 years in 2002, families supporting a child with an intellectual disability were 42% more likely to be living in poverty, 70% more likely to have no savings and to worry about money "all the time", and over twice as likely to be in debt and experience material hardship (Emerson and Hatton, 2007).

For people with intellectual disabilities, living in specific residential settings and participating in day programmes, such as those in schools, worksites and group activity programmes can affect their health status. As an example, in the U.S. adults living in the least restrictive community settings have the highest rates of obesity and low intake of fruits and vegetables (Hsieh et al, 2014; Sisirak et al, 2007).

Limited social support, disruption of personal ties, loneliness, violence against people with intellectual disabilities, and conflicted interactions with peers and supports can be major stressors for this group (Hartley and MacLean, 2009; Petroutsou et al, 2018). Quantity and quality of social relationships affect mental and physical health, as well as health behaviours and mortality risk (Umberson et al, 2010; Umberson and Montez, 2010). Supportive social connections and intimate relations are vital sources of emotional strength and can have a positive effect on health status (Umberson et al, 2010).

ADVOCATE, ENABLE, AND MEDIATE

For people with intellectual disabilities, health promotion leaders are in the early stages of rethinking health as a positive concept emphasising social and personal advocacy and situating health as a resource for everyday life. The Ottawa Charter statement that "health is created and lived by people within the settings of their everyday life, such as, where people with intellectual disabilities learn, work, play and love" (WHO, 1986), creates a foundation for creating supportive spaces to implement tailored health promotion strategies (Dooris, 2006). Enabling, or empowering, people to take control of their advocacy efforts for health promotion broadens the focus beyond individual behavioural change to mediating or facilitating stakeholders' involvement in the socio-environmental, cultural, and access constraints that impact people with intellectual disabilities and their supports. Enabling requires greater sensitivity to power relations, whereas mediating has a central role in bridging the interests of stakeholders (Saan and Wise, 2011). As personal health practices are just one of the determinants of health, the *Ottawa Charter for Health Promotion* guides the global practice of health promotion for people with intellectual disabilities and provides a strategy that incorporates the following five essential actions: 1) build healthy public policy; 2) create supportive environments; 3) strengthen community action; 4) develop personal skills; and 5) reorient health services.

ECOLOGICAL FRAMEWORK TO OPTIMISE HEALTH OUTCOMES

With the development of evidence-based health promotion programmes for people with intellectual disabilities, implementation and sustainability on a large-scale remain tremendous challenges for providers and practitioners. Meeting the programmatic demands for health promotion presents unique opportunities in multiple community settings, such as schools, day programmes, work and residential settings. Some of the ways of addressing this are introduced here, explored and operationalised in Chapter 10.

Building a healthy public policy

Building healthy public policy for people with intellectual disabilities can combine a variety of complementary approaches including legislative approaches, fiscal measures, tax policy, organisational change, and community support. For example, addressing the rising economic concerns related to health needs of this group is critical. Health care cost estimates for people with intellectual disabilities across developed countries can vary substantially depending on a range of factors compared to their non-disabled peers (Ervin and Merrick, 2014; Lunsky et al, 2019). Efforts to address the high costs of this healthcare, while concomitantly achieving high-quality care and outcomes, are emerging with mixed models such as health care homes, managed care and Federally Qualified Health Centers in the U.S. that incorporate legislative, fiscal, policy, and social services changes (Ervin and Merrick, 2014). The overall aim is to *make the healthier choices for people with intellectual disabilities and their supports the easiest choice.* As noted by Williamson and Carr (2009), people need "health stocks," otherwise known as their health resources, to be productive citizens. The value of health is noted by the positive role it plays in facilitating people's abilities to fulfil their roles and responsibilities (WHO, 1986).

Create supportive environments

Creating supportive environments for people with intellectual disabilities requires an understanding that communities are unique, complex, and interrelated, and that health is interrelated with other goals. The links between people and their environments provide a foundation for including a socioecological approach to health. Just as homes, work, and leisure activities are sources of health for people without disabilities, creating accessible environments that are inclusive of people with intellectual disabilities requires universally designed health promotion strategies to ensure that living, working, and recreational conditions are safe, stimulating, satisfying and enjoyable. The evidence-based *HealthMatters Program Scale-Up Initiative* aims to support community organisations to build policies that support *health-friendly services and environments* across community sectors and local and state municipalities (Sisirak et al, 2016b). The *HealthMatters Initiative* is a multi-state research project in the U.S. that is identifying the facilitating "drivers" and processes to scale-up health promotion programming in each state, building health promotion capacity within participating community-based organisations (CBOs), and training CBO staff to implement the evidence-based 12-week *HealthMatters Program* for people with intellectual disabilities (Marks et al, 2010).

Many health promotion programmes developed for people with intellectual disabilities and their supports only focus on individual level behaviour change, such as, exercise, diet, nutrition, physical activity, skills and participation, and stress education (Scott and Havercamp, 2016). To improve health status among people with intellectual disabilities and mitigate the early onset of multiple chronic conditions or associated disability-related conditions, health promotion programmes need to incorporate a range of social and environmental frameworks using a settings-based approach. Enabling people with intellectual disabilities and community stakeholders to increase control over, and improve their health through action in their schools, homes, and work places, is the essential aim of health promotion (Bloch et al, 2014). Through community participation, partnership, and empowerment and equity, sustainable health activities are promoted, action across risk factors in community sectors is integrated, and inequities for people with intellectual disabilities are decreased (World Health Organization (WHO), 2020).

Strengthening community actions

Strengthening community actions is another opportunity that can achieve improved health outcomes through ongoing priority-setting, decision-making, strategic planning, and implementation. For people with intellectual disabilities, who are often socially isolated, emerging research documents the benefits of social prescribing to do the following: 1) improve people's health and wellbeing; 2) potentially reduce the need for secondary care with a healthcare provider who provides specialised services; and, 3) decrease healthcare professionals' workload (Drinkwater et al, 2019). Ownership and control are central to community empowerment efforts. Community development leverages existing community human and material capital to enhance self-care and social support. Active involvement requires all stakeholders, including people with intellectual disabilities and their supports, to have full, continuous, and equitable access to information, learning opportunities for health, and funding support.

Neighbours International engages communities of practice for healthy communities supporting the full participation and contributions of all of its members (Neighbours International, 2020). Using videos, such as "5 Valued Experiences and the 5 Accomplishments," Neighbours International presents ways to support people with intellectual disabilities outside of institutional care to achieve a person-centered life which allows people to contribute to their communities (Neighbours International, 2019).

English pop and theatre group MiXiT describe themselves as "an inclusive pop group trying to show EVERYONE that people can work together and create fantastic things" (Facebook, 2020). In 2018 they produced a film 'for front line staff' advocating the need to stop overmedication, particularly with psychotropic drugs, to help people stay well and have a good quality of life. This personifies the NHS England (2017) campaign STOMP (STopping Over Medication of People with a learning (intellectual) disability, autism or both), itself linked to children and young people via STAMP (Supporting Treatment and Appropriate Medication in Paediatrics; NHSE, 2018).

Developing personal skills

Developing personal skills among people with intellectual disabilities and their supports can occur through health promotion activities, such as awareness raising, health literacy, health education, and targeted life skills. The *HealthMessages Program* in the United States is a peer-to-peer programme led by health coaches who have intellectual disabilities and their mentors, which has demonstrated significant changes in self-efficacy scores, and peer participants had significant changes in physical activity and hydration knowledge, social supports, and total health behaviours (Marks et al,

2008). By developing personal and social skills, people with intellectual disabilities can have more options and control over their own health and their environments enabling them to make actual "choices" that are conducive to health. Because personal control and choice are often challenging for this group, developing advocacy skills is imperative for not only them, but also their supports, as it can be helpful to develop positive health behaviours in partnership.

Lifelong learning can support people with intellectual disabilities to make plans and decisions throughout all stages across the life course and to manage their disability, chronic conditions, illnesses, and injuries as they age. Facilitating lifelong learning must incorporate a settings approach in school, home, work, and community settings. Clear health communication using multi-modal strategies to ensure access needs to be increased among people with intellectual disabilities, their supports, and health services providers (Selden et al, 2000). Improving health literacy among people with intellectual disabilities has the potential to increase knowledge about one's body and the relationship between lifestyle factors (e.g., food choices, physical activity) and health outcomes and to recognise the need to seek care (Marks and Sisirak, 2013).

Reorientation of health services

Shared responsibility for health promotion and the pursuit of health among people with intellectual disabilities and their supports, community groups, health professionals, health service institutions and governments requires a *reorientation of health services*. Within the health sector, the interprofessional team must advocate for the inclusion of health promotion activities and move beyond its restricted focus on providing clinical and curative services. In order to reorient health services and provide holistic care for people with intellectual disabilities, changes are required in professional education and training to shift attitudes among health care professionals and the organisation of health services. *The Health Care for Adults With Intellectual and Developmental Disabilities: Toolkit for Primary Care Providers* is an example of an excellent tool for providers and caregivers to address the cascade of health disparities among people with intellectual disabilities (Vanderbilt Kennedy Center, 2020). This toolkit provides guidelines for people with intellectual disabilities experiencing any of the following: 1) complex or difficult-to-treat medical conditions; 2) difficulty accessing health care; 3) inadequate health care; 4) difficulties expressing symptoms and pain; and, 5) lack of access to wellness, preventive care, and health promotion. Engagement of community advocates is also critical for people with intellectual disabilities and their supports across all settings.

MULTISECTORAL STAKEHOLDERS

As previously mentioned, people with intellectual disabilities are living longer – a great success attributed to advances in medical care, education, and social environment (British Psychological Society/Royal College of Psychiatrists, 2015; Heller et al, 2018). With this increased longevity comes an increasing range of complex issues that health care providers need to address including men and women's reproductive health, sexuality, relationships, abuse issues, and violence (Addlakha et al, 2017; Merrick et al, 2014). The health sector, community, and regulatory environment can complement each other in efforts to address these needs and other social determinants of health (National Academies of Sciences, Engineering and Medicine, 2019). Stakeholders across all sectors need to incorporate a guiding principle that in each phase of planning, implementation and evaluation of health promotion activities, people with intellectual disabilities should become equal partners.

Health is not created within a medical model approach based on illness care, rather health is fulfilled and lived by people within their everyday life. Contemporary health promotion initiatives must continue to expand beyond exercise and diets through systematic studies examining technology such as internet, social media, and cell phone usage patterns among children and adults with intellectual disabilities (Jenaro et al, 2018). Opportunities and risks associated with technology have implications for community engagement through education, employment, recreation, health behaviours, and health outcomes. This demands that people with intellectual disabilities and health professionals are prepared to work with companies to help expand these.

The action areas outlined by the Ottawa Charter continue to provide a structure for implementing health promotion initiatives through actions that build healthy public policy, create supportive environments, strengthen community actions, develop personal skills, and reorient health services. As health promotion for people with intellectual disabilities moves beyond the health sector, key stakeholders and policy makers across many sectors and system levels will become more aware of how their decisions impact health outcomes. With more direct involvement of key stakeholders, they may be more likely to assume greater responsibility for the health of all populations, including people with intellectual disabilities.

CONCLUSION

This chapter has been designed to support the reader in an understanding of health conceptualisations and challenges for people with intellectual disabilities. Health is an everyday resource that enables people to live, learn, work, recreate, and thrive in their communities.

In order to improve health outcomes for individuals the social determinants of health and illness for people with intellectual disabilities must be identified and addressed. The challenge for the reader throughout this chapter was to consider health not as a single amorphous condition but a complex state of multiple levels of wellness.

A focus on ecological frameworks to optimise health outcomes through engagement with people with intellectual disabilities and a focus on capacity building within supportive systems has been discussed, whilst highlighting the need for the promotion of health- and disability-friendly communities. The Ottawa Charter (WHO, 1986) describes key collaborative activities to encourage everyone, including people with intellectual disabilities, to be engaged in maintaining optimal health through mediation, enablement and advocacy.

Dustin's experience (Figure 9.1) considered the connection of health with physical environments and the need to create more supportive, enabling environments as advocated in the Sundsvall Statement of 1991. Discussion of the social determinants of health and the triple burden of disease has been highlighted contemporarily for people with intellectual disabilities by the impact of COVID 19. The global pandemic has illustrated already established issues associated with health challenges, life expectancy and equitable access to primary and secondary health care for people with intellectual disabilities.

Moving forward practitioner training to facilitate access to and improvements in health for people with intellectual disabilities is even more pertinent today as discussed within this chapter (Box 9.1). The impact of unmet need on the health of people with intellectual disabilities (Box 9.2) allows us to consider the social, economic and environmental factors that require health promotion leaders to rethink health as a positive concept, a resource for everyday life that emphasises social and personal advocacy for people with intellectual disabilities.

REFERENCES

ADA. (1990). *Americans With Disabilities Act of 1990.* Available at: https://www.ada.gov/. [Accessed 23 December 2020].

Addlakha, R., Price, J., & Heidari, S. (2017). Disability and sexuality: claiming sexual and reproductive rights. *Reproductive Health Matters, 25*(50), 4–9.

Albuquerque, C. P., & Carvalho, A. C. (2020). Identification of needs of older adults with intellectual disabilities. *Journal of Policy and Practice in Intellectual Disabilities.* https://doi.org/10.1111/jppi.12325.

Ali, A., Scior, K., Ratti, V., et al. (2013). Discrimination and other barriers to accessing health care: perspectives of patients with mild and moderate intellectual disability and their carers. *PLoS One, 8*(8) e70855.

Awofeso, N. (2004). What is the difference between 'primary care' and 'primary healthcare'? *Quality in Primary Care, 12,* 93–94.

Battaglia, A., Bianchini, E., & Carey, J. (1991). Diagnostic yield of the comprehensive assessment of developmental delay/mental retardation in an insitute of child neuropsychiatry. *American Journal of Medical Genetics, 82,* 60–66.

Baur, C. (2007). Health literacy and adults with I/DD: achieving accessible health information and services. Paper presented at the State of Science in Aging with Developmental Disabilities, Atlanta, GA.

Bittles, A., & Glasson, E. (2004). Clinical, social, and ethical implications of changing life expectancy in Down syndrome. *Developmental Medicine & Child Neurology, 46*(4), 282–286.

Bloch, P., Toft, U., Reinbach, H., et al. (2014). Revitalizing the setting approach – supersettings for sustainable impact in community health promotion. *The International Journal of Behavioral Nutrition and Physical Activity, 11,* 118.

Bodde, A. E., & Seo, D. C. (2009). A review of social and environmental barriers to physical activity for adults with intellectual disabilities. *Disability & Health Journal, 2*(2), 57–66.

Bolton, J. M., Morin, S. N., Majumdar, S. R., et al. (2017). Association of mental disorders and related medication use with risk for major osteoporotic fractures. *JAMA Psychiatry, 74*(6), 641–648.

Bowers, B., Webber, R., & Bigby, C. (2014). Health issues of older people with intellectual disability in group homes. *Journal of Intellectual & Developmental Disability, 39*(3), 261–269.

Bowring, D. L., Totsika, V., Hastings, R. P., et al. (2017). Prevalence of psychotropic medication use and association with challenging behaviour in adults with an intellectual disability. A total population study. *Journal of Intellectual Disability Research, 61*(6), 604–617.

British Psychological Society/Royal College of Psychiatrists. (2015). Dementia and people with intellectual disabilities. In *Guidance on the assessment, diagnosis, interventions and support of people with intellectual disabilities who develop dementia.* Leicester, UK: British Psychological Society.

Cardell, B. (2015). Reframing health promotion for people with intellectual disabilities. *Global Qualitative Nursing Research, 2.*

Carmeli, E., & Imam, B. (2014). Health promotion and disease prevention strategies in older adults with intellectual and developmental disabilities. *Frontiers in Public Health, 2.*

Centers for Disease Control and Prevention. (2018). Social determinants of health: know what affects health. Available at: https://www.cdc.gov/socialdeterminants/index.htm. [Accessed 23 December 2020].

Cooper, S. A., McLean, G., Guthrie, B., et al. (2015). Multiple physical and mental health comorbidity in adults with intellectual disabilities: population-based cross-sectional analysis. *BMC Family Practice, 16*(1), 110.

Cummins, R., & Lau, A. (2003). Community integration or community exposure? A review and discussion in relation to people with an intellectual disability. *Journal of Applied Research in Intellectual Disabilities, 16*(2), 145–157.

Debenham, L. (2020). *What is person-centred planning?* Available at: http://www.aboutlearningdisabilities.co.uk/what-personcentred-planning.html. [Accessed 23 December 2020].

Disability Rights Pennsylvania. (2020). *DRP successfully advocates for exceptions to hospital COVID-19 visitation policies for patients with intellectual disability.* Available at: http://www.disabilityrightspa.org/spotlights/drp-successfully-advocates-for-exceptions-to-hospital-covid-19-visitation-policies-for-patients-with-intellectual-disability/. [Accessed 12 January 2021].

Dooris, M. (2006). Healthy settings: challenges to generating evidence of effectiveness. *Health Promotion International, 21*(1), 55–65.

Drinkwater, C., Wildman, J., & Moffatt, S. (2019). Social prescribing. *BMJ, 364,* l1285.

Emerson, E., & Hatton, C. (2007). Poverty, socio-economic position, social capital and the health of children and adolescents with intellectual disabilities in Britain: a replication. *Journal of Intellectual Disability Research*, *51*(Pt 11), 866–874.

Ervin, D., & Merrick, J. (2014). Intellectual and developmental disability: healthcare financing. *Frontiers in Public Health*, *2* 160–160.

Esbensen, A. (2010). Health conditions associated with aging and end of life of adults with Down syndrome. *International Review of Research in Mental Retardation*, *39*(C), 107–126.

Facebook. (2020) MiXiT. Available at: https://www.facebook.com/pg/MiXiTmusic/about/?ref=page_internal. [Accessed 27 December 2020].

Flood, B. (2018). De-prescribing of psychotropic medications in the adult population with intellectual disabilities: a commentary. *Pharmacy (Basel)*, *6*(2).

Gustavson, K. H., Hagberg, G., & Sars, K. (1977). Severe mental retardation in a Swedish county. I. Epidemiology, gestational age. birth weight and associated CNS handicaps in children born 1959–1970. *Acta Paediatrica Scandinavica*, *66*, 373–379.

Hartley, S., & MacLean, W. (2009). Stressful social interactions experienced by adults with mild intellectual disability. *American Journal on Intellectual and Developmental Disabilities*, *114*(2), 71–84. https://doi.org/10.1352/2009.114.71-84.

Havercamp, S. M., & Scott, H. M. (2015). National health surveillance of adults with disabilities, adults with intellectual and developmental disabilities, and adults with no disabilities. *Disability & Health Journal*, *8*(2), 165–172.

Heller, T., Scott, H., & Janicki, M. (2018). Caregiving, intellectual disability, and dementia: report of the Summit Workgroup on Caregiving and Intellectual and Developmental Disabilities. *Alzheimer's & Dementia: Translational Research & Clinical Interventions*, *4*, 272–282.

Hemm, C., Dagnan, D., & Meyer, T. (2015). Identifying training needs for mainstream healthcare professionals, to prepare them for working with individuals with intellectual disabilities: a systematic review. *Journal of Applied Research in Intellectual Disabilities*, *28*(2), 98–110.

Holder, M., Waldman, H., & Hood, H. (2009). Preparing health professionals to provide care to individuals with disabilities. *International Journal of Oral Science*, *1*(2), 66–71.

Hsieh, K., Rimmer, J., & Heller, T. (2012). Prevalence of falls and risk factors in adults with intellectual disability. *American Journal of Intellectual and Developmental Disabilities*, *117*(6), 442–454.

Hsieh, K., Rimmer, J., & Heller, T. (2014). Obesity and associated factors in adults with intellectual disability. *Journal of Intellectual Disability Research*, *58*(9), 851–863.

Institute of Medicine (IOM). (1996). In S. Molla, K. Donaldson, D. Yordy, et al. (Eds.), *Primary care: America's health in a new era. Report of a study by a Committee of the Institute of Medicine.* National Academy Press.

Javaid, A., Nakata, V., & Michael, D. (2019). Diagnostic overshadowing in learning disability: think beyond the disability. *Progress in Neurology and Psychiatry*, *23*(2), 8–10.

Jenaro, C., Flores, N., Cruz, M., et al. (2018). Internet and cell phone usage patterns among young adults with intellectual disabilities. *Journal of Applied Research in Intellectual Disabilities*, *31*(2), 259–272.

Koh, H. K., Oppenheimer, S. C., Massin-Short, S. B., et al. (2010). Translating research evidence into practice to reduce health disparities: a social determinants approach. *American Journal of Public Health*, *103*(S1), S72–S80.

Krahn, G., Hammond, L., & Turner, A. (2006). A cascade of health disparities: health and health care access for people with developmental disabilities. *Mental Retardation and Developmental Disabilities Research Reviews*, *12*, 70–82.

Krahn, G. L., & Fox, M. H. (2014). Health disparities of adults with intellectual disabilities: what do we know? What do we do? *Journal of Applied Research in Intellectual Disabilities*, *27*(5), 431–446.

Krahn, G. L., Walker, D. K., & Correa-De-Araujo, R. (2015). Persons with disabilities as an uncrecognized health disparity population. *American Journal of Public Health*, *105*(Suppl 2), S198–S206.

Kumar, S., & Preetha, G. (2012). Health promotion: an effective tool for global health. *Indian Journal of Community Medicine*, *37*(1), 5–12.

Kuper, H., & Heydt, P. (2019). *The missing billion: access to health services for 1 billion people with disabilities.* Available at: https://www.lshtm.ac.uk/TheMissingBillion. [Accessed 23 December 2020].

Lennox, N. (2002). Health promotion and disease prvention. In V. Prasher, & M. Janicki (Eds.), *Physical health of adults with intellectual disabilities* (pp. 230–251).

Lennox, N., Van Driel, M., & van Dooren, K. (2015). Supporting primary healthcare professionals to care for people with intellectual disability: a research agenda. *Journal of Applied Research in Intellectual Disabilities*, *28*(1), 33–42.

Lewis, S., & Stenfert-Kroese, B. (2010). An investigation of nursing staff attitudes and emotional reactions towards patients with intellectual disability in a general hospital setting. *Journal of Applied Research in Intellectual Disabilities*, *23*(4), 355–365.

Lunsky, Y., De Oliveira, C., Wilton, A., et al. (2019). High health care costs among adults with intellectual and developmental disabilities: a population-based study. *Journal of Intellectual Disability Research*, *63*(2), 124–137.

Majnemer, A., & Shevell, M. (1995). Diagnostic yield of the neurologic assessment of the developmentally delayed child. *Journal of Pediatrics, 127*, 193–199.

Marchildon, J. (2018). *5 Facts about living with a disability in the developing world*. Available at: https://www.globalcitizen.org/en/content/disability-in-the-developing-world/. [Accessed 12 January 2021].

Marks, B., & Sisirak, J. (2013). Community health promotion programmes. In L. Taggart & W. Cousins (Eds.), *Health promotion for people with intellectual and developmental disabilities* (pp. 138–148). Maidenhead, UK: Open University Press.

Marks, B., Sisirak, J., & Donohue Chase, D. (2008). Pilot testing of a health promotion capacity checklist for community-based organization. paper presented at the IAASID 13th World congress, People With Intellectual Disabilities: Citizens of the World, Cape Town, South Africa.

Marks, B., Sisirak, J., & Heller, T. (2010). *Health matters: the exercise and nutrition health education curriculum for adults with developmental disabilities*. Philadelphia: Brookes Publishing.

Melville, C., Finlayson, J., Cooper, S. A., et al. (2005). Enhancing primary health care services for adults with intellectual disabilities. *Journal of Intellectual Disability Research, 49*(3), 190–198.

Merrick, J., Morad, M., & Carmeli, E. (2014). Intellectual and developmental disabilities: male health. *Frontiers in Public Health, 2*, 208.

Minihan, P. M., Robey, K. L., Long-Bellil, L. M., et al. (2011). Desired educational outcomes of disability-related training for the generalist physician: knowledge, attitudes, and skills. *Academic Medicine, 86*(9), 1171–1178.

MiXiT. (2018). *STOMP Stop The Over Medication of People with learning disabilities and autism or both*. Available at: https://www.youtube.com/watch?v=Cqbd2QsJmFw. [Accessed 23 December 2020].

Muldoon, L., Hogg, W., & Levitt, M. (2006). Primary care (PC) and primary health care (PHC). What is the difference? *Canadian Journal of Public Health, 97*(5), 409–411.

National Academies of Sciences, Engineering, and Medicine. (2019). *Investing in interventions that address non-medical, health-related social needs: Proceedings of a workshop*. Washington, DC: The National Academies Press. https://doi.org/10.17226/25544.

National Center for Education Statistics. (2003). *National assessment of adult literacy*. Available at: https://nces.ed.gov/naal/. [Accessed 12 January 2021].

Neighbours International. (2019). *5 Valued experiences and the 5 accomplishments*. Available at: https://www.youtube.com/watch?v=p5iMTSF938I. [Accessed 23 December 2020].

Neighbours International. (2020). Available at: https://www.neighbours-international.com/communities-of-practice.html. [Accessed 23 December 2020].

NHS England. (2017). *Stopping over medication of people with a learning disability, autism or both (STOMP)*. Available at: https://www.england.nhs.uk/wp-content/uploads/2017/07/stomp-gp-prescribing-v17.pdf. [Accessed 24 December 2020].

NHS England. (2018). *Supporting Treatment and Appropriate Medication in Paediatrics (STAMP)*. Available at: https://www.england.nhs.uk/learning-disabilities/improving-health/stamp/. [Accessed 23 December 2020].

NHS England and NHS Improvement. (2019). *Learning Disability Mortality Review (LeDeR) Programme*. Leeds: NHS England and NHS Improvement.

O'Dwyer, M., Peklar, J., McCallion, P., et al. (2016). Factors associated with polypharmacy and excessive polypharmacy in older people with intellectual disability differ from the general population: a cross-sectional observational nationwide study. *BMJ Open, 6*(4) e010505.

O'Dwyer, M., Peklar, J., Mulryan, N., et al. (2017). Prevalence, patterns and factors associated with psychotropic use in older adults with intellectual disabilities in Ireland. *Journal of Intellectual Disability Research, 61*(10), 969–983.

Office of Disease Prevention and Health Promotion. (2016). Determinants of health. In *Healthy People 2020*. Available at: https://www.healthypeople.gov/2020/topics-objectives/topic/heart-disease-and-stroke. [Accessed 23 December 2020].

Office of Disease Prevention and Health Promotion. (2020). *Determinants of health*. Available at: www.healthypeople.gov/2020/about/foundation-health-measures/Determinants-of-Health. [Accessed 6 March 2020].

Ong, N., McCleod, E., Nicholls, L., et al. (2017). Attitudes of healthcare staff in the treatment of children and adolescents with intellectual disability: a brief report. *Journal of Intellectual & Developmental Disability, 42*(3), 295–300.

Oulton, K., Gibson, F., Carr, L., et al. (2018). Mapping staff perspectives towards the delivery of hospital care for children and young people with and without learning disabilities in England: a mixed methods national study. *BMC Health Services Research, 18*(1), 203.

Pelleboer-Gunnink, H., Van Oorsouw, W. J., Van Weeghel, J., et al. (2017). Mainstream health professionals' stigmatising attitudes towards people with intellectual disabilities: a systematic review. *Journal of Intellectual Disability Research, 61*(5), 411–434.

Perry, B. I., Cooray, S. E., Mendis, J., et al. (2018). Problem behaviours and psychotropic medication use in intellectual disability: a multinational cross-sectional survey. *Journal of Intellectual Disability Research, 62*(2), 140–149.

Petroutsou, A., Hassiotis, A., & Afia, A. (2018). Loneliness in people with intellectual and developmental disorders across the lifespan: a systematic review of prevalence and interventions. *Journal of Applied Research in Intellectual Disabilities n/a-n/a.* https://doi.org/10.1111/jar.12432.

Phillips, A., Morrison, J., & Davis, R. W. (2004). General practitioners' educational needs in intellectual disability health. *Journal of Intellectual Disability Research, 48*(2), 142–149.

Reichard, A., Stolzle, H., & Fox, M. H. (2011). Health disparities among adults with physical disabilities or cognitive limitations compared to individuals with no disabilities in the United States. *Disability and Health Journal, 4*(2), 59–67.

Rimmer, J., Yamaki, K., Lowry, B., et al. (2010). Obesity and obesity-related secondary conditions in adolescents with intellectual/developmental disabilities. *Journal of Intellectual Disability Research, 54*(9), 787–794.

Rimmer, J. H., Yamaki, K., Davis, B. M., et al. (2011). Obesity and overweight prevalence among adolescents with disabilities. *Preventing Chronic Disease, 8*(2), A41.

Robertson, J., Hatton, C., Emerson, E., et al. (2015). Prevalence of epilepsy among people with intellectual disabilities: a systematic review. *Seizure - European Journal of Epilepsy, 29*, 46–62.

Roll, A. E. (2018). Health promotion for people with intellectual disabilities – a concept analysis. *Scandinavian Journal of Caring Sciences, 32*(1), 422–429.

Roll, S., Moulton, S., & Sandfort, J. (2017). A comparative analysis of two streams of implementation research. *Journal of Public & Nonprofit Affairs, 3.* https://doi.org/10.20899/jpna.3.1.3-22.

Royal College of Nursing (RCN). (2018). *Learning disability care facing crisis.* Available at: https://www.rcn.org.uk/news-and-events/news/learning-disability-care-facing-crisis. [Accessed 6 March 2020].

Saan, H., & Wise, M. (2011). Enable, mediate, advocate. *Health Promotion International, 26*(Suppl 2), ii187–i193.

Scheepers, M., Kerr, M., O'Hara, D., et al. (2005). Reducing health disparity in people with intellectual disabilities: a report from Health Issues Special Interest Research Group of the International Association for the Scientific Study of Intellectual Disabilities1. *Journal of Policy and Practice in Intellectual Disabilities, 2*(3–4), 249–255.

Scott, H. M., & Havercamp, S. M. (2014). Race and health disparities in adults with intellectual and developmental disabilities living in the United States. *Intellectual & Developmental Disabilities, 52*(6), 409–418.

Scott, H. M., & Havercamp, S. M. (2016). Systematic review of health promotion programs focused on behavioral changes for people with intellectual disability. *Intellectual & Developmental disabilities, 54*(1), 63–76.

Segal, M., Eliasziw, M., Phillips, S., et al. (2016). Intellectual disability is associated with increased risk for obesity in a nationally representative sample of U.S. children. *Disability and health journal, 9*(3), 392–398. https://doi.org/10.1016/j.dhjo.2015.12.003.

Selden, C. R., Zorn, M., Ratzan, S., et al. (2000). *Health literacy, January 1990 through October 1999.* Bethesda, MD: National Library of Medicine.

Shanahan, P. J., Palod, S., Smith, K. J., et al. (2019). Interventions for sleep difficulties in adults with an intellectual disability: a systematic review. *Journal of Intellectual Disability Research, 63*(5), 372–385.

Sisirak, J., Marks, B., Heller, T., et al. (2007). Dietary habits of adults with intellectual and developmental disabilities residing in community-based settings. In Paper presented at the American Public Health Association, 135rd Annual Meeting & Exposition, Washington, DC, 6 November.

Sisirak, J., Marks, B., Heller, T., et al. (2016a). People with IDD: health and wellness for all. In *Critical issues in intellectual and developmental disabilities: contemporary research, practice, and policy.* Washington, DC: AAIDD.

Sisirak, J., Marks, B., Mullis, L., et al. (2016b). *Health matters for people with intellectual and developmental disabilities: building communities of practice for health.* Washington, DC.

Starfield, B. (1998). *Primary care: balancing health needs, services and technology* (2nd ed.). New York and Oxford: Oxford University Press.

Supportive environments for health: The Sundsvall Statement. *Health Promotion International, 6*(4), 297–300.

The Jakarta Declaration on health promotion in the 21st century. *Health Millions, 24*(1), (1998), 29–30 35.

Thierer, T., & Meyerowitz, C. (2005). Education of dentists in the treatment of patients with special needs. *Journal of the California Dental Association, 33*(9), 723–729.

Traci, M. A., Seekins, T., Szalda-Petree, A., et al. (2002). Assessing secondary conditions among adults with developmental disabilities: a preliminary study. *Mental Retardation, 40*(2), 119–131.

Turk, M. A., & McDermott, S. (2020). The COVID-19 pandemic and people with disability. *Disability and Health Journal, 13*(3), 100944.

UK Equality Act 2010. (2010). Equality Act 2010. Available at: https://www.gov.uk/guidance/equality-act-2010-guidance. (Accessed 23.12.2020)

Umberson, D., Crosnoe, R., & Reczek, C. (2010). Social relationships and health behavior across life course. *Annual Review of Sociology, 36*, 139–157.

Umberson, D., & Montez, J. (2010). Social relationships and health: a flashpoint for health policy. *Journal of Health and Social Behavior, 51*(Suppl), S54–S66.

United Nations General Assembly. (2006). *Convention on the Rights of Persons With Disabilities, 13 December 2006, A/RES/61/106, Annex I.* Available at: https://www.refworld.org/docid/4680cd212.html. [Accessed 12 January 2021].

University of Bristol. (2013). *Confidential inquiry into premature deaths of people with learning disabilities (CIPOLD).* Available at: http://www.bristol.ac.uk/cipold/reports/. [Accessed 23 December 2020].

University of Wisconsin Population Health Institute. (2014). *County health rankings model.* Available at: https://www.countyhealthrankings.org/explore-health-rankings/measures-data-sources/county-health-rankings-model. [Accessed 12 January 2021].

Vanderbilt Kennedy Center. (2020) Available at: https://vkc.vumc.org/vkc/. [Accessed 23 December 2020].

Ward, R. L., Nichols, A. D., & Freedman, R. I. (2010). Uncovering health care inequalities among adults with intellectual and developmental disabilities. *Health & Social Work, 35*(4), 280–290.

White-Scott, S. (2007). Health care and health promotion for aging individuals with intellectual diabilities. Paper presented at the State of Science in Aging With Developmental Disabilities, Atlanta.

Williamson, D. L., & Carr, J. (2009). Health as a resource for everyday life: advancing the conceptualization. *Critical Public Health, 19*(1), 107–122.

Wilson, N., Jaques, H., Johnson, A., et al. (2017). From social exclusion to supported inclusion: adults with intellectual disability discuss their lived experiences of a structured social group. *Journal of Applied Research in Intellectual Disabilities, 30*(5), 847–858.

World Health Organization. (1978). Declaration of Alma-Ata. In *International Conference on Primary Health Care.* Alma-Ata, USSR: World Health Organization.

World Health Organization. (1998a). *Health promotion glossary.* Available at: https://www.who.int/healthpromotion/about/HPR%20Glossary%201998.pdf.

World Health Organization. (2005). The Bangkok Charter for Health Promotion in a Globalized World. In *6th Global Conference on Health Promotion.* Bangkok, Thailand: Paper presented at the WHO.

World Health Organization. (1998b). *Fact sheet No.171: Health promotion: milestones on the road to a global alliance – revised.* Geneva: WHO.

World Health Organization. (2003). Health systems: principled integrated care. In *World health report 2003.* Geneva, Switzerland.

World Health Organization. (1986). *The Ottawa charter for health promotion.* Available at: https://www.who.int/healthpromotion/conferences/previous/ottawa/en/. [Accessed 23 December 2020].

World Health Organization. (2020). *Healthy settings.* Available at: http://www.who.int/healthy_settings/en/. [Accessed 6 March 2020].

10

Enabling good health

Kim Lorraine Scarborough and Sharon Paley

KEY ISSUES

- To be effective, strategies for promoting health require the people working with those with intellectual disabilities to combine their knowledge of the individual and their families, with a sound understanding of the communities in which they live.
- A range of person-centred strategies exist to encourage positive health behaviours among people with intellectual disabilities.
- Ensuring access to health interventions is a key role of health and social care providers, with effective communication a core component of this process.

- Reasonable accommodation (United Nations (UN), 2006a), sometimes known as reasonable adjustments, adaptions or measures (UN, 2006b), are essential in achieving positive health outcomes for people with intellectual disabilities, and reducing discriminatory practices.
- Education of the wider health and social care workforce, combined with effective co-working between specialist intellectual disabilities professionals, positively impacts on health outcomes for people with intellectual disabilities.

CHAPTER OUTLINE

INTRODUCTION

The previous chapter explored the concept of health and the reasons why people with intellectual disabilities may experience poorer health than the general population. However, poor health is not inevitable, and this chapter presents a range of practical interventions to address the health needs of people with intellectual disabilities that can be employed by professionals working in conjunction with families and carers. Within the chapter there are discussions related to improving health in people with intellectual disabilities. Topics include autonomy, reasonable accommodations, staff training, public health interventions, health checks, health action planning and behavioural change.

PRINCIPLES UNDERPINNING HEALTH CARE INTERVENTIONS

There are some general principles for reducing health inequalities and supporting people with intellectual disabilities to have healthier lives. The first principle is acknowledging that people with intellectual disabilities have a right to make choices about their health. The second is that working in partnerships, that include people with intellectual disabilities, their families, paid staff and healthcare professionals is vital, and finally that staff in all services need to understand how to effectively reduce health inequalities for people with intellectual disabilities.

Promoting autonomy: capacity and consent

Recognition that people with intellectual disabilities have decision making capacity is not an internationally accepted concept, resulting in the rights and autonomy of people being undermined (European Union Agency for Fundamental Rights, 2013). However, countries including the United Kingdom (Mental Capacity Act (MCA), 2005), Northern Ireland (MCA, 2016), Scotland (Adults with Incapacity Act, 2000), Canada (Bach and Kerzner, 2010) and Australia (Australian Law Reform Commission, 2013) agree that a founding principle when supporting people with intellectual disabilities is the assumption of their capacity to make decisions. In these countries capacity legislation has been implemented to change the behaviour of staff providing services to ensure they uphold the fundamental rights of people with intellectual disabilities to make life choices. At a societal level legislation has added legal sanctions to uphold the principle that people with intellectual disabilities have the same rights and entitlements as everyone else, including making unwise decisions.

Whilst individual territories, states or countries have different, often complex, legislative frameworks there are similarities, for example, that individuals with intellectual disabilities should be supported to make their own decisions. Also, that a health mental capacity assessment is about one decision, so capacity should be re-considered for each health decision to uphold an individual's rights. Reflecting international capacity frameworks, mental capacity legislation across the UK state that practical steps should be taken to present information in an accessible format to individuals with intellectual disabilities to promote understanding. This might be through the use of augmentative and alternative communication methods (see Chapter 5) and by implementing reasonable accommodations (Box 10.1). Giving personalised health information is the basis for informed consent. If understanding is compromised because poor quality information is provided, an individual's autonomy and rights are undermined. People who know the individual need to advocate for accessible information to support understanding and promote health autonomy.

If it is suspected that the individual lacks capacity, health professionals should consult with the individual and their family, or advocate to ensure a capacity assessment is completed (see online Useful resources for an example). If an assessment confirms a lack of capacity then everything must be done in the least restrictive way, and in the best interests of the individual. It is therefore important that those making best interest decisions are themselves informed and this requires knowledge of the person, their wishes, and knowledge of treatment options. The involvement of an independent advocate can help validate best interest discussions and, in some countries, an advocate is formally appointed. If a best interest decision is challenged, a judge can be called on to make decisions.

Developing staff skills and knowledge

There is evidence that poor partnership working can result in terrible consequences for people with intellectual disabilities including preventable death (Office of the Public Advocate, 2016; New South Wales (NSW) Ombudsman, 2018; Heslop et al, 2018). Partnership working is focused on the person with an intellectual disability, their family or advocate and paid staff, alongside the professionals involved in managing health. As discussed in Chapter 9 healthcare professionals may have had limited or no training in caring for people with intellectual disabilities and reports by Lewis and Stenfert-Kroese (2010), Nagarajappa et al (2013) and The Arc (2019) have identified poor knowledge and negative attitudes about supporting the health needs of this group. An example is when Do Not Attempt Resuscitation (DNAR) is recorded in a person's hospital notes (see Lucy's story 10.1). This reflects how clinicians' negative biases towards people with intellectual disabilities impacts on how they judge people's quality of life and make major healthcare decisions, often without consultation. Learning Disability England (LDE) completed a survey in April 2020 during the COVID pandemic and found DNAR was being recorded in the hospital notes of people with intellectual disabilities without consent. It is everyone's responsibility to ensure this does not happen, and to challenge if DNAR has been recorded (LDE, 2020).

BOX 10.1   Reasonable Accommodations

General

- Do not make assumptions, ask what the person needs to access your service.
- Check communication needs, be flexible and use easy to understand jargon free language.
- Identify the person's support needs, discuss confidentiality and sharing information.
- Talk directly to the person with an intellectual disability and check understanding.
- Work with carers to ensure successful health outcomes.
- Ensure carers are supported, e.g. breaks, refreshments, parking permit, sleeping arrangements.
- Where available, work with specialist intellectual disabilities staff to maximise success.
- As far as possible, ensure consistency of personnel and environment.

Strategic

- Provide mandatory intellectual disability, autism and communication training to *all* staff.
- Have people with intellectual disabilities audit signage and information and support training.
- Improve signage e.g. use of symbols/pictures alongside words.
- Challenge poor attitudes towards people with intellectual disabilities e.g. provide retraining.
- Develop policy and procedure to ensure hospital passports are used including flagging (to indicate an individual has a recorded need, prompting staff to take appropriate action).
- Have a range of communication support objects e.g. pictures, objects of reference, models.
- Have a range of accessible resources available e.g. letter templates, ward booklets.
- Have access to a sign language interpreter.

Appointments

- Give at least a double appointment but be prepared to need another; important so as not to overload the person with information.
- Offer an appointment time that reduces stress, e.g. fits with person's routine, medication, when support is available or to limit waiting time.
- Consider if the person needs a quieter area not a busy waiting room, could you give them a pager or telephone them so they can return and not miss their appointment?

Admissions

- Offer a home visit to plan admission, write hospital passport, reasonable accommodation plan, and if needed, a desensitisation plan, pre-visit, sedation if in person's best interest.
- Give sufficient time to ensure person and, where appropriate, the carer can contribute and understands what will happen.

Ward stays

- Where possible, plan if the person needs a quiet area, single room, or close to other people.

Discharge

- Plan ahead and include the person and the people supporting them.
- Give accessible information about medication changes, aftercare or future appointments, also about self-monitoring with contact details if specific symptoms occur.

Developed from work by Giraud-Saunders (2009, p.32), Royal College of General Practitioners (2010), Tuffrey-Wijne et al (2014), MacArthur et al (2015), Mencap (2018)

LUCY'S STORY 10.1

Lucy is a happy, 27-year old who loves going out. Lucy has a profound intellectual disability, uses a wheelchair, and when distressed cries loudly and bites herself. She recently had an infection resulting in high levels of distress and was taken to hospital. Her mother was anxious because of the risks of Lucy acquiring COVID in hospital. Lucy was moved from Accident & Emergency (A&E) to a hospital ward, and due to her disability her mother was permitted to go with her. As part of being admitted to the ward a student nurse went through the documents and commented that Lucy was recorded as DNAR. Lucy's mother questioned what this meant as it had not been discussed in A&E. She was infuriated and insisted it was removed.

Research by the Disability Services Commissioner (2018), NSW Ombudsman (2018) and Heslop et al (2013) highlighted that the lack of specialist intellectual disability training contributes to poor health outcomes for people with intellectual disabilities. These findings suggest the need for mandatory intellectual disabilities training for all healthcare staff, something Paula McGowan in England, Jayne Nicholls in Wales and Kim Creevey in Australia have fought for following the untimely deaths of their family members. Family led campaigns increase awareness of the health inequalities and discrimination experienced by people with intellectual disabilities. This sort of change is 'bottom-upwards' but when successful, influences a 'top-down' response, for example, in the UK mandatory intellectual disabilities training for healthcare staff is now being piloted (Health Education England (HEE), 2020). Many training opportunities have been evaluated including face-to-face awareness sessions for nurses and doctors (MacArthur et al, 2015), and the development of electronic training packages with people with intellectual disabilities (Kleinert et al, 2007). These evaluations found that both electronic and face-to-face training co-produced with people with intellectual disabilities improves attitudes, skills and knowledge. With so many staff needing to be trained, offering a range of learning opportunities will increase access to the much needed education. Therefore, all healthcare staff, from cleaners to senior clinicians, should receive training that involves people with intellectual disabilities as trainers (HEE, 2020). User led organisations like People First and The Arc are delivering training which evaluates well (The Arc, 2019). Achieving effective co-teaching needs people with intellectual disabilities and their carers to work in partnership with training providers.

Health is not only about care provided in traditional healthcare settings, it is also the inclusion of people with intellectual disabilities in community healthy lifestyle projects such as healthy eating, weight loss and exercise groups. Inclusion in community-based activities can be successful in improving people's health (Shoneye, 2012). This demonstrates that when thinking about workforce development we need to look beyond health professionals to staff in our communities that can support healthy lifestyles (who these people might be is discussed later in this chapter).

Providing a basic level of training to staff is important. However, having more knowledgeable staff in key areas is valuable. Jennings (2019) discussed the development of intellectual disability champions. This entailed comprehensive training of staff who did not have a background in working with people with intellectual disabilities, resulting in staff being enabled to deliver training and support to peers, make reasonable accommodations, and improve the experience of people with intellectual disabilities in hospital. Where there are limited specialists in intellectual disabilities this is a model that could be considered across a range of community organisations.

Reasonable accommodations

Reasonable accommodations are defined by the UN (2006a) as the modifications needed to ensure the rights and freedoms of people with disabilities are upheld. Where reasonable accommodations are not employed, discrimination can occur (UN, 2006a). The Canadian Charter of Rights and Freedoms, Part 1 of the Constitution Act, 1993 endorses that reasonable accommodation in the form of actions promoting equality is essential to upholding human rights. Where reasonable accommodations such as those in Box 10.1 are implemented they promote anti-discriminatory practices such as equality of physical access, appropriate environments, mindful involvement and accessible information leading to person-centred care.

Reasonable accommodations are crucial if services are committed to improving health outcomes for people with intellectual disabilities (MacArthur et al, 2015). The breadth of reasonable accommodations (Box 10.1) indicate that adjustments need to be implemented at a strategic level, workforce level, and at individual person level to reduce discrimination, promote autonomy and tackle health inequality. However, even when hospitals have reasonable accommodation/adjustment policies Tuffrey-Wijne et al (2014) and Heslop et al (2013) agree (as was discussed earlier in the chapter), that staff need intellectual disabilities training to implement the policy.

📋 READER ACTIVITY 10.1

Think of a person you know who has an intellectual disability. You are supporting this person to access a healthcare appointment

- Reflect upon what you need to consider in relation to this individual's capacity to make decisions
- Reflect on the reasonable accommodations you could make to support the person at the appointment
- Reflect on the reasonable accommodations the healthcare practitioner should make to ensure the person receives person-centred care that enhances their capacity to make healthcare decisions

Accessible information

The use of accessible information has already been mentioned as a reasonable accommodation. The language of health and illness is varied, sometimes colloquial and jargon filled. People with intellectual disabilities may appear to understand the language used, however health problems such as constipation can go undetected when individuals do not understand the consequences, language or are embarrassed (Coleman and Spurling, 2010). This has become a major concern with early death linked to manageable constipation (Heslop et al, 2018, 2019). Working with individuals to build their health language and understanding helps identify misunderstandings, highlighting areas for health education. There are a number of activities that facilitate the exploration of health knowledge and language, for example

- use of a body outline and asking people with intellectual disabilities to lay images or models of body parts in the correct place–this helps people learn about their bodies and health language. Having the individual lay down and drawing around them may engage a person to talk about their own body
- gather a box of health-related items as a resource to encourage discussion, this might be actual items or photographs
- run a first aid session to help develop language, knowledge and skills, including how to contact emergency services.

Helping people make healthy lifestyle choices means providing accessible health information to enable understanding, including the impact of making an unhealthy choice. Where meaningful health education materials do not exist, staff need to develop resources that are person-centred. Accessible resources can be used to prepare for a health appointment, during an appointment, and after an appointment to reinforce understanding. This aids memory, understanding and supports decision making and compliance with agreed treatment plans.

The Accessible Information Standard (National Health Service UK, 2017), and Access for All (Australian Human Rights Commission, 2016) indicate that people with intellectual disabilities should expect access to understandable health information. Where accessible information exists (see online Useful resources) people with intellectual disabilities may find it confusing (Glaysher, 2005). The use of symbols to support words is used to improve understanding. Although Poncelas and Murphy (2007) found little evidence to support this they identified that when information was read through with the person with intellectual disabilities, it better aided understanding and memory.

Another type of accessible health information is a Patient Held Record. This is a document which the person with an intellectual disability, or their carer, takes to health appointments (Council for Intellectual Disability, 2020). It contains detailed information for health professionals and easily understandable information for the individual who owns it. Patient held records help people remember health history and outcomes of health appointments. They are useful when someone accesses secondary care settings (Talkback, 2019), for example, outpatient appointments. They contain details of medication, allergies, treatments and records of health symptoms that are being monitored. Importantly, health professionals write in them at all appointments ensuring a more holistic view of a person's health when multiple healthcare professionals may be involved.

READER ACTIVITY 10.2

Use the internet to identify at least four pieces of accessible health information for a person you know with an intellectual disability.
- Of the resources you found, following review, which do you consider are accessible to the individual in mind?
- Reflect on how you might improve the resources to meet the individual's needs.

DOMAINS OF INTERVENTION FOR IMPROVING HEALTH CARE DELIVERY

Health and wellbeing are influenced by a range of people, each offering their own level of support based on their resources, knowledge and relationship to the person with an intellectual disability. The concentric circles in Figure 10.1 show that primary support is closest to the person and encompasses enduring relationships. Families, direct support staff and volunteers will have more knowledge of the person's communication needs. People in the secondary level circle might have access to resources or specialist knowledge but need to work in partnership with the individual, families and support staff to ensure health and wellbeing interventions are appropriate and successful. In the outer circle,

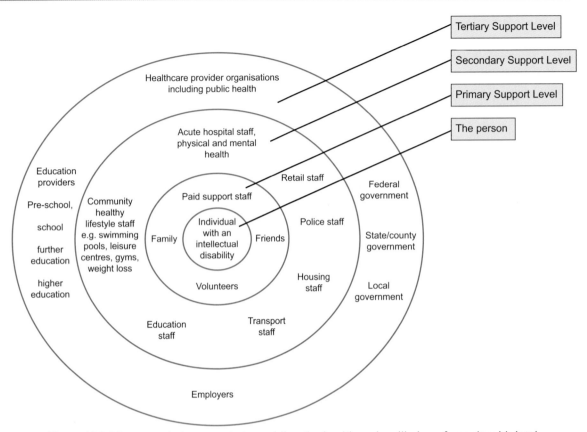

Figure 10.1 Many people have a role in enabling the health and wellbeing of people with intellectual disabilities

organisations need to develop an environment which supports health equality through anti-discriminatory policy and practice, knowledgeable staff, and access to resources that enable reasonable accommodations. The people in Figure 10.1 have differing roles to enable people with intellectual disabilities to make and enact their health choices.

Primary support level: hands on giver of care

Those closest to the person with an intellectual disability have a significant role in enabling good health. Families influence people's lifelong attitudes to health, and healthy lifestyles and can have a positive impact in establishing healthy habits (Nauert, 2018). Primary carers are well placed to make activities meaningful for the individual, for example, in Peter's story 10.2 family involvement in finding a meaningful activity for Peter resulted in physical health gains including weight loss

and mental health gains including building confidence and making friends.

PETER'S STORY 10.2

Peter's activity levels had reduced over the last 20 months since being bullied when out for a walk. He had gained 14 kilos due to becoming sedentary and snacking whilst watching his TV. Peter had played Pokémon when younger and his cousin Paul has started playing Pokémon Go. Peter's mum talked to Peter, downloaded the game and Paul was happy to have a Pokémon buddy to walk with. With rewards for kilometres walked, collecting Pokémon and badges it was an engaging game for Peter, and he felt safe with Paul. Peter gained confidence, made friends and lost weight. For Peter it was walking with a purpose with people who had the same interest as him.

Shoneye (2012) advocates that support staff set a healthy lifestyle example when working with people e.g. having healthy snacks, being active, role modeling structured eating habits such as meals at a table. This is everyday health education and enables the development and maintenance of a healthy lifestyle. In the USA, Dixon-Ibarra et al (2016) report how obesity in adults with intellectual disabilities is 1.5 times higher than the general population and highlighted how, due to more co-morbidities and problems accessing healthcare, the issue of preventing or managing obesity is an area where resources should be focused. However, their work on implementing a physical activity programme in residential services proved unsuccessful due to the failure of staff engagement. This highlights the important role that support staff play in achieving positive outcomes for the people they support. Staff engagement in healthcare programmes could be improved through targeted staff development (Windley and Chapman, 2010). Training should include the implications of unhealthy lifestyles and barriers to healthcare encountered by people with intellectual disabilities, and build staff knowledge, skills and understanding of their responsibilities in supporting people to develop healthy lifestyles and ensuring equitable access to healthcare services (Tracy and McDonald, 2014).

There is evidence to support that organisations should develop staff by adopting approaches based upon coaching and practice leadership to increase positive outcomes for people (Beadle-Brown and Bigby, 2015; Bould et al, 2018). Beadle-Brown et al (2014) explain that the elements of practice leadership should focus on the quality of life for people with intellectual disabilities providing modelling and supervision of staff and involving staff in reviewing their practice. They state that leaders should allocate and organise appropriate support for people with intellectual disabilities. This should include ensuring an appropriate skill mix when appointing staff, with required skills being focused on the people receiving the service as achieved in Mary's story 10.3. There is evidence that the quality of support is higher when a service embeds practice leadership principles and practice leaders are present and engaged with staff and the people they support (Bould et al, 2018).

Secondary support level: working and co-ordinating care through others

Health and wellbeing spans multiple community services and is not focused simply in traditional healthcare. Professional Codes of Practice state that healthcare

MARY'S STORY 10.3

Mary managed a home for people with intellectual disabilities. She identified a lack of activities outside the home and asked people who lived there what they would like to do. Some said they wanted to get out, two spoke of how they enjoyed cycling. Mary appointed two new support staff who were also enthusiastic cyclists. They worked with experienced staff to explore how residents could go cycling. They identified a specialist cycle hiring company, completed risk assessments and established regular cycle trips for eight people. The residents loved being out in the fresh air and staff felt engaged and valued.

professionals must collaborate with people in their care and work effectively by consulting and taking advice from colleagues. As previously discussed, staff inexperienced in providing healthcare to people with intellectual disabilities need support, and specialised practitioners should enhance and expand their role by supporting the development of colleagues from dissimilar backgrounds. This includes embracing the principle that investing time in developing collaborative relationships with other community and health workers is an investment that is as important as the relationships they have developed with people with intellectual disabilities and carers. Below are examples of the range of community-based services that can improve the health and wellbeing of people with intellectual disabilities.

Transport

To engage with community activities is essential whether attending health appointments, participating in activities or attending education or work. Transport includes accessible vehicles, understandable timetables and signage as well as trained facilitative transport staff and supportive processes (Gervais, 2020). Government backed schemes that enable access to free public transport are available in many countries and should be used where possible. Travel buddy schemes have developed to help people with intellectual disabilities to develop local travel plans, but also to experience international holidays (see online Useful resources).

Social prescribing

This is where health professionals refer an individual to community groups to engage people with healthy lifestyle activities such as walking or weight loss (Hsu et al, 2016; The King's Fund 2017). This requires staff training and accessible facilities.

Housing

This should be affordable, safe, accessible and connected to services (The Health Foundation, 2017). The American Association of Intellectual and Developmental Disability (2012) made a position statement calling for people to be free from housing discrimination, and highlighted the reduction in institutional care and lack of affordable and accessible housing. The need for appropriate accommodation affects many countries, for example, in England the NHS (2015) are working with local councils and the Directors of adult services to improve housing for people with intellectual disabilities. This is another example where partnership working can improve people's health.

Community Police

These have a role in relation to keeping people safe and dealing with hate crime, with hate crime impacting on both physical and mental wellbeing (Her Majesty's Inspectorate of Constabulary and Fire Rescue Service 2018). Developing ways for the police and people with intellectual disabilities to build relationships and skills is important (Sheikh, 2011). In some areas 'Safe Places' schemes have been developed where police work in partnership with retailers and local authorities to provide clearly identified areas in the community where people with intellectual disabilities who feel anxious when in the community can go to for support (see online Useful resources). Developing partnership working builds trust and communication skills (Sheikh, 2011), and learning together can develop the communication skills of both police and people with intellectual disabilities, see Box 10.2 for an example of a partnership project.

READER ACTIVITY 10.3

Use an internet search engine to find schemes related to traveling, housing, safe havens, travel buddies, healthy living activities, support groups and more.

Reflect on how your findings could enhance community involvement for a person with an intellectual disability that you support.

Providing care in acute hospital settings

There is a need for national policy change to improve care for people with a range of disabilities when

BOX 10.2   Example of a Partnership Project

A project completed in the UK involved community police working with education staff and people with intellectual disabilities to develop intellectual disabilities community champions. The programme involved role play where a man steals a woman's handbag. The people with intellectual disabilities witnessed the role play and then reported the incident. The incident reports lacked essential information. The police were made aware of the language needs of the group and by working together new knowledge and skills developed in all participants improving communication and relationships.

attending hospital (Cumella and Martin, 2004). Policies and practice aimed at increasing access for all people to global healthcare services includes people with intellectual disabilities (Maltaise et al, 2020).

As well as the previously mentioned detailed Patient Held Record, the use of Hospital Passports (in some countries called health passports) has been found to improve health care experiences (MacArthur, et al 2015). Hospital Passports are succinct, usually 2–3 pages long (see online Useful resources). They aim to provide readily accessible essential information to doctors and nurses of the person's current medication, allergies, important health history, essential communication needs, and behaviour support needs, including essential reasonable accommodations that need to be implemented. The Hospital Passport should be shared immediately a person accesses an emergency appointment. This helps healthcare staff understand their role in enabling access to healthcare for the person they are assessing. When combined with a pain and distress recognition tool such as the Disability Distress and Discomfort Assessment Tool (DisDAT) (see online Useful resources) healthcare staff can monitor for pain and distress. As you will not know when you will need these documents it is good practice to write them in advance, update them regularly, and for the person with an intellectual disability and all carers to know where they are kept.

When planning an appointment or admission having a Patient Held Record, Hospital Passport and DisDAT document is an excellent starting point for developing a person-centred healthcare experience. Reasonable accommodation can be planned and staff can be supported to ensure holistic care. In healthcare settings this may be called patient-centred care which focuses on the individual's needs and circumstances, adopts a holistic, culturally appropriate approach, to support care giving and informed healthcare decisions (Epstein et al, 2010). Research by Kitson et al (2012) reinforces how person-centered care requires staff to involve the person with an intellectual disability in decisions that affect them, consulting with carers and building relationships. This reduces any unforeseen difficulties that might cause anxiety for the person. Whenever possible, care should be coordinated by a named person. Many hospitals employ intellectual disability specialists or nurse navigators who co-ordinate the patient journey. The navigator or liaison nurse is effective at increasing positive health outcomes for people with intellectual disabilities in acute settings (MacArthur et al, 2015). Therefore, when supporting a person to access an acute hospital setting, whether an emergency, outpatients or planned admission, carers should ask if the hospital employs a specialist intellectual disability member of staff and request their involvement. As well as supporting acute hospital care staff to provide person-centred care, work should be undertaken to prepare the individual for what will happen. For a good practice example read John and Daniel's story 10.4 about the pre-admission workshop. Discharge planning is equally important, the person with an intellectual disability alongside their carers will need to be included in planning to promote recovery at home, and this might include additional visits from community nurses or their primary healthcare team.

PRE-ADMISSION WORKSHOP: JOHN AND DANIEL'S STORY 10.4

The pre-admission workshop is an initiative developed by the Intellectual Disability Nursing Team at the School of Nursing and Midwifery, University College Cork, Ireland. The idea to develop the workshop came about as a result of discussions between the team and local intellectual disability support services regarding difficulties people with intellectual disabilities and their carers encountered when they attend hospital. Hospital appointments were a source of anxiety and worry for the person with an intellectual disability and their carers. Entering an unfamiliar environment with lots of new people was overwhelming. Medical equipment, health assessments and medical procedures added to the trepidation. The busy environment and tightly scheduled appointments were not conducive to the needs of people with intellectual disabilities. The fear and anxiety consequent to these experiences limited the extent to which individuals could be involved in their appointments and assessments. The pre-admission workshop aimed to support the person with an intellectual disability to become familiar with the processes and procedures of attending a hospital appointment.

John and Daniel, his support worker, attended one pre-admission workshop. John was due to have a tonsillectomy in the following weeks and Daniel was to accompany him. John has a moderate intellectual disability and autism. On the day of the workshop John attended the Clinical Skills Simulation Resource Centre (CSSRC) in the School of Nursing and Midwifery. The CSSRC was set up to replicate a typical ward situation. John had the opportunity to go through the admission process at his own pace. A nurse greeted him at the nurses' station and explained what would be happening. She completed the admission form with John explaining why the questions are asked and the importance of the information he provided. John had time to ask questions and express his perspective. Moving through the process, the nurse slowly went through the procedure for taking John's vital signs. He explored the equipment including thermometers, sphygmomanometers, especially the cuff which he did not like. He saw how the bed raises, lowers and adjusts. The process for going for the procedure and meeting different professionals was explained and role-played.

Daniel accompanied John through each stage of the workshop. Knowing what to expect in terms of processes and procedures placed him in a better position to support John. Daniel could remind John of the procedures in the intervening period. He knew how John reacted during the workshop and heard his questions, helping him to learn more about John's concerns.

As a result of participating in the workshop both John and Daniel were more prepared and informed about the processes. Their anxiety was reduced as there were less unknowns. The individualised pace of the workshop supported learning and inclusion of the individual, their supporter and services as concerns and worries expressed during the workshop informed supports put in place in the intervening period. The workshop supported John's inclusion in his appointment as he had more information about what is involved. He learned what questions he would be asked and had time to gather information and prepare his answers. This increased the extent to which he could be included.

With thanks to Anne-Marie Martin, University College Cork, Ireland

Tertiary support level: planning services at societal level

To support anti-discriminatory practice, organisations must develop appropriate policies and procedures, and ensure access to resources that enable reasonable accommodations can be made. This includes accessible population-based health promotion. Health promotion aims to encourage positive changes in the health of communities and individuals through people taking more control of their environment and lifestyle. There are four main approaches to health promotion. These are radical, educational, preventative and self-empowering (Bright, 1997). Radical health promotion is a systems approach usually taken by government which seeks to make social and economic changes to improve health and might include housing. The educational approach is about providing information to enable informed health choices, an example is healthy eating campaigns. Preventative approaches include health screening and vaccinations, and self-empowering approaches include changing behaviours to prevent illness and disease. However, Roll (2018) points out that for people with intellectual disabilities we need to adapt health promotion to promote inclusion. An issue with these programmes is inaccessibility due to language, method of delivery, identifying who is eligible to participate or how invitations to participate are presented (Public Health England (PHE) 2016a,b). Health education and promotion activities in the area of healthy lifestyles were found to be common activities in the analysis by Roll (2018). Roll identified that when working in partnerships with the individual, carers, public health staff and intellectual disabilities staff, people with intellectual disabilities achieved positive health outcomes. This means it is imperative we adapt health promotion to make it accessible.

Public health initiatives: vaccination

Public health initiatives focus on national campaigns to promote good health across populations. This includes vaccination schedules recommended by the World Health Organisation (2020) which differ between countries depending on risk. With respiratory disease being a major cause of death in people with intellectual disabilities (Heslop et al, 2013), ensuring people have influenza and pneumonia immunisations is a key public health drive in many countries. For example, influenza vaccination for vulnerable people is covered by the Affordable Care Act (2010) in the USA, and all people with intellectual disabilities in the UK are able to have an influenza vaccination at their doctor's surgery. However, in 2014–15 only 41% of people with intellectual disabilities had their yearly influenza vaccination (NHS Digital, 2016). This failure in uptake might be due to poor information being sent from surgeries, including inaccessible appointment letters, limited understanding about what vaccinations are, and how they are given and not making reasonable accommodations to promote uptake (PHE, 2018). The uptake of vaccination programmes is an area where staff can support people with intellectual disabilities by ensuring healthcare providers know the reasonable accommodations needed to promote attendance (Box 10.1), and ensuring they work with healthcare colleagues to explore reasonable accommodations that could be made. Staff could also review information with the individual to help them understand risks and benefits and make an informed decision.

Public health initiatives: health screening

Health screening is a population-based initiative which the WHO (2019) defines as a process where 70% of a country's asymptomatic population are tested and those with the disease are treated. Whilst screening programmes differ by country depending on healthcare resources, most countries have them (WHO, 2019). PHE (2016a) have produced a reasonable adjustments website to promote the successful involvement of people with intellectual disabilities in cancer screening programmes, however figures from 2014–15 (NHS Digital, 2016) identified that for people with intellectual disabilities, colorectal screening had an uptake of 69%, breast screening uptake was 68% and cervical cancer screening uptake was 30%. As previously discussed not making reasonable accommodations reduces uptake, and where non-attendance can result in being removed from the screening programme (PHE, 2016a) there are long term consequences. However this is not the only barrier in cancer screening programmes. Carers can be a barrier if they consider screening is not required or would be too difficult or traumatic for the person they support. Negative attitudes and poor knowledge of cancer screening may also be present amongst people with intellectual disabilities compounded by screening staff lacking knowledge on supporting this group (PHE, 2016a). The appropriateness of any health screening programme should be discussed with the individual, carers, screening professionals and if appropriate, an intellectual disability specialist to reduce barriers and enable participation. It is important that carers are aware of the screening programmes in their country and advocate that the person they support is included. Exclusion from a screening programme needs to be a person-centred decision and not a default position because a person has an intellectual disability.

Occasionally a person with an intellectual disability is considered unable to participate in health screening due to problems associated with comprehension, cooperation in testing, physical disability or emotional state, for example, previous abuse. Should a decision be taken that attending screening is in the person's best interest, a risk assessment may need to be completed with the healthcare professional doing the health screening. In these circumstances it is likely that a healthcare professional would argue that sedation for a routine health screening test was not in the person's best interest. In this situation, or if the person has made a decision not to attend screening, then monitoring for possible early symptoms should be discussed, and an individual plan developed to ensure any health changes are identified as soon as possible and acted on. Where symptoms are identified that require diagnostic tests then a new capacity and risk assessment would be completed reflecting the change in health status.

Annual health checks

The increased risk of people with intellectual disabilities having significant undiagnosed, unmet or poorly managed health problems is discussed in Chapter 9. In recent years, statutory bodies across Australia and Mencap (2012) in the UK have explored issues related to inequity in healthcare and the impact on people with an intellectual disability. The Office of the Public Advocate (OPA) Queensland (2016), reviewed the deaths of 73 people with intellectual disabilities highlighting the importance of annual health checks for this group. In the UK similar recommendations have been made with family doctors being paid to deliver annual health checks for people with intellectual disabilities (Department of Health (DH), 2007). Annual health checks are a reliable way of identifying and reinforcing healthy habits, whilst also recognising new health problems, monitoring changes in a person's health and improving health outcomes through early diagnosis and treatment (Glover, 2016; Royal College of General Practitioners, 2010).

The annual health check should cover basic health monitoring but also screening related to a person's specific intellectual disability, for example thyroid function in people who have Down syndrome. Health professionals can also engage in health promotion and develop positive communication and relationships with people with intellectual disabilities with an aim to improve uptake of healthcare. There are barriers to accessing an annual health check, for example, in the UK not all family doctors offer them, and beyond the UK many countries do not provide specific annual health checks for people with intellectual disabilities. In the USA, the Affordable Care Act (2010) makes provision for healthcare insurance to provide one Periodic Health Examination a year for all people. This includes basic health monitoring, also vaccinations and immunisations where indicated, and health screening based on risk factors and age not disability. These checks are usually provided within the insurance plan and do not need additional payments.

Checklists have been developed to standardise annual health checks for people with intellectual disabilities including the *Cardiff Health Check* (Kerr, 2001) and the Australian *Comprehensive Health Assessment Programme* (CHAP) (Lennox et al, 2007). Having standardised checklists ensures healthcare professionals provide a comprehensive assessment. Because people with intellectual disabilities may experience difficulties in remembering and communicating their health history, the involvement of a health advocate who is well informed about the person's past and current health status is important. This role should be undertaken by someone who knows the person with an intellectual disability and who can offer support to improve how the health professional and individual communicate. Lennox et al (2007) identified how high staff turnover negatively impacts on knowledge of an individual's health history, reinforcing the need for a patient held record discussed previously. Where people have complex health and/or communication needs, the DH (2007) recommends partnership working between primary care staff and specialist intellectual disabilities staff to promote health equity. Some UK family doctors' practices have taken this one step further and employed specialist intellectual disability professionals (learning disability nurses). Where these professional roles do not exist, the development of intellectual disability champions within health teams might improve services

📄 **BOX 10.3   Top Tips for Conducting Health Checks**

- Communicate – check how the person communicates, use easy language, provide easy-read information, show and tell.
- Speak to the person – ask questions in different ways to check whether they have understood.
- Check whether carers have something to add – they may have important information.
- Use simple words to explain what will happen, what the health test is for, what equipment is for. Let the person see and if possible touch equipment.
- See the person, not the disability – don't allow assumptions about capacity or what is 'normal' to colour your judgement about investigations or treatment. Think about your unconscious biases.
- Be flexible – be prepared to change the way you usually do things; be creative in offering reasonable accommodations that go beyond physical access.
- Involve local people with intellectual disabilities in carrying out equality impact assessments (See Equality and Human Rights Commission, 2017, for more on this) and service audits to check that your services do not discriminate against people with intellectual disabilities and improve reasonable

accommodations if any discriminatory issues are identified.
- Offer your staff training so they are confident in supporting people with intellectual disabilities and involve people with intellectual disabilities and family carers as trainers.
- Be aware that the skills developed in getting it right for people with intellectual disabilities will also help people with dementia and people who find written and spoken language difficult.
- Capture and use data about people with intellectual disabilities to improve your services – use clinical coding and 'flags' to track uptake.
- Get to know the local services for people with intellectual disabilities (where they exist) and find out what support they can offer you to improve your services.

An annual health check identifies current health status. Whilst a doctor would act on any major health issue identified there are often opportunities for carers to work with the person they support to improve their health through setting health goals that are important for the person with intellectual disabilities.

(as discussed earlier in the chapter). Box 10.3 provides some top tips for getting the most out of the annual health check appointment.

SETTING HEALTH GOALS: A HEALTH ACTION PLAN

Health Action Planning (HAP) is a key strategy for health improvement in the UK and is written or updated following an annual health check (DH, 2007, 2009). Key times when HAPs are important are transitions including
- child to adult services
- leaving and moving home
- changes in health status
- retirement
- for those living with older family carers (DH, 2001, p. 64)

Identifying who is responsible for ensuring HAPs are appropriate for the individual and kept up to date is something intellectual disability practitioners working

in partnership with people with intellectual disabilities and carers need to agree (Joseph and Wood, 2008). Whilst the DH (2002) stated that HAPs should be individualised, standardised formats for HAPs have been developed, often with accessible words and graphics (see online Useful resources). Evaluations by Joseph and Wood (2008) indicated satisfaction with HAP documents but queried how relevant set formats are for people with severe and profound disabilities or for people who are literate. This indicates HAPs should be person-centred, whether amending a standard format or developing a bespoke format.

People with intellectual disabilities may smoke, use drugs, drink alcohol and, as discussed in Chapter 9, have a higher risk of obesity and do not exercise as much as is recommended. Therefore, people need access to health education about these topics to ensure equality of health outcomes. Accessible health resources have been developed by an increasing number of organisations, often free or inexpensive (see online Useful resources).

Behaviour change

When a person understands their current health status and set health goals, the next stage is to support behaviour changes that improve health. PHE (2016b) introduced the *Making Every Contact Count* initiative. This initiative aims to reduce health risks through encouraging all contacts with patients to be seen as opportunities for health conversations, education, or referrals to lifestyle change activities such as to weight loss programmes. An example would be, you visit primary care for a medication review and walk away having had a flu immunization and a referral to the local leisure centre for a course aimed at improving core stability to prevent falls. This section considers how health behaviour changes can be initiated and maintained.

Health education

Health education is often supported with written and audio-visual materials including campaigns aimed at populations such as television commercials and leaflets. A specific example is the health education message being promoted by the Ministry of Health in New Zealand (2019) campaign about reducing the use of antibiotics. However, an important consideration of national health education programmes is how clear the message is for people with intellectual disabilities (see Box 10.4 for an example).

Goal setting

Behaviour change can be supported by the process outlined in Figure 10.2 (DH, 2008).

When a person is supported to work through these stages, the individual can develop self-efficacy through developing confidence in their own ability to successfully make changes in their life (see Bandura, 1995, for more about self-efficacy). To maximise opportunities for success, SMART goals can be developed:

S Specific
M Measurable
A Achievable
R Realistic
T Time limited

In Julie's story 10.5, Julie was attending a healthy eating group. In addition, she had one-to-one coaching to help her consider her own health and agree an area to improve. Julie's coach helped her develop SMART goals and worked with her to make an accessible diary so

 BOX 10.4   Example of Healthy Eating Group

When working with a group of people with intellectual disabilities, the facilitator suggested an activity to plan a healthy day's food and drink. The group produced posters about meals, drinks and snacks. When talking about their posters it became apparent that four people felt it was *essential* to drink probiotic drinks every day (misunderstanding a TV commercial), with one person believing this prevented cancer. Despite a public health campaign about eating 5 portions of fruit and vegetables a day only one person understood what a 'portion' meant. Two people believed you should never eat any fat, cheese or milk or you got fat. No one understood about food groups. Doing this activity provided an opportunity to identify misunderstandings and learning needs for future sessions.

Julie could monitor and share her progress. Julie coped with setbacks because she had developed strategies. The group celebrated successes, and rewards were built in. Frey et al (2005) identified that recognising achievement helped sustain motivation in people with intellectual disabilities. As Julie developed belief in her ability to succeed, the goals became harder. Working in this way can help motivate people to succeed, and overcome setbacks which helps develop self-efficacy (Bandura, 1995).

Accessible recording systems contribute to action plans and are useful in evaluation. Food diaries can improve an individual's understanding of food consumption, however keeping such diaries can be difficult for people with intellectual disabilities. Humphries et al (2008) involved people with intellectual disabilities photographing their food intake, the photographs helped people remember what they had eaten and improved communication between the interviewer and the person with an intellectual disability.

Good nutrition is an important aspect of improving and maintaining health reducing obesity linked disease. To improve your knowledge of nutrition and menu planning access the online Reader activity 10.4 and complete the additional reading and activities.

Motivational interviewing

Another approach to helping people change health behaviours is motivational interviewing. Rollnick et al

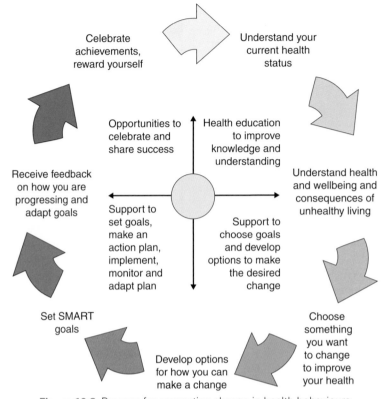

Figure 10.2 Process for supporting change in health behaviours

JULIE'S STORY 10.5

Julie does not meet the *5-a-day* (see online Useful resources) target, limits her variety of fruit and vegetables, and is unsure of how to prepare and cook new things. Having discussed healthy eating Julie would like to improve her diet. Julie has set herself SMART goals, and has discussed what to do on difficult days when she needs to eat more fruit and vegetables. Julie will be honest in her food diary and start again the next day even if she did not eat as well as hoped the previous day. Julie can telephone the coach between 10am and 3pm if she needs support achieving her goals.

Week 1
1. Julie will eat two portions of vegetables and one piece of fruit for 4 out of 7 days.
2. Julie will choose a type of fruit she has not eaten before at the healthy eating session, she will prepare it and then will eat it during the session.

Week 2
1. Julie will eat two portions of vegetable and two pieces of fruit for 4 out of 7 days.

2. Julie will choose a salad vegetable she has not eaten before at the healthy eating session, she will prepare it and will eat it during the session.

Week 3
1. Julie will eat two portions of vegetable and two pieces of fruit for 5 out of 7 days
2. Julie will choose a vegetable she has not eaten before at the healthy eating session, she will learn how to cook it and will eat it during the session.

It is helpful to have an accessible recording system and Julie will complete a pictorial food diary so she can monitor how she is progressing with her goals (see Figure 10.3).

Julie succeeded in her goal with support and was rewarded verbally, with recognition of her success by other group members and, in week 4, with a visit to a hotel where the group were shown how to make a vegetable curry.

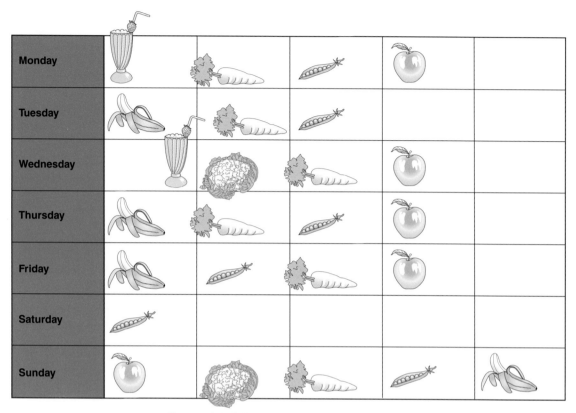

Figure 10.3 Julie's completed food diary, Week 3

(2008) refer to motivational interviewing as conversations that are based on collaboration and support for individual autonomy. Rollnick et al (2008, pp. 7–10) use four principles represented by RULE:

R Resist the righting reflex – you can't and should not try to put things right

U Understand your patient's motivations

L Listen to the person

E Empower the person

Motivational interviewing is not about judging people or telling them what to do or developing a relationship where they feel a need to justify their position. It is about active listening, understanding the individual and helping them identify their motivations and guiding them to make choices. The use of motivational interviewing has been shown to produce positive outcomes in relation to weight management, diet and activity levels and alcohol consumption in the general population (Rubak et al, 2005), with growing evidence that modified motivational interviewing is successful with people with intellectual disabilities (Frielink and Embregts, 2013).

Motivational interviewing is carried out either on a one-to-one basis or in groups with an aim to support people to change their behaviour. It usually requires repeated sessions where a therapeutic relationship is developed. Mendel and Hipkins (2002, p.155) used a FRAMES model to decide structure and content of sessions:

F Feedback personal to the individual

R Responsibility of the individual for changing their own behaviour

A Advice given non-confrontationally about health risks

M Menu of possible goals and ways to achieve

E Empathy raising self-esteem

S Self-efficacy in developing self-belief

The need to support individuals to develop a belief in their own abilities, and effect change in their health behaviours, requires skill not only in communication but also in goal setting that enables successes and develops coping strategies for setbacks. To review your learning about supporting goal setting and behaviour change access the online Reader activity 10.5 about Paul and answer the questions.

CONCLUSION

This chapter has described some of the strategies that might help to improve health outcomes for people with intellectual disabilities. These strategies are not the prerogative of intellectual disability specialists but of all health and social care staff and the wider community. Practitioners inexperienced in working with people with intellectual disabilities must recognise that this group are entitled to the same level of service as the rest of the population. This may mean reasonable accommodations that are person centred are needed. Specialist practitioners need to liaise with other services in order to educate, train and support colleagues from dissimilar backgrounds, with an aim to upskill the wider workforce and embrace the principle that investing time in developing collaborative relationships with other health and social care workers is an investment in the health of people with intellectual disabilities and family carers.

The key points to bear in mind from this chapter are as follow:

- Practitioners need to develop partnerships with the communities they work with as well as the individuals that they provide care for
- Equitable treatment and anti-discriminatory practice are professional and legal requirements requiring reasonable accommodations that are both strategic and individual
- People with intellectual disabilities need accessible information to be supported to make their own health decisions
- The use of a detailed Patient Held Record, alongside a 2–3 page Hospital Passport and a Distress and Discomfort assessment recognition tool like DisDAT can improve access to healthcare services
- Be SMART, remember RULE, and do not forget FRAMES.

REFERENCES

Adults with incapacity (Scotland) Act. (2000). London: The Stationery Office.

Affordable Care Act. (2010). US Department of Health and Human Services. Available at: https://www.hhs.gov/healthcare/index.html. [Accessed 17 September 2020].

American Association of Intellectual and Developmental Disability. (2012). *Joint Position Statement of AAIDD and The Arc*. Available at: https://www.aaidd.org/news-policy/policy/position-statements/housing. [Accessed 20 September 2020].

Australian Human Rights Commission. (2016). *Access for All: improving accessibility for consumers with as disability*. Available at: https://humanrights.gov.au/our-work/employers/access-all-improving-accessibility-consumers-disability. [Accessed 19 September 2020].

Australian Law Reform Commission. (2013). *Equality, capacity and disability in commonwealth laws – capacity and decision-making*. Available at: https://www.alrc.gov.au/publication/equality-capacity-and-disability-in-commonwealth-laws-ip-44/equality-capacity-and-disability-in-commonwealth-laws/capacity-and-decision-making/. [Accessed 14 September 2020].

Bach, M., & Kerzner, L. (2010). *A new paradigm for protecting autonomy and the right to legal capacity*. Available at: https://www.lco-cdo.org/wp-content/uploads/2010/11/disabilities-commissioned-paper-bach-kerzner.pdf. [Accessed 14 September 2020].

Bandura, A. (1995). *Self-efficacy in changing societies*. Cambridge: Cambridge University Press.

Beadle-Brown, J., Mansell, J., Ashman, B., et al. (2014). Practice leadership and active support in residential services for people with intellectual disabilities; an exploratory study. *Journal of Intellectual Disability Research*, 59, 838–850.

Beadle-Brown, J., & Bigby, C. (2015). Observing practice leadership in international and developmental disability services. *Journal of Intellectual Disability Research*, 59(1), 1081–1093.

Bould, E., Beadle-Brown, J., Bigby, C., et al. (2018). The role of practice leadership in active support: impact of practice leaders' presence in supported accommodation services. *International Journal of Developmental Disabilities*, 64(2), 75–80.

Bright, J. (1997). *Health promotion in clinical practice*. London: Baillière Tindall.

Canadian Charter of Rights and Freedoms, Part 1 of the Constitution Act, 1993 amendment, being Schedule B to the Canada Act 1982, c 11. Available at: http://www.efc.ca/pages/law/charter/charter.text.html. [Accessed 14 September 2020].

Coleman, J., & Spurling, G. (2010). Easily missed? Constipation in people with learning disability. *British Medical Journal*, 340, c222. Available at: http://www.bmj.com/cgi/content/full/340/jan26_1/c222. [Accessed 12 September 2016].

Council for Intellectual Disability. (2020). *Personal health records*. Available at: https://cid.org.au/wp-content/uploads/2019/10/25-Personal-health-records.pdf. [Accessed 19 September 2020].

Cumella, S., & Martin, D. (2004). Secondary healthcare and learning disability; results of consensus of development conferences. *Journal of Learning Disabilities*, 8(1), 30–40.

Department of Health. (2001). *Valuing people: a new strategy for learning disability for the 21st century*. Available at: https://assets.publishing.service.gov.uk/government/uploads/system/uploads/attachment_data/file/250877/5086.pdf. [Accessed 1 November 2019].

Department of Health. (2002). *Health action plans. What are they? How do you get one? A booklet for people with learning disabilities*. Available at: https://www.jpaget.nhs.uk/media/186362/health_action_plans.pdf. [Accessed 20 October 2019].

Department of Health. (2007). *Primary care service framework: management of health for people with learning disabilities in primary care*. Available at: http://debramooreassociates.com/Resources/Primary%20care%20service%20framework%20-%20Learning%20disability.pdf. [Accessed 1 September 2019].

Department of Health. (2008). *Improving health: changing behaviour. NHS health trainer handbook*. Available at: https://core.ac.uk/download/pdf/18619054.pdf. [Accessed 28 October 2020].

Department of Health. (2009). *Health action planning and health facilitation for people with learning disabilities: good practice guidance*. London: Department of Health.

Disability Services Commissioner. (2018). *A review of disability service provision to people who have died 2017–18*. Melbourne.

Dixon-Ibarra, A., Driver, S., VanVolkenburg, H., et al. (2016). Formative evaluation on a physical activity health promotion programme for the group home setting. *Evaluation and Programme Planning*, 60, 81–90.

Epstein, R., Fiscella, K., Lesser, C., et al. (2010). Why the nation needs a policy push on patient centered health care. *Health Affairs*, 8, 1489–1495.

Equality and Human Rights Commission. (2017). *Equality impact assessment*. Available at: https://www.equalityhumanrights.com/en/advice-and-guidance/equality-impact-assessments. [Accessed 10 October 2020].

European Union Agency for Fundamental Rights. (2013). *Legal capacity of persons with intellectual disabilities and mental health problems*. Available at: https://fra.europa.eu/en/publication/2013/legal-capacity-persons-intellectual-disabilities-and-persons-mental-health-problems. [Accessed 10 September 2020].

Frey, G., Buchanan, A., & Rosser Sandt, D. (2005). 'I'd rather watch TV': an examination of physical activity in adults with mental retardation. *Mental Retardation*, 43(4), 241–254.

Frielink, N., & Embregts, P. (2013). Modification of motivational interviewing for use with people with mild intellectual disabilities and challenging behavior. *Journal of Intellectual and Developmental Disabilities*, 38(4), 279–291.

Gervais, D. (2020). *Accessible transport solutions: also for the intellectual disability!* Available at: https://www.inclusivecitymaker.com/transport-accessibility-intellectual-disability/. [Accessed 27 September 2020].

Giraud-Saunders, A. (2009). *Equal access? A practical guide for the NHS: creating a single equality scheme that includes improving access for people with learning disabilities*. Available at: http://www.dh.gov.uk/dr_consum_dh/groups/dh_digitalassets/documents/digitalasset/dh_109751.pdf. [Accessed 23 March 2010].

Glover, G. (2016). *Annual health checks for people with learning disabilities*. Available at: https://webarchive.nationalarchives.gov.uk/20160704145757/http://www.improvinghealthandlives.org.uk/projects/annualhealthchecks. [Accessed 2 November 2019].

Glaysher, K. (2005). Making hospitals friendlier and easier to use for people with learning disabilities: a project looking at service-users' perspectives. In T. Shaw & K. Sanders (Eds.), *Foundation of nursing studies dissemination series* (Vol. 3 pp. 1–4).

Health Education England. (2020). *Oliver McGowan mandatory training in learning disabilities and autism*. Available at: https://www.hee.nhs.uk/our-work/learning-disability/oliver-mcgowan-mandatory-training-learning-disability-autism. [Accessed 12 September 2020].

Her Majesty's Inspectorate of Constabulary and Fire Rescue Service. (2018). *Hate crime: what do victims tell us?* Available at: https://www.justiceinspectorates.gov.uk/hmicfrs/wp-content/uploads/hate-crime-what-do-victims-tell-us.pdf. [Accessed 28 September 2020].

Heslop, P., Blair, P., Fleming, P., et al. (2013). *Confidential inquiry into premature deaths of people with learning disabilities (CIPOLD). Final report*. Available at: http://tinyurl.com/lkfgemq. [Accessed 29 September 2019].

Heslop, P., Calkin, R., Huxor, A., et al. (2019). *The learning disability mortality review: annual report 2018 (LeDeR) Programme*. Norah Fry Centre for Disability Studies, University of Bristol.

Heslop, P., & LeDeR team. (2018). *The learning disability mortality review: annual report 2017 (LeDeR) Programme*. Norah Fry Centre for Disability Studies University of Bristol.

Hsu, C., Hertel, E., BlueSpruce, J., et al. (2016). Connecting primary care patients to community resources: lessons learned from the development of a new lay primary care team role. *Journal of Patient-Centered Research and Reviews*, 3, Art. 10.

Humphries, K., Traci, M. A., & Seekins, T. (2008). Food on film: pilot test of an innovative method for recording food intake of adults with intellectual disabilities living in the community. *Journal of Applied Research in Intellectual Disabilities*, 21, 168–173.

Jennings, G. (2019). Introducing learning disability champions in an acute setting. *Nursing Times*, 115(4), 44–47.

Joseph, K., & Wood, S. (2008). *An evaluation of health action planning in Northamptonshire.* Northampton: Healthcare NHS Trust and Northamptonshire Primary Care Trust.

Kerr, M. (2001). *Cardiff health check.* Cardiff: Cardiff University.

The King's Fund. (2017). *What is social prescribing?* Available at: https://www.kingsfund.org.uk/publications/social-prescribing. [Accessed 20 October 2019].

Kitson, A., Marshall, A., Bassett, K., et al. (2012). What are the core elements of patient centered care? A narrative review and synthesis of the literature from health policy, medicine and nursing. *Journal of Advanced Nursing, 69*(1), 4–15.

Kleinert, H., Fisher, S., Sanders, C., et al. (2007). Improving physician assistant students' competencies in developmental disabilities using virtual patient modules. *Journal of Physician Assistant Education, 18*(2), 20–27.

Learning Disability England. (2020). *Do not resuscitate notices and people with learning disabilities.* Available at: https://www.learningdisabilityengland.org.uk/wp-content/uploads/2020/05/DNAR-Survey-Final-Report-13052020.pdf. [Accessed 28 September 2020].

Lennox, N., Bain, C., Rey-Conde, T., et al. (2007). Effect of a comprehensive health assessment programme for Australian adults with intellectual disability: a cluster randomised trial. *International Journal of Epidemiology, 36,* 139–146.

Lewis, S., & Stenfert-Kroese, B. (2010). An investigation of nursing staff attitudes and emotional reactions towards patients with intellectual disability in a general hospital setting. *Journal of Applied Research in Intellectual Disabilities, 23*(4), 355–365.

MacArthur, J., Brown, M., Mckechanie, A., et al. (2015). Making reasonable and achievable adjustments: the contributions of learning disability liaison nurses in 'getting it right' for people with learning disabilities receiving general hospitals care. *Journal of Advanced Nursing, 71*(7), 1552–1563.

Maltaise, J., Morin, D., & Tasse, M. (2020). Healthcare services utilization among people with intellectual disability and comparison with the general population. *Journal of Applied Research in Intellectual Disabilities, 33*(3), 552–564.

Mencap. (2012). *Death by indifference: 74 lives and counting. A progress report 5 years on.* Available at: https://www.mencap.org.uk/sites/default/files/2016-08/Death%20by%20Indifference%20-%2074%20deaths%20and%20counting.pdf. [Accessed 10 November 2019].

Mencap. (2018). *Treat me well: reasonable adjustment for people with learning disabilities.* Available at: https://www.mencap.org.uk/sites/default/files/2018-06/Treat%20me%20well%20top%2010%20reasonable%20adjustments.pdf. [Accessed 21 November 2019].

Mental Capacity Act. (2005). England. Available at: https://www.legislation.gov.uk/ukpga/2005/9/contents. [Accessed 12 August 2020].

Mental Capacity Act. (2016). Northern Ireland. Available at: https://www.legislation.gov.uk/nia/2016/18/contents/enacted. [Accessed 12 August 2020].

Mendel, E., & Hipkins, J. (2002). Motivating learning disabled offenders with alcohol-related problems: a pilot study. *British Journal of Learning Disabilities, 30,* 153–158.

Ministry of Health in New Zealand. (2019). *Resources for antibiotic awareness.* Available at: https://www.health.govt.nz/our-work/diseases-and-conditions/antimicrobial-resistance/resources-antibiotic-awareness. [Accessed 25 November 2019].

Nagarajappa, R., Tak, M., Sharda, A., et al. (2013). Dentists' attitudes to provision of care for people with learning disabilities in Udaipur, India. *The Scandinavian Journal of Caring Science, 27,* 57–62.

National Health Service (UK). (2017). *Accessible information standard specifications – version 1.1.* Available at: https://www.england.nhs.uk/publication/accessible-information-standard-specification/. [Accessed 1 October 2019].

Nauert, R. (2018). *Family and peers have big impact on health.* Available at https://psychcentral.com/news/2011/10/07/family-and-peers-have-big-impact-on-health/30146.html. [Accessed 27 September 2020].

NHS England. (2015). *Building the right support.* Available at: https://www.england.nhs.uk/wp-content/uploads/2015/10/ld-nat-imp-plan-oct15.pdf. [Accessed 12 August 2020].

NHS Digital. (2016). *Health and care of people with learning disabilities.* Available at: https://webarchive.nationalarchives.gov.uk/20180328130852tf_/http://content.digital.nhs.uk/catalogue/PUB22607/Health-care-learning-disabilities-2014-15-summary.pdf/. [Accessed 10 October 2019].

New South Wales Ombudsman. (2018). *Report of reviewable deaths in: 2014 and 2015, 2016 and 2017. Deaths of people with disability in residential care.* Sydney.

Office of the Public Advocate. (2016). *Upholding the right to life and health for people with a disability.* Brisbane: Department of Justice and Attorney General.

Poncelas, A., & Murphy, G. (2007). Accessible information for people with intellectual disabilities: do symbols really help? *Journal of Applied Research in Intellectual Disabilities, 20,* 466–474.

Public Health England. (2016a). *Cancer screening, making reasonable adjustments.* Available at: https://www.gov.uk/government/publications/cancer-screening-and-people-with-learning-disabilities/cancer-screening-making-reasonable-adjustments. [Accessed 1 November 2019].

Public Health England. (2016b). *Making every contact count.* Available at: https://www.gov.uk/government/publications/making-every-contact-count-mecc-practical-resources. [Accessed 20 November 2019].

Public Health England. (2018). *Flu vaccinations: supporting people with learning disabilities.* Available at: https://www.gov.uk/government/publications/flu-vaccinations-for-people-with-learning-disabilities/flu-vaccinations-supporting-people-with-learning-disabilities. [Accessed 19 September 2020].

Roll, A. (2018). Health promotion for people with intellectual disabilities: a concept analysis. *Scandinavian Journal of Caring Sciences, 30,* 422–429.

Rollnick, S., Miller, W., & Butler, C. (2008). *Motivational interviewing in health care: helping patients change behaviour.* Guilford Press.

Royal College of General Practitioners. (2010). *A step by step guide for GP practices: annual health checks for people with a learning disability.* Available at: http://www.rcgp.org.uk/learningdisabilities. [Accessed 1 November 2019].

Rubak, S., Sandboek, A., Lauritzen, T., et al. (2005). Motivational interviewing: a systematic review and meta-analysis. *British Journal of General Practice, 55,* 305–312.

Sheika, S. (2011). *The impact of hate crime against disabled people is far reaching: police responses need to be more consistent.* Available at: https://blogs.lse.ac.uk/politicsandpolicy/hate-crime-disabled/. [Accessed 28 September 2020].

Shoneye, C. (2012). Prevention and treatment of obesity in adults with learning disabilities. *Learning Disability Practice, 13*(3), 32–36.

Talkback. (2019). *Health passports.* Available at: https://talkback-nclude.com/. [Accessed 15 October 2019].

The Arc. (2019). *2018 Support needs of people with I/DD and co-occurring mental health challenges and their families.* Available at: https://thearc.org/wp-content/uploads/forchapters/FSRTC-Focus-Group-Brief-Final.pdf. [Accessed 17 September 2020].

The Health Foundation. (2017). *How does housing influence our health?* Available at: https://www.health.org.uk/infographic/how-does-housing-influence-our-health. [Accessed 20 September 2020].

Tracy, J., & McDonald, R. (2014). *The importance of health to social inclusion; submission to Family and Community Development Committee Inquiry, Social Inclusion and Victorians With a Disability.* Available at: https://www.parliament.vic.gov.au/images/stories/committees/fcdc/inquiries/57th/Disability/Submissions/108_Centre_for_Developmental_Disability_Health.pdf. [Accessed 19 September 2020].

Tuffrey-Wijne, I., Goulding, L., Giatres, N., et al. (2014). The barriers to and enablers of providing reasonable adjusted health services to people with intellectual disabilities in acute hospitals: evidence from a mixed methods study. *British Medical Journal Open, 4,* 4. Available at: https://bmjopen.bmj.com/content/4/4/e004606. [Accessed 24 November 2019].

United Nations. (2006a). *Convention on the rights of persons with disabilities.* Available at: https://www.un.org/development/desa/disabilities/convention-on-the-rights-of-persons-with-disabilities.html. [Accessed 14 September 2020].

United Nations. (2006b). *The concept of reasonable accommodation in selected national disability legislation.* Available at: https://www.un.org/esa/socdev/enable/rights/ahc7bkgrndra.htm. [Accessed 14 September 2020].

Windley, D., & Chapman, M. (2010). Support workers within learning/intellectual disability services perception of their role, training and support needs. *British Journal of Learning Disabilities, 38*(4), 310–318.

World Health Organisation. (2019). *Cancer: screening.* Available at: https://www.who.int/cancer/prevention/diagnosis-screening/screening/en/. [Accessed 1 January 2019].

World Health Organisation. (2020). *Summary of WHO positional papers; recommendations for routine immunizations.* Available at: https://www.who.int/immunization/policy/Immunization_routine_table1.pdf?ua=1. [Accessed 18 September 2020].

11

Physical health

Caroline Dalton O'Connor, Maria Caples and Jillian Pawlyn

KEY ISSUES

- People with intellectual disabilities can experience co-existing physical disabilities and co-morbid health conditions.
- These physical disabilities can significantly impact an individual's quality of life.
- Associated issues include disorders of movement, pain assessment and management, nutrition and hydration, oral health, bladder and bowel function, skin integrity and postural care.

- Appropriate assessment and management of these conditions can significantly increase the quality of life of people with intellectual disabilities.
- It is imperative that people with intellectual disabilities and their families are central to all aspects of care planning and delivery.

CHAPTER OUTLINE

INTRODUCTION

People with intellectual disabilities may experience physical disabilities and co-morbid health conditions which impact their quality of life. The purpose of this chapter is to develop the reader's awareness of these physical disabilities and co-morbid health conditions and their impact on individuals across the lifespan. Best practice in optimising the health status of those with intellectual disabilities utilising contemporary evidence to support a range of appropriate interventions will be introduced. Emphasis will also be placed on managing the complexities of physical health conditions among people with intellectual disabilities in a person-centred manner which promotes the human rights of these individuals.

While 'physical disability' is an umbrella term encompassing a wide range of conditions, this chapter will specifically focus on disorders of movement, pain assessment and management, nutrition and hydration, oral health, bladder and bowel function, skin integrity and postural care.

PHYSICAL DISABILITIES: AN OVERVIEW

Many causes of physical disabilities impact on individuals with intellectual disabilities to a greater or lesser degree. Physical disabilities such as disorders of movement and co-morbid health conditions relating to skin integrity, for example, may be more prevalent in those with cerebral palsy. Environmental factors can also play a role in causing and exacerbating physical disabilities such as complications associated with prematurity, birth trauma, adverse domestic and social circumstances as well as accidental injury and infection (Gates, 2019).

While understanding the cause of an individual's physical disability is important, understanding how physical disability impacts on the individual and how best to ameliorate its impact also requires full consideration. Physical disabilities, in addition to an intellectual disability, can have a marked impact on an individual's quality of life and their capacity to exercise control over it. It is imperative, therefore, that people with intellectual disabilities are actively involved in, and central to the development of, all aspects of supports provided to them.

Supports must be cognisant of the rights of individuals to respect, dignity, choice, autonomy, self-determination and independence. Most importantly, these supports must be fit for purpose and meet the needs of individuals who require them.

DISORDERS OF MOVEMENT

There are two systems in the body concerned with movement: the skeletal system and the muscular system, often referred to together as 'the musculoskeletal system'. The musculoskeletal system is comprised of bones, muscles, joints, cartilage, tendons, ligaments and connective tissue. The bones provide structure and support to the body and protect vital organs such as the heart and brain. Bone is continually regenerating throughout the lifespan; as an individual ages, the 'building up' process slows down. After the age of 30, it is easier to lose bone than to build it up. Between the ages of 40 and 50, more bone mass is lost than is produced.

Normal movement occurs only if there is an intact musculoskeletal system. Other body systems that are involved in normal movement include the respiratory, nervous and circulatory systems (Scanlon and Sanders, 2018). Moreover, movement and positioning of the body are possible through the joints and associated voluntary skeletal muscles which are under the conscious control of the person.

The impact of musculoskeletal problems experienced by an individual with an intellectual disability varies from slight problems with balance which may necessitate the use of walking aids, to partial or total dependence on a wheelchair. Significantly, those with cerebral palsy and profound and multiple intellectual disabilities commonly experience variations in muscle tone, spasticity and gait problems (such as lack of balance and muscle coordination) and tremors or involuntary movements (Mayo Clinic, 2019).

When musculoskeletal disorders are evident, the risk of skin breakdown, aspiration (inhalation of food or fluid) and constipation is significantly increased. These factors can be further exacerbated by poor positioning, inadequate/inappropriate seating, or equipment. Additionally, the individual is at a higher risk of developing serious respiratory problems, fractures, osteoporosis, hip and spinal problems including spinal curvatures, all of which ultimately impact on overall functional ability. Inactivity and immobility can cause complications in almost every major body system.

Immobility can further exacerbate the physical health of the individual leading to reduced muscle mass, muscle atrophy, contractures or chronic loss of joint motion and severe muscle weakness (Crawford and Harris, 2016). Significantly, those with cerebral palsy and profound and multiple intellectual disabilities commonly experience spasticity and joint contractures due to their neuromuscular difficulties.

It is important to recognise that disorders of the musculoskeletal system have far reaching implications not only for the physical health of the individual but also on their psychological and social wellbeing, affecting their overall quality of life.

Spasticity

Spasticity is a condition in which some muscles are continuously contracted which causes tightness within the muscles which can affect normal movement, speech, and gait (American Association of Neurological Surgeons, 2019). For many, spasticity leads to the shortening of muscles which can decrease the range of movement within the limbs over time. The condition can be divided into five subcategories depending on muscles and areas of the body affected: monoplegia (one limb

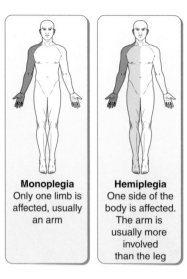

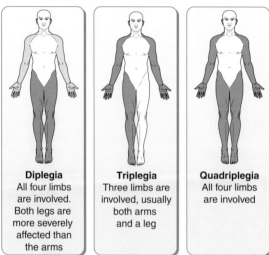

Figure 11.1 Categories of spasticity

positioning, physiotherapy, medication such as muscle relaxants, orthotics, and ultimately surgical interventions. The management of this condition requires the input of a range of professionals dependent on individual needs, and may include nurses, physiotherapists, occupational therapists, family doctor and medical/surgical consultants. Ultimately the cause of, and extent to which spasticity is present will dictate the professional involvement and forms of treatment required.

Curvatures of the spine

The spinal column normally has four spinal curves which are fully developed by the age of 10. At birth there is one slight curve (primary curve) which appears late in fetal development which becomes the thoracic and sacral curve. The secondary curves do not appear until months after birth and consist of the cervical curve which develops with achievement of head control and the lumbar curve which develops when a child begins to stand. For those who do not achieve these milestones, abnormal curvatures of the spine including kyphosis, lordosis and scoliosis can occur.

Kyphosis

Kyphosis is excessive roundness of the upper spine commonly referred to as a humpback. It is also referred to as kypho-lordosis if accompanied by exaggeration of the normal lumbar curve. Known causes include changes in the bones of the vertebrae, congenital deformity, changes in the intervertebral cartilage discs due to loss of bone, or faulty development of supporting muscles of the spine. If muscles are poorly developed, it results in flat foot, rounded shoulders, clumsiness, and lethargy.

Lordosis

Lordosis is an exaggerated lumbar curve in the spine where there is an obvious inward unnatural curvature in the lower back. Lordosis is often seen in obesity, pregnancy and in those with weak muscles. The presentation of symptoms may vary from person to person however the major clinical feature of lordosis is prominence of the buttocks (Children's Hospital of Philadelphia, 2019) (see Figure 11.2).

Scoliosis

Scoliosis is defined as a lateral curvature of the spine and is the most common deformity of the spine (Hresko, 2013). Scoliosis is typically characterised by cause. For

affected), hemiplegia (one side of the body affected), diplegia (spasticity predominately in both legs), triplegia (spasticity in three limbs) and quadriplegia (spasticity in all four limbs) (see Figure 11.1). The consequences of this condition are overall muscle weakness, decreased range of functional ability and impaired coordination. Without appropriate interventions to manage this condition, the physical health of the individual will continue to deteriorate.

There is a broad spectrum of possible interventions available to individuals who experience spasticity ranging from passive movement exercises, correct

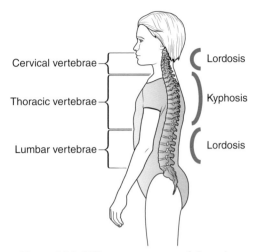

Cervical vertebrae

Lordosis

Thoracic vertebrae

Kyphosis

Lumbar vertebrae

Lordosis

Figure 11.2 Different curvatures of the spine

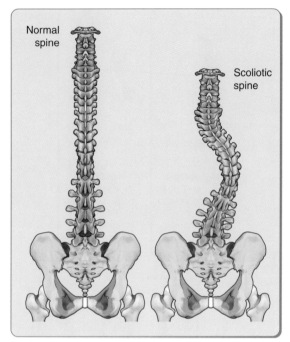

Normal spine

Scoliotic spine

Figure 11.3 Scoliosis

example, congenital scoliosis is an anatomical anomaly associated with failure of the vertebral column to form or segment whereas neuromuscular scoliosis is caused by dysfunction of the central nervous system. For others, the cause of scoliosis may be idiopathic (no known cause) and subclassified as infantile, juvenile, adolescent or adult (Hresko, 2013). The most serious complication of this condition is reduction in the size of the thoracic cavity, compromising the capacity of the lungs and heart to function effectively. With this condition, the person is prone to developing pressure ulcers, back pain and gross deformity of the whole trunk. Early indicators of scoliosis are unequal shoulder heights and slanting of the waist (Hresko, 2013) (see Figure 11.3).

Management of curvatures of the spine

The management of spinal curvatures is highly dependent on the cause and the severity of the condition. For developmental causes such as poor posture, interventions addressing general health, posture and exercise will be warranted. Structural and fixed anomalies are more difficult and at times impossible to treat and correct. However, it is imperative that there is no further structural deterioration so the use of a variety of orthotic aids should be considered including permanent spinal support braces and moulded or supported seating which may slow deterioration.

Developmental dysplasia of the hips

Developmental dysplasia of the hip is the most common skeletal developmental disease, most commonly found in girls, and ranges in severity (Hatzikotoulas et al, 2018). Developmental dysplasia of the hip occurs when the head of the femur (thigh bone) is partially or completely displaced from the hip socket. This condition was previously believed to occur exclusively in the womb; however, it is now recognised that it may occur gradually after birth (Talbot et al, 2017). Early diagnosis is essential as non-surgical management such as a Pavlik harness (a harness which ensures hips are kept in normal alignment) is highly successful in the first 6 months of life. Corrective surgery may be required if non-surgical interventions are unsuccessful.

Dyspraxia

Dyspraxia is referred to as a developmental coordination disorder (DCD), a complex condition with many signs and symptoms. The Dyspraxia Foundation (2019) defines dyspraxia as 'a common disorder affecting fine and/or gross motor coordination in children and adults'.

The person with dyspraxia may present with difficulties with gross motor movement, for example jumping, running, climbing and catching. They may also present with poor posture due to low muscle tone. Additionally, they may experience difficulties with small movements of the fingers including using a pen, knife and fork, tying of shoelaces, buttons or zips. Dyspraxia often affects the ability of the person to process information from the senses and may lead to being over- or under- sensitive to input from any of the senses.

Oversensitivity includes distress at loud noises and fear response on swings due to a lack of awareness of body position in space and spatial relationships. Under sensitivity includes low response to pain and perhaps not responding to their name being called. Such responses are explored in more detail in Chapter 13. Those with dyspraxia may also have poor body awareness and may appear to be clumsy and bang into objects.

Early diagnosis and intervention are important if difficulties are evident in these areas. Therefore, a comprehensive assessment needs to be undertaken inclusive of the individual themselves, family members, support staff and the multi-disciplinary team such as the family doctor, psychologist, occupational therapist, speech and language therapist and physiotherapist.

Osteoporosis

Osteoporosis is a disease characterised by low bone mass and structural deterioration of bone tissue caused by an imbalance between calcium reabsorption and bone formation. As a result, bones become fragile, resulting in a high risk of fractures, especially of the hip, spine and wrist, although any bone may be affected. Osteoporosis is often called a 'silent disease' as it occurs without symptoms and is often diagnosed initially because of a break in a bone.

However, for some, localised pain may present as an early indication of a break. In people with intellectual disabilities, it is beginning to occur more frequently than previously observed as many are now living longer and presenting with age-related conditions. Significantly, women with intellectual disabilities occasionally present with late onset of menstruation (menarche) and early onset of menopause, limiting oestrogen production which is a factor known to increase the risk of osteoporosis (Boschitsch et al, 2017). Other risk factors for osteoporosis are outlined in Table 11.1.

Early diagnosis is paramount, and it is the family doctor who is often required to carry out a detailed health history of the individual, family history and lifestyle factors as part of the initial assessment. A bone mineral density test is also required for a definitive diagnosis.

TABLE 11.1   Risk factors for osteoporosis

Risk	Related to
Lifestyle	Cigarette smoking Excessive alcohol consumption Inadequate calcium intake Little or no weight bearing exercise Low body weight
Non-modifiable risk factors	Genetics – genes determine size and strength of skeleton Ageing
Medication/ Chronic Diseases	Rheumatoid arthritis Endocrine disorders e.g. underactive thyroid Seizure disorders, e.g. epilepsy
Gender (women)	Lack of oestrogen caused by: Early menopause (before age of 45) Early hysterectomy (before age of 45) especially when both ovaries have been removed i.e. oopherectomy Missing periods for six months or more, excluding pregnancy, but as result of over exercising/over dieting
Medications	Glucocorticoid tablets if taken for more than 3 months Anti-epileptic medications Some medications used to treat breast cancer e.g. aromatase inhibitors

Upon diagnosis, an intervention can slow down or arrest the progression of this disease. Numerous interventions are available including advice on weight-bearing exercises such as walking or lifting weights. Indeed, lost bone can be replaced in most people if treated correctly (Compston et al, 2019). Such treatments are aimed at strengthening bone, reducing the risk of fractures, managing pain relief, maintaining bone density, stopping or slowing the rate of calcium reabsorption, reducing discomfort, maintaining a satisfactory lifestyle, preserving physical function and promoting healthy eating. The management of osteoporosis is outlined in Table 11.2.

Meeting the recommended daily requirements for calcium intake can be achieved through the

TABLE 11.2	**Management of Osteoporosis**		
Exercise	Family doctor to be consulted prior to commencing any exercise regimes. Exercise to promote bone and muscle strength. Weight-bearing exercises including walking and jogging are recommended to build and maintain bone mass. Muscle strengthening (resistance) exercises targeting legs, arms and spine 2-3 non-consecutive days per week. It is best to exercise for approximately 30 minutes daily.		
Lifestyle Factors	Be careful of being underweight as this decreases bone density and increases the risk of osteoporosis. Diet rich in calcium and vitamin D is essential as it helps the absorption of calcium. Safe sunlight exposure promotes the manufacture of vitamin D. Reduce smoking, caffeine and alcohol intake.		
Diet and Nutrition	The following calcium intake is recommended for all people, with or without osteoporosis:		
	Children	1-3 years	700mg/day
	Children	4-8 years	1,000mg/day
	Children	9-12 years	1,300mg/day
	Teenagers	14-18 years	1,300 mg/day
	Adults	19-50 years	1,000mg/day
	Adult men	51-70 years	1,000mg/day
	Adult women	51-70 years	1,200 mg/day
	Adults	71 years and over	1,200 mg/day

(National Institutes of Health, 2019)

consumption of a varied diet that includes foods such as dairy products, some green vegetables such as kale and broccoli, tinned fish with soft bones, fortified foods such as breakfast cereals, fruit juices, bread and bottled water.

Medications

Pharmacological intervention may be required, particularly in post-menopausal women, with bisphosphonates considered as first line treatment. For some women, hormone replacement may also be considered (National Osteoporosis Guideline Group, 2018). Hormone replacement therapy (HRT) restores levels of oestrogen to pre-menopausal levels thus slowing bone loss and maintaining bone level. The risks and benefits of HRT need to be assessed individually and carefully discussed due to risks and side effects including breast cancer (Collaborative Group on Hormonal Factors in Breast Cancer, 2019).

Both men and women with intellectual disabilities are at risk of osteoporosis due to inactivity because of impaired mobility and long-term use of antiepileptic and antipsychotic medication classes, with women at an increased risk because of the menopause. Specific attention must be paid to other medications being taken in addition to calcium such as bisphosphonates, phenytoin and levothyroxine as calcium can decrease

their absorption (National Institutes of Health, 2019). Osteoporosis itself is not painful, however analgesics may need to be prescribed and taken as directed to relieve pain following a fracture.

PAIN ASSESSMENT AND MANAGEMENT

Numerous reports such as *Treat me Right!* (Mencap, 2004), *Death by Indifference* (Mencap, 2007), *Learning disabilities and CQC inspection report: Research and analysis* (Public Health England (PHE), 2018a) have identified that pain experienced by people with intellectual disabilities is poorly recognised by professionals thus impacting on the health and wellbeing of this population.

> *"Pain is whatever the experiencing person says it is existing whenever he says it does."*
> McCaffery, 1968, p. 95, *cited in Dougherty and Lister, 2008*

Pain is subjective and multi-dimensional, impacting differently on everyone, the individual's experience of pain is worsened when they experience barriers when communicating their discomfort. Assessment and treatment of pain is often complex. For people with intellectual disabilities, communicating the location of their

---

BOX 11.1 Signs and symptoms of pain

- Aggression directed towards themselves or others;
- Changes to how the person holds or moves their body, including altered facial expression;
- Changes to mobility or balance;
- Change in behaviour, such as tearfulness, irritability or withdrawal;
- Changes to appetite or vocalisation;
- Confusion;
- Restlessness or changes in their sleep patterns; (Public Health England, 2017)

BOX 11.2 Pain assessment tools

- Non-Communicating Children's Pain Checklist-Revised (NCCPC-R) (Breau et al, 2003);
- Non-Communicating Adults Pain Checklist (NCAPC) (Lotan et al, 2009);
- The Paediatric Pain Profile (PPP) (Institute of Child Health, University College, London and Royal College of Nursing Institute, 2003–2011);
- Pain and Discomfort Scale (PADS) (Bodfish et al, 2001).

---

pain and explaining how pain is impacting on their daily lives can be a significant barrier to its successful management. Often people with intellectual disabilities may rely on the observations and actions of others to ensure effective pain management.

However, it is evident that underdiagnosis of pain, under utilisation of pain assessments and the misconception that people with intellectual disabilities have higher pain thresholds than the general population limit effective management of pain (Kerr et al, 2006; Beacroft and Dodd, 2010). Failure of health and care staff to recognise and respond to pain and distress in this population remains a concern (Mencap, 2012), with the quality of pain relief indicated as one of the potential contributory factors to untimely death (LeDeR, 2019).

For those individuals who have the capacity to self-assess and identify their personal level of pain, augmentative and alternative communication devices can be used and include easy-read assessment tools or visual analogue pain scales e.g. Wong-Baker FACES Pain rating scale (Wong and Baker, 1983).

Stages of the pain assessment

1. The assessment begins with the carer or supporting person asking themselves 'is the person showing any of the signs and symptoms which indicate they might be in pain?' These might include all those signs and symptoms listed in Box 11.1 plus additional ones specific to the individual.

After your observations, ask the person to tell you about their pain (use words and pictures they will understand). If the person communicates non-verbally,

talk to them in a way they will understand (ask to see their communication passport – see also Chapter 5 and Chapter 10 for more information on this); also talk to the person who knows them best.

2. Carry out a clinical assessment of pain (with consent), this would include;

- Mental status examination, noting any changes to the person's usual mental state;
- Checking vital signs, temperature, pulse and respirations to notice changes from the person's norm, or signs of infection;
- Inspection, asking the person to tell or show you where the pain is, observing for changes in posture, guarding injuries, colour and pigment changes, sweating, hair and nail changes, swelling and oedema, atrophy, poor healing;
- Musculoskeletal examination, to detect for temperature changes, oedema, muscle tenderness or discomfort in joints;
- Neurological examination may also be undertaken in consultation with a pain specialist (Richeimer, 1998; Painaustralia, 2016).

3. For those who are dependent on others to identify the presence or absence of pain, effective management requires the use of appropriate pain assessment tools such as those in Box 11.2.

A further tool which is useful for assessing distress, which may be a contributory factor in a person's pain, is the Disability Distress and Discomfort Assessment Tool (DisDAT) (St Oswald's Hospice and Northumberland Tyne & Wear NHS Trust v22-2021).

Additionally, observation of the individual and knowledge of any general health issues are fundamental to successful pain management. Information from family and significant others relating to how the individual expresses pain is also vitally important. An electronic healthcare 'passport' or similar document that contains a description about how a person expresses pain or distress is useful for ascertaining what is normal for that person (LeDeR, 2019, p. 59). Examples of tools which can assist with this include My Pain Profile (Del Toro, 2009) or a Person-centred Pain Picture (Moulster and Jones, 2015).

Regardless of which tool is used, it is essential that the information is used to inform the person's care and to manage their pain. It is also important to review the clinical assessment of the person's pain as the presenting signs and symptoms will change, therefore, as with all assessments the pain assessment needs to be updated to reflect these changes and inform changes in treatment. To test your knowledge and understanding of pain assessment undertake Reader Activity 11.1 in the accompanying online resource.

NUTRITION AND HYDRATION

Nutritional issues impact significantly on the quality of life of all people, including those with intellectual disabilities, from both a physical and social perspective. Food plays an essential role in the lives of individuals; not only does it ensure adequate nutrition and hydration, it is also a means of sensory stimulation (see Chapter 13) and can promote social engagement. However, for many people with intellectual disabilities and their families, mealtimes can be a source of stress and anxiety as those who experience difficulties with eating and drinking can be affected by slow growth, inadequate weight gain, dehydration and malnutrition (Royal College of Physicians and British Society of Gastroenterology, 2010). Conversely, obesity can also negatively impact on a person's wellbeing contributing to health issues relating to mobility, gastrointestinal disorders and cardiorespiratory conditions. Obesity is considered a significant determinant of ill health in an ageing population (Melville et al, 2011).

Individuals with mild to moderate intellectual disabilities are at a greater risk of obesity in comparison to those with severe to profound intellectual disabilities (McCarron et al, 2017). Table 11.3 provides key definitions relating to nutrition and hydration.

Obesity

The World Health Organisation (2018) has identified obesity as a major health concern for all individuals. It

TABLE 11.3   Definitions of nutrition and hydration

Term	Definition
Underweight or overweight	An individual can be defined as being under- or overweight when they weigh less or more than the recommended weight as identified by body mass index (BMI) (Freshwater and Maslin-Prothero, 2005). An individual is deemed to be underweight if he or she has a BMI below 18.5 (WHO, 2019).
Malnourished	The state of being poorly nourished which may be caused by inadequate food or essential nutrients either from poor absorption, eating and drinking difficulties and metabolic disorders (Freshwater and Maslin-Prothero, 2005).
Dehydrated	Loss or removal of fluid where fluid intake fails to replace fluid lost from the body due to excessive sweating, polyuria (excessive urination), vomiting, diarrhoea and eating and drinking difficulties (Freshwater and Maslin-Prothero, 2005).
Obesity	The accumulation and excessive storage of fat on the body. Caused by excessive calorie intake. Level of obesity is calculated using body mass index (Freshwater and Maslin-Prothero, 2005). Morbid obesity is classified when a person has a BMI of above 30 (WHO, 2019).

is generally accepted that the level of obesity in people with intellectual disabilities is higher than the general population (Spanos et al, 2013). Effective management of obesity is required to reduce the development of hypertension, type 2 diabetes, cardiovascular disease, cerebrovascular accidents and coronary heart disease (Rimmer et al, 2010).

Several determinants of obesity in the population of people with intellectual disabilities include level of intellectual disability. People with mild to moderate intellectual disabilities have greater levels of obesity (87.5%) in comparison to those with severe to profound intellectual disabilities (64.3%). Women (83.1%) have a higher prevalence of obesity when compared to their male counterparts (75.9%) (McCarron et al, 2017). Obesity also becomes a more significant issue as people age. Therefore, given the increased longevity of people with intellectual disabilities, obesity is a significant health issue which must be addressed (Melville et al, 2011).

Research has indicated that reducing calorie intake, increasing physical activity and being intrinsically motivated and supported by family members can positively impact the management of obesity in the population of people with intellectual disabilities (Martinez-Zaragoza et al, 2016). Reader Activity 11.2 encourages consideration of a personalised approach to Kate's situation.

DISORDERS OF EATING AND SWALLOWING

There are three phases of normal swallowing: oral (mouth), pharyngeal (swallowing reflex is triggered) and oesophageal (movement of food along the oesophagus into the stomach) (Dalton, 2019). When eating, food is placed in the mouth. Effective lip closure is essential to prevent spillage. Food is then chewed, sucked and mixed with saliva to create a bolus (ball) which is then swallowed. Biting and chewing reduces the size of food to manageable lumps which is pushed by the tongue into the oesophagus and onwards to the stomach for digestion. Food is prevented from entering the airway through the actions of the epiglottis (see Figure 11.4).

While for the majority of people with intellectual disabilities, eating and drinking are automatic social activities, for some, disorders of eating and swallowing are more prevalent due to reduced or heightened oral sensation, abnormalities of the mouth such as cleft lip or palate, uncoordinated and involuntary movements as a result of conditions such as cerebral palsy or behaviour problems that interfere with one's ability to participate appropriately at mealtimes, for example hyperactivity. Some common features of these disorders include excessive drooling, difficulty with chewing, difficulty or delay with swallowing, tongue thrust, pocketing of food, coughing, choking and regurgitation.

 READER ACTIVITY 11.2

Kate is a 56-year-old lady who has a mild intellectual disability and is living independently in the community. She is responsible for her own dietary intake and describes her love for takeaway meals. She also works in a local cafeteria with access to food all day long. She is very vocal about her dislike of exercise and tries to avoid it if possible. Over the years she has progressively gained weight and currently her anthropometrics are height 5′ 4″ (163 cm) and weight 170 pounds (77 kg). There is a family history of high cholesterol and Type 2 diabetes. Kate recently attended her family doctor who took routine bloods for screening. Her HbA$_1$C was 6.1% and her total serum cholesterol was 8.1mmol/L. Her family doctor has recommended that she loses weight as her blood readings indicate she has pre-diabetes and high cholesterol. Whilst Kate recognises the need for change, she has reported a lack of motivation to do so.

It is important to recognise that Kate's lack of motivation will require a health promotion approach that adopts a mix of risk communication and behavioural change. The focus for Kate needs to be centred around motivating her to want to make lifestyle changes for herself. Therefore, psychological concepts such as self-regulation, habituation and stages of change are important in addressing the issue of sustained change for Kate. Self-regulation also warrants attention as it relates to a person's ability to alter in response to social cues and involves goal setting and sticking to those goals. It is important for Kate that achievable goals are set to ensure she succeeds in her efforts and is not disappointed.

- Calculate Kate's Body Mass Index (Body Mass Index is calculated as your weight (in kilograms) divided by the square of your height (in metres)).
- What health issues is Kate at increased risk of developing?
- What dietary/exercise changes would you recommend for Kate?
- What social norms do you envisage to be influencing factors to Kate's lifestyle behaviours?
- Identify what you would consider to be achievable goals for Kate.

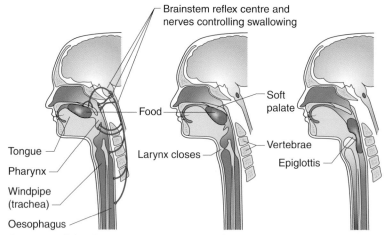

Figure 11.4 Structure of the throat and the mechanics of swallowing. Purves et al., 2007

Gastro-oesophageal reflux disease (GORD)

GORD is a condition which involves the backward flow of stomach contents into the oesophagus (throat) resulting in a burning sensation in the chest (Seeley et al, 2010). Signs include chest pain, vomiting, refusal or fear of eating, recurrent wheezing and heartburn. Stomach contents entering the airway may cause coughing and choking, potentially leading to recurrent episodes of aspiration pneumonia (Pawlyn and Carnaby, 2009); consequently, GORD causes irritation and distress making mealtimes an uncomfortable experience.

According to Van Timmeren et al (2016), GORD is one of the most commonly diagnosed gastrointestinal (GI) health issues amongst adults and older adults with intellectual disabilities. Those with severe to profound intellectual disabilities experience a higher incidence of GORD. Galli-Carminati et al (2006) estimate that up to 70% of people with intellectual disabilities could potentially experience GORD and as such is a significant area of concern. Indeed, the presence of an intellectual disability may often lead to under diagnosis of this condition as some individuals may be unable to express symptoms of discomfort. Additionally, GORD can be exacerbated as a result of coexisting conditions such as cerebral palsy, postural abnormalities (scoliosis) and enteral (tube) feeding where correct upright positioning of an individual is not maintained for an adequate amount of time post administration of the enteral feed.

It is imperative that GORD is promptly treated as inappropriate management of this condition can lead to significant respiratory conditions, including pneumonia.

In some instances, treatment with proton pump inhibitors (a group of medicines that work on the cells that line the stomach, reducing the production of acid) may be appropriate. In other cases, nasogastric (NG) nutrition or the insertion of a percutaneous endoscopic gastrostomy (PEG) may be required for tube feeding.

Dysphagia

Dysphagia is a disorder of swallowing where problems can occur during any phase of swallowing from the point where food is taken into the mouth, the bolus is prepared and is pushed into the stomach via the oesophagus (Rubin and Crocker, 2006). Dysphagia is potentially a life-threatening condition that can cause dehydration, malnutrition, asphyxiation and aspiration, ultimately causing respiratory tract infections, a leading cause of mortality among people with intellectual disabilities (Howseman, 2013). There is a far greater incidence of dysphagia amongst the population of people with intellectual disabilities when compared to the general population.

Therefore, the importance of providing support to those with eating and swallowing difficulties cannot be underestimated and it is essential that the signs and symptoms are recognised and taken seriously. Some of the more common signs of dysphagia include coughing while eating, choking, obvious distress, drooling, spillage of food and saliva, pocketing of food in the cheeks, difficulty with chewing, coughing when not eating, tiring during eating and regurgitation. Changes in speech pattern may also be noted (Dalton et al 2011). All people identified as poorly nourished or at risk of malnutrition should have a nutritional assessment completed as a matter of urgency. While there are many nutritional assessment tools available, the Malnutrition Universal Screening Tool (MUST) (British Association for Parenteral and Enteral Nutrition, 2011) is often used to identify these individuals.

Aspiration pneumonia

Aspiration pneumonia occurs when food is aspirated (inhaled) into the lungs (Pawlyn and Carnaby, 2009). The signs of this include coughing and choking, gagging, wheezing, lengthy feeding times, recurrent chest infections, high temperature and change of facial colour. The individual may appear flushed, pale or cyanosed (bluish discolouration of the skin as there is not enough oxygen in the blood). It should be noted that 'silent' aspiration may occur where the above signs are absent, but the individual experiences recurrent episodes of chest infections or pneumonia and further investigations are warranted. These investigations may include some or all of the following: arterial blood gases (checks for levels of oxygen, carbon dioxide and acidity levels in the blood), chest X-rays, computerised tomography (CT) of the chest, and swallowing studies (Sanivarapu and Gibson, 2019). At this stage, referral to a physiotherapist, speech and language therapist and dietician would be warranted for assessment of needs.

Management of disorders of eating and swallowing

The management of conditions relating to eating and drinking difficulties requires the input of the multidisciplinary team, to include the individual themselves, family members, speech and language therapist, nurse, occupational therapist, physiotherapist and support staff. Concerns relating to the management of disorders of eating and swallowing should be dealt with promptly through appropriate assessment. If any of the aforementioned signs are evident, a referral to a speech and language therapist (SLT) who has expertise in dysphagia is the first line of intervention. Once the SLT carries out the assessment, a planned intervention will be identified and implemented to support the individual.

Any intervention must be planned in conjunction with the individual, significant others and members of the multidisciplinary team. Interventions are dependent on the severity of the presenting condition and can vary from simple modifications to diet to enteral feeding. All eating and swallowing interventions should have at their core the potential to minimise the risk of aspiration and facilitate adequate nutrition and hydration. Such interventions may include the use of medication, correct positioning during

and after meals, the use of appropriate eating utensils and adaptation of eating utensils as required. In addition, attention should be paid to the presentation of meals and to ensure a choice of food is available to optimise the person's appetite for and enjoyment of food.

Of specific importance are strategies that include changes to the texture and consistency of food ranging from pureed, minced, ground, chopped and modified regular foods. Fluids may also need to be thickened and there are many products available on the market for this purpose. Fluid textures range from 'thin' such as water, teas and coffee to naturally 'thick' fluids such as milk (see Figure 11.5). For comprehensive information on the appropriate management of the diet of those with dysphagia please refer to the International Dysphagia Diet Standardisation Initiative framework (2019) (see Figure 11.5).

Prior to any planned intervention, including enteral feeds, the person must be made comfortable in an environment that is conducive to eating and drinking with specific emphasis on the social aspect of eating. This can be achieved through effective communication, gaining trust and consent using a person-centred approach where the needs and requirements of the individual are central to the care planning process. This section of the chapter should equip you to help Peter and his mother in Reader Activity 11.3.

 READER ACTIVITY 11.3

Peter is 5 years old and has a severe intellectual disability and cerebral palsy which affects all four of his limbs. He communicates non-verbally. He is unable to walk and uses an adapted wheelchair to mobilise independently. He lives at home with his parents and his mother is his primary carer. Peter has dysphagia and experiences difficulties chewing and swallowing. Symptoms experienced include episodes of coughing and choking when eating and drinking. Peter has been hospitalised on two occasions with aspiration pneumonia.

Recently, mealtimes have become stressful for both Peter and his mother and they are seeking support to minimise the risk of aspiration and to facilitate adequate food and fluid intake.

How would you minimise the impact of dysphagia?

How would you ensure adequate food and fluid intake?

What other actions might you consider to support Peter and his mother?

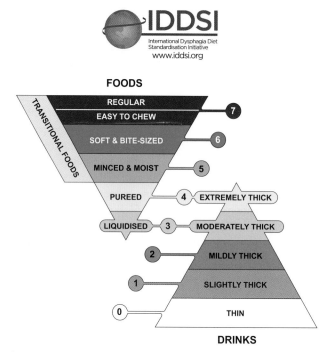

Figure 11.5 International Dysphagia Diet Standardisation Initiative framework (2019)

ORAL HEALTH

People with intellectual disabilities often experience poorer oral health than the general population (Yoshihara et al, 2005). They have a higher prevalence and greater severity of periodontal disease when compared to the general population. They also have higher levels of untreated dental caries, have more missing teeth and less filled teeth when compared to those without intellectual disabilities (Anders and Davis, 2010). According to Mac Giolla Phadraig et al (2015) 34.1% of people with intellectual disabilities have no teeth in comparison to 14.9% of the general population in Ireland. This study also found little evidence that people with intellectual disabilities who had no teeth were benefiting from dentures.

Research indicates that people with intellectual disabilities have higher levels of plaque and poorer oral hygiene than the general population (Anders and Davis, 2010). It is suggested that issues such as a lack of manual dexterity to effectively remove plaque when brushing contribute to this.

The importance of the role of carers in supporting people with intellectual disabilities to effectively care for their teeth has been repeatedly highlighted in ensuring effective oral care (Pradhan et al, 2015). Chapter 12 promotes the ability of many people with intellectual disabilities to develop such skills themselves. Regrettably, oral disease has not been prioritised when compared with other complex medical conditions identified in this population despite the severity of its impact on the overall health of the individual. A comprehensive oral assessment should be undertaken, and an individualised oral care plan should be developed to meet each individual's needs in consultation with a dentist and dental hygienist.

BLADDER AND BOWEL FUNCTION

Elimination is a private and independent bodily function of the bladder and bowel and is not usually a cause of concern until difficulties arise. The embarrassment often associated with discussing these functions can lead to non-disclosure of problems and their presence can negatively impact on both the person and their family through social isolation. At times, even if problems are recognised, difficulties in accessing appropriate professional support may often occur (Pawlyn and Carnaby, 2009). Bowel and bladder problems are an important general health issue that often goes unrecognised for many reasons including diagnostic overshadowing.

TABLE 11.4 Normal process of elimination

Urinary elimination	Bowel Elimination
Urine collects in the bladder (1500mls per day on average per adult)	Faeces pass along the intestine towards the rectum
Pressure activates nerve endings stimulating the urge to urinate	Sensory nerves in the rectum are activated stimulating the urge to defaecate
Urethral sphincter muscle relaxes	Anal sphincter muscle relaxes
Person passes urine	Person passes faeces

Diagnostic overshadowing is where symptoms arising from physical health problems are misattributed to the person's intellectual disability and can result in delays to diagnosis and treatment (Ali et al, 2013).

The elimination process is very subjective and varies from person to person. People usually urinate up to five times a day and some people will have one bowel movement a day whilst others may have a bowel movement between three times a week to several times a day (Burton and Ludwig, 2014). Knowing the norm for an individual can assist in recognising irregularities. The normal process of elimination is outlined in Table 11.4.

Urinary incontinence

Urinary incontinence is an involuntary leakage of urine and it occurs when there is an abnormality in the bladder or the bladder neck (Gibson et al, 2016). Normally, an individual is aware of the urge to pass urine, but in the case of polyuria (excessive production of urine), infection, constipation and reduced mobility and manual dexterity, this ability is impaired. Neurogenic bladder is the name given to urinary conditions where people lack bladder control as a result of neurological damage, for example people with spina bifida (Mixon et al, 2018). The bladder becomes flaccid, distended or spastic with frequent involuntary urination.

For those with intellectual disabilities who are trying to achieve urinary continence, the issue can be further compounded by reduced mobility and cognitive impairments. In this instance, there can be a failure to recognise signals which indicate the bladder needs to be emptied.

Urinary incontinence is individual and not all cases can be cured but can successfully be managed. The prerequisites for achieving urinary continence include the ability to store urine, sit properly on the toilet and pass urine voluntarily. However, in order to achieve continence, people with intellectual disabilities need support from the multi-disciplinary team specifically in relation to education of healthy bladder and bowel, diet, nutrition and exercise as the first line of intervention. It is not advisable to immediately resort to using incontinence pads or aids as these can lead to dependence and learned helplessness.

Those caring for people with intellectual disabilities who are experiencing continence issues should strive for excellence in care via a continence management plan which places continence assessment at the core (Keenan et al, 2018). The ability to achieve continence will vary from person to person depending on the severity of their intellectual disability and associated conditions. Chapter 12 considers a range of practical strategies to support people with intellectual disabilities to develop their skills in this area. Environmental adaptations such as raised toilets, grab rails, foot supports and hoists can be used to support continence. Appropriate continence wear may also be considered to ensure the dignity and comfort of the individual.

Urinary retention

Urinary retention is the inability to empty the bladder at all or the inability to completely empty the bladder (Burton and Ludwig, 2014). Factors that contribute to urinary retention may include obstruction of the urethra (bladder stones), enlargement of the prostate (a walnut-sized gland located between the bladder and the penis), nerve damage (spina bifida and multiple sclerosis), embarrassment or fear and weak bladder muscles. Additionally, cystocele (where the bladder drops into the vagina), constipation, narrowing of the urethra and surgery also contribute to this condition.

The signs and symptoms include an inability to urinate, discomfort or pain in the lower abdomen, abdominal distension, leakage of urine between trips to the toilet and feeling of incomplete emptying of the bladder (National Institute of Diabetes and Digestive and Kidney

Disease, 2014). Management of urinary retention varies from person to person and can include conservative methods such as correct positioning of the individual, promoting relaxation and avoiding delay when the urge to empty their bladder arises. If these approaches fail, the use of cholinergic drugs to stimulate the bladder may be required. Additionally, urinary catheterisation may be necessary and types of catheterisation may range from intermittent self-catheterisation to an indwelling Foley catheter and ultimately long-term suprapubic catheterisation depending on the severity of the condition.

Intermittent self-catheterisation

Intermittent self-catheterisation is carried out by the individual at 3–4-hourly intervals throughout the day to maintain dryness, promote comfort, prevent infection and improve quality of life. This method is the approach of choice for those who can understand the technique and who have the capacity to self-catheterise. Those with spina bifida or impaired bladder function benefit from this intervention.

It is important that the person uses the toilet prior to catheterisation as this technique is used to completely empty the residual urine from the bladder, further promoting normal bladder function. As this technique requires the introduction of a catheter (hollow tube used to remove urine) to the bladder, it is essential that excellent personal hygiene is maintained. This must include washing of hands with warm water and soap, washing of the labia from front to back for women, tip of the penis for men using baby wipes or plain soap and water (British Association of Urological Surgeons, 2017). There is a possible risk of tissue damage, pain and urinary tract infection during catheterisation. In this event the person needs to seek medical attention to resolve any of these issues.

Faecal incontinence

Faecal incontinence is a sign or symptom of an underlying condition relating to neuromuscular conditions, physical disabilities, spinal cord trauma, behavioural difficulties, failure to recognise the urge to defecate and difficulties with dressing or undressing. There is a loss of voluntary ability to control the exit of faeces from the bowel, therefore it is imperative that the cause (or causes) for each individual is diagnosed promptly as many factors are relatively simple to reverse (National Institute

for Clinical Excellence (NICE), 2007). Moreover, faecal incontinence has remained a largely hidden problem due primarily to the embarrassment and shame experienced by individuals. Faecal incontinence is further compounded by the presence of an intellectual disability with a clear association between IQ level and rates of incontinence, with people who have severe or profound intellectual disabilities being particularly affected (von Gontard, 2015). For some, treatment is often not prioritised or even considered as there can be a perception that faecal incontinence is symptomatic of an intellectual disability as opposed to a skill that can be taught (see Chapter 12 for further information on the development of skills associated with continence).

Thus, the management of this condition needs to be prompt, appropriate and include members of the multi-disciplinary team including a continence advisor to identify appropriate treatment strategies. These may include use of skills training programmes, education, appropriate and accessible toileting facilities, changes to diet and lifestyle and use of appropriate continence aids (Nazarko, 2018). A comprehensive assessment of bowel pattern needs to be undertaken to establish the extent of the problem and, following this, interventions can be planned and implemented accordingly. The process begins with identifying reversible factors such as clothing, diet and exercise, progressing to the use of specialised continence aids with surgery being the last.

SKIN INTEGRITY

It is a function of the skin to prevent infection, regulate body temperature, maintain fluid and chemical balance and produce vitamin D. In addition, one's ability to respond to pain, temperature and touch is regulated by nerve endings in the skin (Flanagan, 2013). If skin integrity is compromised, infections and decubitus ulcers (pressure ulcers) may occur. Common factors of pressure ulcer risk include limited mobility, loss of sensation, history of a previous pressure ulcer, nutritional deficiency, the inability of people to reposition themselves, underlying medical conditions e.g. diabetes and significant cognitive impairment (NICE, 2014). Table 11.5 outlines those groups greatest at risk of skin breakdown.

Considering the risks presented, personal hygiene and attention to skin integrity are of paramount importance. As part of a person-centred care approach, assessment of the skin should be undertaken to determine an

TABLE 11.5	Patient groups at risk of skin breakdown (Wounds UK, 2018, p. 5)	
Patient group	**Skin changes**	**Potential problems**
Older adults	Becomes thinner, loses elasticity, reduced blood supply, subcutaneous fat decreases, skin hydration decreases.	Skin tears, pressure damage, infection, inflammation, dryness/flaking; possible related issues with nutrition/patients with dementia, cellulitis.
Spinal cord injury/paralysis	Alterations to vascular supply, temperature control, maceration/moisture, loss of collagen, lack of muscle/atrophy, impaired sensation due to damaged nerves in the skin (Rappl, 2008).	Skin tears, pressure damage, infection, inflammation.
Critically ill and injured children	Intrinsic changes due to pressure duration, shear and friction, poor perfusion and maceration (Inamadar and Palit, 2013).	Nappy dermatitis, skin tears, pressure damage.
Patients with spina bifida and cerebral palsy	Decreased skin perfusion, cutaneous reaction to drugs, perineal dermatitis and inflammation due to incontinence (Inamadar and Palit, 2013).	Pressure damage.
Bariatric patients	Altered epidermal cells, increased water loss, dry skin, maceration, increased skin temperature, and reduced lymphatic flow and perfusion (Shipman and Millington, 2011).	Pressure damage, skin tears, diabetic ulcers, psoriasis, moisture lesions.
Oncology patients	Radiation leads to inflammation, epidermis damage, decreased perfusion (NHS, 2010).	Pressure damage, reduced wound healing, skin infections, cellulitis.

individual's level of risk. Jones (2017) advocates that a holistic assessment is undertaken; this should include taking a medical history assessing medication, continence, nutrition and fluid intake, mobility and mental capacity.

Given the intimate nature of such an assessment, the personal integrity and dignity of the individual is a foremost concern. In addition, to ensure appropriate person-centred care, the individual's cultural and religious beliefs must be addressed. Discretion in undertaking this assessment and discussion of outcomes is paramount in maintaining the respect and dignity of the individual. This is amongst the approaches operationalised in the next chapter.

When undertaking an assessment of the skin, clinical guidance (NICE, 2014) advocates the use of pressure ulcer risk assessment scales (PURAS) such as the Braden Scale (Braden and Bergstrom, 1989), the Norton risk-assessment scale (Norton et al, 1962) or the Waterlow Score (Waterlow, 2005). These scales examine features such as skin type, skin integrity, continence, mobility, activity, nutrition and cognitive awareness. In the event of an identified risk to skin integrity, care should include a balanced diet, adequate fluid intake, good personal hygiene, use of appropriate skin care products, changes in positioning, correct use of and adaptation of equipment and clothing made from natural fibres such as cotton.

POSTURAL CARE

Postural care is a method of positioning that aims to preserve and restore body shape and tonus for people with movement difficulties (Public Health England, 2018b). People with profound and multiple intellectual disabilities often sit and lie in limited positions, resulting in a high risk of body shape distortion. Using correct equipment and positioning techniques the body shape in people with movement difficulties can be protected. The distortion of body shape due to poor postural care is preventable. Reader Activity 11.4 applies an experiential approach to better understand the positional challenges and discomfort felt by many people with intellectual disabilities.

Position yourself in a chair in a seated position. Place your hands in your lap or if your chair has armrests place your arms along the armrests. If possible, place your feet flat on the floor, if the chair is too tall, you may be on the tips of your toes.

Remain in this seated position for as long as you can without it becoming uncomfortable.

While you are seated, turn your awareness to the sensation of pressure on the soles of your feet, your tiptoes, the backs of your legs, your buttocks, your back and shoulders, your neck. Does your head hang forward or are you concentrating on holding your head upright? Concentrate on the sensations in your arms and hands.

Make a mental note of any sensations which encourage you to adjust your position. As you sit contemplating your own postural comfort, consider how it might feel for you if you could not adjust your own position and relied on other people to assist you.

For many of us we take it for granted that we can adjust our position to meet our own comfort needs whether it is lifting our feet, moving, raising our hand, or just shifting the pressure on our buttocks, but for some people they are entirely reliant on others to help them adjust their position.

According to Hill and Goldsmith (2009), the protection of body shape can be achieved through using a 24-hour approach to postural care. The approach is applied to all body positions which the individual adopts during their day. It includes the provision of adaptive seating, positioning equipment to support the person in lying, including at night, moving and handling techniques, advice and training for family carers and professionals across all settings (Crawford and Curran, 2014).

Postural care is essential for our comfort and is a key component in attaining good health. Failure to protect body shape can result in health complications (Mencap and Postural Care Action Group, 2011). For example:

- contractures – where the muscles tighten up and the person can't straighten their limbs;
- scoliosis – where there is asymmetry in the curvature of the spine;

- difficulty breathing–where the space within the chest cavity is compromised;
- poor digestion–where the space within the abdomen is compromised;
- constipation–this may be due to the position of the organs in the gut being compromised, or due to the person not having the correct seating position for digestion and bowel emptying;
- pressure on internal organs–where the space within the body is compromised.

There are also social consequences of incorrect postural care, the person may have reduced eye contact due to their head not being adequately supported. They may have difficulties participating in activities if their trunk/torso is not appropriately supported. They may have poor quality sleep due to pain or discomfort due to inadequate or inappropriate support at night. The consequences of failing to provide incorrect postural care are illustrated in Figure 11.6.

With the right approach to postural care, the person and their family can benefit from overall improvement in their quality of life with improved daily functioning and participation.

CONSTIPATION

Constipation is one of the most common digestive complaints experienced by people with intellectual disabilities; prevalence is higher than amongst the general population (Carey et al, 2016). A variety of factors can cause constipation including poor fluid and fibre intake, lack of physical activity, side effects of medication and stress (Brown, 2019).

Arguably, sedentary lifestyles, lack of exercise and increased longevity among people with intellectual disabilities (Marsh et al, 2010), over reliance on laxatives, inability to communicate the urge to defecate, issues with correct positioning on the toilet and lack of understanding amongst carers can further increase the risk of developing constipation (Brown, 2019). Symptoms of constipation include straining, hard stools, halitosis (bad breath), infrequent defaecation and the Bristol stool scale (Lewis and Heaton, 1997) can be utilised to classify faeces according to the amount of time spent in the colon.

Management of constipation

Given the personal and subjective nature of this condition, the person must be at the centre of any

What are the consequences of failing to provide postural care?

The figure below describes how severe changes in body shape can come about and how this can lead to premature death.

Failure to provide postural care – the consequences

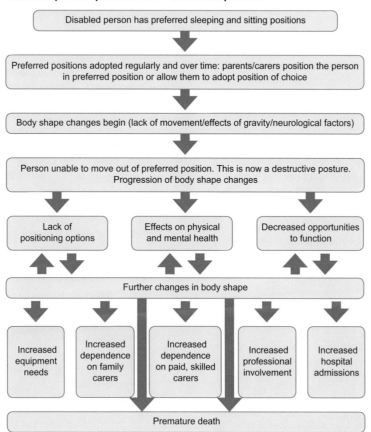

Figure 11.6 What are the consequences of failing to provide postural care? (NHS Scotland, 2018, p. 35)

intervention supported by significant others and members of the multi-disciplinary team including the nurse, physiotherapist, the family doctor and the dietician. In this instance, referral to the dietician is the first action as the dietician will carry out a nutritional assessment, identify a planned intervention and consider the appropriate support required to promote a healthy bowel. Any interventions are dependent on the severity of the condition and can vary from simple modifications to diet and lifestyle to medical interventions. Intervention plans are multifactorial and should include some or all the following aspects, beginning with increasing

fibre and fluid in the diet: correct positioning as this is required to ensure comfort; full emptying of the bladder and bowel. If aids such as continence pads are required, it is advisable to liaise with a continence advisor in relation to the selection of appropriate pads and the correct disposal of them. Additionally, physical activity and the use of medications also need to be addressed as part of the intervention.

People with intellectual disabilities are frequently prescribed many medications and constipation is a notable side effect. It is essential that those supporting this population are aware of this and take appropriate action to combat these side effects. Luke's situation in Reader Activity 11.5 provides an opportunity to consider helpful approaches.

READER ACTIVITY 11.5

Luke is a 30-year-old man with a moderate learning disability and Down syndrome. He lives in a community home with three of his peers with the support of social care workers. He has good communication skills and enjoys interacting with people. Luke has poor muscle tone (hypotonia), is slightly overweight and does not like to participate in regular exercise. From a dietary perspective he needs encouragement to eat fruit and vegetables and to take drinks during the day. Recently, Luke has been experiencing constipation. He is stressed about this and he is reluctant to leave the house unless assured he can access a bathroom.

- How would you identify the impact of constipation on Luke?
- How would you support Luke to manage his constipation?
- What other actions might you consider to support Luke?

CONCLUSION

Physical disabilities impact significantly on the lives of people with intellectual disabilities. This chapter has sought to raise overall awareness of the reader to the key issues relating to physical disabilities and has offered guidance to support people who experience difficulties relating to disorders of movement, eating and swallowing and nutritional difficulties as well as issues relating to the bladder and bowel. The provision of appropriate person-centred supports identified in this chapter can positively impact on an individual, not only by minimising the impact of physical disabilities on the person's physical, mental and social well-being, but by significantly improving their overall quality of life.

REFERENCES

Ali, A., Scior, K., Ratti, V., et al. (2013). Discrimination and other barriers to accessign health care: perspectives of patients with mild and moderate intellectual disability and their carers. *PLoS One, 8*, e70855. https://doi.org/10.1371/journal.pone.0070855.

American Association of Neurological Surgeons. (2019). Spasticity. Available at: https://www.aans.org/Patients/Neurosurgical-Conditions-and-Treatments/Spasticity. [Accessed on 21 November 2019].

Anders, P. L., & Davis, E. L. (2010). Oral health of patients with intellectual disabilities: a systematic review. *Special Care in Dentistry, 30*(3), 110–117.

Beacroft, M., & Dodd, K. (2010). Pain in people with learning disabilities in residential settings – the need for change. *British Journal of Learning Disabilities, 38*(3), 201–209.

Bodfish, J. W., Harper, V. N., Deacon, J. R., et al. (2001). *Identifying and measuring pain in persons with developmental disabilities: a manual for the Pain and Discomfort Scale PADS.* Morganton, NC: Western Carolina Center.

Boschitsch, E. P., Durchschlag, E., & Dimai, H. P. (2017). Age-related prevalence of osteoporosis and fragility fractures: real-world data from an Austrian menopause and osteoporosis clinic. *Climacteric, 20*(2), 157–163.

Braden, B., & Bergstrom, N. (1989). Clinical utility of the Braden scale for predicting pressure sore risk. *Decubitus, 2*(3), 50–51 44–46.

Breau, L. M., Camfield, C. S., McGrath, P. J., et al. (2003). The incidence of pain in children with severe cognitive impairments. *Archives of Pediatrics and Adolescent Medicine, 157*(12), 1219–1226.

British Association for Parenteral and Enteral Nutrition (BAPEN). (2011). *The 'MUST' explanatory booklet. A Guide to the 'Malnutrition Universal Screening Tool' 'MUST' for Adults.* Available at: https://www.bapen.org.uk/pdfs/must/must_explan.pdf. [Accessed 27 January 2020].

British Association of Urological Surgeons. (2017). *Self-catheterisation in women.* Available at: https://www.baus.org.uk/_userfiles/pages/files/Patients/Leaflets/ISC%20female.pdf. [Accessed 29 November 2019].

Brown, M. (2019). Constipation. In O. Barr & B. Gates (Eds.), *Oxford handbook of learning and intellectual disability nursing* (pp. 188–190). Oxford University Press.

Burton, M., & Ludwig, L. (2014). *Fundamentals of nursing care: concepts, connections and skills.* Philadelphia: F.A. Davis.

Mac Giolla Phadraig, C., Guerin, S., & Nunn, J. (2015). Should we educate care staff to improve the oral health and oral hygiene of people with intellectual disability in residential care? Real world lessons from a randomized controlled trial. *Special Care in Dentistry, 35*(3).

Carey, I. M., Shah, S. M., Hosking, F. J., et al. (2016). Health characteristics and consultation patterns of people with intellectual disability: a cross-sectional database study in English general practice. *British Journal of General Practice, 66*(645), e264–e270.

Children's Hospital of Philadelphia. (2019). Lordosis. Available at: https://www.chop.edu/conditions-diseases/lordosis. [Accessed 21 November 2019].

Collaborative Group on Hormonal Factors in Breast Cancer. (2019). Type and timing of menopausal hormone therapy and breast cancer risk: individual participant meta-analysis of the worldwide epidemiological evidence. *Lancet, 394*(10204), 1159–1168.

Compston, J. E., McClung, M. R., & Leslie, W. D. (2019). Osteoporosis. *Lancet, 393,* 364–376.

Crawford, A., & Harris, H. (2016). Caring for adults with impaired physical mobility. *Nursing, 46*(12), 36–41.

Crawford, S., & Curran, A. (2014). 24-Hour postural management for community dwelling adults with learning disabilities. *Posture and Mobility: The Journal of the Posture and Mobility Group, 31*(Winter), 15–19.

Dalton, C. (2019). Dysphagia. In B. Gates & O. Barr (Eds.), *Oxford handbook of learning and intellectual disability nursing* (pp. 196–197). Oxford: Oxford University Press.

Dalton, C., Caples, M., & Marsh, L. (2011). Management of dysphagia. *Learning Disability Practice, 14*(9), 32–38.

del Toro, G. (2009). *My pain profile.* Available at: https://www.dyingmatters.org/sites/default/files/user/images/pain%20assessment%20tool%20Notts%20final%20doc.pdf. [Accessed 19 December 2019].

Dougherty, L., & Lister, S. (2008). *The Royal Marsden Hospital manual of clinical nursing procedures.* Oxford: Wiley.

Dyspraxia Foundation. (2019). *Dyspraxia at a glance.* Available at: http://dyspraxiafoundation.org.uk/about-dyspraxia/dyspraxia-glance/. [Accessed 15 May 2020].

Flanagan, M. (2013). *Wound healing and skin integrity: principles and practice.* Chichester, UK: John Wiley & Sons.

Freshwater, D., & Maslin-Prothero, S. E. (2005). *Blackwell's nursing dictionary.* Oxford: Blackwell.

Galli-Carminati, G., Chauvet, I., & Deriaz, N. (2006). Prevalence of gastrointestinal disorders in adult clients with pervasive developmental disorders. *Journal of Intellectual Disability Research: JIDR, 50*(10), 711–718.

Gates, B. (2019). Causes and manifestations of intellectual disability. In O. Barr & B. Gates (Eds.), *Oxford handbook of learning and intellectual disability nursing* (pp. 14–15). Oxford University Press.

Gibson, W., Wagg, A., & Hunter, K. F. (2016). Urinary incontinence in older people. *British Journal of Hospital Medicine, 77*(2), C27–C32.

Hatzikotoulas, K., Roposch, A., Shah, K. M., et al. (2018). Genome-wide association study of developmental dysplasia of the hip identifies an association with GDF5. *Communication Biology, 1*(56), 1–11.

Hill, S., & Goldsmith, L. (2009). Mobility, posture and comfort. In J. Pawlyn & S. Carnaby (Eds.), *Profound intellectual and multiple disabilities. Nursing complex needs* (pp. 328–347). Oxford: Wiley-Blackwell.

Howseman, T. (2013). Dysphagia in people with learning disabilities. *Learning Disability Practice, 16,* 14–22.

Hresko, M. T. (2013). Idiopathic scoliosis in adolescents. *The New England Journal of Medicine, 368*(9), 834–841.

Inamadar, A. C., & Palit, A. (2013). *Critical care in dermatology.* Delhi: Jaypee Medical Publishing.

International Dysphagia Diet Standardisation Initiative. (2019) Complete IDDSI Framework. Available at: https://iddsi.org/IDDSI/media/images/Complete_IDDSI_Framework_Final_31July2019.pdf

Institute of Child Health, University College, London. Paediatric Pain Profile. Available at: https://ppprofile.org.uk/. [Accessed 19 December 2019].

Jones, M. L. (2017). Fundamentals of tissue viability, 1.2. Skin care: assessment. *British Journal of Healthcare Assistants, 11*(2), 72–73.

Keenan, P., Fleming, S., Horan, P., et al. (2018). Urinary continence promotion and people with an intellectual disability. *Learning Disability Practice, 21*(3), 28–34.

Kerr, D., Cunningham, C., & Wilkinson, H. (2006). *Responding to the pain experiences of people with learning difficulty and dementia.* Available at: https://www.jrf.org.uk/sites/default/files/jrf/migrated/files/9781859354599.pdf. [Accessed 19 December 2019].

LeDeR. The Learning Disability Mortality Review Programme. (2019). *Annual Report 2018.* Bristol: University of Bristol Norah Fry Centre for Disability Studies. Available at: http://www.bristol.ac.uk/media-library/sites/sps/leder/LeDeR_Annual_Report_2018%20published%20May%202019.pdf. [Accessed 19 December 2019].

Lewis, S. J., & Heaton, K. W. (1997). Stool Form Scale as a useful guide to intestinal transit time. *Scandinavian Journal of Gastroenterology, 32*(9), 920–924.

Lotan, M., Moe-Nilssen, R., Ljunggren, A., et al. (2009). *Appendix 1 Non-Communicating Adult Pain Checklist NCAPC.* Available at: http://bora.uib.no/handle/1956/3726. [Accessed 19 December 2019].

Marsh, L., Caples, M., Dalton, C., et al. (2010). Management of constipation. *Learning Disability Practice, 13*(4), 26–28.

Martínez-Zaragoza, F., Campillo-Martínez, J. M., & Ato-García, M. (2016). Effects on physical health of a multicomponent programme for overweight and obesity for adults with intellectual disabilities. *Journal of Applied Research in Intellectual Disabilities, 29*(3) 2500–2265.

Mayo Clinic. (2019). *Cerebral palsy*. Available at: https://www.mayoclinic.org/diseases-conditions/cerebral-palsy/symptoms-causes/syc-20353999. [Accessed 28 September 2020].

McCaffery, M. (1968). *Nursing practice theories related to cognition, bodily pain and man environment*. Los Angeles: Student store, UCLA.

(2017). Health, wellbeing and social inclusion: ageing with an intellectual disability. In M. McCarron, M. Haigh, & P. McCallion (Eds.), *Wave 3 IDS-TILDA*. School of Nursing and Midwifery, Trinity College Dublin.

Melville, C. A., Boyle, S. L., Miller, S., et al. (2011). An open study of the effectiveness of a multi-component weight-loss intervention for adults with intellectual disabilities and obesity. *The British Journal of Nutrition*, *105*(10), 1553–1562.

Mencap & Postural Care Action Group. (2011). *Postural care: protecting and restoring body shape*. Available at: https://www.mencap.org.uk/sites/default/files/2016-11/Postural%20Care%20booklet.pdf. [Accessed 19 December 2019].

Mencap. (2004) Treat me right! Available at: https://www.mencap.org.uk/sites/default/files/2016-08/treat_me_right.pdf. [Accessed on 19 December 2019].

Mencap. (2007). *Death by indifference*. Available at: https://www.mencap.org.uk/sites/default/files/2016-06/DBIreport.pdf. [Accessed 19 December 2019].

Mencap. (2012). *Death by indifference: 74 deaths and counting*. Available at: https://www.mencap.org.uk/sites/default/files/2016-08/Death%20by%20Indifference%20-%2074%20deaths%20and%20counting.pdf. [Accessed 19 December 2019].

Mixon, A. C., Mandzak Fried, K., & Guy, W. (2018). Understanding and treating neurogenic bladder. *Journal of Life Care Planning*, *16*(3), 13–16.

Moulster, G., & Jones, M. (2015). Biophysical aspects of learning disability nursing: pain assessment and recognition. In B. Gates, D. Fearns, & J. Welch (Eds.), *Learning disability nursing at a glance*. Chichester: Wiley.

National Institute for Clinical Excellence. (2007). *Faecal incontinence. The management of faecal incontinence in adults*. London: NICE.

National Institute for Health and Care Excellence. (2014). *Pressure ulcers: prevention and management*. Available at: www.nice.org.uk/guidance/cg179. [Accessed 12 December 2019].

National Institute of Diabetes and Digestive and Kidney Disease. (2014). *Urinary retention*. United States Department of Health and Human Services. Available at: https://www.niddk.nih.gov/health-information/urologic-diseases/urinary-retention#sec5. [Accessed 29 November 2019].

National Institutes of Health. (2019). *Calcium fact sheet for consumers*. Available at: https://ods.od.nih.gov/factsheets/Calcium-Consumer/. [Accessed 3 January 2021].

National Osteoporosis Guideline Group. (2018). *NOGG 2017: clinical guideline for the prevention and treatment of osteoporosis*. Available at: https://www.sheffield.ac.uk/NOGG/NOGG%20Guideline%202017.pdf. [Accessed 27 November 2019].

Nazarko, L. (2018). Faecal incontinence: investigation, treatment and management. *British Journal of Community Nursing*, *23*(12), 582–588.

NHS. (2010). *Skincare of patients receiving radiotherapy*. Scotland: NHS Quality Improvement Scotland.

NHS Scotland. (2018). *Learning byte: postural care*. Available at: https://www.nes.scot.nhs.uk/media/4090964/postural_care_learning_byte.pdf. [Accessed 12 December 2019].

Norton, D., McLaren, R., & Exon-Smith, A. (1962). *An investigation of geriatric nursing problems in hospital*. London: Churchill Livingstone.

Painaustralia. (2016). Clinical assessment of pain: factsheet 3. Available at: https://www.painaustralia.org.au/static/uploads/files/painaust-factsheet3-jan-16-wfksvufhgrzc-wfyaoehyvpzw.pdf. [Accessed 15 May 2020].

Pawlyn, J., & Carnaby, S. (Eds.). (2009). *Profound intellectual and multiple disabilities: nursing complex needs*. Oxford: Wiley-Blackwell,

Pradhan, A., Keuskamp, D., & Brennan, D. (2015). Pre-and post-training evaluation of dental efficacy and activation measures in carers of adults with disabilities in south Australia–a pilot study. *Health and Social Care in the Community*, *24*(6), 739–746.

Public Health England (PHE). (2017). Recognising and managing pain in people with learning disabilities. Available at: https://www.slideshare.net/PublicHealthEngland/social-care-staff-pain-management/1. [Accessed 19 December 2019].

Public Health England. (2018a). Learning disabilities and CQC inspection report: research and analysis. Available at: https://www.gov.uk/government/publications/learning-disabilities-and-cqc-inspection-reports/learning-disabilities-and-cqc-inspection-reports. [Accessed 19 December 2019].

Public Health England. (2018b). Postural care and people with learning disabilities: guidance. Available at: https://www.gov.uk/government/publications/postural-care-services-making-reasonable-adjustments/postural-care-and-people-with-learning-disabilities. [Accessed 19 December 2019].

Purves, W. K., Sadava, D., Orians, G. H., et al. (2007). *Life: the science of biology* (4th ed.). Sinauer Associates.

Rappl, L. M. (2008). Physiological changes in tissues denervated by spinal cord injury tissues and possible effects on wound healing. *International Wound Journal*, 5(3), 435–444.

Richeimer, S. H. (1998). The assessment of the patient with pain. In M. E. Gershwin & M. E. Hamilton (Eds.), *The pain management handbook. Current clinical practice*. Totowa, NJ: Humana Press.

Rimmer, J. H., Yamaki, K., Davis, B., et al. (2010). Obesity and obesity-related secondary conditions in adolescents with intellectual/developmental disabilities. *Journal of Intellectual Disabilities Research*, 54(9), 787–794.

Royal College of Physicians and British Society of Gastroenterology. (2010). *Oral feeding difficulties and dilemmas. A guide to practical care, particularly towards the end of life. Report of a working party*. London: Royal College of Physicians and British Society of Gastroenterology.

Rubin, L., & Crocker, A. (2006). *Medical care for children and adults with developmental disabilities*. Canada: Paul H Brookes.

Sanivarapu, R. R., & Gibson, J. (2019). *Aspiration pneumonia*. In *StatPearls*. Treasure Island, FL: StatPearls Publishing. Available at: https://www.ncbi.nlm.nih.gov/books/NBK470459/. [Accessed 15 May 2020].

Scanlon, V. C., & Sanders, T. (2018). *Essentials of anatomy and physiology* (8th ed.). Philadelphia: F. A. Davis Company.

Seeley, R., VanPutte, C., Reagan, J., et al. (2010). *Seeley's anatomy and physiology* (9th ed.). New York: McGraw Hill.

Shipman, A. R., & Millington, G. W. M. (2011). Obesity and the skin. *The British Journal of Dermatology*, 165(4), 743–750.

Spanos, D., Melville, C. A., & Hankey, C. R. (2013). Weight management interventions in adults with intellectual disabilities and obesity: a systematic review of the evidence. *Nutrition Journal*, 12(132).

St. Oswald's Hospice and Northumberland Tyne and Wear NHS Trust (v22) (2021). Disability Distress and Discomfort Assessment Tool DisDAT. Available at: https://www.stoswaldsuk.org/media-new/5181/disdat-22.pdf.

Talbot, C., Adam, J., & Paton, R. (2017). # Late presentation of developmental dysplasia of the hip: a 15-year observational study. *The Bone and Joint Journal*, 99-B(9), 1250–1255.

The International Dysphagia Diet Standardisation Initiative. (2016). Available at: https://iddsi.org/framework/. [Accessed 27 January 2020].

Van Timmeren, D., Van der Putten, A. A. J., Van Schrojenstein Lantman-de Valk, H. M. J., et al. (2016). Prevalence of reported physical health problems in people with severe or profound intellectual and motor disabilities: a cross-sectional study of medical records and care plans. *Journal of Intellectual Disability Research*, 60(11), 1109–1118.

von Gontard, A. (2015). Nocturnal enuresis, daytime urinary and faecal incontinence in children with special needs. *Australian and New Zealand Continence Journal*, 21(2), 54–58.

Waterlow, J. (2005). *The Waterlow Score*. Available at: http://www.judy-waterlow.co.uk/waterlow_score.htm. [Accessed 12 December 2019].

Wong, D., & Baker, C. M. (1983). *Wong-Baker FACES Pain Rating Scale*. Available at: http://wongbakerfaces.org/. [Accessed 19 December 2019].

World Health Organisation. (2018). *Obesity and overweight*. Available at: https://www.who.int/news-room/fact-sheets/detail/obesity-and-overweight. [Accessed 19 January 2020].

World Health Organisation. (2019). *Body mass index*. Available at: http://www.euro.who.int/en/health-topics/disease-prevention/nutrition/a-healthy-lifestyle/body-mass-index-bmi. [Accessed 19 January 2020].

Wounds UK (2018). *Best practice statement: maintaining skin integrity*. London: Wounds UK. Available at: https://www.wounds-uk.com/download/resource/7571. [Accessed 12 December 2019].

Yoshihara, T., Morinushi, T., Kinjyo, S., et al. (2005). Effects of periodic preventative care on the progression of periodontal disease in young adults with Down's syndrome. *Journal of Clinical Periodontology*, 32(6), 556–560.

12

Empowerment through skill development

Jo Lay and Zuzana Matousova-Done

KEY ISSUES

- Skill acquisition develops self-confidence and self-belief.
- Interdependence promotes skill development based upon individual choice and competence.

- A focus on Activities of Daily Living supports functional assessment and person-centred planning in learning and developing new skills
- There are a range of teaching skills and strategies that encourage and facilitate skill development.

CHAPTER OUTLINE

INTRODUCTION

This new chapter explores strategies for the promotion of skills teaching towards the development of activities of daily living to support and enable people who have intellectual disabilities. Self-care skills, a series of routine activities that are performed on a day-to-day basis such as personal care needs, dressing, eating and drinking, maintaining continence and moving around (mobility), are referred to as basic Activities of Daily Living (ADLs). Developing skills is essential in maximising an individual's competence and independence, but also in providing self-worth and confidence. The aim of skills teaching is not necessarily to make someone fully independent in a task or activity; indeed, it can be argued that most of us are never fully independent, and so support from others promotes an interdependent relationship. The psychology of interdependence recognises the importance of therapeutic relationships in establishing our self-identity and giving value to our skills and attributes by recognising how they promote the well-being of others. Interdependence also encourages us to see each other as equals. We do not all need the same skills and attributes but appreciate the strengths of others and what they provide to us. This chapter will therefore consider these issues within the exploration of skills including personal care, dressing, eating and drinking, promoting continence, and mobility. Use of personal illustrations will consider the diversity of skill development based upon individual competence.

The recognition of human rights alongside changes in societal attitudes towards disabilities throughout the 20th century to the current day has challenged individuals and services to develop teaching practices which promote an ordinary life model of care and support. This has been influenced by the work of Wolfensberger (1972) who developed the principles of 'Normalisation' and 'Social Role Valorisation' (see also Chapter 3), advocating that people with intellectual disabilities want, and have the right to, the same life opportunities as others. During the 1970s and 1980s a number of skills teaching frameworks and models were established to support children and adults with intellectual disabilities such as the Bereweeke Skills Teaching System (Felce et al, 1983) and Conductive Education (Rowley, 2019). These are still in use today and will be discussed in more detail later in this chapter. These strategies were based upon teaching frameworks which recognised that individuals with intellectual disabilities may not have followed the same developmental milestones as others or have been able to process the same learning experiences due to their cognitive impairment. Their success therefore depends on an individual approach. In the UK community care initiatives and legislation have recognised the key pillars of rights, independence, choice and inclusion as the driving forces behind a person-centred approach to care and promotion of individual competence (Department of Health (DH), 2001). The key features of a person-centred approach are shown in Box 12.1.

Person centred approaches have led to the development of the personalisation agenda where services are based upon the individual's preferences and choices, and therefore personal to them. Although person-centred care is seen as a global approach to health and wellbeing, the implementation of this has been faster in some countries (World Health Organisation (WHO), 2015). People with intellectual disabilities may need a range of support strategies to exercise this decision making as well as support in living the life they want, as independently as they can. This chapter seeks to identify communication and teaching frameworks, and strategies which will facilitate decision making as well as promoting skills development.

SKILLS TEACHING

Care or support plans which focus on skills teaching need to be positive and motivational. We must find

> ### 📄 BOX 12.1   Key features of a person-centred approach
>
> - the person is at the centre of the approach. This may involve creative strategies to promote involvement by focusing on what the individual likes and environments that minimise anxiety.
> - family and friends are full partners. The individual should be in control of this but the key message is that the approach is not purely service led.
> - it reflects the person's capacities, what is important to them and the support they need to make a valued contribution within their community.
> - it incorporates a shared vision and commitment to action that upholds the rights of the person at the centre.
> - It leads to continuous listening, learning and action that supports the person at the centre to live the life they choose (Department of Health, 2002).

the aspects of learning that resonate with the person to engage a desire for achievement. This involves taking the time to get to know an individual and ensuring that a person-centred approach is at the heart of this. We must recognise that what works well for one person may not for another. Learning approaches which focus on our strengths are important in giving us self-confidence to recognise the skills that we already have, and the belief in our potential to develop these further, however difficult that may be. Whilst this chapter does not focus on the development of communication skills (issues relating to these are comprehensively covered in Chapter 5) we acknowledge that this is an essential aspect of skills development.

The nature of intellectual disabilities leads to a diversity of need and ability in developing skills and competence. Supporters of people therefore need skills, knowledge and access to a wide range of professionals who can help to promote learning. This knowledge and skill may come from different sectors of support services and professionals including health, education and psychology but may also be supported by the experience and expertise of others including family and friends. The key is to provide an inclusive and inter-professional approach to learning which recognises and respects the contributions of all but focuses on the uniqueness of the individual (Sanderson et al, 2015). Personalisation provides benefits to all, not just the learner, in promoting positive values.

Skills teaching can utilise specific methods of learning through assessments and frameworks but can also be part of a wider educational pedagogy or intervention. Perhaps the most prominent teaching approaches stem from the theories of social constructionism, behaviourism and social learning theory.

Social constructionism

Conductive Education (CE) was developed in the 1940s by Dr András Peto in Hungary to support young people with cerebral palsy, and other neurological and motor disabilities, to develop their independence, motor skills and competence using a goal setting approach based on social constructionist theory (Rowley, 2019). CE is based upon the values of human potential, that is the recognition that if we are motivated and supported, we can all learn to develop our competence and skills. CE utilises group activities to provide peer support and instructor coaching which promotes the development of interpersonal relationships and provides a motivational base for the development of individual goals. Coaching provides affirmation and the recognition of progress in achieving goals that have been set (Rowley, 2019). Trained teachers, known as conductors, provide the coaching support. There are a number of coaching models used to enhance this process which could also be utilised to facilitate other learning opportunities. One popular coaching model is GROW developed by John Whitmore (Leadership Foundation for Higher Education, 2018), outlined in Table 12.1.

CE is still widely used in many countries and links to this can be found in the accompanying online resource.

Behaviourist perspective

The most common teaching approach/behavioural intervention used from a behaviourist perspective is Applied Behavioural Analysis (ABA) (see also Chapter 17). Ivan Pavlov (1849–1936) (Classical conditioning) and Burrhus. F. Skinner (1904–1990) (Operant conditioning) are credited as the founders of this approach which recognises that behaviour is learnt from experience and interaction with our environment (Morris et al, 2005). Learning is broken down into antecedents (what occurs prior to an activity/behaviour), the action/behaviour itself and finally consequence of the action.

TABLE 12.1		The Grow Model
G	Goal	Setting meaningful targets for the individual or team
R	Reality	Understanding what is happening now. Be concrete in language used. Facilitators need to be skilled in questioning to determine the current reality, e.g. What works well now and what doesn't? What are the strengths of the individual?
O	Options	Generating ideas that focus on problem solving
W	Will	The individual or team choose the option they want to create into an action plan

Prompting and fading

Techniques that can be used for skill development at the antecedent stage include prompting and fading. Prompting provides cues to encourage an individual to take a particular action and is helpful when usual antecedents don't help. For example, part of developing skills in dressing may be wearing weather related clothing. If the individual is going for a walk on a cold day, they may need a verbal or physical prompt to wear a coat or jacket. To promote independence the technique of fading can then be used to reduce the prompts until the individual has learnt to recognise the impact of weather on the clothes they choose. In this example prompting and fading may involve;

1. Prompting
   - It's cold outside, here is your coat.
2. Fading
   - Do you think you need a coat?
   - What is the weather like outside?

ABA uses reinforcement to promote desired outcomes, and in the past has been criticised for having a focus on the behaviour and consequence as opposed to considering the meaning that the behaviour held for the individual (Kelly and Barnes-Holmes, 2014). Millman (2020) suggests that there are still criticisms of ABA as a method which again seeks to fix and control, rather than empathetically support the development of competence. Positive Behavioural Support (PBS) is a framework which seeks to improve quality of life and skill development through person-centred values (PBS Academy, 2016). Support can incorporate strategies such as reinforcement but within a framework of choice, inclusion and participation.

Reinforcement

Reinforcement recognises that the consequences of an action/specific behaviour can increase or decrease the likelihood of that behaviour happening again. Positive reinforcement is where something is added following successful completion of a task. Negative reinforcement is where something is taken away. This is not the same as punishment as it could be removing something from the environment that is causing distress, i.e. reinforcing a positive outcome for the individual.

Shaping

Shaping, or use of successive approximations (Shrestha, 2017), provides a way of encouraging and reinforcing a skill until a person becomes competent. It recognises that there may be a number of stages that a person needs to accomplish before they reach their end goal. By reinforcing any aspect of learning that is a step towards completing the final task, the individual has an increased chance of reaching their goal (Shrestha, 2017).

Task analysis

Task analysis is a process frequently used within ABA but can also be used as a standalone tool to facilitate skill development. It involves breaking down a task or learning activity into small steps. Task analysis was developed specifically for supporting people with intellectual disabilities in residential settings as the 'Bereweeke Skills Teaching System' (Felce et al, 1983). It provided a systematic way of teaching skills based on development of competence and independence. Tasks are broken down into component parts (see Reader activity 12.1).

Breaking the task into steps supports the learner to understand the logic of a process as well as ensuring more manageable components, considering the individual needs of the learner such as age and concentration ability (Pratt and Steward, 2018). If this person-centred focus is not considered it can lead to unrealistic expectations which may disengage the person or cause distress. The task can be implemented as a logical process known as forward chaining, i.e. you start teaching the skills from the beginning of the task; or you may use backward chaining. Backward chaining involves starting with the

READER ACTIVITY 12.1   Task analysis

Consider a day-to-day activity that you undertake e.g. making a cup of tea.

Write down the list of steps that you make to do this until you get to the desired outcome.

Your list may look something like this:

1. Unplug the kettle
2. Take it to the sink
3. Fill with water
4. Switch the kettle on
5. Wait for the kettle to boil
6. Put a tea bag into the cup
7. Add the boiling water to the cup
8. Wait 2 minutes
9. Remove the tea bag into the bin
10. Add milk and sugar to the cup

However, you may have started at a different point. Your task analysis may look different based on the equipment and set up of your kitchen, e.g. you may have a stove top kettle. Other considerations may include safety awareness, e.g. a risk assessment of managing boiling water. How do you know how much water to put in?

end point of a task and working backwards which can be more motivational as the individual will consistently achieve the goal e.g. getting the cup of tea. You can test your understanding and reflect on techniques introduced in this section by completing Reader activity 12.2 in the accompanying online resource.

Social learning theory

Bandura (1977) further developed behavioural learning theories into Social Learning Theory. In this he added two new aspects to the way people learn; recognising the mediating processes which happen between experiencing a stimulus and having a response, and secondly the importance of observational learning (McLeod, 2016). The four mediating processes are

1. Attention – How much notice do we take of the behaviour? How conscious are we of it?
2. Retention – How much do we remember of the behaviour? What can help us to remember?
3. Reproduction – To be able to reproduce or copy behaviour. What is our level of competence?

TABLE 12.2	**Frameworks and models of skills teaching**
Portage	Home visiting education service for pre-school age children (National Portage Service, 2019). Portage practitioner will work with families to promote involvement in family life & community; seek to minimise & remove barriers which impact on inclusion & learning and support the development of local services which promote inclusion & positive opportunity. https://www.portage.org.uk/
TEACCH (Treatment and Education of Autistic and Communication-Handicapped Children)	Began in 1966 as child research project in Department of Psychiatry of School of Medicine at University of North Carolina, USA. Not a single teaching method/approach, but a framework that provides structure for teaching. Its principles include understanding culture of autism, i.e. truths & realities of autism experience; developing individualised person/family centred plan for each person as opposed to fixed curricula; structuring physical environment; using visual supports & prompts to make timetables & plans predictable & understandable; using visual supports for individual tasks. https://teacch.com/ (see also Chapter 15)
SPELL	Designed to understand and respond to needs of children & adults on autistic spectrum. Can be used in combination with other strategies & teaching frameworks. Emphasises ways to change environments and support using person centred values. The focus is on Structure (S), Positive Approaches and Expectations (P), Empathy (E), Low Arousal (L) and Links (L) between all the individual's needs and services they use. https://www.autism.org.uk/what-we-do/professional-development/training-and-conferences/support-spell (see also Chapter 15)
Social Stories	A social learning tool which promotes meaningful and safe communication through a shared narrative that recognises the different perceptions of others. Gray (2018) provides a ten-step process of defining criteria to guide authors in developing a story which focuses on an idea, concept, skill or achievement. This includes a focus on the individual, a clear structure and a clear goal https://carolgraysocialstories.com/ (see also Chapter 15)

4. Motivation – To want to reproduce the behaviour.

Subsequent models and frameworks of learning have sought to consider these and provide a systematic way of recognising the impact of environment and culture on learning for people with intellectual disabilities and/or autism. Table 12.2 provides an overview of some of these, but the list is not exhaustive.

ACTIVITIES OF DAILY LIVING

Activities of Daily Living (ADLs) are very personal and play a major part in people's confidence, independence, overall functional or developmental growth, motivation and sense of achievement (Ardic and Cavkayter, 2014). Being able to look after oneself, and to fulfil basic needs, can be complex for someone who may have underlying problems including impairments in the area of sensory integration, vision, cognition, communication, swallowing, fine and/or gross motor skills, co-ordination, mobility and health (Swapna and Sudhir, 2016; Weis, 2014) or simply living where adaptation, space, resources or obtaining appropriate food or drink may be a major issue. In addition, a person with disabilities, impaired cognitive ability or poor motor planning may have difficulty in sequencing, timing and grading motor activities which can lead to signs of distress or anxiety and prevent them attempting or completing the task. Teaching ADLs in order to increase independence can be challenging (Ardic and Cavkayter, 2014). Age, culture and personal interest may further play a role in choosing to complete individual tasks or the importance of the essential ADLs.

There are many definitions of the essential ADLs but the agreed common categories are shown in Table 12.3 (Edemekong et al, 2020).

Activities of Daily Living encompass the basic or essential needs we use to function. As we grow, we develop life skills to live independently or with assistance and services

TABLE 12.3   Common categories of ADLs

ADL	Examples
Personal care needs	Washing oneself (bathing, showering, sponge down or wipe down by a sink or using a small container); Grooming, oral and intimate care.
Dressing	Being able to physically dress/undress oneself and to make decisions regarding clothing and/or accessories.
Eating and drinking	Being able to drink or feed oneself using appropriate utensils or assistive devices.
Promoting continence	Having the mental and physical capability and capacity to use a toilet and/or continence aids; Getting on/off the toilet and maintaining hygiene.
Mobility	Getting in and out of bed; Ability to move oneself from seated to standing and move around; Abilities in internal and external environments; Managing aids and support required.

READER ACTIVITY 12.3   How independent am I?

Consider your home environment and whether you live on your own or with family.
- Do you consider yourself independent?
- What influences this decision?

Looking at the list of ADLs in Table 12.3 and examples of IADLs that follows, can you identify any areas where you need support or help?

At the beginning of the chapter we noted the importance of human interdependence. However independent we feel, most of us rely on strengths and skills of others to support this whether that be in ADLs or IADLs such as money management, home improvement etc.

Consider that your needs have changed, and you may now need support or further support to complete ADLs. What would be most important to you in maintaining as much independence as you can?

that we may require throughout our lives. Those skills are referred to as Instrumental Activities of Daily Living (IADLs). IADLs require complex thinking and organisational skills (Edemekong et al, 2020). They include:
- Basic communication skills using any means of communication with others (for example telephone, mobile telephone, internet, media or email)
- Meal preparation including menu planning, cooking, cleaning afterwards, safe use of kitchen equipment and utensils
- Housework including laundry, mopping, washing dishes, vacuuming, dusting and making bed
- Managing medications (where applicable) including taking medication when prescribed, correct dosage and managing refills
- Shopping including an ability to decide what to buy and where
- Transportation including ability to arrange own transport, driving oneself or use public transport
- Managing personal finances including using a card, transactions, living within a budget and paying bills.

Dr Sidney Katz is credited with first using the term Activities of Daily Living in 1950 (Edemekong et al, 2020). Katz developed ADLs as part of a functional assessment for older people who wanted to maintain independence (Wallace and Shelkey, 2007). A simple scoring system was used to determine whether the individual was fully independent or if they needed assistance (dependent). For example, in dressing, independence was viewed as being able to retrieve clothes from cupboards and being able to put them on without assistance. The Barthel ADL Index, published in 1965, sought to introduce levels of support e.g. slight, moderate, severe or total dependency (Mahoney and Barthel, 1965). This encourages us to think about how we define or measure independence, and how that definition impacts on choices and rights (see Reader activity 12.3).

An individual approach to ADLs and skills teaching is essential in promoting and maintaining a person-centred focus. What skills does the individual want to learn? What are their priorities? This should underpin the involvement of any members of a multi-disciplinary team working with a person who has an intellectual disability. ADLs were introduced as a nursing model/theory by Roper et al in 1980 (Roper et al, 1996). They

BOX 12.2 Roper Logan and Tierney's Activities of Living

- Maintaining a safe environment
- Communication
- Breathing
- Eating and drinking
- Elimination
- Washing and dressing
- Controlling temperature
- Mobility
- Working and playing
- Sleeping
- Sexuality
- Death and dying

advocated that their Activities of Living model provided an approach and organisation of care and support toward increasing independence and quality of life based upon 12 ALs (see Box 12.2).

This model extends the view of what essential ALs are towards a more holistic view of quality of life, recognising the impact that they have on our physical and emotional development. It encourages us to develop opportunities for people to explore their needs and preferences within each AL (Roper et al, 1996). However, it has been critiqued as simply becoming a checklist (O'Connor, 2002). Roper et al (1996) were clear that its success relied upon using it within a systematic process of assessment, planning, implementation and evaluation. In this chapter, we focus on the ADLs outlined in Table 12.3 but consider the influence of factors such as dependence/independence promoted by Roper et al (1996), and explore these in relation to choice, best interests, human rights, privacy and dignity and safety including use of assistive devices.

PERSONAL CARE NEEDS

Whether we are getting ready for bed or getting up in the morning, there are a series of routines that we all like to complete in a certain sequence to feel refreshed and relaxed. If our routine is disturbed for a variety of reasons our state of mind may change, it may affect the way we appear to others and our overall general attitude. Good personal and intimate hygiene and self-care may include:

- washing our body (bathing, showering, bed bath or washing with a flannel)

- drying
- skin care (application of prescription or personal creams and lotions)
- brushing teeth and oral hygiene
- grooming (hair, make up, nail care, shaving, foot care)
- where required, managing a wound, stoma or catheter bag care.

Following personal care routines requires a set of physical, communication (Klein, 1983) and cognitive skills (Weis, 2014) including being able to read social cues e.g. appropriate time of day or place (Swapna and Sudhir, 2016). Assessments and care plans (detail of need and how this will be supported) which recognise personal and health orientated goals focus on consent and capacity, promote independence and can determine an appropriate level and intensity of support in each area (Wenar and Kerig, 2006; Wehman and Targett, 2004). Consistent use of care plans through effective team working is essential in supporting the individual to help manage any emotional distress involved in introducing change and develop coping strategies.

Washing our body, including intimate care and hygiene, should be part of our daily routines and helps us feel dignified and good about ourselves (World Health Organisation [WHO] and United Nations Children's Fund [UNICEF], 2019). Drying our body after a wash is essential as it prevents multiplication of any remaining bacteria in a moist environment. Washing and drying is a process that involves multiple tasks and subtasks and people with intellectual disabilities may require assistance (Gill et al, 2006). A checklist for supporting personal care is provided in Box 12.3. Teaching and creating plans that provide a positive experience play a vital role in promoting independence and self-care (De-Rosende-Celeiro et al, 2019).

Skin care is an integral part of personal care. Washing, drying and moisturising (including under any folds or breasts and between the toes) contributes to healthier skin presentation and appearance, as well as prevention of infections and skin related diseases. Lack of attention to skin care can lead to discomfort, dryness and skin conditions. This includes poor manual handling; excessive washing; high water temperature; not drying properly, tight or non-breathable materials; and poor sun care. One resultant issue, pressure ulcers, has been further discussed in Chapter 11 but can also include eczema, psoriasis, ulcers, sun damage, dandruff, allergic reactions and irritations and cellulitis (Morris-Jones, 2019). Person centred care plans should include any family skin issues, allergies and seasonal effects, as well as appropriate application of skin care products, amounts and frequency.

Oral and dental hygiene contribute to our general health and overall well-being. Having strong teeth and being able to smile, talk and chew without pain contributes to an increase of self-esteem, confidence, good nutrition, and quality of life (Wilson et al, 2019). People with intellectual disabilities experience poorer oral hygiene (see Box 12.4) and current research seeks ways to improve it and to prevent oral disease (Waldman and Perlman, 2012).

It is important that oral hygiene as part of the care plan is developed with the individual and reflects not only their medical history but also daily oral assessments,

any difficulties such as pain or discomfort, and step by step instructions on oral hygiene. The assessment should include for example: the state of the gums (firm, healthy, inflamed or bleeding), mouth ulcers, any damaged and loose teeth or cavities and the margins of the buccal (oral) cavity (lips, on or below tongue, cheeks and palate). Several assessment tools are easily accessible to support with this (Australian Institute of Health and Welfare, 2009; Chalmers et al, 2004). People with feeding devices, such as a nasogastric or gastrostomy tube, or dentures also require good oral hygiene and care. It is vital to be mindful of medication, as some types of medication are linked to gingival overgrowth (antiepileptic medication), dry mouth and may contain sugar (syrups).

When we are supporting someone with an intellectual disability with personal and intimate care it is vital that we are sensitive to their needs e.g. cultural and religious background (Department of Health, 2009) including any necessary rituals that happen during personal and intimate care. For example, in Hindu, Muslim and Sikh religions the preference is to wash under running water and in Muslim religion, the genitals are washed with the left hand (Attum et al, 2020). Person centred planning tools can provide support in helping an individual to explore their choices, likes and dislikes. One example is Essential Lifestyle Planning (ELP) which was introduced as a guided process to help people get the lives they want (Smull, 1996); initially used to support people moving from hospital support to new environments it is now commonly used in developing wider opportunities and choices (Social Care Institute for Excellence (SCIE), 2005). It is essential to learn what is important to the person. For us to understand this it can be useful to reflect on our own choices and the importance they play in our lives. ELP asks what a good day and a bad day looks like for an individual, to help them focus on likes and dislikes; it then gives further opportunity to consider the level of importance e.g. is it preferred or is it essential (see Reader activity 12.4 and Personal illustration 12.1 (Clive).

DRESSING

Dressing involves a variety of steps in a sequence either to put clothes on or take them off; each item of clothing has its place in the sequence. The acts of dressing and undressing give people with intellectual disabilities an opportunity to develop or master many skills including self-awareness, movement, balance, stereognosis (recognising and identifying objects without any visual cues using tactile manipulation), body schema (series of processes registering where body parts are in space),

communication and fine and gross motor skills (Werner, 2018; Holmes and Spence, 2004). Carers may believe it is easier to dress a person than teach them to do it independently, as this may decrease any frustration and behaviours of concern that are usually linked with dressing and sequencing (Freeman Watson et al, 2010), especially in instances where there are deficits in perceptual-motor coordination as well as hand movements and visual inputs (Carmeli et al, 2008). Teaching individuals to master skills in dressing independently can greatly improve their self-esteem, confidence, outlook on life, dignity, self-realisation and potential (Pestana, 2014) (see Personal illustration 12.2, Glynis).

Individual choice of clothing is essential to promote identity and self-expression regardless of financial resources. What is sometimes underestimated is the physical and emotional protection clothing provides. From an emotional perspective it may positively alter the state of mind of the individual, especially when a compliment is paid and there is positive attention from others. A good choice of clothing and fabric can further

---

 READER ACTIVITY 12.4

Explore Essential Lifestyle Planning further through a web-based search.

Now think about how you could apply the concepts to yourself.

What happens in the first half hour of a typical day for you?

Think about everything that you do and the choices that you make. You should think about the time that you spend, e.g.

7.00 Alarm goes off (radio because I don't like the beeping). Has to be BBC Radio 2. Press snooze.

7.05 Alarm goes off again. Get up, go to the toilet etc.

How did you wake up? What routines do you have? Is the sequence important? Are products or brands important? How would you feel if the routine was changed?

PERSONAL ILLUSTRATION 12.1   Providing personal care

Clive is a 41-year-old male who has a diagnosis of a moderate intellectual disability, sensory needs and cerebral palsy (triplegia); he prefers an electric wheelchair to mobilise. He has difficulties communicating verbally which make him frustrated and can lead to him becoming agitated and hitting out at others, especially during personal and intimate care, impacting on his relationship with carers. The primary carer used Essential Lifestyle Planning (Smull and Sanderson, 2005) to support his other carers to appreciate the importance of enabling Clive to identify his own choices and take control of his care, even though he needed support with this. His carers subsequently formulated a care plan with Clive that recognised that:

- Clive prefers a bed bath twice a day; in the morning before breakfast and in the evening at 7pm;
- He requests a shower once a week and could inform staff when this should be.
- He likes to be hoisted with an electric hoist using a parachute sling with a headrest.
- The water for the bed bath has to be luke-warm, with Nivea shower gel already squeezed into the water.
- A sponge should be used to wash Clive's body and a face cloth to wash his face.

- Clive prefers to be assisted by a male carer or two older female carers.
- Clive can use a lifting pole with handle and a cot side to hoist himself up or turn from side to side.
- He likes to be patted dry as opposed to rubbed and uses a prescription cream for his body.
- Clive uses an electric shaver and an electric toothbrush with a timer. He can use these independently if handed to him.
- Clive prefers specific brands of toiletries and keeps a list of these in his shopping file.
- Clive likes to keep his hair short.
- Clive requests to have a manicure and pedicure once a fortnight as part of a relaxation activity.

Clive is more relaxed, interested and engaged in self-care when he recognises that he is in control of his decisions. To help Clive receive consistency in support, staff have developed task analysis summaries with him (see Reader activity 12.1) for each personal care activity using photographs to show staff how to support him with positioning etc. Clive can use this to prompt staff on what support he needs.

protect from stigma and can act as a physical and emotional shield (Howlett et al, 2013; Freeman Watson et al, 2010). It is important to note that whilst shielding a disability may be important to an individual, equally important is to help them develop self-acceptance and self-confidence; a task made easier in a society that accepts us all as individuals.

Clothing accessories such as fastening buttons, zips, poppers, laces or hooks may present a challenge for some people with intellectual disabilities therefore it is essential that those difficulties are reflected in the person-centred plan. Many companies and retailers (including Marks & Spencer, Tommy Adaptive, Nike and SpecialKids.Company) have started designing clothing for people with different types of disabilities including sensory issues, with their best interest in mind. It may take some time to find suitable equipment therefore much encouragement, patience, prompts and assistance are important especially at the beginning of learning new skills. If available, the support of an Occupational Therapist (OT) may prove invaluable in provision of aids and equipment. Task analysis can again provide a useful tool for breaking down tasks based on individual need. Each part of the task is called a 'chain' and each chain can be given the time and attention it needs to find the best strategy for the individual (see Personal illustration 12.2, Glynis). Sequence/communication boards may display images, symbols or photographs to communicate needs or wants in an ordered way and can be instigated by the individual or carer. This sequence can also be displayed in other formats such as Social Stories and Talking Mats (see Chapters 15 and 5 respectively). Further support can be given through factors to consider when supporting dressing (Box 12.5).

EATING AND DRINKING

Developing skills in eating and drinking are essential for developing good eating habits that promote health and social wellbeing. This includes the functional development of biting, chewing, swallowing and even preparation for learning to speak, facial formation and social interaction. For people with intellectual disabilities, who have difficulties, sensitivities or intolerances, mealtimes must create a pleasant experience that minimises anxieties or upsets. During drinking and mealtimes, carers can observe any difficulties that cause concern e.g. difficulties chewing or swallowing and consider

> ### 👤 PERSONAL ILLUSTRATION
> #### 12.2   Dressing
>
> Glynis is a 35-year-old female with moderate intellectual disabilities, spastic hemiplegia of her right side, limited communication, slight visual impairment and mental health issues. Glynis loves to choose her clothes and shoes. She goes shopping 6-monthly for her clothing. This routine is important to Glynis and highlights the link between ADLs and IADLs in developing skills to engage in activities which promote quality of life. She loves cotton and stretchy materials without any fastenings as she finds them difficult and this makes her extremely frustrated. She buys elastic waist trousers, and her preferred underwear are sport bras and brief style underpants. She loves orthopaedic sturdy shoes with hook and loop touch fastening. Glynis has a favourite shop where she buys most of her garments. The shop assistants know her well and support her with shopping and payment. Glynis has limited understanding of the value of the money and can get upset if the received change appears less in volume. The assistants learnt to break the change into smaller notes/coins when giving her change back. Glynis uses pictorial prompts to aid her with her dressing sequence. These include photos of her and her clothing and are hanging on the wall by her bed. They do not look like a plan, rather social photos, but Glynis likes to follow the sequence and will talk through her routine, particularly those steps that require more concentration such as her shoes. She requires one carer to assist her. Glynis may need assistance with choosing clothes to wear on the day especially if she is going out, attending a party or has a visitor.

how these must be investigated and addressed. One useful assessment is the Malnutrition Universal Screening Tool (MUST) (British Association for Parenteral and Enteral Nutrition (BAPEN), 2011). Other health issues and behaviours that may be observed in relation to eating and drinking include back arching or squirming, poor coordination, oral issues, postural and skeletal issues, congestions or 'wet voice' or vocal quality (these can be especially observed after meals) or reflux (Government of South Australia, 2020; Riquelme et al, 2016). Dysphagia, a specific disorder of swallowing that

BOX 12.5 Factors to consider when supporting dressing

- Type and styles of clothing including colours, materials, shapes and fastening options. This includes shoe size and appropriate styles.
- Adaptive aids for each step if necessary.
- Person's position. This may include sitting on the floor, against a wall (if balance is poor), on the chair or bed with feet being supported. If the person has severe physical disabilities the comfortable position may be either on their side or on their back facing up; a pillow can be used to alter the position and to add extra support.
- Position of the carer. Either in front, by the side or behind the person. It is also important to add the number of carers if strenuous physical support is involved.
- The chosen sequence and techniques that must be followed consistently and precisely. This includes visual support and prompts. If for example a person has a weaker arm, dressing this arm should be first in the sequence.
- Communication. Describing the actions, body and clothing parts as well as the sequence.
- Consent.

PERSONAL ILLUSTRATION 12.3 Eating and drinking

Charles is a 58-year-old male with a mild intellectual disability, autism, communication difficulties, coordination issues and sensory sensitivities. Mealtimes can be challenging for him. He has a sequence board with pictures including how to set up and clean the table, how to sit up (trunk control and facing the food) and how to eat and drink. Charles' support staff use his board as a prompt, keeping a record of what prompts are needed so his care plan can be updated as he develops skills. He sits by the window, has a melamine plate with a plate guard, a melamine cup with 2 handles and a scoop spoon with an adjusted handle. This routine is important to Charles and therefore a key part of his plan that all carers need to be aware of. If Charles has a meal outside of his home, following these principles can greatly reduce his anxiety. He prefers softer texture of food and needs to be reminded to slow down and to chew his food. At home he prefers to sit with 3 other residents he knows well who make minimal noise and little conversation. His sequence board contains visual cues for Charles and guidance for carers on communication and coping strategies should he become upset.

occurs more commonly in people with more profound intellectual disabilities was discussed in Chapter 11.

People with intellectual disabilities may be obese or malnourished (McGuire et al, 2007) which can further impact on their eating and drinking habits and overall health. Nutrition support such as healthy eating plans (NHS, 2017) are effective interventions (Guerra et al, 2019). A person with an intellectual disability may not feel thirsty or may not know how to communicate thirst so dehydration and a lack of fluid intake must be considered as part of the assessment and intervention. A lack of fluid may cause health issues including urinary tract infection and constipation. It is important to keep in mind, however, the difference between providing assistance and hindering the individual's progression towards independence.

The eating and drinking activity itself is crucial in promoting a positive social experience (Sari and Bahceci, 2012). As previously mentioned, mealtimes can be an anxiety and distress provoking activity if the whole process, or parts of it, are unenjoyable and unpleasant (see Personal illustration 12.3, Charles). Schedules, rotation, preparation, and visual cues used as prompts can be adopted to support the overall experience. This

includes preparation, eating and drinking activity itself and cleaning up (Choi and Panko, 2016; Liu et al, 2015). Factors to support eating and drinking are highlighted in Box 12.6. Involving the individual is key, regardless of the support they need. People with profound and multiple disabilities can commonly experience physiological difficulties such as the aforementioned dysphagia however choice and decision making should be recognised in approaches to eating and drinking alongside nutritional need and safety (Fairclough et al, 2011). Best (2019) provides an overview of commonly used enteral feeding tubes (also referred to in Chapter 11) which usually place food directly into the stomach or small intestine. Enteral feeding is a last resort and handfeeding techniques should be utilised as an approach or a prompt before this occurs (Batchelor-Murphy et al, 2017). This could involve supporting someone to eat directly (the carer holds the utensil), under the hand (the carer holds the utensil but places this hand under the person's hand

BOX 12.6 Factors to support eating and drinking

- Involvement in the shopping, meal planning, cooking and setting up the table and environment (learning and understanding new words/pictures/signs and instructions, sequencing, naming the food and utensils, colour, locations, interactions, communication and smells).
- Teaching to sit at the table, to point, to pick up the plate, to clean up, turn taking and listening, eating with others or in noisy and different environments.
- Identifying the appropriate assistive devices such as slip mats, cutlery and crockery, trays, clothes protectors, straws and holders.
- Adjusting the environment may include different styles of chairs and tables, specialised cushions, desensitising programmes and level of the person's sensory tolerance.
- Playing games related to eating and drinking.
- Oral-motor exercises.
- Chosen teaching technique to promote independence.
- Consistency and preference of the food.
- Observation; changes in behaviours and attitudes such as playing with the food, taking food from others, showing frustration, withdrawn, eating more or less than usual and no eating.
- Time is important, no rushing the person through the courses can ensure proper chewing and concentration and can prevent choking.
- When supporting a person to eat; sit at eye level, in front of the person, communicate the steps, give the person time to chew and swallow, do not rush and relax, small portions (we must be mindful of the jaw and mouth control, teeth and movements of the tongue), use the right utensils and technique.
- Inclusion in routine of cleaning up and tidying by either physically guiding them, modelling, sequencing, planning, let them tell you what to do or explain what you are doing whilst you are doing it and let them observe and use it as an interactive activity.

so they still feel involved in the process) or over hand (the person holds the utensil but the carer guides their hand). The person-centred care plan should include a detailed guideline on how to support the person to eat, as well as maintaining equipment.

PROMOTING CONTINENCE

It is understood that good and regular bladder and bowel functions are an important factor at any stage of life as they contribute to our overall wellbeing.

Difficulties with continence can have multiple causes. Some individuals may be unable to master the functions and learn to use the toilet independently due to the nature of disabilities, failure to recognise signals, associated health, behavioural and emotional issues. However, if the person is unable to achieve an independent toileting regime, it is still important to continue with going to the toilet and continence management as this promotes long term learning and independence. Equipment and assistive devices that promote dignity, independence and support include grab rails and transfer equipment. Assessments and plans should include health promotion, education strategies, and step by step interventions reflecting human rights, privacy, essential needs, wishes and realistic aspirations and goals. Involving a continence advisor and other professionals from a multidisciplinary team, where available, may further enhance the journey in successful toileting and continence management.

It is recognised that people with intellectual disabilities have a higher prevalence of incontinence than the general population (Calveley, 2019; NHS England, 2018). In addition, they may have difficulties communicating their needs effectively and early signs of difficulties with bowel or bladder control and discomfort may be missed. Assumptions may exist that incontinence may be part of the diagnosis of the person with an intellectual disability (Rogers and Patricolo, 2014), therefore it may appear easier and less stressful to use continence products. Even if the person uses products, changing them in the bathroom helps them to associate changing with the toilet. It is important to persist and be consistent across all environments (for example home, school, after care, relatives' houses) for toilet training to be successful. The increase in levels of self-esteem and the sense of accomplishment once this aspect of self-care is reached or maintained is rewarding for both individual and supporter. Before toilet training is introduced, there are factors to be considered to ensure that the person is ready (see Box 12.7)

Toilet training should be focused on developing a healthy routine that is centered on positive, individualised and consistent approaches (see Personal illustration 12.4, Derek). These could include

- Multidisciplinary approach i.e. a coordinated approach from a range of different professionals and services.

BOX 12.7 Key features of promoting continence

- Bladder and bowel control (usually better during the day than night. It may take up to several years before nighttime dryness is achieved).
- Readiness (physical, emotional and social); it must be a positive experience.
- Communication (able to indicate "the need to go" verbally or otherwise).
- Ability to cope with setbacks and regressions which are a normal part of toilet training.
- Accessibility of toilet and equipment.

- Environment and toilet modification – e.g. equipment that supports independence, safety, correct posture and stability (for example insert seats, step stools or toilet surround frame).
- Sensory issues – avoid smells, touch, sounds, light or any movement or body awareness that is upsetting for the person (for example deodorants, air fresheners, flushing the toilet, fans, bright lights, texture of toilet paper).
- Clear communication and cues – e.g. use or adapt teaching strategies that are familiar to the person to help them to understand what is expected of them – video, modeling, signs, pictures, gestural prompts, visual cues such as a toilet bag, visual boards and task management (indicating the breaking down of the tasks into small sequences for example pull pants down, sit and do 'wees' and 'poos', get some toilet paper and wipe your bottom etc.), a toy to learn and practice the sequence (a teddy bear or a doll) or short and clear language; statements are better than questions (for example "toilet time" rather than "do you need to go to the toilet?")
- Develop a daily toilet routine that is predictable and consistent e.g. toilet record charts and stool consistency (using Bristol Stool Chart; Lewis and Heaton, 1997); use of signs or pictures to support any verbal prompt where required; watch for any cues (verbal or behavioural) indicating the need for the toilet for example shifting, facial expression, crossing legs, or using words or sounds for the needs of going to the toilet.
- Management of accidents (wetting and soiling) e.g. always take the person to the toilet and support them to sit on the toilet; staying positive, encouraging and calm is an important factor.

 PERSONAL ILLUSTRATION 12.4 Developing continence

Derek was a 7-year-old boy diagnosed with Autistic Spectrum Condition, Attention Deficit Hyperactivity Disorder (ADHD) and Sensory Processing Disorder. Derek still wore nappies and his mother reported that they tried on numerous occasions to toilet train him but all the attempts were unsuccessful. He did not express the need to go to the toilet and was biting his arms when he was "forced to use the toilet". Initial assessment and observations indicated that Derek was constipated most of the time and did not like the environment or the toilet seat as it was cold. A combination of poor nutrition and fluids as well as side effects of medication were further identified as additional causes. Derek's mother indicated that she could not cope with the stress of toilet training therefore his father and one of the siblings stepped in. Nutrition was adjusted and a chart was introduced, both family members were trained in monitoring the stool using the Bristol Stool Chart and the family doctor prescribed a stool softener. The toilet environment was adjusted by eliminating all the noises and smells at home and Derek seemed comfortable with 100% cotton boxer shorts (a few styles of underpants were initially introduced). The toilet seat was covered with a cloth and a small bright step for under Derek's feet for better positioning was introduced. His father identified signs and times when Derek needed the toilet and a schedule with pictures was introduced. He recorded every step that was positive and made a video for Derek. Derek seemed to like the video and watched it all the time. The combination of the learning tool showing calm Derek and achievements in every step, adjustments to the environment, nutrition and the introduction of the stool softener, as well as giving Derek a choice of underpants achieved successful toilet training at home. Different environments were gradually introduced using the same techniques and steps.

- Positive reinforcement – Star charts or any other reward system may help to support the person.
- Food and fluid intake – it is vital that the individual has good nutritional meals and snacks full of fibre and fluids in order to maintain a healthy bladder and bowel function. Including the person in meal, snack

and drinks preparation may help to establish healthy eating habits even for those with sensory issues.

Pads, pants, nappies in young children, catheters or stoma bags are used to aid continence management and to stay dry and comfortable as well as promote elimination of urine and stools in a dignified and respectful manner. People with profound and multiple intellectual disabilities who have weaker bladder and bowel function are amongst those that use continence aids. It is very important for health and social wellbeing to take good care of skin and maintain good intimate hygiene and toileting routines (changing pads or emptying the catheter bag regularly). This can prevent skin breakdown and the development of pressure ulcers.

Good menstrual care and intimate and personal hygiene for girls and women with intellectual disabilities must also be maintained. Teaching strategies to change feminine products are similar to toilet training and must be person centred and individualised.

MOBILITY

It is thought that by 2050 there will be an increase in mobility issues for people in the over-60 age group (Manini, 2013). There will be many factors contributing to this, including illnesses and diseases, sensory and physiological impairments, poorer quality of life and lifestyle, barriers in the built environment and social exclusion (Iezzoni, 2003). People with intellectual disabilities may experience issues with mobility because of their disability or associated conditions e.g. cerebral palsy. Other causes of mobility issues include injuries from falls, long-term side effects of medication, decreased levels of physical activity, obesity, poor posture control, and other factors (Bell, 2019). The ability to move around freely and feel the freedom of movement, is important for people's emotional and physical well-being, and socio-economic status. Barrier-free living is only achieved through universal access in the built environment, using universal design principles. This, in turn, provides autonomy, dignity, inclusion, realising potential and control over one's life.

Person-centered management plans need to address risk assessment and the use of appropriate assistive aids and equipment (see Personal illustration 12.5, Joseph). These may include

- Correct seating, seating and mobility systems, and postural management: correct body posture where

PERSONAL ILLUSTRATION
12.5 Mobility

Joseph is a 30-year-old man who has profound and multiple intellectual disabilities, experiences incontinence, and requires a specialised and adjustable wheelchair. He weighs 30kg, has allergies and very delicate skin. Joseph has been unable to go out as no transport was available to meet his moving and handling needs; he loves outings and socialising. An adapted car in which Joseph could be transported in his wheelchair would have been ideal but was not financially feasible. Unfortunately, taxis or public transport are scarce. Whenever he needed to go out the home was using a standard car into which he was physically transferred from his wheelchair into the car and vice versa. It was identified that equipment was needed to transfer Joseph in and out of the motor vehicle on his trips to the local shopping mall or other facilities. The home purchased a portable hoist and a parachute-style sling with head support. The OT trained all the staff including Joseph in safe practices in manually handling during transfers. This not only improved the carers' physical health and well-being but also decreased Joseph's anxiety while the hoist was being used. Photographs of the hoist and sling were used to reinforce learning and added to plans to provide a visual reference. Joseph rests on a large bean bag or on a couch in various positions when at home. This keeps him mobilised, physically active, and aware. His physiotherapist and personal trainer designed an exercise routine and trained the carers and Joseph. This routine was recorded as a visual care plan for Joseph, which documents the sequence of events using pictures. This acts as a prompt for Joseph and his supporters. Joseph is now also being hoisted onto a chair (for upper-body strength exercises) and his bed.

hips and all joints of the body are centered and aligned; trunk positioning; feet correctly positioned on the floor or on wheelchair footplates; and sitting position is at 90°degrees (unless otherwise specified). Some people with intellectual disabilities, especially those with profound and multiple disabilities, rely on their carers for daily repositioning, mobilisation, and minimising discomfort, to prevent further deformities, physical ill-health, breathing difficulties, and pressure ulcers.

- Good postural management in general to prevent any physical ill-health issues or complications. This should be supported by an appropriate professional such as a physiotherapist.
- Improving or maintaining everyday functional skills including drinking, eating and continence.
- Foot health, including podiatry services and purchasing good quality and supportive footwear.
- Access to medical check-ups, medication reviews, physical and mental health services, addressing visual and auditory issues, all of which play a major role in increasing mobility and confidence.
- Promoting physical fitness in collaboration with professional partners.
- Good quality beds and mattresses to ensure quality sleep, which is important in maintaining cognitive, mental, emotional, and physical well-being.
- Assistive devices including splints, braces, wheelchairs, hoists with slings, standing frames, boards, cushions, handrails and walkers. An Occupational Therapist or a designated professional will be able to advise and train.

It is crucial that care givers are trained in manual handling and transferring to promote good practice. During manual handling, it is important that the carer has a good rapport with the person, is empathetic, and encourages empowerment and autonomy of the person, supporting them to maximise their potential and independence.

CONCLUSION

The fundamental rights of an individual who has an intellectual disability must be paramount in promoting their quality of life and respecting their wishes to live the life they choose, regardless of level of need. Recognition of ADLs and IADLs provide a framework from which to explore choices and opportunities; and identify specific assessment tools to support this. Through person-centred approaches the individual and carers can harness local professionals and services to utilise their expertise and experience in promoting an individualised plan to develop skills and competence. These approaches stimulate creativity and positive expectations for an individual's life journey.

REFERENCES

Arciuli, J., & Brock, J. (2014). *Communication in autism.* Amsterdam: John Benjamin Publishers.

Ardic, A., & Cavkayter, A. (2014). Effectiveness of the modified intensive toilet training method on the teaching toileting skill to children with autism. *Education and Training in Autism and Developmental Disabilities*, 49(2), 263–276.

Attum, B., Hafiz, S., Malik, A., & Shamoon, Z. (2020). *Cultural competence in the care of muslim patients and their families.* Available at: https://www.ncbi.nlm.nih.gov/books/NBK499933/. [Accessed 8 December 2020].

Australian Institute of Health and Welfare (AIHW). (2009). *Caring for oral health in australian residential Care.* Available at: https://www.nice.org.uk/Media/Default/Oral%20health%20toolkit/Oral_health_assessment_tool.pdf. [Accessed 25 November 2020].

Bandura, A. (1977). *Social learning theory.* Englewood Cliffs, NJ: Prentice Hall.

British Association for Parenteral and Enteral Nutrition. (BAPEN). (2011). *Malnutrition universal screening tool.* Available at: https://www.bapen.org.uk/pdfs/must/must_full.pdf. [Accessed 2 January 2021].

Batchelor-Murphy, M., McConnell, E., Amella, E., et al. (2017). Experimental comparison of efficacy for three hand feeding techniques in dementia. *Journal of the American Geriatric Society*, 65(4), 89–94.

Bell, T. (2019). Physical health and wellbeing: people with profound and multiple learning disabilities. In O. Barr & B. Gates (Eds.), *Oxford handbook of learning and intellectual disability nursing* (2nd ed.). Oxford: Oxford University Press.

Best, C. (2019). Selection and management of commonly used enteral feeding tubes. *Nursing Times Online*, 3(115), 43–47.

Calveley, J. (2019) Continence. In O. Barr & B. Gates (Eds.) *Oxford handbook of learning and intellectual disability nursing* (2nd ed., pp. 216–217). Oxford: Oxford University Press.

Carmeli, E., Bar-Yossef, T., Ariav, C., et al. (2008). Perceptual-motor coordination in persons with mild intellectual disabilities. *Journal of Disability and Rehabilitation*, 30(5), 323–329.

Chalmers, J., Johnson, V., Tang, J. H., et al. (2004). Evidence-based protocol: oral hygiene care for functionally dependent and cognitively impaired older adults. *Journal of Gerontological Nursing*, 30(11), 5–12.

Choi, S. S., & Panko, L. (2016). *Practice and patience: strategies to address feeding problems in early childhood.* Pittsburgh, PA: Children's Hospital.

Department of Health. (2001). *Valuing people – a new strategy for learning disability for the 21st century.* London: HMSO.

Department of Health. (2002). *people - a new strategy for learning disability for the 21st century: planning with people towards person centred approaches: guidance for implementation groups.* London: HMSO.

Department of Health (DH). (2009). *Religion or belief: a practical guide for the NHS.* London: DH.

De-Rosende-Celeiro, I., Torres, G., SeoaneBouzas, M., et al. (2019). Exploring the use of assistive products to promote functional independence in self-care activities in the bathroom. *PLoS ONE, 14*(4). Available at: https://doi.org/10.1371/journal.pone.0215002. [Accessed 27 November 2019].

Edemekong, P., Bomgaars, D., & Levy, S. (2020). *Activities of daily living.* Available at: https://www.ncbi.nlm.nih.gov/books/NBK470404/. [Accessed 7 December 2020].

Fairclough, J., Burton, S., Craven, J., et al. (2011). *Home enteral tube feeding for adults with a learning disability.* Available at: https://www.choiceforum.org/docs/enteral.pdf. [Accessed 14 December 2020].

Felce, D., Jenkins, J., Dell, D., et al. (1983). *The Bereweeke Skill-Teaching System: system administrator's handbook.* Windsor: NFER-Nelson.

Freeman Watson, A., Blanco, J., Hunt-Hurst, P., et al. (2010). Caregiver's perception of clothing for people with severe and profound intellectual disabilities. *Perceptual and Motor Skills, 110*(3 Pt 1), 961–964. Available at: https://www.researchgate.net/publication/45492820_Caregivers'_perceptions_of_clothing_for_people_with_severe_and_profound_intellectual_disabilities. [Accessed 3 December 2019].

Gill, T. M., Allore, H. G., & Han, L. (2006). Bathing disability and the risk of long-term admission to a nursing home. *Journal of Gerontology: Medical Sciences, 61A*(8), 821–825.

Government of South Australia: Department of Education. (2020). *Oral eating and drinking procedure.* Available at: https://www.education.sa.gov.au/sites/default/files/oral-eating-drinking-procedure.pdf?v=1589176578. [Accessed 10 September 2020].

Gray, C. (2018). The social story philosophy. *Social Stories, 10.2.* Available at: https://carolgraysocialstories.com/wp-content/uploads/2018/12/Social-Stories-10.2-Criteria.pdf. [Accessed 3 January 2021].

Guerra, N., Neumeier, W. H., Breslin, L., et al. (2019). Feedback and strategies from people with intellectual disability completing a personalized online weight loss intervention: a qualitative analysis. *Intellectual and Developmental Disabilities, 57*(6), 527–544.

Holmes, N. P., & Spence, C. (2004). The body schema and the multisensory representation(s) of peripersonal space. *Cognitive Processing – International Quarterly of Cognitive Science, 5*(2), 94–105.

Howlett, N., Pine, K. L., Orakcioglu, I., et al. (2013). The influence of clothing on first impression: rapid and positive responses to minor changes in male attire. *Journal of Fashion Marketing & Management, 17*(1), 38–48.

Iezzoni, L. (2003). *When walking fails: mobility problems of adults with chronic conditions.* CA: University of California Press.

Kelly, M., & Barnes-Holmes, D. (2014). Measuring implicit and explicit acceptability of reinforcement versus punishment interventions with teachers working in ABA versus mainstream schools. *The Psychological Record, 65*, 251–265.

Klein, M. D. (1983). *Pre-dressing skills: skills starter for self-help development.* Communication Skills Builders.

Leadership Foundation for Higher Education. (2018). *John Whitmore – the grow model.* Available at: https://www.lfhe.ac.uk/download.cfm/docid/8AED4DD6-31EE-46F9-B97A6EEB1750B22E. [Accessed 7 December 2020].

Lewis, S. J., & Heaton, K. W. (1997). Stool Form Scale as a useful guide to intestinal transit time. *Scandinavian Journal of Gastroenterology, 32*, 920–924.

Liu, W., Galik, E., Nahm, E. S., et al. (2015). Optimizing eating performance for long-term care residents with dementia: testing the impact of function-focused care for cognitively impaired. *Journal of the American Medical Directors Association, 16*(12), 1062–1068.

Mahoney, F., & Barthel, D. (1965). Functional evaluation: the Barthel Index. *Maryland State Medical Journal, 14*, 56–61.

Manini, T. M. (2013). Mobility decline in old age: a time to intervene. *Exercise and Sports Science Reviews, 41*(1), 2. Available at: https://www.ncbi.nlm.nih.gov/pmc/articles/PMC3530168/#R4. [Accessed 30 November 2020].

McGuire, B. E., Daly, P., & Smyth, F. (2007). Lifestyle and health behaviours of adults with an intellectual disability. *Journal of Intellectual Disability Research, 51*(7), 497–510.

McLeod, S. (2016). *Albert Bandura social learning theory.* Available at: https://www.simplypsychology.org/bandura.html. [Accessed 2 January 2021].

Millman, C. (2020). *Why autism ABA goes against everything B.F. Skinner believed in.* Available at: https://neuroclastic.com/2020/03/04/why-autism-aba-goes-against-everything-b-f-skinner-believed-in/. [Accessed 2 January 2021].

Morris, E., Smith, N., & Altus, D. (2005) B.F. Skinner's contributions to applied behaviour analysis. *Behaviour Analysis, 28*(2), 99–131.

Morris-Jones, R. (2019). *ABC of dermatology* (7th ed.). West Sussex: Wiley.

National Portage Service. (2019). *What is portage?* Available at: https://www.portage.org.uk/about/what-portage. [Accessed 31 October 2020].

NHS. (2017). *Managing weight with a learning disability.* Available at: https://www.nhs.uk/live-well/healthy-weight/managing-weight-with-a-learning-disability/. [Accessed 12 December 2020].

NHS England. (2018). *Excellence in continence care. Practical guidance for commissioners and leaders in health and social care.* Leeds: NHS England.

O'Connor, M. (2002). *Using the Roper, Logan and Tierney model in a neonatal ICU.* Available at: https://www.nursingtimes.net/roles/childrens-nurses/using-the-roper-logan-and-tierney-model-in-a-neonatal-icu-01-05-2002/. [Accessed 8 December 2020].

Pestana, C. (2014). Exploring the self-concept of adults with mild learning disabilities. *British Journal of Learning Disabilities, 43,* 16–23.

PBS Academy. (2016). *PBS competence framework.* Available at: http://pbsacademy.org.uk/. [Accessed 1 November 2020].

Pratt, C., & Steward, L. (2018). *Applied behavior analysis: the role of task analysis and chaining.* Available at: https://www.iidc.indiana.edu/irca/articles/applied-behavior-analysis.html. [Accessed 2 January 2021].

Public Health England. (2019). *Oral care and people with learning disabilities.* Available at: https://www.gov.uk/government/publications/oral-care-and-people-with-learning-disabilities. [Accessed 16 April 2020].

Riquelme, L. F., Benjamin, R. D., Tahhan, H. J., et al. (2016). Feeding/swallowing disorders: maintaining quality of life in persons with intellectual disability. *Journal of Intellectual Disability Diagnosis and Treatment, 4(2),* 81–93.

Rogers, J., & Patricolo, M. (2014). Addressing continence in children with disabilities. *Nursing Times, 110(43),* 22–24.

Roper, N., Logan, W., & Tierney, A. (1996). *The elements of nursing* (3rd ed.). Edinburgh: Churchill Livingstone.

Rowley, E. (2019). The Conductive Group. A social basis for learning in the modern world. *Conductive College Journal, 1(2).*

Sanderson, H., Goodwin, J., & Kinsella, E. (2015). *Personalising education: a guide to using person centred practices in schools.* Available at: http://helensandersonassociates.co.uk/papers/using-person-centred-practices-schools/. [Accessed 2 January 2021].

Sari, H., & Bahceci, B. (2012). Nutritional status of children with an intellectual disability. *International Journal on Disability and Human Development, 11(1),* 17–21.

Shrestha, P. (2017). *What is shaping a behaviour?* Available at: https://www.psychestudy.com/behavioral/learning-memory/operant-conditioning/what-is-shaping-behavior. [Accessed 7 December 2020].

Smull, M. (1996). *Overview of essential life planning.* Available at: http://www.allenshea.com/brochure.pdf. [Accessed 2 January 2021].

Smull, M., & Sanderson, H. (2005). *Essential lifestyle planning for everyone.* Available at: http://allenshea.com/wp-content/uploads/2017/02/Essential-Lifestyle-Planning-for-Everyone.pdf. [Accessed 2 January 2021].

Social Care Institute for Excellence (SCIE). (2005). *Adult placements and person-centred approaches –erson-centred planning.* Available at: [Accessed 3 August 2021].

Swapna, K. S., & Sudhir, M. A. (2016). Behaviour modification for intellectually disabled students. *Journal of Humanities and Social Science, 21(2),* 35–38.

Waldman, B., & Perlman, S. (2012). Ensuring oral health for older individuals with intellectual and developmental disabilities. *Journal of Clinical Nursing, 21(7–8),* 909–913.

Wallace, M., & Shelkey, M. (2007). *Katz Index of Independence in Activities of Daily Living.* Available at: https://www.alz.org/careplanning/downloads/katz-adl.pdf. [Accessed 8 December 2020].

Wehman, P., & Targett, P. S. (2004). Principles of curriculum design: road to transition from school to adulthood. In P. Wehman & J. Kregel (Eds.), *Functional curriculum for elementary, middle, and secondary age students with special needs* (2nd ed., pp. 1–36). Austin, TX: Pro-Ed.

Wenar, C., & Kerig, P. (2006). *Developmental psychopathology: from infancy through adolescence.* London: McGraw-Hill.

Werner, D. (2018). Dressing. In D. Werner (Ed.), *Disabled village children: a guide for community health workers, rehabilitation workers, and families.* Berkeley, CA: The Hesperian Foundation. Available at: https://www.dinf.ne.jp/doc/english/global/david/dwe002/dwe00239.html. [Accessed 3 December 2019].

Weis, R. (2014). *Introduction to abnormal child and adolescent psychology.* SAGE.

World Health Organisation (WHO). (2015). *WHO global strategy on person-centred and integrated health services.* Geneva: WHO.

World Health Organisation. (2019). Water, sanitation and hygiene. in health care facilities: from resolution to revolution. Available at: https://www.youtube.com/watch?v=Su53NTLFkdA&feature=youtu.be. [Accessed 27 November 2019].

Wilson, N. J., Lin, Z., Villarosa, A., et al. (2019). Countering the poor oral health of people with intellectual and developmental disability: a scoping literature review.

BMC Public Health, 19, 1530. Available at: https://bmcpublichealth.biomedcentral.com/track/pdf/10.1186/s12889-019-7863-1. [Accessed 4 December 2019].

Wolfensberger, W. (1972). *The principle of normalisation in human services*. Toronto: National Institute on Mental Retardation.

13

Expanding sensory awareness

Linda Diane Parham and Debbie Crickmore

KEY ISSUES

- Five basic sensory systems - visual, auditory, olfactory, gustatory and tactile – are well known.
- A further three sensory systems – vestibular, proprioception and interoception – are attracting interest.
- Where sensory integration has developed, sensory data is received and processed without apparent effort.

- Differences may be experienced by children and adults with intellectual disabilities in single or multiple systems with physical, psychological and/or social effects on daily life.
- Expanded sensory awareness can improve how people with intellectual disabilities are supported to enjoy a healthy, sensory-friendly lifestyle.

CHAPTER OUTLINE

INTRODUCTION

Sensory awareness was introduced in the previous (6th) edition of this book, focusing on the five basic sensory systems of visual, auditory, olfactory, gustatory and tactile. You may recognise these better as sight, hearing, smell, taste and touch. This revised and developed chapter will extend readers' knowledge and understanding of a further three sensory systems; vestibular, proprioception, and the most recently discussed set of sensations, interoception (STAR Institute for Sensory Processing Disorder, 2020). Whilst it may be artificial to discuss a sense in isolation, we sometimes adopt this approach within the chapter for clarity, for example, by use of section headings and in summary Table 13.1 (for the five basic sensory systems) and Table 13.7 (for the further three sensory systems). The eight senses are clearly

represented in these summary tables by Widgit Symbols (2002–2022), reproduced with kind permission. Two senses from the basic group (hearing and touch) and one from the further group (interoception) are explored in exemplar tables within the chapter (Tables 13.3, 13.6 and 13.10 respectively) with tables for all other senses appearing in the accompanying online resource.

Each of us has a unique sensory profile, our experiences are individual and subjective, we have preferences and our abilities vary. Where sensory integration has developed, we receive and process sensory data without apparent effort not only from the (five basic and three further) individual senses, but also in complex combinations. As will be elaborated upon in this chapter, issues with sight and hearing are recognised as being more commonly experienced by people with intellectual disabilities than people without. Whilst issues with smell, taste and touch, vestibular, proprioceptive and interoceptive senses may be experienced by people with intellectual disabilities, they may be more difficult to identify, define and enumerate. We suggest the physical, psychological and social health of individuals with intellectual disabilities can be adversely impacted by sensory sensitivities and differences. They may be considered anecdotal and not be responded to constructively or consistently. Particularly where people have difficulty articulating their experiences, supporters should hone their skills of observation to contribute toward construction of individual sensory profiles, enabling interpretation of observable behaviours in environmental contexts and subsequent testing of helpful responses; this not only minimises negative effects but also serves to capitalise on preferences and abilities.

Focusing on a developing area of interest in relation to people with intellectual disabilities, this chapter is intended to extend sensory awareness by providing 'entry level' knowledge and suggesting supportive rather than prescriptive responses. This recognises the diversity of sensory experience, including personal profiles that mix hypo- and hyper-sensitivity to different senses.

To illustrate a relationship between sensory awareness and intellectual disability, we begin by briefly considering two conditions, CHARGE syndrome and congenital rubella syndrome, which both affect multiple sensory channels and can co-exist with intellectual disabilities.

CHARGE syndrome is determined genetically, though of course each person living with it will experience it uniquely. Box 13.1 (from the Charge Syndrome Foundation, 2021) identifies CHARGE features relevant to this discussion.

Sense International (2021), a global charity supporting and campaigning for children and adults affected by *deafblindness*, describes it as 'a combination of vision and hearing impairment' (not necessarily meaning total deafness or blindness), as in the case of CHARGE above.

It may also be referred to as *dual sensory loss* (Deafblind UK, 2021).

When someone is born with combined sight and hearing difficulties, this is called *congenital* deafblindness. Maternal infection with German measles during pregnancy, though much less common in countries where a vaccination against the virus is available, can lead to babies born with congenital rubella syndrome who may have deafness (see Table 13.3 later in the chapter), cataracts and other eye conditions (see Table 13.2 in the accompanying online resource) (Sense 2019). Maternal infection with cytomegalovirus during pregnancy is also linked to babies born with dual sensory loss and intellectual disabilities (CMV Action 2021).

Hearing and sight problems developed in child or adulthood are called *acquired* deafblindness. This may be due to an accident, illness or as a result of ageing in later life.

FIVE BASIC SENSORY SYSTEMS

The first part of the chapter will focus on the five basic sensory systems; sight, hearing, smell, taste and touch, as represented in Table 13.1.

Sight

Visual processing, from photoreceptors in the retina of the eye, through the optic nerve, to the visual centre of the brain, is briefly depicted in Table 13.1. Some people with intellectual disabilities, whose eyes appear normal, experience difficulties attributed to *cerebral* or *cortical blindness* or *cortical visual impairment* (damage to the visual area in the occipital lobes at the rear of the brain). Eyes are designed to function as a pair, enabling binocular (literally meaning two-eye) vision. For example, whilst it is possible to *see* with only one eye (monocular vision), three-dimensional vision is impaired, especially in relation to judgement of distances. The external parts of the eye (right of Figure 13.1) are the

- pupil – the 'black dot' in the centre of the eye that allows light to pass into the eye, normally becoming smaller in bright light (constricting) and bigger (dilating) in dim light
- iris – the ring surrounding the pupil that provides the colour of our eyes (the white of the eye is the sclera), consisting of tiny muscles that adjust the size of the pupil, as described above

> **BOX 13.1   Features of CHARGE syndrome relevant in a multi-sensory context**
>
> - vision loss
> - decreased or absent sense of smell
> - low muscle tone
> - hearing loss
> - facial palsy leading to difficulties eating
> - absent or reduced balance

TABLE 13.1   How the five basic sensory systems work (Senses represented by Widgit Symbols © Widgit Software 2002–2022 www.widgit.com)

Sense	Stimulus	Pathway; sense organ to brain	Areas of brain receiving & integrating nerve impulses into sensation
visual	Light rays bounce off objects, enter eyes	- **photoreceptors** (rods and cones) in retina convert light rays into impulses that travel via **optic nerve** (see Figure 13.1) to **occipital lobe** for interpretation of image	i.
hearing	Sound waves collected by outer ears	- outer ear passes sound waves inward; middle ear carries to oval window - inner ear (see Figure 13.2); fluid in **cochlea** carries waves of pressure - **mechanoreceptors** (hair cells) transmit nerve impulses that travel via **auditory nerve** to **temporal lobe** [i.] for interpretation of what the sound is or what it means - final sound processing performed by **parietal** [ii.] and **frontal lobes** [iii.]	ii. iii.
smell	Chemical particles released by odorous material, float through air, enter the nose	- **chemoreceptors** (olfactory nerve cells) in nose stimulated - carry impulses to **olfactory bulbs** below **frontal lobes** [iv.] to **olfactory cortex**, located on underside of **temporal lobe** [v.] (see Figure 13.3) - **temporal lobe** interprets smell information - recognition of smell usually involves parts of frontal lobe	iv. v.
taste	Chemicals from food, drinks or other materials dissolve in saliva on tongue	- molecules from food enter taste buds (tiny bumps on tongue), where **chemoreceptors** detect molecules (see Figure 13.3) - impulses traverse **cranial nerves** to **brainstem** - gustatory pathway carries information to gustatory area in **parietal lobe** where conscious perception of taste arises	
touch	Skin touched, cooled, heated, or injured	- **mechanoreceptors** activated (see Figure 13.4), touch pressure messages move up spinal cord to thalamus & **parietal lobe** of brain - **thermoreceptors** detect temperature; **nociceptors** detect pain, sensations travel up spinal cord using different route than touch pressure - messages relayed to several areas in primitive parts of brain, brainstem, parietal lobe	

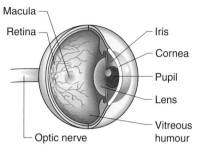

Figure 13.1 Cross section of the human eye

- cornea – the transparent membrane that covers the iris and pupil and merges into the sclera, through which light passes to enter the pupil and reach the retina at the back of the eye (left of Figure 13.1).

The externally visible accessory structures of eyebrows, eyelashes and eyelids have important protective functions, with each eye sitting in a bony socket (known as the orbit) occupied by fatty tissue designed to reduce the risk of injury. Blinking cleans and lubricates the eye using fluid secreted by glands including the tear (lacrimal) glands.

Directly behind the pupil of the eye is the lens (left of Figure 13.1). Tiny muscles inside the eye adjust the shape of the lens to bend (refract) light that bounces off objects and enters the eye. Light then passes through the vitreous body of the eye (the jelly-like filling within the eyeball) to the retina at the back of the eye where two types of specialised cells (rods and cones) begin the process of converting light rays into nerve impulses that travel via the optic nerve to the brain. The brain then interprets the visual image to make sense of it.

The macula is a spot on the retina that is located at the back of the eye. When we directly focus on looking at something, we adjust the position of the eye so that incoming light strikes the macula. The central point of the macula contains only cones, which provide us with highly detailed colour vision. Rods, which provide black-and-white vision, are dominant in the rest of the retina. Rods allow sight of shades of grey in dim light, for example moonlight, whereas cones are sensitive to blue, green and red light, combining to produce different colours. An absence or deficiency in one of the three types of cones leads to inability to distinguish some colours from others, known as colour blindness (Tortora and Derrickson, 2010).

A further mechanical process involving the function of the eye relates to the action of six muscles that co-ordinate the eyeball in vertical, horizontal and rotational movements. This is essential to enjoy the benefits of binocular vision described earlier, and to adjust to seeing things at different distances which allows us to have depth perception (use of vision to know how far away objects are). Imbalance in the eye muscles may manifest as strabismus (squint) that can be bilateral (affecting both eyes), unilateral (affecting one), divergent (eyes pointing away from each other) or convergent ('crossed eyes'). Around 20% of children with Down syndrome have a squint (Woodhouse and Charlton, 2018).

Impact of sight on personal experiences and behaviour

Vision helps us develop and maintain our independence; communicate with others; embark on and nurture relationships; move safely around and make sense of our world. Difficulties are likely to encroach on areas of life including leisure, skills, education and work. UK charity SeeAbility (2020) conveys in an Easy read factsheet that

- adults with intellectual disabilities are 10 times more likely to have serious sight problems than other adults
- children with intellectual disabilities are 28 times more likely (as sight problems are comparatively rare in the general population of children)
- people with intellectual disabilities who have very high support needs are most likely to have sight problems
- 6 in 10 people with intellectual disabilities need glasses.

Range of conditions affecting sight

General risk factors for eye disease include advancing age (over 60) and being a member of a family with a history of eye disease; eye health may be neglected because eyes do not usually hurt when something is wrong (Vision Matters, 2010). A range of visual issues that can occur is shown in Table 13.2 in the accompanying online resource, from more temporary and treatable conditions to permanent, with suggested interventions.

Identifying sight issues

Where universal child health surveillance programmes exist, for example in England (National Health Service (NHS), 2019), a physical examination is conducted within the first 72 hours of life and continues at intervals in childhood. This should establish whether there are congenital, peri-natal (for example, retinopathy of prematurity, see Hartnett and Penn, 2012) or early childhood issues affecting sight and enable referral to appropriate services for treatment or vision aids.

Indicators of developing problems, such as sore, blood-shot or cloudy eyes and changes in behaviour or response to activities, can be readily observed by family members and caregivers. These concerns should be explored by seeking advice at a primary level from a pharmacist, family doctor or eye specialist such as an optometrist. Using an ophthalmoscope to shine a small beam of light into the eye, it is possible for a professional to examine different parts of the eye, including the retina and the surfaces of the cornea and lens (see Figure 13.1). This might lead to recognition of a correctable sight impairment, for example, near-sightedness remedied by lenses prescribed by the optometrist and made by the optician. Some individuals have very mild strabismus that may not be obvious to others but affects vision. To improve vision through remediating eye muscle difficulties, specialists called orthoptists may provide a programme of eye muscle exercises. There may also be a need for further inquiry by referral to an ophthalmologist (a physician who specialises in eye conditions).

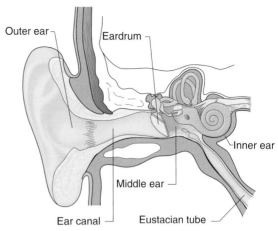

Figure 13.2 Structure of the ear

- the inner ear – contains receptors for hearing and balance.

The part of the ear that is external to the head is known as the auricle or pinna. Its shape (like the flared end of a trumpet) is designed to collect sound waves and pass them into the ear canal, a curved tube extending from the side of the head toward the eardrum. The ear canal contains hairs and ceruminous glands that secrete wax (cerumen) to help prevent dust and dirt from entering the ear. The eardrum (tympanic membrane) is a thin, semi-transparent partition between the outer and middle ear that vibrates when sound waves enter the ear.

The middle ear is a small, air-filled cavity between the eardrum and inner ear. An opening leads directly to the eustachian tube (see Figure 13.2) connecting with the upper part of the throat. Its function is to allow air into the middle ear to keep pressure even on both sides of the eardrum, so the risk of rupture is reduced. Infection or trauma, for example, caused by self- or non-accidental injury, can also cause tearing of the eardrum known as perforation. Three tiny bones are attached to, and extend across, the middle ear, taking their names from their shapes – hammer (malleus), anvil (incus) and stirrup (stapes). Together they are known as ossicles. Tiny muscles control the amount of movement of these bones to prevent damage from excessively loud noises. The stirrup bone fits into a small opening between the middle and inner ear known as the oval window. This apparatus can be seen in Figure 13.2. The condition otosclerosis can cause severe conductive hearing loss as excess bone growth prevents the ossicles in the middle ear from moving freely.

 READER ACTIVITY 13.1

Identify someone with an intellectual disability that you know well, who is happy for you to observe the way they use their sight.

Read Introduction and How to use the FVA tool in SeeAbility's (2019) Functional Vision Assessment (FVA) available online at https://www.seeability.org/fva then download and complete pages 4-14 with the individual identified.

Hearing

Auditory processing, where sound travels from the ear to the auditory centre of the brain via mechanoreceptors in the cochlea and auditory nerve, is briefly depicted in Table 13.1. Hearing loss can result from damage to the primary auditory area in the temporal lobes at the sides of the brain. The structure of the ear is divided into three main regions, shown at Figure 13.2.
- the outer ear – collects sound waves and passes them inward
- the middle ear – carries sound vibrations to the oval window

The inner ear contains semi-circular canals and the cochlea (appearing in Figure 13.2 resembling a snail's shell). The semi-circular canals are the sense organs for balance (also referred to as the vestibular apparatus, discussed in the second part of this chapter) and the cochlea is the sense organ for hearing. When sound waves enter the ear canal, they cause the ear drum to vibrate. In turn, this vibration is passed to the hammer, anvil and stirrup bones to the oval window. Fluid in the cochlea carries waves of pressure that are transmitted into nerve impulses by hair cells and carried to the primary auditory area in the temporal lobe of the brain via the auditory nerve. Auditory information is further distributed to the parietal and frontal lobes of the brain, which contribute to the interpretation of sounds – particularly speech sounds – so that they are meaningful in the context of the person's immediate life situation.

There are two main types of hearing loss and these are displayed in Table 13.3.

Impact of hearing on personal experiences and behaviour

For the population of people with intellectual disabilities, the Foundation for People with Learning Disabilities (FPLD) (2021) estimates around 40% experience *moderate* to *severe hearing loss*, (particularly people with Down syndrome), that occurs more frequently as people grow older. The most common cause of hearing loss in older adults is presbycusis, which is typically gradual, progressive and bilateral (Spiby, 2014) due to degeneration of inner ear structures.

Range of conditions affecting hearing

Tinnitus is a constant ringing sound in the ears, which may grow louder over time, interfering with hearing. It often results from frequent exposure to loud sounds, such as very loud music, sitting too close to speakers or exposure to very strong vibration or loud construction noises; it is also associated with normal ageing.

Hyper- or hyposensitivity to sounds (also called hyper- or hypoacusis) refers to over- or under-reactivity to sound. The person who is hyposensitive or hyporeactive does not have a hearing loss but may not notice or be alert to many sounds that most people would immediately notice. In over-reactivity or hyperacusis, ordinary sounds that do not bother most people (such as the sound of a flushing toilet) may be very irritating, painful, or frightening. The person who is hypersensitive/hyper-reactive to sound may put their hands over their ears in response to a loud sound or avoid noisy places such as busy restaurants or large gatherings. Many individuals with auditory hyper-reactivity find

TABLE 13.3 **Types and characteristics of hearing loss**			
Types of hearing loss	**Possible causes**	**Effects in daily life**	**Management suggestions**
Sensorineural; accounts for over 80% of deafness			
Damage to ear drum, (sensory) hair cells and/or Damage to auditory nerve (neural)	- genetic - age related (hair cells naturally die off, eardrum loses elasticity, tiny bones stiffen) - excessive noise (distorts and damages hair cells)	Changes ability to hear quiet sounds, reduces quality of sound, will often struggle to understand speech. Prelingual deafness impacts ability to acquire language.	Currently irreversible, use technological/augmentative support, e.g. - hearing aids - objects of reference (see Chapter 5)
Conductive			
Sounds unable to pass freely to inner ear	Blockage or abnormality in outer or middle ear, e.g. - excess ear wax - fluid from infection - ruptured eardrum	Sounds become quieter, although not usually distorted.	Can be temporary or permanent; risk increases with history of middle ear disease. Medical management, e.g. - drops - minor surgery
Mixed; sensorineural and conductive hearing losses present at same time			

it helpful to wear earphones designed to muffle environmental sounds, when going to places where sounds are bothersome. Auditory hyper-reactivity is common among individuals who have autism (see Chapter 15).

Identifying hearing issues

In addition to detecting sound, the cochlea can produce sounds (otoacoustic emissions) that can be recorded by a sensitive microphone placed next to the eardrum. This vibration of the hair cells is absent or greatly reduced in deaf babies and can be detected quickly and non-invasively by a screening test (Tortora and Derrickson 2010), such as that provided in England (NHS, 2018). A cochlear implant, often referred to as a bionic ear, is a surgically implanted electronic device that provides a sense of sound to a person who is profoundly deaf or severely hard of hearing.

Contrasting with hearing loss is hearing hypersensitivity, which may be evident in infants, children, or adults. Infants and children may cry, scream, or try to get away from sounds that are sharp, abrupt, or at a loud volume – even if others are not bothered by these sounds. Adolescents and adults with auditory hyper-sensitivity also display these behavioural reactions and may additionally verbalise that they organise their life to avoid loud or noisy environments, including social situations such as parties or activity groups. For others, attempting physical escape may be the immediate response. This can be perceived as a challenge to services and limit people's access to their local communities (see Chapter 17). Use Reader activity 13.2 to help you reflect on the experiences of people you support.

Auditory hyper- or hypo-reactivity is identified through observable behaviours in everyday life, which may be formally assessed using sensory questionnaires, such as the Sensory Profile-2 (Dunn, 2014) for infants and children, the Adolescent-Adult Sensory Profile (Brown and Dunn, 2002), and the Sensory Processing Measure (2nd edition) (SPM-2) (Parham et al, 2021). The Sensory Profile-2 instruments classify individuals into categories related to presence and severity of under- and over-reactivity. Users must examine item ratings to determine which sensory systems may be involved. In contrast, the SPM-2 provides norm-referenced T scores for 7 sensory systems, (not including interoception). If a score is elevated (indicating problems) for a given sensory system, such as the auditory system, users of the SPM-2 need to examine the questions that received high scores to identify whether hyper-reactivity, hypo-reactivity, perceptual problems, or a combination of these are involved. The SPM-2 questionnaires cover the lifespan from infancy, beginning at 4 months old, through to older age (90+ years old).

Smell and Taste

Olfactory processing (sense of smell), from the nose to the brain is briefly depicted in Table 13.1. Olfactory processing involves the detection of chemical molecules floating in the air. As these chemical particles given off by odorous materials are inhaled, chemoreceptors in the nose are stimulated. The chemical message is then transported via olfactory nerves from the nose to the olfactory bulbs below the frontal lobes of the brain. From here, the olfactory information is delivered to other areas of the brain; the primary olfactory area in the temporal lobe where conscious awareness of smell begins, and the limbic system and hypothalamus, where emotional and memory-evoked responses to odours are generated.

Gustatory processing (sense of taste), from the tongue to the brain is briefly depicted in Table 13.1. As food is dissolved in saliva, chemoreceptors are stimulated. Impulses from the taste buds traverse cranial nerves to the medulla oblongata in the brain. From here, the gustatory pathway carries information to other areas of the brain; the primary gustatory area in the parietal lobe where conscious perception of taste arises, and the limbic system, hypothalamus and thalamus (Tortora and Derrickson, 2010), accounting for memories, interpretations and emotional reactions to taste. This is a sense difficult to separate from others; food has temperature and texture, stimulating thermoreceptors and mechanoreceptors for tactile sensations, and chemoreceptors for aroma. Taste is especially influenced by the sense of smell. When affected by a cold, it is the blocked nose that makes food lack flavour. It is for this reason that smell and taste are considered together here, being co-presented in Figure 13.3. However, taste is considered much simpler than smell, as only five primary tastes can be distinguished; sour, sweet, bitter, salty and umami (described as 'meaty' or 'savoury'), with all other flavours being a combination of these and accompanying smells and tactile sensations.

📑 READER ACTIVITY 13.2

Watch and listen to this online video that was created to help people understand how auditory hyper-reactivity can lead to overall "sensory overload," resulting in impaired ability to function:

https://www.youtube.com/watch?v=K2P4Ed6G3gw

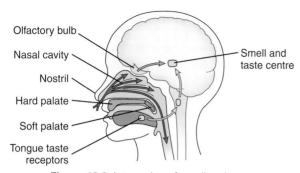

Figure 13.3 Interaction of smell and taste

Impact of smell and taste on personal experiences and behaviour

With ageing the sense of smell deteriorates, olfactory receptors reducing from around age 50. A sense of smell can enhance quality of life for an individual, particularly where fragrances are emotionally associated with events, people or memories; conversely, loss of smell can bring anxiety and lead to depression (Erskine and Philpott, 2020). The sense of smell can be positively harnessed to assist people who are visually impaired for example, by supporters who always use the same perfume to aid recognition. Fragrant objects of reference (see Chapter 5), for example soap or shampoo can be offered to indicate bath or shower time, and the opportunity can be provided to make menu choices by smelling food and drink.

Community practitioners should be aware that adaptation (decreasing sensitivity to frequently encountered odours), occurs rapidly (Tortora and Derrickson, 2010). This is apparent when the curry we cooked last night 'hits' us when we open the front door arriving home from work, yet we were (relatively) unaware of it at breakfast. So, people living with more pungent smells, for example blocked drains or local industry (or more dangerous, for example leaking gas), may become accustomed to them, not identifying them as potentially detrimental to health. In some cases, this may have been perceived as indicative of individuals lacking skills to keep themselves healthy and safe.

As the number of taste buds declines with age, older people might derive less enjoyment from foods they previously favoured. They may indicate a preference for more strongly seasoned foods. Complete adaptation (loss of sensitivity) to a specific taste can occur in one to five minutes of continuous stimulation (Tortora and Derrickson, 2010), possibly contributing to persistent ingestion by some people with intellectual disabilities of substances others might find noxious (for example pica,

see Chapter 17, and the voracious appetite associated with Prader-Willi syndrome). Conversely, there may be occasions where we are encouraging people to take substances they find unpleasant, for example medication. Practitioners should be guided by their professional codes and the invaluable support of their local pharmacist in addressing this and the dry mouth (xerostomia) that is a side effect of some medications.

Taste has links to pleasant and unpleasant emotions (you may find this in Reader activity 13.3), with even new born babies reacting positively to sweet foods and expressing disgust at bitter tastes (Tortora and Derrickson, 2010). Statistics from 2017–18 (NHS Digital, 2019) point to less people with intellectual disabilities receiving screening for breast and colorectal cancer. A possible consequence of this is more advanced conditions requiring more aggressive treatments. Chemotherapeutic agents and radiation treatments can cause nausea and gastrointestinal upset regardless of what the individual tries to eat, leading to loss of appetite due to development of taste aversion. So, people might avoid food if it has previously made them unwell, even if the root cause is the treatment. This can be hugely difficult for carers, for whom food may be inextricably linked to nurture.

READER ACTIVITY 13.3

To illustrate that the sense of smell is not just about detection of odour, try to identify your most favourite and least favourite smells.

Are they present in your life today or are they from another time, perhaps childhood?

When you recall – or smell – them, do they evoke memories?

If you had hyposmia or anosmia, do you think you could as easily summon up any memories and emotions associated with them?

Range of conditions affecting smell and taste

Anosmia is loss of the sense of smell and can have a detrimental effect on the ability to taste leading to potential loss of appetite or seeking out highly flavoured foods. In those living alone, inability to detect rotten food could lead to food poisoning. Inability to smell gas leaking, or smoke from a fire in the house, may also have fatal consequences.

Hyposmia is a reduced ability to smell, affecting half of those over 65 and 75% of those over 80, though this exceeds the median age of death for people with intellectual disabilities in the 2018 Learning Disabilities

Mortality Review (LeDeR) (University of Bristol, 2019a). However, hyposmia can also be caused by neurological changes, such as a head injury or Alzheimer's disease, certain drugs (including over-the-counter medications such as antihistamines in the form of nasal sprays or gels, analgesics or steroids) and the damaging effects of smoking (Cedars Sinai, 2020). Consequently, it is a condition that those supporting people with intellectual disabilities should be aware of. A range of taste and/or smell issues is shown in Table 13.4 in the accompanying online resource, with possible responses.

Identifying issues with smell and taste

Sensory questionnaires described in the Hearing section of this chapter may be useful in identifying smell or taste characteristics that are very different from most people in the same age bracket (Dunn, 2014; Parham et al, 2021). When specialist referral is indicated for smell and taste disorders, a complete health history and physical examination will be undertaken. Alongside of this are other tests that may include measuring the lowest strength of a chemical that can be recognised, comparing tastes and smells of different chemicals, "scratch and sniff" tests and "sip, spit, and rinse" tests where chemicals are placed on certain parts of the tongue (Cedars Sinai, 2020). Such a battery may disadvantage individuals with intellectual disabilities who are non-verbal or lack appropriate vocabulary and understanding. They are also likely to have been dependent upon support to identify potential issues and convince a primary health professional to make a specialist referral. In recent years, smell training programmes (McClelland, 2019) have been developed that may prove, with further research, to be helpful for some individuals with intellectual disabilities.

Topically, loss or change to sense of smell or taste has been prominent during the COVID-19 pandemic due to the frequency with which it is reported as a symptom of infection. Early indications are that most people affected can expect substantial improvement within a short period (Walker et al, 2020).

Touch

Tactile processing is briefly depicted in Table 13.1. This involves the transmission of tactile information from the receptors in the skin to the thalamus of the brain, which filters and integrates the tactile information, and then relays this refined tactile information to the limbic system and the parietal lobe of the brain. Tactile information that is relayed to the limbic system may evoke emotion immediately, and then be incorporated into long-term memory as a meaningful experience (either positive or negative). When the parietal lobe receives the tactile information, it further analyses and organises this information, and interprets the meaning of the incoming sensations of touch in combination with proprioceptive sensations (discussed in the second part of this chapter), while drawing from memory of past tactile experiences. The parietal lobe then distributes the processed tactile information to other areas of the brain that specialise in vision, hearing and organisation of action, so that tactile information is integrated with other sensory information. When the person's neural systems are working well, this complex process occurs effortlessly.

The skin is the organ for touch (tactile) sensations. Touch receptors are embedded in the skin across the entire body, as well as within the lining of many internal structures such as the inside of the mouth, on the surface of the tongue, and in the lining of internal organs in the digestive system. Many types of tactile receptors are distributed across the body, and stimulation of these receptors provides important information required to
- identify and locate objects without using vision
- manipulate objects, such as tools, precisely and skilfully
- experience sustained comfort and pleasure in ordinary non-threatening situations
- avoid or minimise injury from burning, heavily pressing, or cutting/breaking the skin
- perform many tasks efficiently without relying on vision, such as dressing oneself.

For many individuals with impaired or absent vision, touch sensations are relied upon extensively to compensate for visual loss. Further, tactile sensations often evoke emotional responses such as pleasure, irritation, disgust, excitement, calming, or pain, particularly when combined with other sensations such as smell, taste and body awareness (proprioception).

Different types of tactile receptors are highly specialised for detecting different types of stimuli on the skin as illustrated in Figure 13.4. Tactile receptors may be specialised to detect very light touch, or to respond only to heavier touch (called deep pressure). Some receptors respond mainly to static (steady, not moving) touch, while others are very sensitive to the direction and speed of touch stimuli that are moving rapidly across the skin. Still others only respond when there is damage to the skin (pain sensations).

Impact of touch on personal experiences and behaviour

Touch experiences are necessary for health and sustaining close relationships. Decades of research has shown that nurturing touch is critical in infancy but also supports health and well-being throughout life (Field, 2014). Tactile sensitivity (also called tactile responsiveness, reactivity or modulation) refers to whether a person tends to over- or under-react to tactile sensations. In tactile hyposensitivity, the person is not affected by a tactile stimulus that would bother or upset most people. Individuals who are hyposensitive to touch sensations are sometimes at risk for danger or injury because they do not readily notice important tactile messages, such as those involving pain from cuts or from extreme pressure, or the presence of objects contacting the skin that could produce injury, such as something very hot or producing a chemical burn. This is sometimes called a "sensory registration" problem, meaning that the brain does not register or notice the stimulus in a timely fashion (or at all). An example from clinical practice is of a young child with autism who walked into a lake, heading into deep water while noticing neither the tactile nor the visual sensations of water

rising up over their chest and neck. Fortunately, they were rescued and did not drown as a consequence of their under-reactivity to tactile sensations. A range of tactile hyposensitive issues is shown in Table 13.5 in the accompanying online resource, with suggested interventions.

Tactile over-reactivity (also called hyper-reactivity or tactile defensiveness) is much more common than tactile under-reactivity and involves excessive or extreme responses to touch sensations. This term is used when an ordinary tactile stimulus that most people would not notice, or would perceive as unthreatening or even pleasant, is perceived as very irritating, painful, and/or distressing. Tactile defensiveness leads to avoidance of many touch sensations, particularly those involving light moving touch, such as the sensation of clothing moving or brushing across the skin. Consequently, many individuals with tactile defensiveness affecting the entire body will be able to tolerate only particular types of clothing and particular fabrics. They may actively withdraw from being touched by another person, and consequently others may misinterpret them as personally rejecting when the withdrawal was in response to the touch sensation, not the person. Some individuals with tactile defensiveness experience it within the mouth,

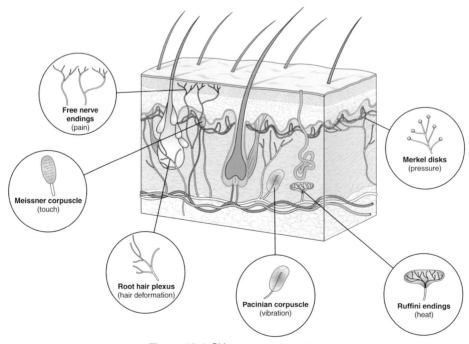

Figure 13.4 Skin sensory receptors

resulting in their tolerance for only a few types of food textures. They may easily gag, choke, or be unable to tolerate chewing food or thick drinks with particular textures. In extreme cases, they may have a very small repertoire of foods that they can tolerate, which may have negative consequences for nutrition. A range of tactile hypersensitive issues is shown in Table 13.6, with suggested interventions.

With combined visual and hearing impairments, touch may be the primary source for information (Hampson, 2013). However, touch should not be something supporters simply 'administer' to people with intellectual disabilities during delivery of care, it should be (appropriately) reciprocated. For example, it may be used by children and adults who are deafblind to identify supporters (perhaps by a watch or a more intentional identifier, for example a particular key fob around their neck), to seek and give reassurance, convey emotion and so on. Further, ample opportunities for safe and appropriate tactile exploration should be provided, for example, manipulation of objects with a wide variety of textures and pliability, including functional use of tools as well as play, crafts or other creative activities involving materials with varying textures and resistance. It is usually most helpful to start with tactile activities or materials that are acceptable, and then gradually expose the person to more challenging tactile experiences. Using heavy materials or asking the person to push or pull heavy items such as moving furniture is often helpful for both under-responsiveness and over-responsiveness in the tactile system.

Range of conditions affecting touch

Loss of the sense of touch may occur due to a peripheral neuropathy, which is a condition in which the sensory nerves that detect touch have been damaged or have not functioned normally from birth. The most common causes of peripheral neuropathy are accidental injuries or work-related stress on joints, that damage the nerves conveying tactile and other sensations. One common cause of peripheral neuropathy that has emerged in recent decades is excessive use of computer keyboards. In this condition, wrist tendons continuously press against sensory nerves, eventually damaging them. In severe cases, the loss of the senses of touch and proprioception in the hand may be permanent and disabling.

Individuals with spinal cord injury or disease may lose the senses of touch, pain and proprioception in the areas of the body that cannot send sensory messages up to the brain, due to the injury in the spinal cord which puts up a "road block" that the sensory messages cannot go around.

Some conditions that block the tactile and proprioceptive messages from moving up the spinal cord to the brain may be seen at birth, for example, in a condition called spina bifida (National Institute of Neurological Disorders and Stroke (NINDS), 2021). In spina bifida, the tail end of the spinal cord did not develop normally, and nerves affecting the lower body often are damaged. Where there is loss of movement and sensation in the legs (paraplegia), individuals may rely on supporters to anticipate potential effects of impaired touch. For example, the temperature of bath water should be checked to avoid burns or chills, body positions should be altered frequently to reduce risk of pressure ulcers, and particular care should always be taken where skin is breached in affected areas (see Chapters 11 and 12).

Identifying touch issues

Tactile difficulties are often invisible and overlooked. If tactile perception difficulties are suspected, then screening by a physician may be appropriate. A more in-depth assessment may be provided by an Occupational Therapist (OT) with training in this area. Standardised questionnaires that address tactile processing (Brown and Dunn, 2002; Dunn, 2014; Parham et al, 2021) are often particularly helpful in identifying touch issues. These questionnaires gather information about how well tactile perception, and especially tactile reactivity, are functioning in everyday life. Standardised tests may also be used such as the Sensory Integration and Praxis Tests (SIPT) (Ayres, 1989). These typically examine how precisely the person can identify points on the skin where they are touched, while their vision is blocked. In these tests, the person's performance is compared to research indicating the average performance of people in a similar age group (infants through to adults). Additionally, the OT will observe for behavioural signs of tactile over- or under-reactivity during tactile testing.

Having explored the five basic sensory systems, the second part of the chapter will now introduce the further three sensory systems illustrated in Table 13.7.

THREE FURTHER SENSORY SYSTEMS

Body Sense: Proprioception

Although most people are not aware of the proprioceptive sensory system, the sensations from it have a profound effect on everyday activities. In fact, if this sensory system is not working normally, your movement will be

TABLE 13.6   A range of issues with tactile hypersensitivity (high-, over-sensitivity)

What you might see	Effects in daily life	What could you do to help?
Withdraws from being touched, as if gentle or light touch is painful	May be misinterpreted as rejecting or disliking the person who touched them.	Use very firm, steady contact when touch is necessary, teach person to ask for firmer touch when appropriate
Certain food textures cause discomfort due to heightened sensitivity	Food refusal, limits self to bland ('beige' or 'white') foods	Offer range of flavours and textures, starting with what person tolerates, very gradually expanding toward more challenging textures
May only eat foods with smooth textures, like well-mashed potatoes or ice cream (without additions such as sprinkles or chopped nuts)	If food repertoire very limited, anorexia (refusal of most food) may result, which can seriously compromise health and well-being. Excessive weight loss (if avoids most food) or weight gain (if eats only calorie rich food) may result	Rotate foods to avoid restrictive diet. Monitor nutritional content of food to ensure adequate nutrition. Liaison with dietetics and/or dentistry if indicated. Use of vitamin and mineral supplements, under guidance of dietician or physician
Rejects clothing that slides or flutters or bunches up against skin; wants clothes to fit tightly against skin (e.g., wants to wear clothing too small, heavy jackets even when warm outside), or belt very tightly cinched	May be misinterpreted as merely trying to get attention, or trying to control others, when the person actually is irritated and distracted by tactile sensations of clothing	Work with person to identify tolerable, socially acceptable clothing
Likes and may seek out very firm touch or pressure, such as squeezing objects firmly, or seeking very firm hugs	Seeking firm hugs may be misinterpreted as sexual or aggressive. May damage objects unintentionally due to grasping too firmly	Acknowledge person most comfortable with firm pressure on skin, educate others
		Work with person and caregivers to find appropriate ways to frequently obtain this sensory input

TABLE 13.7 How the further three sensory systems work (Senses represented by Widgit Symbols © Widgit Software 2002-2022 www.widgit.com)

Sense	Stimulus	Pathway: sense organ to brain	Areas of brain receiving & integrating nerve impulses into sensation
body	Muscles & tendons stretch	- activates **mechanoreceptors** in muscles & joints - mechanoreceptors detect stretch of muscle and tendons - **nociceptors** detect pain in joints - proprioceptive information carried to **parietal lobe** for body awareness	
balance	Movement of head through space	- activates **mechanoreceptors** in inner ear (**semi-circular canals & otolith organs**, see Figure 13.5) - mechanoreceptors detect pull of gravity on head & movement of head through space, send vestibular messages into **brainstem** to activate automatic responses to loss of balance - vestibular information further relayed to **parietal lobe** for integration with proprioceptive and visual information to influence planned movement	
organs	Internal tissues & organs change/ activate in response to changing internal events	- mechano- & chemoreceptors within internal organs detect pain, pressure & chemical molecules - interoceptive information sent to **brainstem centres**, then to **hypothalamus, anterior insula & anterior cingulate gyrus** (located deep in brain on inside surface of each side of brain)	

affected so much that you may not be able to get dressed, climb stairs or eat unaided. Proprioceptive sensations are essential for smooth and accurate movement coordination. For example, they allow you to move your arm the precise distance needed to successfully pick up an object with your hand, without over- or undershooting.

The word "proprioception" is derived from the Latin word "proprio," meaning "one's own." So, proprioception means the perception of one's own body. Specifically, this term refers to the sensations arising from the stretch of joints and muscles, the organs for proprioception. Joints are the places in the body where different bones meet, and muscles are attached to bones in a manner that makes movement possible. Examples of locations of joints in the body include the knee, ankle, elbow and wrist, shoulders, neck, jaw, spine (back bones), and each place within a toe, finger or thumb where you can make smaller movements (for example, throwing or kicking a ball, or using a keyboard). Special receptors embedded in the muscles and joints tell the brain whether a body part is moving (or not) and, if so, exactly how far, fast, and in what direction. This is possible because the proprioceptive receptors are sensitive to the stretching of muscles and joints. Messages about these sensations are constantly flowing into the parietal lobe of the brain, and most of the time we are not consciously aware of this complex sensory processing of messages from body parts. We just "know" how we are positioned when sitting, standing or moving without having to think about it.

Proprioceptive receptors are the fastest sensory receptors – they send information to the brain much more quickly than vision, hearing, smell, taste, touch or vestibular receptors (discussed in the next section of this chapter). This makes it possible to adjust your body or arm/leg position while moving, even if very quickly, for example, while running up stairs or making a fast sports move. The quick processing of proprioceptive sensations is also protective, so we don't overstretch muscles or joints unnecessarily.

Proprioceptive receptors send messages to the brain via the same route used by tactile messages. When tactile and proprioceptive messages reach the brain, they are integrated seamlessly to provide awareness of how the body is positioned and how it is moving, based on the incoming sensations from the skin, muscles, and joints. Although vision also contributes to this awareness in everyday life, most of our body awareness comes from tactile and proprioceptive sensations. This is why we can move in a coordinated manner, or position ourselves safely while in a completely dark room. Proprioception also allows you to know if part of your body has been moved by an external force, even if you did not initiate any movement. For example, if a person moved your hand while you were awake but your eyes were closed, you would know the direction your hand had been moved. Sometimes the term "somatosensory" ("somato" means body) is used to refer to these two systems (tactile and proprioceptive) working together in synchrony.

Impact of proprioception on personal experiences and behaviour

Good proprioception is necessary to effectively position ourselves (for example, sit down without falling over) and influences every action we make. Specifically, it regulates the timing of when the action begins and ends, and guides the movement of each body part involved including the direction of the action, the forcefulness of the action, and any adjustments that need to be made during the action to ensure accuracy.

Proprioception also seems to play an important role in self-regulation of alertness and attention (arousal level) as well as emotion regulation. Activities that supply a lot of proprioceptive sensations include heavy work activities such as pushing, pulling, lifting, or carrying packed boxes or moving furniture. The muscle work needed to manage the heavy weight during these activities tends to have a focusing effect for many people. Activation of proprioceptive messages from the jaw muscles also seems to have a calming effect. This may be why many people like to chew gum while under stress. Often young children who have difficulty processing sensory information may chew on their clothes (e.g., the collar or sleeve of their shirt) or on rubbery objects, which often seems to be calming. Where this is seen in adults with intellectual disabilities we should also 'think sensory', whilst maintaining awareness that there may be other explanations, for example an attempt to communicate or relieve a sore mouth.

If proprioception is not working well, the person will have difficulty organising and timing actions with precision. Even activities that are done almost every day may be challenging, and the person may perform tasks in ways that seem odd to other people. Proprioception may also influence social relationships. For example, if a person does not have precise proprioception and tends to hold objects with too much force, squeezing too hard and sometimes breaking them, they may be viewed as someone who is deliberately destructive, when the breakage was not intended. The opposite may also occur; the person may not hold objects with enough force, so that objects sometimes fall out of their hand accidentally, resulting in breakage which others may misinterpret as careless.

When proprioception is poor, motor coordination, often postural control and balance, are areas of difficulty. Many individuals have low muscle tone, affecting posture, which can adversely affect seated activities such as handwriting, as well as gross motor activities such as climbing stairs. Individuals may have difficulty participating in activities requiring physical coordination such as playing hopscotch with other children or participating in sports with other adolescents or adults.

Range of conditions affecting proprioception

Difficulty with proprioception may affect people with a wide range of conditions. For example, it is common among people with sensory processing or intellectual disabilities, but it may also affect others without any known disability. Poor proprioception affects many individuals with autism spectrum conditions (see Chapter 15) and some individuals with Down syndrome. Proprioceptive difficulties can also result from neurological injuries or diseases, depending on exactly where the damage occurs in the nervous system. Examples include brain or spinal cord injury, stroke and multiple sclerosis. Additionally, in situations where injury to a joint (for example, a sprained ankle) has damaged the proprioceptors within that joint, the result of the injury may include loss of proprioception at that joint. A range of issues with body awareness (proprioception) is shown in Table 13.8 in the accompanying online resource, with possible responses.

Identifying proprioception issues

As for tactile difficulties, proprioception issues are often invisible and overlooked. If proprioception difficulties are suspected, then screening by a physician may be appropriate. A more in-depth assessment may be provided by an OT or Physical (Physio-) therapist with training in this area. Typically, assessment will involve the therapist moving the person's finger, toe, wrist, ankle, arm or leg up or down while vision is occluded, holding it for a few seconds, and then returning the limb to a resting position. The person is then asked to move the body part into the position where the therapist had previously moved it. Therapists with special training in sensory integration may also use a standardised test of proprioception (e.g., Ayres, 1989), and questionnaires

that provide scores on proprioceptive processing that compares to the typical functioning of most people in the same age range (Parham et al, 2021). These questionnaires gather information about how well proprioception is functioning in everyday life. Additionally, the therapist will observe for behavioural signs of proprioceptive over- or under-reactivity during testing.

Ian Waterman's famous personal story (Reader activity 13.4 in the accompanying online resource) provides an example of how loss of proprioception impacts daily life.

Balance Sense: Vestibular Processing

The vestibular system is another most people have never heard of – but as for proprioception, damage to this system may be devastating. This is because the vestibular system is responsible for detecting the pull of gravity – specifically the relationship of gravity to the position of the head as one is moving around. This is a fundamental sensory system because we need to manage the constant effects of gravity on our bodies, in order to move functionally. The position of the head is critical in this system because the vestibular sensory receptors are located in the inner ear. This location allows the system to precisely detect the angle and speed at which the head is moving through space. It alerts the rest of the brain about the direction and velocity of head movement, and this information is constantly used to maintain balance, whether moving or staying still. Vestibular sensations also affect arousal level: they can either increase alertness (imagine riding a very fast roller coaster or going down a speed elevator in a super high building) or generate feelings of calmness or drowsiness (imagine gently and rhythmically rocking in a rocking chair).

Below is the figure we used earlier in the section on hearing. We have relabelled it to draw your attention to the vestibular receptors, which are attached to the cochlea (containing sound receptors) but send entirely different kinds of sensory messages to the brain. The structures in this figure that contain vestibular receptors are (1) the semi-circular canals, and (2) the otilith organs, the utricle and saccule, located inside the bulge at the base of the semi-circular canals.

The semi-circular canals are responsible for detecting "angular movement" of the head. Angular movement is any movement that is changing direction (not in a straight line). Examples of angular movement include spinning around, turning the head to look beside or behind you, walking or running on a curving path, or turning a corner

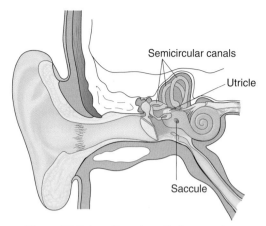

Figure 13.5 Location of vestibular receptors

while in a moving vehicle. Three interconnected semi-circular canals are located on each side of the head.

Whenever your head changes direction while moving, tiny hair-like cells (embedded in a flap of tissue within each semi-circular canal) bend in opposition to the movement. For example, if you are turning toward the right, the hair cells bend toward the left. When the hair cells bend, they relay messages to the brainstem. From there, messages about change in head velocity (speed and direction of head movement through space) are relayed downward to activate muscles needed to keep balance, to maintain a stable head position, and to protect the head and body from injury. Simultaneously, messages about the head movement travel upward to the parietal lobe, where vestibular information is integrated with proprioceptive and visual information.

Messages about head movement are also relayed to eye muscles, causing the eyes to move in opposition to the head movement. For example, when the head moves toward the right, the eyes automatically shift toward the left. This allows us to have a "stable visual field" when moving through the world. In other words, eye movements continually correct their position relative to head movement, so that that the world does not seem to be jiggling or whirling around whenever the head moves.

The otolith organs are a separate set of vestibular receptors adjacent to the semi-circular canals, consisting of two structures on each side of the head, the utricle and the saccule, located within the bulge at the base of the semi-circular canals. Unlike the semi-circular canals, which detect relatively fast angular movements, the otolith organs detect linear movements of the head, including

slow movement and the pull of gravity. A unique feature of each otolith organ is that they contain a band of sensory neurons that have tiny hair-like extensions which led to their being called "hair cells." Resting on top of the hair cells is a layer of tiny calcium carbonate crystals (called otoliths or otoconia) that roll across the hair cells when there is acceleration or deceleration of head movement in a straight line, which can be upward, downward, forward, backward, or diagonally through space. When the head moves forward, for example, the otoliths roll backward. As these crystals roll across the hair cells they bend them causing the cell bodies of these neurons to fire and send messages about the direction and velocity of the linear motion into the brain.

The otolith organs additionally play an important role in maintaining optimal posture. For example, if a person becomes tired, bored or drowsy, the body starts to slump and shift off-balance. As this happens proprioceptors in the muscles and joints throughout the body, along with vestibular receptors that detect poor head alignment, signal the brain to correct posture (including head position) so that the person does not slump further or fall over.

Because the vestibular system works so closely with parts of the brain that activate body movements, vestibular sensations are integrated not only with vision, but also with tactile and proprioceptive sensations arriving in the parietal lobe of the brain. This integrated sensory information constantly 'streams' information to the brain's centres for planning, organising and producing movement, which are located in the frontal lobe.

If a head movement signals danger (for example, changes in head position while tripping and losing balance), the vestibular centres in the brainstem send out messages to activate automatic protective movement patterns. This normally happens very quickly – much more quickly than if you initiated the movements consciously. For example, imagine slipping on ice. As you begin to fall, your arms extend and your legs may activate to try to catch your balance. As you continue to fall toward the ground, your head and shoulders will lift away from the ground to protect the brain, because the vestibular system detects the direction of the fall and activates neck muscles to lift the head away from the ground.

Impact of vestibular processing on personal experiences and behaviour

When the vestibular system is working well, we are able to do many kinds of activities – both sedentary and physically active – without having to think about keeping our balance. As noted earlier, vestibular and proprioceptive processing work very closely with each other in order to maintain postural stability and balance while sedentary and also while moving, whether the movement is very slight as when adjusting posture, or whether it involves very large movements, such as when dancing or participating in sports. In addition, maintaining balance of our physical body plays a role in being able to coordinate actions involving the right and left sides of the body in a well-synchronised manner. This is because the vestibular-proprioceptive systems make major contributions to our unconscious ability to be centred in our body.

If the vestibular system is not developing optimally, posture and movement are affected. For example, postural control (maintaining a centred and stable position while sitting), balance while moving, motor coordination in general, and/or ability to synchronise actions of the right and left sides of the body may be poor compared to most peers. When these challenges are seen in children, adults often assume the child is not paying attention, is lazy, or not putting in enough effort. Telling the child to "sit up straight" or pay more attention is generally ineffective and may contribute to the child developing a view of self as incompetent.

Typically, children tend to actively seek out intense vestibular experiences more than adults. Although this tends to diminish with age, some individuals have a lifelong inclination to frequently engage in intense vestibular-stimulating activities. Examples include running and rock climbing (which have strong proprioceptive aspects), trampoline jumping, dancing, riding motorcycles, driving cars fast (ideally on a safe track designed for that purpose), bungee-cord jumping and so on. For lifelong vestibular-seeking individuals, it is helpful to build frequent intense vestibular experiences into their daily or weekly routines, with careful consideration of safety, affordability and feasibility.

Other people are overly sensitive to vestibular stimulation and may go out of their way to avoid vestibular experiences that would not bother most people, such as riding on an elevator or stepping onto an escalator or walking up stairs. In general, avoiding anxiety-provoking experiences in daily life is adaptive, unless it is so extreme that it limits or negatively affects the person's work or personal life. Young children with extremely over-reactive vestibular systems may be so anxious about moving across different surfaces, that their motor development is compromised. In extreme cases, the child may refuse to step from a hard floor onto a gymnastics mat, or to step from a firm sidewalk onto a grassy lawn.

Range of conditions affecting vestibular processing

As described earlier, difficulty processing vestibular sensations may lead to over- or under-reactivity to vestibular sensations. These differences in vestibular processing may accompany a specific medical condition, but often they do not. In many cases, they seem to be an aspect of the person's temperament or general level of sensitivity to stimuli, so it is plausible they may have genetic origins.

At any age, infection affecting the inner ear may result in dizziness due to inflammation of the vestibular receptors, interfering with their function. For example, labyrinthitis is inflammation of the semi-circular canals, which can impair the ability of the vestibular receptors to signal accurate changes in head position or movement. This often results in dizziness, which may be so severe that the person cannot maintain balance while standing or walking. Vestibular neuritis (inflammation of the nerve that carries vestibular messages into the brain) may similarly impair vestibular functioning.

As the antibiotic gentamicin is toxic to the vestibular system at any dosage (Ahmed et al, 2012), it should be avoided entirely. Decades of research clearly indicate that severe and permanent loss of balance very often affects those who have taken this prescription medication, although hearing is not affected.

Ageing usually introduces challenges to vestibular processing. For example, vestibular receptors may no longer work very efficiently due to age-related changes in vestibular structures, which in some cases is a result of reduced blood flow to vestibular receptor neurons. Loss of balance causing injury from falling can happen at any age, but becomes a greater concern with age, particularly after about 60 years of age. A range of issues with vestibular sensations is shown in Table 13.9 in the accompanying online resource, with possible responses. An excellent source of additional information regarding vestibular conditions is provided online by the Vestibular Disorders Association (VeDA) (2021).

Identifying vestibular issues

If any sudden changes in balance or tolerance for movement occur, for example, dizziness or nausea with ordinary movement, evaluation by a physician should be made as soon as possible. Referral to an ear specialist such as otolaryngologist may be appropriate. In cases where vestibular receptor damage is suspected, further referral to a vestibular physiologist may be made for detailed testing to verify whether the problem is in the peripheral vestibular system (i.e. the semi-circular canals or the otolith organs – the utricle and saccule) or whether the problem is in the central nervous system (the vestibular centres in the brainstem and parietal lobe). Methods used to evaluate the vestibular system may include placing electrodes around the eyes to detect, record and evaluate eye movements as the person sits in a rotating chair, or using the electrodes to evaluate eye movements as a circular screen with vertical lines rotates around the person who is sitting still.

Physical (Physio-) therapists or OTs with special training in sensory integration or in vestibular rehabilitation may also conduct evaluations to determine the extent to which vestibular difficulties are affecting everyday-life functioning. Tests of balance such as standing on one foot or walking with heel-to-toe are usually involved, and sometimes tests of bilateral coordination as well (Ayres, 1989). Standardised questionnaires such as the Sensory Processing Measure-2 (Parham et al, 2021) may also be helpful. This information may be used to plan a therapy programme supporting recovery of vestibular functioning, as far as possible. More information about interventions for vestibular difficulties is provided by the Vestibular Disorders Association (VeDA) (2021).

Internal Organs Sense: Interoception

Interoception involves the brain's awareness and interpretation of sensations arising from internal organs, such as the stomach, intestines, heart, and lungs. More specifically, interoception involves giving meaning to internal organ functions and activities, such as heart rate, respiration (breathing), satiety (fullness after eating), need to urinate or defecate, and autonomic nervous system activity such as sweaty palms, associated with "fight or flight" reactions (Price and Hooven, 2018). It provides a "moment by moment mapping of the body's internal landscape" (Khalsa and Lapidus, 2016, p. 2). The cerebral cortex receives these sensory messages and interprets their meaning, often in terms of emotions. For example, sweaty palms along with a rapid heart rate may be interpreted by the brain as a fear experience, which may lead the cerebral cortex to decide to escape the situation or stop doing a particular activity.

This is a relatively new area of discussion and study in the field of sensory integration and processing, as well

as in psychotherapy, clinical psychology, nursing and mindfulness meditation. Because our knowledge on this topic is just emerging, we provide a brief overview here.

Impact of interoception on personal experiences and behaviour

Although much is not yet fully understood about interoception, emerging evidence strongly suggests that it has a significant influence on how we interpret our personal situation and emotional state moment-by-moment; this in turn strongly influences our relationships and our decisions for action. Interoception may influence ability to assess risk accurately and to establish and maintain relationships, including interpretation of nonverbal cues from others and from our own bodies. Interoceptive awareness is thought to make important contributions to self-regulation (Price and Hooven, 2018), as it is a primary contributor to awareness and interpretation of our emotions (Craig, 2003). Additionally, it is essential for managing basic physiological processes such as eating, drinking, using the toilet and sleeping, as these processes generate feelings such as hunger, thirst, need to urinate or defecate and sleepiness.

Range of conditions affecting interoception

At the time of writing, interoception difficulties have not been studied enough to determine how prevalent they are across different conditions. Thus far, it seems likely that interoception difficulties may affect people of all ages, across a wide range of conditions, including psychiatric diagnoses such as panic disorder, depression, somatic symptom disorders, anorexia nervosa, and bulimia nervosa (Khalsa and Lapidus, 2016), as well as individuals with no known developmental or medical condition. People with developmental conditions or intellectual disabilities may be affected including children with sensory integration difficulties. For example, children who are under-responsive to pressure or pain sensations may routinely hold in faeces or urine when the bowel or bladder is full, because they are not aware of the fullness which creates an urge to empty or void. This may lead to bowel or bladder incontinence when these structures overflow, or bladder infection or impacted bowel. Those who are over-responsive may also retain faeces, but for different reasons: because they experience their passage as painful or very intense, in situations where there is no infection or structural abnormality in the body that would account for the pain. Better understanding of interoceptive difficulties may yet offer an additional tool in preventing premature death in people with intellectual disabilities (see Chapters 9 and 10) as recognised by the University of Bristol's LeDeR Programme (2019b).

Some experts suggest that interoception difficulties may be causal factors in autism as well as in alexithymia. Alexithymia is a condition that involves difficulty with identifying and describing one's own feelings, limited imagination, and difficulties distinguishing between emotional feelings and body sensations (Apfel and Sifneos, 1979). Alexithymia is common among individuals with autism (see Chapter 15), with rates possibly as high as 65% (Bird and Cook, 2013). Currently the research is inconsistent as to whether interoception difficulties are causally related to alexithymia or to autism (Brewer et al, 2016; Nicholson et al, 2018; Hobson et al, 2020). Research into the next decade will likely clarify relationships among interoception, alexithymia, and autism.

Identifying interoception issues

Professionals such as psychiatrists, psychologists, nurses, and OTs may provide assessments of interoception, but in any case special training in this area is required. Assessments generally will involve interviews and questionnaires that focus on interoceptive issues. It is likely that new methods and instruments for assessing interoception will be emerging in the coming years, as knowledge of interoceptive disorders expands. A range of issues associated with interoception is shown in Table 13.10, with possible responses.

PUTTING IT ALL TOGETHER

To draw together the eight sensory systems (five basic plus three further) explored within this chapter, this final section considers the individual, everyday experience of eating and drinking. Figure 13.6 shows each sense overlapping with the identified experience at the centre, which could be substituted for many others, for example dressing, mobilising, working or playing. Whilst the eight senses might also be presented as variously overlapping with each other, this would create a complex image. However, it might serve to emphasise

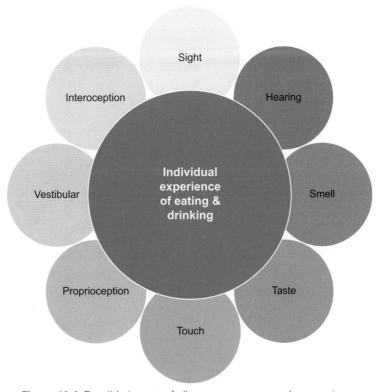

Figure 13.6 Possible impact of all senses on an everyday experience

TABLE 13.10   Issues with interoception (Issues represented by Widgit Symbols © Widgit Software 2002–2022 www.widgit.com)

What you might see	Effects in daily life	Helpful responses
Urinary processing (toilet) May not notice - need to visit toilet, until too late, - pain due to infection or blockage	Avoids social events due to possibility of wetting or soiling Others may avoid them due to wetting or soiling resulting in limited social life May have trouble functioning normally due to infection Medical care may not be sought because not noticed until critical	Plan specific & frequent times to visit toilet, especially after eating or drinking Try continence products Observe for signs that person may be in pain, even if they don't verbalise it, when in doubt, seek medical evaluation
Sleep May not notice when need to sleep, has very erratic sleep schedules, frequent night waking, leaving bed to become active, daytime sleeping	May not be able to function well at home, school, or work due to sleep deprivation Daytime sleeping perpetuates night awakening May try to wake up others while they are sleeping at night	Encourage regular schedule for bedtime at night (if helpful, daytime nap) Seek help from sleep disorder specialists Plan daytime schedule to involve plenty of physical activity, so fatigue sets in at evening time
Emotions May not notice or recognise internal sensations, unable to communicate to others how they feel	Difficulty maintaining relationships due to inability to communicate feelings & emotions accurately Strain placed on relationships because of lack of self-care (result of poor interoception) May misinterpret visceral sensations e.g. may experience hunger but think it is anger (if expressed, could be interpreted as behaviour of concern, see Chapter 17)	Explain alexithymia to others, so they realise person not deliberately manipulative or controlling Seek help from professionals experienced in providing interventions for interoceptive difficulties e.g., Mindful Awareness in Body-Oriented Therapy (MABT) (see Price and Hooven, 2018)

READER ACTIVITY 13.5

Identify someone with an intellectual disability that you know well, and an activity they regularly undertake.

Place the activity at the centre of Figure 13.6 and consider the potential impact on it of the eight surrounding senses for the identified individual.

You may find some senses support the individual to complete the activity very well. Others may provide more of a challenge. For each sense, consider whether it is operating within an adaptive range or whether they may be experiencing hypo- or hypersensitivities. Crucially, where unusual responses are identified, how might they be reduced or overcome?

the complexity of the processes presented within this chapter, the marvel of their unconscious interplay and further understanding of difficulties experienced where functioning of individual senses and their overall integration does not naturally occur.

The individual at the centre of this figure, a fictional young woman with an intellectual disability, might experience eating and drinking as follows, starting with sight and progressing (clockwise) in the order that senses are presented in the chapter. Where Emilia, as we will call her, has difficulty expressing her sensory experience verbally, contributions have been made by supporters who know her well.

- I enjoy cookery programmes on television but with my poor sight rely on verbal descriptions of the dishes
- When I hear the corn popping in the pan I know it's cinema night!
- I don't like food cooked with cheese as even tiny amounts of very mild types smell *really* bad to me
- My favourite meal is pasta cooked (well beyond!) al dente and served with a smooth white sauce
- Please check the temperature of my food and drink as I don't seem to notice if they're too hot or cold
- I'm not deliberately messy, I just find it hard to co-ordinate my cutlery
- I pay better attention to my meal if I can have intense movement experiences beforehand
- I become dehydrated easily as I don't seem to realise when I'm thirsty.

Whilst not claiming to be an objective, comprehensive, professionally administered assessment, such a personalised 'snapshot' of individual experience can be

swiftly and easily translated into helpful supports for a holistically healthy, sensory-friendly approach to eating and drinking for Emilia. Using such a 'building block', it is not difficult to see how this could then be developed into a whole-life approach using, for example, tools outlined in Chapter 4 such as the RIX Wiki.

To consolidate your learning from the chapter, please complete Reader activity 13.5, referring to the tables within the accompanying online resource where appropriate.

CONCLUSION

This chapter has considered the range of functioning of the five basic senses and extended this to include the further three that are attracting interest. When these systems are intact, the overall experience of receiving, regulating and integrating incoming information appears effortless. However, where there are differences in single senses, in the way they combine, and their total interplay with each other, individuals can have unusual, disrupted, sometimes distressing responses that limit their daily lives and their ability to maintain health and wellbeing. Enhanced understanding of sensory issues can enable individuals and supporters to advocate changes in homes, schools and communities; as we continue to learn more, the insights and repertoire of helpful interventions and strategies offered here can only increase.

REFERENCES

Ahmed, R. M., Hannigan, I. P., MacDougall, H. G., et al. (2012). Gentamicin ototoxicity: a 23-year selected case series of 103 patients. *Medical Journal of Australia*, *196*(11), 701–704. Available at: https://www.mja.com.au/journal/2012/196/11/gentamicin-ototoxicity-23-year-selected-case-series-103-patients.

Apfel, R. J., & Sifneos, P. E. (1979). Alexithymia: concept and measurement. *Psychotherapy and Psychosomatics*, *32*(1–4), 180–190.

Ayres, A. J. (1989). *Sensory integration and praxis tests*. Western Psychological Services.

Bird, G., & Cook, R. (2013). Mixed emotions: the contribution of alexithymia to the emotional symptoms of autism. *Translational Psychiatry*, *3*(7), e285.

Brewer, R., Cook, R., & Bird, G. (2016). Alexithymia: a general deficit of interoception. *Royal Society Open Science*.

Brown, C., & Dunn, W. (2002). *Adolescent/Adult Sensory Profile*. Pearson.

Cedars Sinai. (2020). *Smell and taste disorders*. Available at: https://www.cedars-sinai.org/health-library/

diseases-and-conditions/s/smell-and-taste-disorders.html. [Accessed 24 February 2020].

Charge Syndrome Foundation. (2021). *Signs and symptoms.* Available at: https://www.chargesyndrome.org/about-charge/signs-symptoms/. [Accessed 26 February 2021].

Connor, Z. (2016). *Eating.* Available at: https://www.autism.org.uk/about/health/eating.aspx. [Accessed 24 February 2020].

CMV Action. (2021). *Diagnosis and symptoms in babies.* Available at: https://cmvaction.org.uk/what-cmv/diagnosis-symptoms. [Accessed 26 February 2021].

Craig, A. D. (2003). Interoception: the sense of the physiological condition of the body. *Current Opinion in Neurobiology*, *13*, 500–505.

Deafblind, U. K. (2021). What is deafblindness? Available at: https://deafblind.org.uk/information-advice/what-is-deafblindness/. [Accessed 26 February 2021].

Dunn, W. (2014). *Sensory Profile 2.* London: Pearson Clinical.

Erskine, S. E., & Philpott, C. (2020). An unmet need: patients with smell and taste disorders. *Clinical Otolaryngology*, *45*(2), 197–203.

Electronic Medicines Compendium (EMC). (2021). *Chlorpromazine 100mg tablets.* Available at: https://www.medicines.org.uk/emc/product/3476/smpc#UNDESIR-ABLE_EFFECTS. [Accessed 26 February 2021].

Field, T. (2014). *Touch* (2nd ed.). Cambridge, MA: The MIT Press.

Foundation for People with Learning Disabilities (FPLD). (2021). *Hearing loss.* Available at: https://www.learning-disabilities.org.uk/learning-disabilities/a-to-z/h/hearing-loss. [Accessed 26 February 2021].

Hampson, A. (2013). *Sense factsheet 11. Sensory integration and CHARGE.* London: Sense.

Hartnett, M. E., & Penn, J. S. (2012). Mechanisms and management of retinopathy of prematurity. *New England Journal of Medicine*, *367*, 2515–2526.

Hobson, H., Westwood, H., Conway, J., et al. (2020). Alexithymia and autism diagnostic assessments: evidence from twins at genetic risk of autism and adults with anorexia nervosa. *Research in Autism Spectrum Disorders*, 73. https://doi.org/10.1016/j.rasd.2020.101531.

Khalsa, S. S., & Lapidus, R. C. (2016). Can interoception improve the pragmatic search for biomarkers in psychiatry? *Frontiers in Psychiatry*, *7*, 121.

McClelland, L. (2019). *Smell and taste disorders.* Available at: https://www.uhb.nhs.uk/Downloads/pdf/PiSmellTaste Disorders.pdf. [Accessed 25 February 2021].

Mason, I., & Stevens, S. (2010). Instilling eye drops and ointment in a baby or young child. *Community Eye Health*, *23* *(72)*, 15.

National Health Service (NHS). (2019). *Eye tests for children.* Available at: https://www.nhs.uk/conditions/eye-tests-in-children/. [Accessed 25 February 2021].

National Health Service (NHS). (2018). *Hearing tests for children.* Available at: https://www.nhs.uk/conditions/hearing-tests-children/. [Accessed 25 February 2021].

NHS Digital. (2019). *Health and care of people with learning disabilities, experimental statistics: 2017 to 2018.* Available at: https://digital.nhs.uk/data-and-information/publications/statistical/health-and-care-of-people-with-learning-disabilities/experimental-statistics-2017-to-2018. [Accessed 26 February 2021].

National Institute of Neurological Disorders and Stroke (NINDS). (2021). *Spina bifida fact sheet.* Available at: https://www.ninds.nih.gov/DISORDERS/PATIENT-CAREGIVER-EDUCATION/FACT-SHEETS/SPINA-BIFIDA-FACT-SHEET. [Accessed 25 February 2021].

National Autistic Society (NAS). (2018). *Pica.* Available at: https://www.autism.org.uk/about/behaviour/challenging-behaviour/pica.aspx. [Accessed 24 February 2020].

Nicholson, T. M., Williams, D. M., Grainger, C., et al. (2018). Interoceptive impairments do not lie at the heart of autism or alexithymia. *Journal of Abnormal Psychology*, *127*(6), 612–622.

Parham, L. D., Ecker, C., Kuhaneck, H. M., et al. (2021). *Sensory Processing Measure-2.* Torrance, CA: Western Psychological Services.

Price, C. J., & Hooven, C. (2018). Interoceptive awareness skills for emotion regulation: theory and approach of mindful awareness in body-oriented therapy (MABT). *Frontiers in Psychology*, *9*, 798.

SeeAbility. (2019). *Functional vision assessment (FVA).* Available at: https://www.seeability.org/fva. [Accessed 23 February 2020].

SeeAbility. (2020). *Eye care messages for people with learning disabilities. Easy read factsheet.* Liverpool: SeeAbility.

Sense. (2019). *Rubella and sensory impairment.* Available at: https://www.sense.org.uk/get-support/information-and-advice/conditions/rubella/. [Accessed 26 February 2021].

Sense International. (2021). *About deafblindness.* Available at: https://www.senseinternational.org.uk/about-deafblindness. [Accessed 19 February 2021].

Spiby, J. (2014). *Screening for hearing loss in older adults.* London: NSC.

STAR Institute for Sensory Processing Disorder. (2020). *Your 8 senses.* Available at: https://www.spdstar.org/basic/your-8-senses. [Accessed 17 February 2020].

Tortora, G., & Derrickson, B. (2010). *Essentials of anatomy and physiology* (8th ed.). John Wiley & Sons.

University of Bristol. (2019a). *2018 Learning disabilities mortality review (LeDeR).* Bristol: Norah Fry Centre for Disability Studies.

University of Bristol. (2019b). *Constipation: Dying for a poo.* Available at: https://www.bristol.ac.uk/media-library/

sites/sps/leder/ConstipationJANnewsletter.pdf. [Accessed 27 February 2021].

Vestibular Disorders Association (VeDA). (2021). Available at: https://vestibular.org/vvcreplay/. [Accessed 25 February 2021].

Vision Matters. (2010). *A sight test is a vital health check.* Vision Matters.

Walker, A., Pottinger, G., Scott, A., et al. (2020). Anosmia and loss of smell in the era of COVID-19. *British Medical Journal, 370.* https://doi.org/10.1136/bmj.m2808.

Woodhouse, M., & Charlton, P. (2018). *Eye conditions in children.* London: Down's Syndrome Association.

14

Epilepsy

Christian Brandt

KEY ISSUES

- Epilepsy is a frequent neurological disorder caused by a disturbed balance between excitatory and inhibitory processes in the brain.
- Prevalence of epilepsy amongst people with intellectual disabilities is generally higher than in the general population.
- Holistic assessment should take into account the impact of epilepsy on the overall health and wellbeing of an individual.

- Treatments vary and may include drug therapy, surgery, rehabilitation, psychotherapy and other non-pharmacological interventions.
- Seizure management should focus on achieving seizure freedom; when not possible a reduction in seizure frequency without intolerable side effects should be the goal.

CHAPTER OUTLINE

INTRODUCTION

Epilepsy is not synonymous with intellectual disabilities, however, people with intellectual disabilities form an important and unique subgroup of all people living with epilepsy. A diagnosis of epilepsy in someone with an intellectual disability gives rise to an array of special implications in terms of investigations and management. Treatment should be multimodal and multiprofessional. This is because the constellation of epilepsy and intellectual disabilities is associated with a range of complex comorbidities and psychosocial implications that will require intervention from a range of professional disciplines. Such disciplines will include not only specialists in the care of people with intellectual disabilities and neurologists and psychiatrists but also possibly physicians from other disciplines, generic specialist epilepsy nurses and other health and social care providers. These professionals play equally important roles and their involvement may be greater than that experienced when working with people with epilepsy but without intellectual disabilities. This chapter will introduce the reader to the basic principles of epileptology (the study of epilepsy) and special implications for the diagnosis and treatment of epilepsy in people with intellectual disabilities.

WHAT IS EPILEPSY?

Epilepsy is a disorder characterised by recurrent epileptic seizures. This seems to be a simple fact but it is nevertheless important to keep in mind. A person with epilepsy is healthy in between the epileptic seizures, at least with regards to the epilepsy. If they are not healthy between the seizures, then this is due to other comorbid disorders or conditions. Generally speaking, epilepsy is a consequence of a disturbed balance between excitatory and inhibitory processes in the brain. Important players are the hormones glutamate (excitatory transmitter) and GABA (inhibitory transmitter) but also ion channels (especially sodium and potassium channels). A person may develop epilepsy for different reasons. Typical aetiologies are focal brain lesions, for instance due to a perinatal cerebral infarction, tumours or malformations of cortical development, e.g. focal cortical dysplasias or subependymal periventricular heterotopias. Diffuse brain-damage can be caused for instance by perinatal hypoxia, for instance in preterm delivery.

Epilepsy and people with intellectual disabilities

The prevalence of epilepsy is significantly higher among people with intellectual disabilities than in the general population, increasing with the degree of disability. In 2001, Lhatoo and Sander estimated that 6% of children with mild learning (sic) disabilities, 24% with severe learning disabilities and 50% with profound learning disabilities experienced epilepsy (terminology reflecting the age of the source). A population-based study of adults with intellectual disabilities in a defined geographical area of the UK (McGrother et al, 2006) identified a prevalence of epilepsy of 26%, at least 26 times higher than in the general adult population.

Many people's epilepsy develops within the first two years of life however, an even higher number develop it after 60 years of age. This latter peak is mainly due to cerebrovascular disorders (for example, strokes), brain tumours and dementias. People with Alzheimer's dementia are at increased risk of developing epilepsy. This is of significance to people with intellectual disabilities, particularly those with Down syndrome, as many develop Alzheimer's much earlier than those without intellectual disabilities, often in their 40s or 50s, and thus may also have epileptic seizures (see below).

There are also differences in incidence between higher- and lower-income countries in that the incidence of epilepsy is higher in the latter, probably because of infectious diseases affecting the brain (Fiest et al, 2017).

DEFINITION AND CLASSIFICATION

Historically, a diagnosis of epilepsy was made after two unprovoked epileptic seizures had occurred. This remains important as many people will have an epileptic seizure without recurrence once in their life. It is important to understand that in many instances a single seizure caused by, for example, an encephalitis, a metabolic disturbance, a brain trauma or alcohol withdrawal does not warrant a diagnosis of epilepsy. Nowadays, however, a diagnosis of epilepsy will be made after a first unprovoked seizure if there is an underlying condition which indicates a high recurrence risk (Fisher et al, 2014). For example, a high risk of recurrence is likely after a cerebral infarction thus a diagnosis of epilepsy should be made at the stage of first seizure and drug treatment initiated. It is important to know in clinical practice, that two seizures within 24 hours are counted as one for this definition.

Classifying seizures and epilepsy types is crucial for identifying the right treatment. The International League against Epilepsy (ILAE) is the world organisation of epilepsy professionals. This institution has recently introduced new classifications of seizures and of epilepsy types (Fisher et al, 2017; Scheffer et al, 2017). Given the transition from the older classification to the new may take several years both classifications may be in use for some time. This chapter therefore will provide not only an overview of the new classification of epilepsy but also a basic overview of the older. Different seizure types under both classifications are summarised in Table 14.1.

Older classification

Under the older classification, epileptic seizures are divided into focal and generalised seizures (see Figure 14.1). Focal (or in other words: partial) seizures are simple or complex. "Simple" just means that consciousness is preserved during the seizure, "complex" that consciousness is impaired. One criticism of these definitions is that the terms "simple" and "complex" are misleading. Furthermore, they are only very rough classificatory terms.

Generalised seizures include generalised tonic-clonic seizures (GTCS), tonic, clonic, myoclonic

TABLE 14.1 Different seizure types under new and older classifications

New Term	Older Term	Outdated term
Generalised Onset Motor	Generalised Tonic Clonic	Grand Mal, Major Motor, Convulsion
Unknown Onset Tonic Clonic	Generalised Tonic Clonic	Grand Mal, Major Motor, Convulsion
Generalised Onset Non-Motor	Generalised Absence	Petit Mal
Focal Aware Motor	Simple Partial	Jacksonian
Focal Aware Non-Motor	Simple Partial/Aura	
Focal Impaired Motor	Complex Partial	Psychomotor, Temporal Lobe
Focal to Bilateral Tonic Clonic	Secondary Generalised	Grand Mal, Major Motor, Convulsion
Focal/Generalised Myoclonic	Myoclonic	Minor Motor
Focal/Generalised Atonic/Tonic	Atonic/Tonic Drop Attack	
Focal/Generalised Clonic/Tonic	Clonic/Tonic	

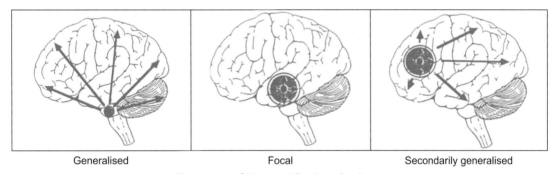

Generalised Focal Secondarily generalised

Figure 14.1 Older classification of epilepsy

seizures and absences. It is important to note that a GTCS may arise within the context of a generalised or of a focal (or partial) epilepsy; in the latter it is termed a secondarily generalised tonic-clonic seizure (see Figure 14.1). An epilepsy can be symptomatic (the aetiology is known), kryptogenic (symptomatic aetiology is assumed but not proven) or idiopathic (a genetic aetiology is assumed).

New classification

In the current classification of epileptic seizures the distinction between focal and generalised seizures has been maintained (Fisher et al, 2017) (see Figure 14.2).

Focal

Focal seizures are separated into "aware" and "impaired awareness". "Aware" means that the person is able to recall the seizure afterwards, "impaired awareness" that they are not. A second distinction is between seizures with and without motor symptoms: "motor onset" or "non-motor onset" seizures. So, in the event that a person can't recall the entire seizure, and there are automatisms like lip smacking or swallowing during the seizure, then it is called a focal non-aware motor seizure with automatisms. This is being called a psychomotor seizure by many and some might argue it is acceptable to keep older terms for colloquial use.

The application of the new classification may lead to terms that seem to be paradoxical. A person who has a seizure which he or she cannot recall entirely but which started with a déjà-vu experience is a focal non-aware cognitive seizure. This déjà-vu experience is known as an 'aura' - a warning that a seizure is about to occur. 'Aura' is another term that has not been retained in the

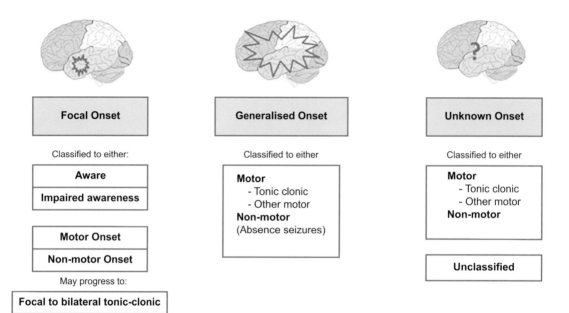

Aware = Awareness during the seizure, knowledge of self and environment, consciousness is intact.
Motor = Movement or motion
Unclassified = Seizures with patterns that do not fit into the other categories or there is insufficient information to classify the seizure

Figure 14.2 Newer classification of epilepsy Source: Redrawn with permission from Epilepsy Action Australia, https://www.epilepsy.org.au/

new classification but may be useful in clinical practice. It is also important to remember that some people with intellectual disabilities will not have the cognitive ability and/or communication skills/vocabulary to describe a seizure, but this should not mean that they are unable to recall having one.

Generalised

Generalised epilepsies typically present with generalised epileptiform activity on an EEG (electroencephalogram) and are associated with a range of seizure types including absence, myoclonic, atonic, tonic, and tonic–clonic seizures (Scheffer et al, 2017). They are often caused by a genetic predisposition and as such are called genetic generalised epilepsies.

Whilst the classification of the epilepsies differentiates between focal and generalised epilepsy types there is also a combined generalised and focal type and an unknown type (Scheffer et al, 2017). Aetiology is subdivided into five (plus unknown) categories: structural, genetic, infectious, metabolic, immune.

Status epilepticus

While a "regular" epileptic seizure terminates by itself after a relatively short time, a status epilepticus is a seizure lasting for more than five minutes or a series of at least two epileptic seizures with no interval during which the affected person regains a normal state of function (Trinka et al, 2015). Every seizure type can occur as a status epilepticus. A non-convulsive (as opposed to convulsive) status epilepticus may only be characterised by blurred consciousness or behaviour changes and often needs an EEG recording (see below) for establishing the diagnosis. However, status epilepticus of tonic-clonic seizures is a life-threatening situation and needs immediate treatment (see later section on rescue medication).

PROGNOSIS

Epilepsy in general is associated with a good prognosis. Around 70% of those affected will become seizure free. On the other hand, this means that around 30% will continue to have seizures. The more antiepileptic drugs have been tried with a person, the more unlikely is a hope for seizure freedom with the next drug. When two drugs have failed – provided they have been appropriately selected, used and tolerated – the epilepsy is called "drug resistant" (Kwan et al, 2010). A cross-sectional examination of 675 residents, described 'as a rule with additional intellectual disabilities of different degrees' in long-term care at the Bethel Epilepsy Centre in Germany identified 35.6% overall as seizure free (Huber et al, 2005). For those with mild intellectual disabilities the seizure free figure was 39.2% dropping to 21.9% in people with the most profound intellectual disabilities. This means the prognosis of epilepsy in people with intellectual disabilities tends to be worse than that found in the general population but seizure freedom may still be achieved in a considerable number; in those who continue to have seizures, it is even more important to avoid the intolerable side effects of drugs and help achieve a good quality of life.

Although epilepsy in general is not life-threatening, mortality rates in those with the condition are higher than the general population. This applies to all people with epilepsy but even more so in those with intellectual disabilities. The relative mortality rates of diseases can be measured by the Standardized Mortality Ratio (SMR). In those with epilepsy it is around 1.6–3 but this rises to between 7–50 if the person also has an intellectual disability (Forsgren et al, 2005). This elevation is in part due to pneumonias, an important cause of death in people with epilepsy and intellectual disabilities, but also to Sudden Unexpected Death in Epilepsy (SUDEP).

Around one in 1,000 people with epilepsy die every year from SUDEP (DeGiorgio et al, 2019); those with frequent sleep-associated tonic-clonic seizures have an increased risk. Therefore, optimising treatment and improving adherence to treatment is the most important preventative step; attending to a person after a tonic-clonic seizure can also limit the risk but this is only possible if the seizures are detected. Seizure detection devices can help but a plan must be made as to who will be alerted and how this person can visit the individual, especially in the case of those living on their own. People with Dravet syndrome (see later section Genetics in diagnosis for further detail about this condition) carry a higher risk of dying from SUDEP. Relatives bereft by SUDEP have demanded in recent years that doctors should inform people earlier about the risks (see Reader activity 14.1).

READER ACTIVITY 14.1

Click on the Epilepsy Society link below and listen to Kerry's story.

Think about how you might communicate the risk of SUDEP in an accessible way to someone with an intellectual disability and their family.

Consider what additional support they may need.

https://epilepsysociety.org.uk/about-epilepsy/personal-stories/kerrys-story

Diagnosis and differential diagnosis

Effective treatment of epilepsy is dependent on an accurate diagnosis of seizure type. A full and person-centred assessment must be undertaken to establish the cause and effect of seizures on any person with an intellectual disability and their quality of life. Where possible, decisions about potential investigations and treatment must be made in partnership with the individual and their relevant others. Particular attention must therefore be paid to the accessibility of these processes (see also Chapter 4).

Regardless of the presence or absence of an intellectual disability, the first approach to a person with a seizure disorder is the same - taking the personal and medical history and completing a physical examination. Taking a history is especially important when epilepsy is suspected compared with other diseases as doctors have rarely the opportunity to directly observe a seizure. This means important details have to be reported either by the person themselves or by relatives and caregivers. Use of epilepsy diaries that record the timing and presentation of seizures can also be useful (see also section on Evaluating treatment). Taking the history and making a diagnosis in epilepsy sometimes resembles detective work. Whilst reports from individuals, relatives, caregivers, teachers, colleagues and so on is the classical way of obtaining information, the possibility to watch and analyse seizures using recording devices such as smartphones has increased in recent years (Pandher and Bhullar, 2016). Relatives and caregivers should be encouraged to record seizures if a firm diagnosis has yet to be made or when new seizure types occur. In the event of recording, it is important to remember that the safety of the person takes precedence.

READER ACTIVITY 14.2

A number of best practice guidelines exist to promote the safety of an individual experiencing a seizure.

Read and make notes on What to do when someone has a seizure provided by the UK charity Epilepsy Action (2020b) at https://www.epilepsy.org.uk/info/firstaid/what-to-do

The taking of routine bloods is necessary when a person with a first seizure presents to the emergency department in order to exclude acute symptomatic seizures occurring with metabolic disorders like hypoglycaemia (low blood sugar) or infections. Examination of the cerebrospinal fluid (which protects the brain and spinal column) by lumbar puncture is necessary when encephalitis (inflammation of the brain) or meningitis (inflammation of the meninges, protective layers around the brain and spinal cord) is suspected. Moreover, lumbar puncture has gained importance in the diagnosis of autoimmune diseases as causes of epilepsy and epileptic seizures. The most important technical examination methods in epileptology are the EEG and neuroimaging with Computed Tomography (CT) and Magnetic Resonance Imaging (MRI) scans. Some people need sedating medication before examinations. In case of an EEG recording, this must be a medication which does not influence the EEG, e.g. a low-potency neuroleptic.

Epileptiform potentials (a special type of brain wave detected by EEG) support the diagnosis of different types of epilepsy; the EEG is also crucial in diagnosing non-convulsive status epilepticus. Despite these benefits, the role of EEG in monitoring the course of epilepsy is normally overestimated. This means, repeated EEG recordings do not normally indicate success or non-success in seizure treatment.

While a CT scan of the brain (and skull and neck) is an emergency examination after a first seizure or when a head injury due to a seizure (drop attack) is suspected, thorough examination for the aetiology of a seizure needs an MRI of the brain which can be distressing because of noise, narrow space and duration of the examination. All people should be prepared for this procedure and there exist a range of online resources that can help support those with intellectual disabilities. In some people with intellectual disabilities, a CT or an MRI scan may only be obtained under general anaesthesia, and therefore the benefit of the examination has to be balanced against the normally minor risks of anaesthesia.

READER ACTIVITY 14.3

Select an online patient information guide that could be used to prepare someone needing an MRI scan.

Using the *Guide to making information accessible for people with a learning disability* published by NHS England (2018) at https://www.england.nhs.uk/wp-content/uploads/2018/06/LearningDisabilityAccessCommsGuidance.pdf

1. Reflect on the extent to which this information would be accessible to someone with an intellectual disability.
2. Consider how any improvements could be made.

Molecular genetics has made major progress in recent years. When the aetiology of a seizure is not known after the steps described here or when a syndrome is suspected, then genetic examination, chromosome analysis, Array-CGH or other genetic examinations, should be considered, normally in cooperation with a geneticist. Making a genetic diagnosis can give guidance for treatment and assist with family planning if desired. Knowing the aetiology of the epilepsy can be helpful for the affected person or for the family. Country-specific legislation applies to the use of genetic diagnostics.

Psychogenic non-epileptic seizures

Psychogenic non-epileptic seizures (PNES) form an important differential diagnosis in seizure disorders. PNES are paroxysmal attacks with symptoms that can resemble epileptic seizures; they are not associated with epileptiform activity in the EEG (LaFrance et al, 2013) however they can also occur alongside epileptic seizures in some people. In a recent study among a group of adults with epilepsy and intellectual disabilities living in a care facility, 7.1% were also found to have PNES. Most of them were female and had mild or moderate intellectual disabilities (van Ool et al, 2018). It is important to differentiate PNES from epileptic seizures otherwise a person will receive unnecessary and potentially harmful anti-epileptic drug (AED) treatment including emergency interventions such as narcosis and mechanical ventilation.

Treatment of choice for PNES in general is psychotherapy. Many people with PNES have a history of psychological trauma (Labudda et al, 2018). Cognitive-behavioural therapy (CBT) with elements of dialectic-behavioural therapy (DBT) and methods of trauma therapy are also in use (Labudda et al, 2020). It can be difficult to obtain freedom from PNES but co-existing psychiatric problems will be ameliorated in many cases. Anecdotal evidence would suggest that psychosocial interventions are often helpful in people with intellectual disabilities and PNES. Seizure-precipitating situations must be analysed with professional help. The loss of a caregiver, a noisy roommate or excessive demands at work may precipitate PNES. In these cases, psychosocial interventions rather than classical psychotherapy are helpful.

Comorbidities

Epilepsy is associated with several comorbidities. The focus here will be on comorbidities in the context of epilepsy and intellectual disabilities. Depression occurs in around 20% of persons with epilepsy (Mula, 2019); the presence of epilepsy is also associated with negative mood symptoms in those with intellectual disabilities (van Ool et al, 2016). This may be due to reactions to stigmatisation and to the psychosocial consequences of epilepsy but there are also other reasons. Scientists have found common aetiologies of and shared pathophysiological pathways between epilepsy and depression (Kanner, 2009). Depression in people with (particularly severe) intellectual disabilities may present atypically. Unspecific symptoms like social withdrawal should arise suspicion (see Chapter 16 for more on this issue). As will be discussed in Chapter 17, behavioural difficulties are often found in people with intellectual disabilities and these are sometimes exaggerated by AEDs (antiepileptic drugs) although this may be overestimated; a comprehensive assessment is therefore essential. Treatment is multi-modal and antipsychotic medication should be administered only if necessary and for a limited period of time. Frequent somatic comorbidities in people with intellectual disabilities and thus also in those with intellectual disabilities and anxiety are shown in Table 14.2. There is a danger that symptoms of a comorbid disorder will be incorrectly attributed to the intellectual disability rather than to a distinct disease ("diagnostic overshadowing"). The consequence is that

TABLE 14.2 Selected somatic comorbidities in people with intellectual disabilities

Physical disabilities
Respiratory infections (pneumonia)
Urinary tract infections
Bone fractures
Constipation
Reflux oesophagitis
Obesity
Nutritional problems with underweight
Dental problems

the comorbid disorder will not be diagnosed and thus not be treated.

TREATMENT

Generally, the aim of antiepileptic treatment is to achieve seizure freedom or if this is not achievable a reduction in seizure frequency without intolerable side effects. If seizure freedom cannot be reached, it is important to focus on other issues affecting quality of life (QoL). In people who continue to have seizures, QoL is mainly affected by the tolerability of AEDs and the presence of comorbid depression. For people with many seizures, a reduction of the seizure frequency may not be a meaningful improvement. Reduction of drop seizures, avoidance of injuries, no occurrence of episodes of status epilepticus and a reduction in presentations to the emergency room may be much more meaningful. Also, a reduction in the frequency of rescue medication administration is an important achievement. Rescue medication is an important tool to interrupt cluster seizures (see below) but may have sedating side-effects lasting for hours and thus impairing daily living.

The pillars of epilepsy treatment are drug therapy, epilepsy surgery, rehabilitation treatment, psychotherapy and other non-pharmacological interventions and these are now discussed. Whatever the combination of treatment, it must be person-centred and agreed, where possible, with the person with an intellectual disability and/or their significant others.

Antiepileptic drugs (AEDs)

All modern AEDs undergo a strictly regulated process of robust trialling and monitoring however it is important to note that research exploring the efficacy and tolerability of antiepileptics amongst people with intellectual disabilities is currently very limited. A recent Cochrane review identified only 14 randomised controlled trials (RCTs) involving a total of 1116 people with intellectual disabilities (Jackson et al, 2015). Whilst this represents a very small number compared to the number of people without intellectual disabilities involved in pivotal studies of modern AEDs, in general the data showed the effectiveness of antiepileptics in this population. The spectrum of side effects was also comparable. However, it must be noted that the quality of this systematic review was low and therefore results should be viewed with caution; only 4 studies reported on seizure freedom, 8 on seizure frequency, also 8 on responder rate, 3 reported data on behaviour monitoring. None of the studies reported data on the cognitive effects of the AEDs used, yet this is important as behavioural and cognitive side effects of epilepsy treatment can have devastating consequences.

Despite there being around 25 available AEDs, none have been found to have superior efficacy as compared to the others (Charokopou et al, 2019). Therefore, it is even more important to adjust the drug regimen to the individual situation, especially to age, gender, comorbidities, life situation and preferences. An "ideal AED" would have the following attributes: efficacious (without losing efficacy over time), tolerable, not teratogenic (i.e. not doing harm to an unborn child when the mother is taking the drug during pregnancy), with low potential for interaction with other drugs (AEDs and comedication) and available for a reasonable price. Additional considerations might be around the different formulations of the drugs and methods of administration. This is particularly important for those who have swallowing difficulties and/or are enterally fed.

To review all available AEDs would be far beyond the scope of this chapter. Nevertheless, a few drugs shall be presented here, especially with regard to their use with people with intellectual disabilities. Those that are indicated for certain syndromes are discussed later in the chapter.

Enzyme inducing antiepileptic drugs (EI-AEDs)

The strongest EI-AEDs are phenobarbital, phenytoin and carbamazepine. Enzyme induction means that the drugs enhance metabolism by the liver and thus have a high potential for interaction with other drugs. Some people with intellectual disabilities may also be being treated with psychotropic drugs, and some of those may show increased metabolism in combination with EI-AEDs. Also, EI-AEDs may have long-term consequences in terms of increased risk for osteoporosis (reduction in bone density often caused by low levels of calcium) or atherosclerosis (the narrowing of arteries caused by the build-up of fats). Despite the potential dangers of these drugs, EI-AEDs are still used in many countries, in some instances for economic reasons. If this is unavoidable, interactions and tolerability must be carefully monitored.

AEDs with behavioural side-effects

Epilepsy is a disorder of the brain, AEDs thus act on the brain, and therefore, they – at least some of them – have a potential to induce behavioural change that can include increased risk of aggression and irritability (Brodie et al, 2016). For example, levetiracetam leads to aggressiveness in around 10% of patients with epilepsy increasing to 30% amongst those who also have intellectual disabilities (Brodtkorb et al, 2004). The structurally related AED brivaracetam seems to be associated with fewer behavioural side effects (Brandt et al, 2016, 2020) but they have been observed in people with intellectual disabilities as well (Andres et al, 2018). Perampanel, licensed in the EU for the add-on treatment of focal onset and tonic-clonic seizures from the age of 12 years (in the US also for monotherapy of focal epilepsy from age 4), is a very potent AED, for instance in tonic-clonic seizures (French et al, 2015). Behavioural changes including severe aggressive and self-injurious behaviour have been reported (Huber, 2014; Andres et al, 2017) for this drug and these need to be monitored.

AEDs with cognitive side-effects

Some AEDs may be associated with cognitive side-effects, for example topiramate and zonisamide may affect cognition, especially word fluency. Significantly, there is some danger that a cognitive decline in a person with an intellectual disability might be incorrectly attributed to a process of ageing rather than to a drug effect. It is therefore important to monitor cognition after a change of the AED regimen, at least when certain drugs are involved. It has been shown that people with mild and moderate intellectual disabilities may experience the same type of side-effects under topiramate that have been described in people without intellectual disabilities (Brandt et al, 2015) and that a subset of widely used neuropsychological instruments can be administered in this group to monitor any changes in cognition (for example see recent study by Meschede et al, 2020).

Sodium channel blocking agents

This is a group of drugs widely used especially in focal epilepsies. Main examples are carbamazepine, oxcarbazepine, eslicarbazepine acetate, lamotrigine and in different ways lacosamide and cenobamate (Krauss et al, 2020). Dizziness is a common side-effect whilst carbamazepine, oxcarbazepine and eslicarbazepine are also associated with hyponatremia (low sodium concentration in the blood).

Valproate

This drug is listed here as a group in its own right. It is a broad spectrum drug, i.e. it can be used in the treatment and management of a range of different seizure types but its use has been restricted by authorities in women of child-bearing age as it is highly teratogenic. It may cause neural tube defects even in low doses and can lead to behavioural problems and impaired intelligence when unborn children are exposed to the drug in utero. Therefore, the use of valproate in women of child-bearing age is limited to cases in which all other efforts have failed. More information about the risk of valproate in pregnancy can be found in the guidance issued by the UK Medicines and Healthcare Products Regulatory Agency (2020).

In clinical practice a careful approach to the prescription of AEDs is necessary in people with epilepsy and intellectual disabilities. One has to assume a higher sensitivity to side effects in comparison to the general population with epilepsy, and therefore observation, especially with regard to subtle cognitive side effects, requires special attention (Harbord, 2000). If possible, doctors should treat epilepsy with monotherapy, i.e. just one AED is administered. If this is not successful, the drug should be changed to another single drug, thus maintaining monotherapy. This may be repeated with other drugs but normally at this point a second drug will be added leading to combination therapy. Two should be the maximum number of AEDs used with

an individual but there may be exceptions where this is increased to three. Indeed, there are still instances where four or more have been prescribed to a person with an intellectual disability however polytherapy like this should be challenged as it can lead to unwanted interactions and potential harmful side-effects. This reflects the disadvantages that people with intellectual disabilities still face today. Sometimes, general neurologists are reluctant to withdraw drugs and families or caregivers fear withdrawal seizures (those that occur as result of stopping the medication). In these cases, individuals should be referred to epilepsy specialists who will advise.

Rescue medication

A single epileptic seizure, as long as not associated with injuries or dangerous behaviour, is not an emergency. People who are present while someone has a seizure should try to protect the affected person by, for example, removing burning cigarettes, sharp-edged furniture or preventing the person from running into traffic. They must not exert force or try to place anything between the teeth. The administration of rescue medication (RM) is an important topic as many people with intellectual disabilities have severe and complex epilepsies that give rise to cluster seizures or status epilepticus. Cluster seizures (repetitive seizures not fulfilling the criteria for status epilepticus) may have a major negative impact on daily living, and status epilepticus – at least a convulsive status – is a life-threatening situation. A drug that can be administered by caregivers enables treatment to start without having to wait for the emergency services to arrive. RM normally belongs to the group of benzodiazepines. Licensed drugs and available preparations that constitute rescue medication differ markedly from country to country therefore, they will not be covered here in detail but some general guidance follows.

Rectal preparations, for instance diazepam, are available and have proven efficacy and safety. Rectal administration of a drug is, however, difficult during a seizure and is nowadays regarded as invasive, potentially comprising a person's dignity. Benzodiazepines for intranasal (via the nose) and buccal (via the mouth, between gums and cheek) are much more convenient but their availability and labelling vary between countries and thus have to be checked. If a seizure cluster or a status epilepticus does not terminate after the administration of RM, then further treatment by the emergency services or in hospital is necessary. Schools, residential homes and places of employment may demand RM to be given after a single seizure. This is normally not necessary however such a decision should be made in advance in partnership with the person, their family and relevant health professionals. Administration of rescue medication should follow the protocol outlined in a person's individual plan of care.

Crises in people with intellectual disabilities can present emergency services with unique challenges. For example, the taking of medical history or a personal examination can be difficult so caregivers must be involved.

Admission to hospital – be it in case of casualty or for a planned in-patient stay – may be distressing for a person with an intellectual disability so reasonable adjustments (accommodations) need to be made to minimise levels of distress and ensure care is person centred (see Chapter 10).

 READER ACTIVITY 14.4

There exist a range of resources that might help people with intellectual disabilities to communicate important issues about their epilepsy and its management to health professionals in the event of, for example, a hospital admission.

Can you identify any?

Consider the extent to which they empower the individual to have maximum control over the situation.

Epilepsy surgery

When two adequate AED trials have failed in a person with focal epilepsy, the patient should be referred to a specialised centre in order to assess them for the option of surgery. People with intellectual disabilities may also benefit from being offered this form of treatment with one retrospective study showing a comparable clinical outcome to those without intellectual disabilities (Davies et al, 2009). Yet numbers of people with a low IQ in this study were small and it has shown that prognosis of resective epilepsy surgery (removal of brain tissue in the area where seizures originate) in people with intellectual disabilities depends on the level of impairment; the milder the intellectual disability, the better the prognosis, and vice versa. Resective surgery is even an option in a multifocal disorder like the Tuberous Sclerosis Complex (TSC, see also below) (Jansen et al, 2007). Corpus callosotomy (CC) is a palliative surgical option in epilepsy for drop attacks. In a small published case series nearly 40% of patients were reported to be free of disabling seizures one year after surgery (Asadi-Pooya et al, 2013). Vagus nerve stimulation may also be considered (Cross et al, 2017). This process involves sending electrical impulses through the vagus nerve to calm irregular brain activity.

Diets

The Ketogenic diet (KD) is the treatment of choice in genetically determined glucose-transporter defects. Ketones can also help improve seizure control, as a KD mimics the metabolic state of fasting by the intake of nutritional fat (Elia et al, 2017). There are different forms of KD including the Modified Atkins Diet. KD is widely used in refractory epilepsies (seizures not controlled by seizure medication) in children. There are also several studies showing its efficacy in adults although there remain questions about long-term efficacy and safety (see also Goswami and Sharma, 2019).

Cannabidiol

Cannabidiol has been recently introduced into the array of options. There is much demand for cannabidiol from individuals and relatives in recent years. It has to be kept in mind that it is not a panacea or an especially "healthy" option because it is derived from a plant but it is a drug like others with proven efficacy for two syndromes, Dravet and Lennox-Gastaut (Epilepsy Action, 2020a), and most recently Tuberous Sclerosis (Tiele et al, 2021). However, like other efficacious drugs, side effects can be expected.

Psychotherapy

Whilst not a treatment for epilepsy itself, psychotherapy is supportive therapy that enables people to cope with the condition and is important for the treatment of comorbid depression and anxiety; this said it can be difficult to find a psychotherapist who is experienced in treating people with intellectual disabilities.

LIVING (WELL) WITH EPILEPSY

It is important to maintain a regular sleep-wake cycle in genetic generalised epilepsy as fragmented sleep can contribute to increased risk of seizure activity (Gibbon et al, 2019) although it is less important in focal epilepsies. Alcohol consumption should also be restricted to very small amounts or even avoided. Many AEDs are associated with cerebellar (from the cerebellum, the area of the brain that controls coordination and balance) side-effects like dizziness and unsteady gait, as is alcohol, therefore alcohol may increase AED toxicity. Moreover, alcohol may provoke seizures in some syndromes. While these simple rules for daily living may be helpful, unnecessary restrictions must be avoided.

Sports

Exercising is important for all of us; it improves not just physical health, e.g. cardiac fitness and muscle strength but also mental well-being and self-esteem. When done together with others, it can lead to better social integration. Exercising is also important as, previously mentioned, some AEDs, especially the enzyme-inducing ones, increase the risk of developing conditions such as osteoporosis. Physical and nutritional problems, living in residential care and the presence of – among other syndromes – Down syndrome contribute also to this risk (Mayer, 2005). Exercising can improve coordination which decreases the risk of falls preventing bone fractures.

Whilst there is no evidence to suggest a positive correlation between increased physical activity and an improvement in seizure management, only in rare exceptions does sport worsen the seizures. Yet people with epilepsy can and do face restrictions on sports which in turn can affect their opportunity to engage with others and be a barrier towards optimising their mental wellbeing, particularly where the epilepsy is accompanied by a diagnosis of depression. Safety of the affected individual is paramount however everything should be done to help facilitate access to sport. Swimming is dangerous for those who are not seizure free therefore they must be accompanied by a person who can rescue them while in the pool or a proven buoyancy aid must be worn. Swimming in open water is to be avoided. A booklet with recommendations for several forms of sport can be found in the online Useful resources (Dröge et al, 2021). Although it is only available in German, the colour-coded tables may be helpful for readers of other languages as well.

Patient empowerment/coping

If epilepsy is resistant to therapy, the focus of treatment changes. Ultimately, this is about achieving the best possible QoL even with persistent epileptic seizures. Patient education, self-management and empowerment are important steps. The Psycho Educative Programme about Epilepsy (PEPE) is a programme designed for people with intellectual disabilities and epilepsy. It is originally a German programme which has been translated into English (see Kushinga, 2007). Trainer courses are available in English.

Evaluating treatment

Every treatment effort must be evaluated; its efficacy must be balanced against side effects, risks and harms of the therapy. The primary goal in epilepsy treatment is to achieve seizure freedom or, at a minimum, an improvement in seizure frequency. This must be monitored. The most important instrument is a seizure diary. The individual or relatives and caregivers must be instructed to document each seizure in the diary, coding different seizure types with different letters or symbols (see online Useful resources). A treatment regimen will sometimes be evaluated after years, and it is not possible to recollect data without written documentation. Although the reliability of individuals' and relatives' recordings may be limited, there is currently no better form of documentation. Seizure detection devices e.g. wrist worn sensors, bed monitors etc. are available but their value is currently more in the field of safety and not of documentation. One reason is that they also have limited use, capturing only certain seizure types, mostly tonic-clonic seizures. In those who cannot keep diaries by themselves, caregivers, e.g. staff in a residential home, have this task.

Adherence to or compliance with a therapeutic regimen is limited in epilepsy (de Mota Gomes et al, 2016), and due to cognitive difficulties including memory and comprehension can present specific challenges when working with people with intellectual disabilities. Therefore, adherence should be monitored, at least in the case of breakthrough seizures occurring after a period of seizure freedom. Measurement of the serum concentrations ("blood level") of AEDs is called therapeutic drug monitoring (TDM). Whilst it has been the mainstay of evaluation for decades, its value has been questioned in recent years, at least for the newer AEDs. The remit of TDM should be clear to all those involved. Besides the control of adherence it can be used when side effects or incorrect administration of a drug or even an intoxication are suspected, also for certain drugs in pregnancy, in renal (kidney) and hepatic (liver) failure (Brandt and May, 2011). When impaired adherence is detected, the patient should not be blamed, but the underlying difficulties identified and solutions sought. Some people may be non-compliant when they do not understand the importance of regular administration. In this case, a patient education course (for example the PEPE programme) is helpful. Some may forget to take their medication. In this case, a weekly dispenser should be recommended, possibly in addition to a helpful smartphone application. If all this does not lead to success, others must take responsibility to remind the person to take their medication.

Another reason for irregular administration may be side effects, i.e. the person feels he or she is not tolerating the medication and therefore does not take it regularly. A doctor may then detect a low blood level and increase the dose. This will lead to even more side effects and in turn to more non-compliance resulting in a vicious circle. Therefore – and for other reasons – the individuals must be asked about and examined for side effects. Individuals and caregivers can give information on sedating side effects whilst simple examinations can reveal symptoms of ataxia (a group of disorders affecting co-ordination, balance and speech), and as previously mentioned, cognitive tolerability must be monitored using neuropsychological instruments.

Safety issues

Although absolute safety of a person with epilepsy cannot be achieved, any attempts to maximise this must be balanced against their autonomy. A seizure protection helmet can prevent skull and brain injury in those with frequent falls. These can be manufactured and tailored to individual needs, with fortifications for the protection of glasses, for instance. Acceptance by patients can be improved by a choice of colours. In case of potential back injuries, protectors may be discussed. The need for close attendance also applies to those with uncontrolled epilepsy taking a bath. A prominent review (Verita,

2015) focusing on the case of Connor Sparrowhawk, a young English man with an intellectual disability and epilepsy who drowned in the bath in an in-patient facility, concluded his death could have been prevented by improved epilepsy risk management.

GENETICS IN DIAGNOSIS

Major advances have been made in the field of genetics in recent years. This has led to improved diagnostic methods and also in some cases to the designation of novel therapeutic approaches that continue to evolve. Care for people with intellectual disabilities in this area is thus progressive although it is interesting to note that for many years it was a neglected area of investigation. Yet the marked variability in the symptoms associated with particular genetic findings mean that there are still many unanswered questions. For example, whilst most people with DEPDC5 gene mutations (an autosomal dominant inherited condition where the affected family members can have different types of focal epilepsies, most frequently frontal lobe epilepsy) are of unaffected intelligence, there are also people with intellectual disabilities among them (Baldassari et al, 2019). The next part of this section considers a number of specific conditions linked to intellectual disabilities that have epilepsy as part of their clinical manifestation. These syndromes show typical symptoms and constellation which have implications for treatment, counselling and prognosis.

Dravet syndrome

With this syndrome the onset of epilepsy is within the first 2 years of life, often within the first year. Initial development is normal. There is a typical seizure tetrad of early infantile febrile clonic seizures, myoclonias, atypical absences (absences that don't follow the same pattern as typical absences e.g. may be longer in duration) and focal non-aware seizures. Heterozygous SCN1A loss-of-function mutations are the most frequent genetic cause. Fever, heat and sports activities are frequent seizure-precipitating factors. With regard to drug treatment, sodium-channel blocking AEDs must usually be avoided. Stiripentol and cannabidiol are in use in Dravet syndrome but other AEDs are also working. There are promising data for fenfluramine, a drug with a serotonergic mechanism (i.e. modifies the effect of serotonin in the body) (Lagae et al, 2020), and the drug has been approved by the European Medicines Agency for the treatment of seizures associated with Dravet syndrome as an add-on therapy to other antiepileptic medicines for patients 2 years of age and older.

Tuberous Sclerosis Complex

Tuberous Sclerosis Complex (TSC) is a neuropsychiatric system disease with – in varying frequency and degrees – epilepsy, intellectual disabilities, autism and social dysfunction (Curatolo et al, 2015). TSC has also typical somatic comorbidities. Tumours of the brain, lung, heart and kidneys may occur. There is a typical appearance with facial angiofibromas and other dermatologic symptoms. Dental enamel defects may be present. Having said all this, it is obvious that treatment should be in the hands of specialists, for instance in TSC centres, who deliver comprehensive care for people with the syndrome. There is, however, evidence that this happens only in a proportion of people (Hamer et al, 2018). Brain MRI shows multiple tubers as structural correlates for TSC. The epilepsy in these patients is focal, and thus AEDs working in focal epilepsies are in use. Some years ago, the mTOR pathway (a signalling pathway in the brain) was detected as the pathophysiological mechanism for TSC. This has led to the discovery of everolimus, an immunosuppressive agent, for the treatment of TSC, first for brain and kidney tumours and meanwhile also for epileptic seizures in TSC (French et al, 2016; Franz et al, 2018). Although there are usually multiple lesions in TSC, successful epilepsy surgery is possible. Therefore, those with TSC and drug refractory epilepsy should be referred to a surgical epilepsy centre.

Lennox-Gastaut syndrome

This syndrome is not that precisely defined in comparison to the aforementioned. A consensus group has fixed criteria for the diagnosis: Lennox-Gastaut syndrome (LGS) is associated with multiple seizure types, to include tonic, atonic, atypical absence seizures with tonic seizures predominantly occurring at night and an abnormal EEG consisting primarily of an interictal (between seizures) pattern of diffuse, slow spike-wave (SSW) complexes at <3Hz, occurring during wakefulness (Cross et al, 2017). LGS occurs mainly in people with intellectual disabilities although intellectual disability is not always present at the onset of the syndrome. Epilepsy in LGS is usually drug refractory. Drugs in frequent use are valproate, lamotrigine, topiramate, zonisamide, levetiracetam, lamotrigine, and recently cannabidiol as a non-exclusive list. Felbamate is a drug of further choice when "all other options" have failed as it can cause life-threatening liver and haematological problems. Rufinamide works in drop seizures associated with LGS.

Down syndrome

This syndrome with a trisomy of chromosome 21 has threefold implications with regard to epilepsy. First, focal epilepsy may develop, mainly in childhood and youth. Second, other paroxysmal symptoms like cardiogenic syncopes and behavioural symptoms have to be differentiated from epileptic seizures. Third, epilepsy may develop within the course of a dementia from Alzheimer type in adulthood, often around 40 – 50 years of age or even earlier. This goes along with myoclonic jerks and tonic-clonic seizures. The term Late Onset Myoclonic Epilepsy in Down Syndrome (LOMEDS) has been coined. Drug treatment has to be chosen and initiated carefully as persons may negatively react with it, behavioural side effects being a specific concern.

READER ACTIVITY 14.5
Consolidation of learning

To consolidate your learning from this chapter, please read **Box 14.1 Elizabeth's story**

Imagining you are supporting Elizabeth, answer the following questions

* How would you gather evidence that Elizabeth may be having epileptic seizures?
* Is there any evidence to support a differential diagnosis?
* How would you advise Elizabeth's sister to gather evidence to aid diagnosis?
* How would you support Elizabeth to take her medication?
* What safety measures would you advise?
* What might be triggering seizures?

Answers may be found in the accompanying online resource.

BOX 14.1 Elizabeth's story

Elizabeth has just turned 47. She celebrates her birthday on New Year's Eve, in earlier times, an excuse for quite a party. Elizabeth was the second of two daughters, born to Bill and Mary. Her father was a landlord and his wife and their girls helped out in the pub. Elizabeth used to reminisce about happy times with her family but she would never talk about her mother's suicide. Many elements of this were kept from her. Bill never talked about Mary after her death and her photographs were quickly taken down. One morning Elizabeth awoke to a group of Bill's friends moving through the flat, taking away Mary's clothes.

Physically, despite having Down syndrome, Elizabeth had been generally healthy. She would have intermittent ear infections and developed a dental abscess in her early thirties. One hot summer's day, aged 16, when collecting glasses at her father's pub, Elizabeth had collapsed without warning. This had been a near miss and she never worked in the pub again.

Now Elizabeth's life is quite different. She has recently moved in with her sister's family. She had begun to display signs of not coping as well in Independent Supported Living. Her bedroom had been at the top of a steep flight of stairs and Elizabeth had been struggling with depth perception. She has become increasingly fearful of crossing the threshold into different rooms. Elizabeth has had frequent episodes of urinary incontinence and also experienced constipation on a regular basis. Care staff coming to help her get ready in the morning noticed her body would jerk when she awoke.

Elizabeth has a recent diagnosis of dementia. Some days she can almost seem like her old self. She gets a twinkle in her eye and her sister sees the old Elizabeth. However, there are days when the old Elizabeth seems lost, gone forever. Elizabeth increasingly refuses medication, causing her sister great anxiety. Recently Elizabeth has had two episodes where her body has stiffened, and all four limbs have intermittently shaken. Her skin goes a grey colour and she gets tinges of blue around the mouth. These episodes lasted about a minute each time. After the episode Elizabeth is confused, can be agitated, tired and needs to sleep. Elizabeth's sister suspects that she may have had some of these episodes at night because she can be very hard to awake and can be very confused in the morning. One morning there was dried blood around Elizabeth's mouth and on her pillow.

With thanks to Edward Jones, Learning Disability Epilepsy Nurse, Humber Teaching NHS Foundation Trust, UK

CONCLUSION

Epilepsy is a complex health condition that can affect different dimensions of health and wellbeing. The higher prevalence of the condition amongst those with intellectual disabilities justifies special consideration of the needs of this group. Without careful management, epilepsy can lead to both a decrease in quality of life and an increase in the possibility of premature death. Epilepsy management may be multi-factorial and a range of options exist to maximise seizure control. Wherever possible, decisions around treatment should be made in partnership with individuals and where appropriate and necessary, significant others.

REFERENCES

Andres, E., Kerling, F., Hamer, H., et al. (2017). Behavioural changes in patients with intellectual disability treated with perampanel. *Acta Neurologica Scandinavica*, *136*(6), 645–653.

Andres, E., Kerling, F., Hamer, H., et al. (2018). Behavioural changes in patients with intellectual disability treated with brivaracetam. *Acta Neurologica Scandinavica*, *138*(3), 195–202.

Asadi-Pooya, A. A., Malekmohamadi, Z., Kamgarpour, A., et al. (2013). Corpus callosotomy is a valuable therapeutic option for patients with Lennox-Gastaut syndrome and medically refractory seizures. *Epilepsy & Behavior*, *29*(2), 285–288.

Baldassari, S., Picard, F., Verbeek, N. E., et al. (2019). The landscape of epilepsy-related GATOR1 variants. *Genetics in Medicine*, *21*(2), 398–408.

Brandt, C., & May, T. W. (2011). Therapeutic drug monitoring of newer antiepileptic drugs. *Laboratoriums Medizin*, *35*(3), 161–169.

Brandt, C., Lahr, D., & May, T. W. (2015). Cognitive adverse events of topiramate in patients with epilepsy and intellectual disability. *Epilepsy & Behavior*, *45*, 261–264.

Brandt, C., May, T. W., & Bien, C. G. (2016). Brivaracetam as adjunctive therapy for the treatment of partial-onset seizures in patients with epilepsy: the current evidence base. *Therapeutic Advances in Neurological Disorders*, *9*(6), 474–482.

Brandt, C., Klein, P., Badalamenti, V., et al. (2020). Safety and tolerability of adjunctive brivaracetam in epilepsy: in-depth pooled analysis. *Epilepsy & Behavior, 103*(Pt A), 106864.

Brodie, M. J., Besag, F., Ettinger, A. B., et al. (2016). Epilepsy, antiepileptic drugs, and aggression: an evidence-based review. *Pharmacological Reviews, 68*(3), 563–602.

Brodtkorb, E., Klees, T. M., Nakken, K. O., et al. (2004). Levetiracetam in adult patients with and without learning disability: focus on behavioral adverse effects. *Epilepsy & Behavior, 5*(2), 231–235.

Charokopou, M., Harvey, R., Srivastava, K., et al. (2019). Relative performance of brivaracetam as adjunctive treatment of focal seizures in adults: a network meta-analysis. *Current Medical Research and Opinion, 35*(8), 1345–1354.

Cross, J. H., Auvin, S., Falip, M., et al. (2017). Expert opinion on the management of Lennox-Gastaut syndrome: treatment algorithms and practical considerations. *Frontiers in Neurology, 8*, 505.

Curatolo, P., Moavero, R., & de Vries, P. J. (2015). Neurological and neuropsychiatric aspects of tuberous sclerosis complex. *The Lancet Neurology, 14*(7), 733–745.

Davies, R., Baxendale, S., Thompson, P., et al. (2009). Epilepsy surgery for people with a low IQ. *Seizure, 18*(2), 150–152.

DeGiorgio, C. M., Curtis, A., Hertling, D., et al. (2019). Sudden unexpected death in epilepsy: risk factors, biomarkers, and prevention. *Acta Neurologica Scandinavica, 139*(3), 220–230.

de Mota Gomes, M., Navarro, T., Keepansseril, A., et al. (2016). Increasing adherence to treatment in epilepsy: what do the strongest trials show? *Acta Neurologica Scandinavica, 135*, 266–272.

Dröge, C., Thorbecke, R., & Brandt, C. (2021). *Sport bei epilepsie*. Bonn: The Michael Foundation.

Elia, M., Klepper, J., Leiendecker, B., et al. (2017). Ketogenicdiets in the treatment of epilepsy. *Current Pharmaceutical Design, 23*(37), 5691–5701.

Epilepsy, Action. (2020a). *Medical cannabis for epilepsy in the UK*. Available at: https://www.epilepsy.org.uk/info/treatment/cannabis-based-treatments. [Accessed 30 December 2020].

Epilepsy Action. (2020b). *What to do when someone has a seizure*. Available at: https://www.epilepsy.org.uk/info/firstaid/what-to-do. [Accessed 30 December 2020].

Epilepsy Society. Kerry's story. Available: https://epilepsysociety.org.uk/about-epilepsy/personal-stories/kerrys-story. [Accessed 30 December 2020].

Fiest, K. M., Sauro, K. M., Wiebe, S., et al. (2017). Prevalence and incidence of epilepsy: a systematic review and meta-analysis of international studies. *Neurology, 88*(3), 296–303.

Fisher, R. S., Acevedo, C., Arzimanoglou, A., et al. (2014). ILAE official report: a practical clinical definition of epilepsy. *Epilepsia, 55*(4), 475–482.

Fisher, R. S., Cross, J. H., French, J. A., et al. (2017). Operational classification of seizure types by the International League Against Epilepsy: position paper of the ILAE Commission for Classification and Terminology. *Epilepsia, 58*(4), 522–530.

Forsgren, L., Hauser, W. A., Olafsson, E., et al. (2005). Mortality of epilepsy in developed countries: a review. *Epilepsia, 46*(Suppl 11), 18–27.

Franz, D. N., Lawson, J. A., Yapici, Z., et al. (2018). Everolimus dosing recommendations for tuberous sclerosis complex–associated refractory seizures. *Epilepsia, 59*(6), 1188–1197.

French, J. A., Krauss, G. L., Wechsler, R. T., et al. (2015). Perampanel for tonic-clonic seizures in idiopathic generalized epilepsy: a randomized trial. *Neurology, 85*(11), 950–957.

French, J. A., Lawson, J. A., Yapici, Z., et al. (2016). Adjunctive everolimus therapy for treatment-resistant focal-onset seizures associated with tuberous sclerosis (EXIST-3): a phase 3, randomised, double-blind, placebo-controlled study. *Lancet, 388*(10056), 2153–2163.

Gibbon, F. M., Maccormac, E., & Gringras, P. (2019). Sleep and epilepsy: unfortunate bedfellows. *Archives of Disease in Childhood, 104*(2), 189–192.

Goswami, J. N., & Sharma, S. (2019). Current perspectives on the role of the ketogenic diet in epilepsy management. *Neuropsychiatric Disease and Treatment, 1*(5), 3273–3285.

Hamer, H. M., Pfafflin, M., Baier, H., et al. (2018). Characteristics and healthcare situation of adult patients with tuberous sclerosis complex in German epilepsy centers. *Epilepsy & Behavior, 82*, 64–67.

Harbord, M. G. (2000). Significant anticonvulsant side-effects in children and adolescents. *Journal of Clinical Neuroscience, 7*(3), 213–216.

Huber, B., Hauser, I., Horstmann, V., et al. (2005). Seizure freedom with different therapeutic regimens in intellectually disabled epileptic patients. *Seizure, 14*(6), 381–386.

Huber, B. (2014). Increased risk of suicidality on perampanel (Fycompa®)? *Epilepsy & Behavior, 31*, 71–72.

Jackson, C. F., Makin, S. M., Marson, A. G., et al. (2015). Pharmacological interventions for epilepsy in people with intellectual disabilities. *Cochrane Database of Systematic Reviews,* (9), CD005399.

Jansen, F. E., van Huffelen, A. C., Algra, A., et al. (2007). Epilepsy surgery in tuberous sclerosis: a systematic review. *Epilepsia, 48*(8), 1477–1484.

Kanner, A. M. (2009). Psychiatric issues in epilepsy: the complex relation of mood, anxiety disorders, and epilepsy. *Epilepsy & Behavior, 15*(1), 83–87.

Krauss, G. L., Klein, P., Brandt, C., et al. (2020). Safety and efficacy of adjunctive cenobamate (YKP3089) in patients with uncontrolled focal seizures: a multicentre, double-blind, randomised, placebo-controlled, dose-response trial. *Lancet Neurology, 19*(1), 38–48.

Kushinga, K. (2007). The Pepe Project: trialling a German epilepsy education programme for English use. *Learning Disability Practice, 10*(5), 10–13.

Kwan, P., Arzimanoglou, A., Berg, A. T., et al. (2010). Definition of drug resistant epilepsy: consensus proposal by the ad hoc Task Force of the ILAE Commission on Therapeutic Strategies. *Epilepsia, 51*(6), 1069–1077.

Labudda, K., Frauenheim, M., Illies, D., et al. (2018). Psychiatric disorders and trauma history in patients with pure PNES and patients with PNES and coexisting epilepsy. *Epilepsy & Behavior, 88*, 41–48.

Labudda, K., Frauenheim, M., Miller, I., et al. (2020). Outcome of CBT-based multimodal psychotherapy in patients with psychogenic nonepileptic seizures: a prospective naturalistic study. *Epilepsy & Behavior, 106*, 107029.

Lagae, L., Sullivan, J., Knupp, K., et al. (2020). Fenfluramine hydrochloride for the treatment of seizures in Dravet syndrome: a randomised, double-blind, placebo-controlled trial. *Lancet, 394*(10216), 2243–2254.

LaFrance, W. C., Jr., Baker, G. A., Duncan, R., et al. (2013). Minimum requirements for the diagnosis of psychogenic nonepileptic seizures: a staged approach: a report from the International League Against Epilepsy Nonepileptic Seizures Task Force. *Epilepsia, 54*(11), 2005–2018.

Lhatoo, S. D., & Sander, J. W. (2001). The epidemiology of epilepsy and learning disability. *Epilepsia, 42*(Suppl 1), 6–9; discussion 19–20.

Mayer, T. (2005). Besondere Bedeutung von Knochenstoffwechselstörungen bei mehrfach–behinderten Menschen mit Epilepsie. *Zeitschrift für Epileptologie, 18*(3), 178–183.

McGrother, C. W., Bhaumik, S., Thorp, C. F., et al. (2006). Epilepsy in adults with intellectual disabilities: prevalence, associations and service implications. *Seizure, 15*, 376–386.

Medicines and Healthcare Products Regulatory Agency. (2020). Valproate use by women and girls. Available at: https://www.gov.uk/guidance/valproate-use-by-women-and-girls. [Accessed 12 December 2020].

Meschede, C., Witt, J. A., Brömling, S., et al. (2020). Changes in cognition after introduction or withdrawal of zonisamide versus topiramate in epilepsy patients: a retrospective study using Bayes statistics. *Epilepsia, 61*(14). https://doi.org/10.1111/epi.16576.

Mula, M. (2019). Developments in depression in epilepsy: screening, diagnosis, and treatment. *Expert Review of Neurotherapeutics, 19*(3), 269–276.

NHS England. (2018). *Guide to making information accessible for people with a learning disability*. Available at: https://www.england.nhs.uk/wp-content/uploads/2018/06/LearningDisabilityAccessCommsGuidance.pdf. [Accessed 30 December 2020].

Pandher, P. S., & Bhullar, K. K. (2016). Smartphone applications for seizure management. *Health Informatics Journal, 22*(2), 209–220.

Scheffer, I. E., Berkovic, S., Capovilla, G., et al. (2017). ILAE classification of the epilepsies: position paper of the ILAE Commission for Classification and Terminology. *Epilepsia, 58*(4), 512–521.

Tiele, E. A., Bebin, E. M., Bhathal, H., et al., & the GWPCARE6 Study Group. (2021). Add-on cannabidiol treatment for drug-resistant seizures in tuberous sclerosis complex: a placebo-controlled randomized clinical trial. *JAMA Neurology, 78*(3), 285–292.

Trinka, E., Cock, H., Hesdorffer, D., et al. (2015). A definition and classification of status epilepticus – report of the ILAE Task Force on Classification of Status Epilepticus. *Epilepsia, 56*(10), 1515–1523.

van Ool, J. S., Haenen, A. I., Snoeijen-Schouwenaars, F. M., et al. (2016). A systematic review of neuropsychiatric co-morbidities in patients with both epilepsy and intellectual disability. *Epilepsy & Behaviour, 60*, 130–137.

van Ool, J. S., Haenen, A. I., Snoeijen-Schouwenaars, F. M., et al. (2018). Psychogenic nonepileptic seizures in adults with epilepsy and intellectual disability: a neglected area. *Seizure, 59*, 67–71.

Verita (2015). *Independent review into issues that may have contributed to the preventable death of Connor Sparrowhawk*. Available at: https://www.england.nhs.uk/wp-content/uploads/2015/10/indpndnt-rev-connor-sparrowhawk.pdf. [Accessed 30 December 2020].

15

Autism spectrum conditions

Tom P. Berney and Mary Doherty

KEY ISSUES

- Our perception of autism is evolving. A part of this is reflected in the different labels we use.
- Diagnosis is a clinical judgement: there is no biological test.
- The presentation of autism varies greatly as does the degree of disability. It is also likely to be accompanied by other disorders and disabilities, particularly intellectual disability. It can be difficult for individuals, families and carers to know what to expect and to adjust their lives to it.
- The common threads are difficulties in coping with people and with uncertainty as well as in social communication.

- The prevalence of autism has increased; evolving concepts, better resources and greater public awareness mean more people are being diagnosed.
- Appropriate supports including the provision of predictability, communicative support and sensory adaptations will reduce stress and improve coping.
- There are many approaches to the management of autism however these are often poorly researched which leave individuals and families open to exploitation.

CHAPTER OUTLINE

INTRODUCTION

Autism is one of a group of *neurodevelopmental disorders,* each of which reflects the impairment of a cluster of specific skills such as the ability to read, write, talk and understand speech, calculate, recognise and remember faces, concentrate, coordinate movement and many more. These clusters form an identifiable pattern, a syndrome, which in about 5% of the population is pronounced enough to affect everyday life (the threshold used to identify something as a disability/disorder). Besides autism, they include attention deficit hyperactivity disorder (ADHD), developmental coordination disorder (DCD), speech and language disorders, tics and a variety of learning disorders such as dyslexia and dyscalculia.

Autism is particularly associated with intellectual disability which is present in 30–40% of autistic people; the greater the degree of intellectual disability, the more likely are they to be autistic, the prevalence ranging from about 20% in mild intellectual disability to 30-40% in severe intellectual disability (Brugha et al, 2016; Bryson et al, 2008). Both conditions affect functional ability and a clinician needs to be familiar with each on its own if they are to disentangle their characteristics and their effects.

This chapter sets out the current concept of autism; what causes it, how it is defined and recognised and some of the approaches that are helpful in supporting people with intellectual disabilities with the condition. Much is unknown in a field that is constantly evolving (Happé and Frith, 2020) and dominated by money, miracle cures and enthusiasm; fertile ground for exploitation by theorists and snake-oil salesmen. We aim to point you towards useful areas to explore and to avoid being side-tracked by the more speculative approaches that promise relief or cure. Our perception of autism is evolving with research and widespread discussion, reflected in the rapid increase in scientific studies, public awareness and the requirement for professional competence.

Contrary to other chapters in this book, when alluding to people with autism we have employed the term 'autistic person' in contrast to person-first language e.g. 'person with epilepsy' that is preferred for other chronic conditions. To understand this further, we direct the reader to Haelle (2019) who clearly presents the discussion.

WHAT CHARACTERISES AUTISM?

The description of this syndrome has been evolving ever since it was identified in 1943 to reach the present international consensus set out by two bodies

- The American Psychiatric Association in its Diagnostic and Statistical Manual (DSM-5) (American Psychiatric Association, 2013)
- The World Health Organisation in its International Classification of Disease (ICD 11) (World Health Organisation, 2018).

While DSM-5 sets out the criteria for a diagnosis, ICD 11 gives a description of autism, a prototype, against which the clinician can match their client.

In the absence of any physical or laboratory test, a diagnosis of autism remains a judgement made by a clinician, familiar with the condition, and the focus is on deficits (rather than assets) including:

Characteristic difficulties with reciprocal social relationships

These very real difficulties can show in many ways. An inability to grasp unwritten social rules, to make conversation or to share interests leave the autistic person the odd one out, particularly in a non-autistic social group (Crompton et al, 2020). Socially awkward, reticent or too familiar, with problems in understanding and managing friendships, they are often bullied. Although less obvious in a group of people with intellectual disabilities, an unwitting lack of awareness of the thoughts or feelings of others allows social mistakes and gives offence, while an apparent lack of concern for others is readily misinterpreted as arrogance and selfishness.

Communication differences and difficulties

These are non-verbal as well as verbal and involve comprehension as well as expression. These modalities are often mismatched so that apparently fluent speech and expressive gestures do not mean that there is good understanding even if words, phrases and gestures are echoed back, particularly where the person has an intellectual disability. This habit of echoing is the regular basis for the mistaken comment 'he understands everything I say.' However, for some it may be that they simply need enough time to decode what they have heard. Appearances are deceptive, a steady smile may indicate anxiety rather than mirth, silence can be an inability to put something into words rather than not wanting to say something. Often there is a lack of fluency or speech may be too even, lacking vivacity, too loud or too quiet or be out of synchrony with gaze and gesture. The underuse of nonverbal communication can make the person appear impassive and robotic.

Restrictive, Repetitive and inflexible patterns of Behaviour (RRB)

These can include interests or activities that are unusual in their intensity, content or the amount of time they absorb (American Psychiatric Association, 2013). There is often a repetitive or ritualistic quality in these which may range from collecting and arranging objects, stereotyped movements (such as rocking) or an adherence to routines and set ways of doing things. These are part of a wider inflexibility making it difficult to cope with uncertainty and unexpected change (American Psychiatric Association, 2013). Although this cluster of characteristics may look like obsessive-compulsive disorder, there is a fundamental difference in that the autistic person finds it a comfort rather than an imposition and would not want it treated.

Unusual sensory responses

The autistic person may be drawn to, or repelled by, a broad variety of sensory stimuli. There is a great variation of these, not just between individuals but within their own sensory profiles, so that someone may be hypersensitive in one modality (e.g. hearing) but hyposensitive in another (e.g. taste), insensitive to the volume of music but averse to unexpected sound. These traits vary over time and in different circumstances. Stimuli which may be so subtle as to pass unnoticed by most (the hum and flicker of neon lighting, the ticking of a clock, the scratchiness of a woollen jersey, the pungency of a smell or the everyday noise of a street or shop) can produce agitation or even overwhelming and incapacitating distress. In some, a heightened awareness of the taste, texture or colour of food may result in a dangerously selective diet (e.g. Avoidant/Restrictive Food Intake Disorder – ARFID). In others, hyposensitivity might show itself in a lack of reaction to sudden or loud noises or to unexpected pain (allowing injury to pass unnoticed). Although not specific to autism, such anomalies occur more frequently with it and unless specifically asked about have an unrecognised impact on everyday life.

Although autism must be present from early childhood (a defining criterion), these difficulties may remain unnoticed where there are limited social demands or the child has been well supported (as in the structure of a well-organised primary school) and only become apparent when they move into a more demanding setting.

Autism takes varied forms and with different intensity so that functional ability (e.g. as described by The Vineland Social Scale) ranges from people who are competent professionals through to those who are almost completely dependent on carers. This is distinct from cognitive ability (measured as IQ); although autism and intellectual disability are associated, most autistic people are of at least normal intellectual ability.

READER ACTIVITY 15.1

Make a list of the main types of sensory input (how you 'feel' the world around you).

Then, list examples of the variety of stimuli that affect each input. Remember to include less obvious examples such as visual depth (which is necessary to catch an object or to cope with stairs).

Think of credible examples of the ways these might present as unusual behaviour. Resist the temptation to find links with non-specific behaviour such as distractibility which, while it might indicate an abnormal awareness of, say, visual stimuli, might equally reflect an innate attention deficit.

List how you might discover reliably whether an abnormal sensory sensitivity is present. Remember that everyone has sensory preferences so your aim is to identify those which are sufficiently unusual to affect the autistic person's behaviour.

You can find examples at https://www.autismeducationtrust.org.uk/sensory-profiles/https://www.autism-westmidlands.org.uk/wp-content/uploads/2019/03/Sensory_Issues_March_2019.pdf

OUR USE OF LABELS

This reflects our perception of autism as a categorical disorder, one of the most clear-cut psychiatric entities in the 1980s. Further research brought the recognition of subtler forms and of concurrent conditions to arrive at our present recognition of a more complex, pervasive and prevalent condition (Mandy and Skuse, 2008; Rapoport et al, 2009). A useful analogy for this search for meaningful pattern in this sea of neurobehavioural characteristics is the way we grouped stars into constellations in the past (see Figure 15.1).

Clear-cut, core autism is relatively simple to identify. However, it is only one end of a continuum of characteristics that become less obvious and less frequent until they fade into the neurotypical traits of the non-autistic general population. The diagnostic threshold is the point on this continuum at which someone's function is sufficiently impaired for them to be identified as autistic. However, diagnosis is a subjective, clinical judgement and the threshold will shift with time, circumstance and fashion. This ambiguity is disguised by the confident use of a

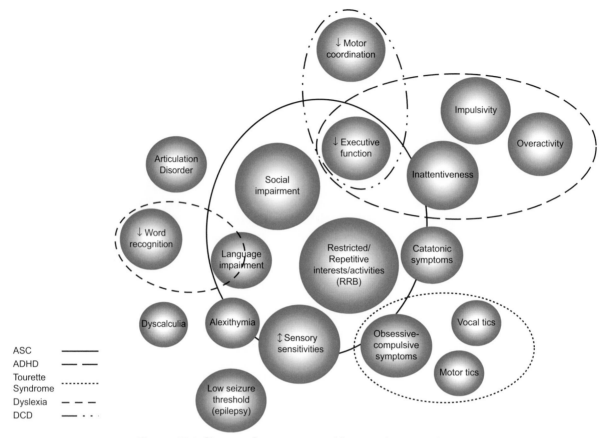

Figure. 15.1 Clusters of symptoms combine to make up syndromes

categorical label, something that is essential to developing a management plan, service access and service planning.

There have been several, unsuccessful attempts to subdivide autism. 'Asperger syndrome' was introduced in 1994 to test the idea that those of normal cognitive ability and with good grammatical speech formed a consistent subgroup. Eighteen years later it was judged to have failed by those revising DSM and it was dropped as a formal diagnosis although the term lives on as a useful identity for many autistic people.

This perception of autism as a 'disability/disorder' identified by impairment contrasts with autism as a 'condition' which also has many positive attributes notably a tendency to a cooler, objective approach to the world and the way it works, better able to perceive patterns and to seek systematic solutions. The diagnostic spotlight, selecting those characteristics that serve as useful criteria, leaves other, more loosely linked features in the shadows such as a photographic memory, pattern recognition, speed reading, perfect pitch, and skills in chess, mathematics and objective thinking; a point brought out by Chris Packham, an English naturalist (Packham, 2016). The resultant profile of ability can be so uneven as to defy any overall descriptor.

It is debatable as to whether autism is a 'condition,' a 'disability' (deserving the support of others) or a clear 'disorder' (requiring treatment). These distinctions are more than semantic for it reflects the extent to which we think that our society should

- make adjustments to offset a disability, a normal variation in the human condition (a social model of disability),
- treat an individual for a psychiatric disorder (a medical model of disability).

Here, we use the neutral, umbrella term 'autism' to embrace a group of people with a common thread of difference and difficulty, whose world requires adaptation if they are to make the most of life.

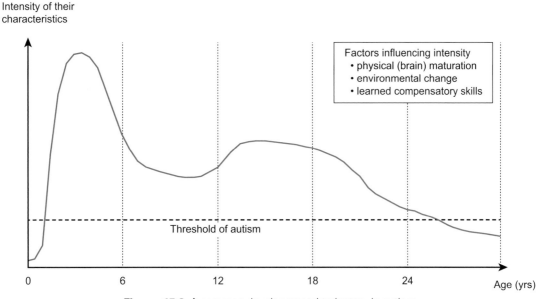

Figure. **15.2** A common developmental trajectory in autism

DEVELOPMENTAL CHANGE

In autistic people, developmental changes occur and while the tendency is overall for this to occur as spurts of improvement (particularly in later childhood and early adulthood), setbacks may come with adolescence, illness and stress (see Figure 15.2). The last is often the consequence of a change in circumstance such as leaving school. Whilst for some this may be an escape from academic demands, teasing and bullying, for others it can be an unwelcome change/move from the predictable certainty of a busy, organised school programme to the chaotic boredom of unstructured adulthood. The presence of intellectual disability may mean that autistic characteristics are perceived as a non-specific behavioural disturbance meaning that they may not get the specialist help they require, while in its absence, additional demands, whether of marriage or occupation, may amplify what were autistic traits.

By adulthood, the combination of physical maturation, a more tolerant environment, acquired compensatory skills, particularly with the confusion that comes from concurrent conditions (notably intellectual disability), means obvious autism becomes something fainter and blurred, making its identification more difficult, especially in the absence of a good description of childhood.

 READER ACTIVITY 15.2

Think of someone you know who has difficulty getting on with people, who appears insensitive to others, goes their own way without checking (attracting comments such as 'not a team player' and 'arrogant').

• What other characteristics do they have that might suggest they are autistic?
• What other characteristics do they have that might suggest other neurodevelopmental disorders?

PSYCHOLOGICAL CHARACTERISTICS

A range of psychological characteristics may be associated with autism and these include:

An impaired 'Theory of Mind'

The ability to recognise that other people might not think the way you do, more vividly labelled 'mind-blindness', is well known. Although neither specific to autism nor invariably present, it can explain much of the apparent egocentricity in the person's approach to the world. However, the consequent identification of autism with impaired empathy has been thrown into question as further research revealed the complexity of the factors involved including, for example, difficulties in the recognition of one's own emotions (alexithymia) and internal physical sensations (interoception) as well as the distinctions between cognitive and affective empathy (Fletcher-Watson and Bird, 2020).

Executive function

This includes a variety of cognitive functions such as the ability to identify a problem, to work out how to tackle it, to start it, to complete it, coping with setbacks and side-issues, and to know when to stop. It involves working memory, impulse control, inhibition and mental flexibility, as well as the initiation and monitoring of action. It is a global concept and difficulties with it are frequent in neurodevelopmental disorders in general as well as often the root of the major difficulties that prevent an autistic person coping with everyday tasks, although its presence may also be attributed to concurrent ADHD (Jones et al, 2018).

Weak central coherence

This means that rather than seeing the bigger picture the individual's mindset leads them to see individual elements, neglecting their wider context, whether looking at a scene or listening to a verbal explanation. It can allow the person, undistracted by the context, to identify detail overlooked by others (Happé and Frith, 2006).

The attraction of a simple, stereotypic description of autism leads to a black and white impression with specific abilities being either present or absent. The reality is that characteristics may be impaired or enhanced and that there is great individual variation, as caught by Wing's analogy with the multicoloured *spectrum* of light (as distinct from the *autistic continuum* described earlier; personal communication 2005).

CONCURRENT CONDITIONS

Autism is a pervasive disorder, affecting not just the nervous system but also the rest of the body and personality. Although there is no consistent pattern, abnormalities of the immune and autonomic system regularly occur while abnormal connective tissue may contribute to problems with joints and heart valves. There is an increase in sleep problems, obesity and diabetes while gastrointestinal symptoms have been described in anything between 17% and 86% of autistic people: these include discomfort, bloating and pain and can range from constipation to diarrhoea.

Epilepsy occurs in 3–5% of autistic people (in the absence of intellectual disability) (Croen et al, 2015; Rydzewska et al, 2019). To set this in context, epilepsy has a population prevalence of about 1% rising where there is intellectual disability to 10–30%, depending on the degree of intellectual disability.

Reduced life expectancy is associated with autism but the relationship appears indirect. Thus, where there is intellectual disability, earlier death results from epilepsy, chest and cardiovascular causes while, in the more able, it is a consequence of suicide and relates to autism's association with depression and bipolar disorder (Hirvikoski et al, 2016).

The neurodevelopmental disorders/disabilities

These come in clusters so that the presence of one is a signal that others may be present. Someone with autism or an intellectual disability is more likely to have other disorders such as

- Inattentiveness,
- poor impulse control,
- overactivity (the cluster of disabilities that make up ADHD)
- the poor coordination of dyspraxia (or developmental coordination disorder (DCD)),
- tics (and Tourette disorder),
- the low seizure threshold that predisposes to epilepsy,
- developmental learning disorders in reading, writing or mathematics,
- a developmental speech or language disorder.

Thus ADHD, present in 4% of children and 3–5% of adults, occurs in 30–40% of autistic people (Polderman et al, 2014); with tics in 10% of autistic children and DCD in 70% (the last two occurring in about 5–6% of the general population). Although there is the suggestion that the incoordination of autism is linked to visual processing and that of DCD to spatial processing (Hannant et al, 2018), our difficulty in disentangling the two conditions exemplifies the problem with thinking of these as categorical disorders.

Psychiatric disorder

This is more frequent in autism and the combination brings the risk that each may be missed or misdiagnosed. Emotional disorders are the most frequent and include a variety of anxiety disorders such as generalised anxiety disorder, agoraphobia, social phobia and obsessive-compulsive disorder (OCD). Intense anxiety may result in panic, freezing, a catastrophic 'melt-down', a psychotic adjustment reaction or catatonia (the last two inviting a mistaken diagnosis of schizophrenia). While depression is more frequent, it may be overlooked as its symptoms can be attributed to a person's autism.

However, estimates of prevalence of psychiatric disorder will depend on the population picked and the methodology used to identify both autism and the disorder (e.g. autism can alter not only the presentation of symptoms, but also the way a person responds to a standard questionnaire). There is often difficulty in describing internal thoughts, emotions and sensations and an account can be vague, talking of a sense of apprehension, 'feeling overwhelmed', 'stressed out' and 'not coping.' Alternately, the person may fall back on concrete expression, for example, describing thoughts as voices which are then misinterpreted as hallucinations. Their difficulty with nonverbal expression may mean that their presentation does not fit with what they are saying (something which is also found in schizophrenia). Impassivity or, even worse a fixed smile, coupled with an unwitting egocentricity, may attract the label of dissocial personality disorder. Unconventional behaviour, emotional lability and an apparently disproportionate response to social relationships and stress may lead the clinician to think of emotionally unstable (borderline personality) disorder. The immediacy of these symptoms makes it easy to overlook the significance of more subtle changes such as an increased sensitivity to the environment, an increase in rituals or a greater degree of planning, preparation and avoidance.

Symptoms are not specific to one disorder. Inattentiveness may indicate ADHD but it may also result from an autistic person's incomprehension of what is going on. Apparently compulsive rituals may be part of OCD but may also reflect an autistic routine which its owner, in contrast with the OCD sufferer, would not want treated.

Autism brings a variety of unusual behaviours which become problematic in excess, whether in intensity or in the time spent on them. Thus a sensory aversion to certain food, an intense dedication to a specific diet or an unwillingness to change can all result in a very restricted, bizarre diet and a potentially dangerous weight loss which, although it also can reduce emotional distress, is distinct from the distortion of body image found in anorexia nervosa (itself associated with autism) (Brede et al, 2020; Westwood and Tchanturia, 2017). In some, repetitive self-stimulation unchecked by a typical awareness of pain may provide the foundation for self-injurious behaviour (SIB). Factors such as distress or the concern of those around may push the individual into a damaging excess which can go on to become habitual and entrenched.

Extreme/Pathological Demand Avoidance (PDA), although not recognised in the international classification systems (ICD and DSM), has been adopted to describe children who present with a behaviour profile characterised by the very abnormal

- avoidance of compliance with everyday demands (using a variety of social strategies, including excuses and distraction),
- anxiety when demands cannot be avoided,
- attempts to control situations,
- impulsivity as well as sudden and extreme changes of mood.

There is debate as to whether this behavioural profile is a variant of autism (and specific to it), whether it might be seen in other conditions, or whether it is a condition in its own right (Green et al, 2018).

LIFE WITH AUTISM

Hidden disability can be more difficult to grow up with than something overt; people are less understanding and individuals often sense that they are somehow different without knowing how or why. Labels such as 'thick' or 'clumsy' combined with the lack of friends and limited social skills make autistic people easy targets to bully and tease. The effect is to erode what self-confidence there is, perpetuating self-isolation and contributing to later underachievement (Balfe and Tantam, 2010). Episodes of distress may be misinterpreted, being attributed to maladaptive training or communication rather than, for example, to misunderstanding or sensory factors. Unrecognised, the disability is seen as the fault of the individual so that for example a wife, initially attracted to the open straightforwardness of her husband, may tire of his lack of intuitive understanding and a failure to respond to her unspoken desire for romance.

The autistic family

Behavioural disturbance is more frequent and more intense in autism than in intellectual disability and may be heightened by intuitive responses on the part of the carer. Compounding this is the association with psychiatric conditions which applies not just to the autistic person but also to near relatives, a link that is not attributable simply to the stress of care (Daniels et al, 2008; Piven and Palmer, 1999). At the same time, the familial pattern of autism means that many parents are autistic, part of a 'lost generation' of undiagnosed adults. For many this brings an intuitive understanding of their autistic child which should be respected and supported even though their parenting style may seem unconventional to the non-autistic observer.

The autistic community

While most autistic people want to have social relationships, they are hampered by their social and communicative limitations and many find it easier to mix with other autistic people. The internet has opened the way to a widespread number of local, national and international networks. The development of these communities has encouraged the shift in perception of autism from a medical disorder to it being one of the range of differences in brain function that go to make up normal variation in the human population (the concept of *neurodiversity*) (Shields and Beversdorf, 2020).

Employment

While many employment issues run across the field of disability (Chapter 23) there are three issues particularly pertinent to autistic people

1. Autism is associated with particular talents, notably in computer sciences, an area that *Specialisterne*, a Danish consultancy company has sought to exploit (see online Useful resources). Looking to work with both autistic people and employers they have established a global network of centres to introduce and support autistic people to areas such as programme testing and data entry

2. Autistic people can be high achievers therefore their condition may only come to light when they run into difficulties at which point the diagnosis often reframes the difficulties and allows their resolution and subsequent support and mentoring. There are many autistic doctors across the world and *Autistic Doctors International* provides peer support for medical staff (see online Useful resources)

3. Many autistic services provide specialist support for people across the whole intellectual range, supporting them into placements similar to those for non-autistic people.

HOW IS AUTISM IDENTIFIED?

With increasing public awareness and readily available online checklists (see Box 15.1) autism is suspected more frequently; indeed, the label is entering popular use.

📄 BOX 15.1   Alerting characteristics where there is substantial intellectual disability

Intellectual disability comes with delayed developmental skills, obscuring the signs of concurrent autism. Recognising this can be difficult and the clinician has to identify skills and behaviour that is out of keeping with the individual's overall level of functioning or, if they have an underlying medical disorder, with its symptomatology.

Difficulties with reciprocal social relationships
- An unusual, one-sided response to contact by others – these may include actively avoiding people, simply ignoring them or moving away after a fleeting contact (which may include a standard routine such as a greeting, kiss or hug). However, the autistic person may engage in some pleasurable physical activities (rough and tumble, tickling games) or be demanding, provocative or disinhibited.
- Few or no sustained relationship with their peers leaving them a 'loner' who stands aloof and who may appear unaware of those around them.

Communication difficulties and differences
- a disproportionate impairment of language relative to their other ability,
- repetitive stereotypic speech which is too loud/soft, or has an unusual quality, rate or pitch and an excessive use of echolalia, neologisms or speech that is just idiosyncratic (in comparison to others of their developmental level),

---

📄 **BOX 15.1   Alerting characteristics where there is substantial intellectual disability—con'd**

- talking at (rather than to) you with little awareness of your response,
- limited use of nonverbal expressions so that there is a rather wooden, impassive appearance with few gestures and underused or poorly coordinated gaze. The effect of the latter is that the person appears either to be avoiding eye contact (misinterpreted as furtive) or else is looking through you (and may appear aggressive).

Restrictive, repetitive and inflexible patterns of behaviour (RRB)

- unusual interests, obsessively pursued which may range from collections of twigs or toys to people's birthdays or car registrations.
- Repetitive stereotypies – finger twiddling, hand flapping, rocking, tapping. A set approach to everyday life that may include unusual routines or rituals. Change is often upsetting.

Unusual sensory responses (Explored in Reader activity 15.1)

- Attracted to and even held by specific sensory stimuli such as patterns, movements or sounds.
- Episodes of sudden emotional arousal which may appear spontaneous but which careful observation find to be in response to a specific sensory trigger. The arousal may present as anxiety/panic, aggression, non-specific distress, repetitive self-injury or simply avoidance of the stimulus (e.g. refusing to wear a garment of a particular material or colour).
- The individual may be unable to say what it is that they like/dislike, let alone explain it.

Diagnosis is only one element of the broader process of assessment which describes a person, their ability and needs as well as addressing more specific questions about, say, the capacity to make a particular decision or the risk of offending. It is a clinical judgement and as such is dependent on the clinician's expertise. In turn, this depends on their training and experience of autism in its varied forms as well as of other, complicating conditions. It requires enough information to match against the accepted definition. Often coming from a blend of questionnaire, rating scale and diagnostic interview, the aim is to get a true picture of the individual across a number of settings, something that is helped by informants who have known the individual reasonably well and over some time. The clinician may use a variety of instruments (for examples see Box 15.2) to gather and organise information, but the process differs from making a research diagnosis where consistency is a priority which is helped by validated algorithms (which have no place in clinical work). The diagnosis is usually clear cut but there are those whose characteristics are subtle, masked by their circumstances or confused by the features of other disorders. It is not easy to disentangle the effects of autism and intellectual disability and experience with those of normal ability is thus essential. Here, the decisions can be a difficult judgement call which is influenced by the purpose of the diagnosis, whether in response to a particular need, service or research programme.

Self-diagnosis is subjective and unreliable but encouraged by the difficulty in accessing a diagnostic service whether because of limited availability (with long waiting times), a fear of assessment/professionals or cost. The availability of self-rating scales and internet information means that it is common and it is something that research and services will need to accommodate (Lewis, 2017; Whitney and Stansfield, 2019).

It is important to note that there is no laboratory test for autism although a variety of irrelevant analyses are on sale. A biological anomaly does not necessarily contribute to the cause of the autism or have any bearing on its management.

WHAT CAUSES AUTISM?

It has become clear that autism is the final common pathway of a wide variety of underlying mechanisms which result in the reorganisation of the brain overall rather than in any specific region or system. It is highly heritable with traits, if not the full-blown syndrome, often present in parents and siblings. While the likelihood of having an autistic child is about 1%, the

BOX 15.2   **Some instruments that might be used to identify autism in the presence of intellectual disability**

Questionnaires

Many are designed for self-completion and require a level of ability which makes them unsuitable for someone with concurrent intellectual disability even when completed by a carer. Those that are useful examine behaviour and are often designed for childhood. The following are some of the parent report questionnaires (Charman et al, 2018)

- *The Social Communication Questionnaire (SCQ)* is a 40-item questionnaire which is primarily aimed at childhood and which derives from the ADI (described below).
- *The Social Responsiveness Scale (SRS)* developed by Constantino & Gruber is a 65-item scale that has an adult as well as a child version.
- *The Children's Communication Checklist (CCC)* is a 70-item scale that asks about language and communication impairment.
- *The Autism Behavior Checklist (ABC)* is a questionnaire to be completed by parents. It has a good statistical basis for identifying ASC in young children (Krug et al, 1988).

Interview Schedules

All of these are well-researched and give numerical scores that can be used in research with a diagnostic algorithm. Most are complex instruments and require formal training of the user. They are complementary to (rather than a replacement for) clinical experience.

- *Childhood Autism Rating Scale* (CARS-2). A 15-item scale that organises and grades information gathered from parents, carers and observation. The simplest of the main instruments, its categories have not been updated to match the evolving diagnostic criteria (Schopler et al, 1988).

- *The Autism Diagnostic Interview (Revised) (ADI(R)).* A 96-item interview that takes a developmental history from parents; a substantial part focuses on the presentation in early childhood. It is a diagnostic instrument that only includes items immediately relevant to a diagnosis and takes about 2–3 hours (Lord et al, 1994).
- *ADOS-2.* The Autism Diagnostic Observation Scale (2nd edition) is a subject interview that complements the ADI history (see above). It takes 30-70 minutes (with an additional 20 minutes scoring) and is designed to elicit the symptoms of ASC using a standard kit. The whole range of age and ability are covered by five modules (Kamp-Becker et al, 2018).
- *The Diagnostic Interview for Social and Communication Disorders (DISCO).* This is a structured interview that gathers and synthesises information from a variety of informants, including the individual, to give a broad assessment of their developmental disabilities. Favoured for general clinical use it takes 2–3 hours to administer (Wing et al, 2002).
- *The Developmental, Dimensional and Diagnostic Interview (3di)* is a parent interview which, designed to be used with a computer and advance questionnaires, allows an assessment to be completed in an hour (Skuse et al, 2004). Designed for childhood, it has been extended for use across the whole range of age and ability.
- *The Scale of Pervasive Developmental Disorder in Mentally Retarded Persons (PDD-MRS).* A well-validated and reliable structured interview of the carers of people with intellectual disabilities across the whole age range. Is being used as a research tool, particularly in Holland where it was developed (Kraijer and de Bildt, 2005).

probability of a second autistic child is at least 13%, rising to about 60% should it be an identical twin. Again, the probability is proportional to the closeness of the genetic relationship, being about 8% for a half sibling and 3% for a cousin. However, the underlying **genetic mechanism** is complex and only partially understood

(Parihar and Ganesh, 2016). What is known is that about 10% of cases originate from rare, disease-causing genes, frequently associated with intellectual disability, such as Tuberous Sclerosis, Fragile X and Down syndromes. More often in autistic people there is an increase in minor gene anomalies, risk alleles, which are

BOX 15.3 Understanding what I'm told

There are some interesting words and it is fascinating how just one word in a sentence can change the whole meaning of that sentence. Even to change an emphasis does that apparently. Here is an example

I can't do that ... implies that I can't, but maybe someone else can.

I *can't* do that ... implies it is not possible.

I can't do *that* ... implies that I can't do that, but may be able to do something else.

I am told that I put an emphasis on the wrong words sometimes and change the meaning when I don't actually want to. This often means that I am misunderstood or misunderstand others (Jackson, 2002).

 BOX 15.4 Thinking visually

I think in pictures. Words are like a second language to me ... when someone speaks to me, his words are instantly translated into pictures ... one of the most profound mysteries of autism has been the remarkable ability of most autistic people to excel at visual spatial skills while performing so poorly at verbal skills (Grandin, 2006).

found across the neurodiverse general population; individually they do not result in autism but interact and increase the individual's susceptibility to the condition and appear to underlie the continuum that runs from autistic traits to shade into the full-blown manifestation of autism.

There is also a substantial **environmental component** which, although it may be sufficient on its own (e.g. prenatal rubella), may simply nudge a genetic predisposition further along the continuum of severity. There is evidence that this occurs with risk factors such as neonatal prematurity and hypoxia, maternal ill health (obesity and diabetes), and parental age at conception (mother over 40 years, father over 50 years). There is no evidence that immunisation, maternal hypertension or smoking or assisted fertilisation are relevant while the

evidence on prenatal exposure to alcohol, pesticide or air pollution is equivocal (Lord et al, 2020).

There is an association between neurodevelopmental disorders and adverse childhood events/trauma. It is unclear where the cause lies but the suspicion is that there is a common, underlying genetic predisposition for such conditions. These include post-traumatic stress disorder (PTSD) and reactive attachment disorder as well as other psychiatric disorders.

While the initial characteristics of autism may be set by this combination of forces - genetic and environmental - the interaction continues throughout development with the brain being shaped by its environment so that the autistic characteristics are amplified or reduced over time. Severe deprivation (as in the Romanian orphanages) in itself can produce an autistic syndrome although having been acquired rather than innate and showing some remission it has been given the clinical label of 'quasi-autism' (Rutter et al, 2007). In summary, autism is a behavioural syndrome with a variety of causes and presentations that are made up of a number of components (such as the domains for 'social responsiveness' and 'a rigid, repetitive, attention to detail'). Research has to cope with this complexity; studies that have approached autism as a single entity have been disappointing, opening the door to untested hypotheses stemming from anecdotal accounts or underpowered studies.

PREVALENCE OF AUTISM

Prevalence of autism has been measured by two distinct methods. These are population-based surveys and surveillance/register studies.

Population-based surveys

In these types of survey researchers systematically assess a population using a combination of questionnaire and interview. From these it has been found that just over 1% of the general childhood population are autistic, of whom about half have a significant intellectual disability. The more severe the degree of disability, the more likely a child is to be autistic (see Tables 15.1 and 15.2).

In adulthood the results are less clear. While the overall prevalence remains the same, adults had a less severe degree of intellectual disability (Brugha et al, 2016). This may reflect some increase in ability with age

TABLE 15.1   **Prevalence of autism in 9 year old children (Baird et al, 2006)**

Overall prevalence		1.1%
Broken down by level of ability	Normal ability	0.51%
	Mild intellectual disability	0.48%
	Moderate/severe intellectual disability	0.17%

TABLE 15.2   **Prevalence of autism in children and adolescents with intellectual disabilities (de Bildt et al, 2003)**

All young people with intellectual disabilities	8-20%
Mild intellectual disabilities	10%
Moderate/severe intellectual disabilities	30%

(Simonoff et al, 2019) as well as a reduced recognition of intellectual disability (it is likely that the demand of an academic setting means that intellectual disability is more consistently identified in childhood).

Surveillance/register studies

These count the number of people that have been identified as autistic by an administrative system such as the number of autistic children registered in special education provision or with their family doctor. These often show a higher prevalence and marked geographical variation as identification is done by different people, using different methods and subject to a variety of pressures, for example, the benefits brought by a diagnosis such as entry to special education. Thus the reported prevalence for the USA in 2016 was 1.3–3.1% of 8 year old children (Maenner et al, 2020) and for Northern Ireland in 2020 it was 1.8–6.9%. of school-age children (Rodgers and McCluney, 2020).

There has been a huge shift in our perception of autism from it being understood in the 1970s as a rare condition (occurring in only 0.04% of the population) of whom 80% had a substantial intellectual disability. Surveillance study results suggest that autism's prevalence is rising (an 'autism epidemic'), but it is better explained by changes in the way autism is defined, labelled and discovered, all furthered by the greater public and professional awareness of autism and an increase in services.

INTERVENTIONS

When poorly understood, autism offers opportunity for a wide range of interventions, many with little to recommend them except a charismatic salesman's heartfelt belief in what he has to sell – which probably did work for someone, somewhere, at least once. Interventions variously offer to cure autism, improve impaired adaptive skills or remove unwanted behaviour. Some treatments target hypothetical biological anomalies (medication, diets and supplements). In considering the evidence of their efficacy, there are some pitfalls. For example, many interventions are recommended on the basis of a series of case reports. However, behaviour changes when people know they are being studied (Hawthorne effect) or if they expect the intervention to work (Pygmalion effect) can occur so there should be a comparison group who are getting a placebo treatment. However, a placebo may improve an autistic child, not because of its actual merit, but because their family, expecting change, may behave differently towards them, thus the efficiency of the actual intervention is difficult to ascertain. Many studies underestimate the difficulty and cost of an adequate double-blind trial in which not only the individual but also the observers are unaware as to whether the intervention is being used or not. Even where there is a blind comparison of two groups, there is the possibility that their selection has been biased or that their allocation to either experiment or control group has not been random. Moreover, the spontaneous variation in autistic features means that the study needs to continue long enough to be sure that the intervention is actually producing a sustained change.

A further issue with respect to measures of effectiveness is when the outcome of the intervention is unclear or poorly defined. For example, an autistic person learning a new skill in one setting may be unable to apply it in other areas of their life; something that might be missed in too specific an outcome (Carruthers et al, 2020). This situation might be compounded by publication bias where there is a preferential acceptance of positive results leaving the reader unaware of how often an intervention has fallen short.

READER ACTIVITY 15.3

Choose a paper reporting a successful autism intervention. Imagine that it has been handed to you by the parents of an autistic child; they want to know what you think of it and whether they should get it for their child. Besides its main findings consider

1) Who wrote the paper, where were they working and what is their previous track record?
2) How reputable is the journal that accepted it? The more prestigious the journal, the harder it is to get acceptance and the more likely it is that the paper has been reviewed by an independent, expert panel.
3) Who might stand to gain from the paper and its implications?
4) How were the subjects found? How reliable are their diagnoses? (if, for example, they are self-diagnosed volunteers, does the paper address this)?
5) Is this a case series or a comparison of two or more groups? If the latter, were the subjects aware of which form of treatment they were getting; were the observers (family and researchers) aware?
6) Does the paper set out its limitations?

   How would you decide:
- Whether the programme was likely to help the individual?
- What were its drawbacks?
- Whether it was worth the cost in time and money?
- What to include in your answer?

Social skills and strategies

The fundamental intervention for autism is education. Involving both home and school/college, it needs to include the social skills that non-autistic people acquire largely informally as they grow up. For example, such training might include how to recognise and respond to the viewpoint and feelings of others, and how to behave in social groups and in different settings. These can cover a wide range of activities and include, for example, which urinal to use in a public toilet, how and when to buy a round of drinks, how to complain to a shop and how to distinguish and relate to different authority figures.

Of particular importance is learning how someone might cope with their emotions. Many have difficulty in identifying and describing their own internal state and need to acquire this *emotional literacy* before they can go on and cope with emotions that include anxiety, anger and depression. Besides learning their acceptable expression, it can include strategies for avoiding and dealing with evocative situations and techniques for reducing emotional arousal.

Teaching must be systematic and based on flexible, personalised plans. Tailored to the autistic person in a way that they can understand, it requires adequate support and structure and should include the education of friends, family, carers and anyone else involved in the person's development.

Communication

Autism implies that the person has some degree of difficulty in communication whether it be their ability to express their needs, to use language in social situations or to understand what someone else means. Their levels of receptive and expressive communication may be very disparate; that someone is non-speaking does not mean that they do not understand what is said. Similarly, fluent phrases do not necessarily mean good comprehension. There can be a similar divorce between verbal and non-verbal communication, and in the end it is essential that each modality is appreciated and augmented communication used where appropriate (e.g. in talking mats, keyboards, sign-language).

Autism brings more subtle barriers. It is not unusual for the autistic person to take the literal meaning of what is said and fail to 'read between the lines'. Some process auditory information very slowly and need time to understand a question or request. A non-autistic person will have difficulty in appreciating what the autistic person is thinking; a problem of double empathy (Milton, 2012) with misunderstanding frequently causing distress. Communication can be helped by employing the following strategies
- Reduce anxiety. Be guided by the autistic person as well as their friends and carers to make the meeting familiar and predictable. Try to ensure that they know what they might expect (why you are meeting them, where, when and for how long) and that the setting is quiet, comfortable and distraction-free. It is worth checking in advance whether they have any specific sensory needs.

- Use language that suits the individual's level of understanding.
  - Keep your language brief, clear and unambiguous, focusing on the main message you are wanting to convey. Do not pad with woolly, unnecessary language.
  - Be specific and use concrete terms, particularly in dealing with abstract concepts such as time and frequency.
  - Be wary of anything that might be misinterpreted (irony, sarcasm, metaphors or idiosyncratic turns of phrase.
  - Check regularly that each of you has understood the other correctly.
- Make sure you have their attention. Even though you are looking and talking to them do not assume they know this is directed at them. Remember some people find it difficult to listen and look at the speaker at the same time since nonverbal signals can confuse and distract; don't insist that they look at you.
- Allow the person enough thinking time to process what has been said and to overcome their initial difficulty of putting their thoughts into words. If you respond too soon or with too much, it may overload the individual's auditory processing; even though they may be able to repeat back what has been said, they may be unable to grasp its meaning (people often echo something as they try to understand it, giving a false impression of comprehension). Verbal fluency may give a misleading impression of comprehension; check that a point has been understood before moving on.
- Be positive when providing instructions. Tell the individual what it is that they should be doing rather than what they should not be doing.
- Adopt a more concrete and structured approach, focusing on practical matters, actual behaviour and specific problems rather than abstract concepts. In helping someone to make a decision, offer a limited number of choices at a time, each with a clear effect.
- Use visual supports. Many autistic people appear to be visual learners, more able to process information that comes visually as compared to verbally. Besides helping to establish and maintain attention, especially where someone is listening selectively, they can pick out the discussion's overall structure and direction.

The structured environment

A well-structured and supported setting is one of the most effective ways of supporting most autistic people;

reducing anxiety and its behavioural disturbance to allow learning. This is a key component of many recognised programmes including **TEACCH** (**T**reatment and **E**ducation of **A**utistic and related **C**ommunication–handicapped **Ch**ildren) from the University of North Carolina (Siu et al, 2019; see online Useful resources) and **SPELL** (Structure, Positive (approaches and expectations), Empathy, Low arousal, Links) developed by the National Autistic Society (Povey, 2015).

The physical setting

Distractibility may be an innate part of autism as well as part of a concurrent disorder and is increased by anxiety and uncertainty. The individual will be helped by clarity, not just in the physical layout but also where and how materials are presented. Some need unusually well-defined designated areas as, for example, 'this is where I eat,' 'this is where I sleep,' 'this is where I play' and are confused and distressed by multifunctional rooms and sensory distractions, particularly where the setting is for work or learning. Many people are at their most comfortable and able, likely to function where

- there is a clear, visual environment with well-marked and consistent areas and boundaries,
- distracting sounds are shut out. Some will need some form of sensory screen such as ear defenders or noise-cancelling headphones with/without background music.
- visual distractors, including people, movement, mirrors, windows and clutter are excluded, perhaps using curtains and dividers (see Figure 15.3).

There is no general recipe for different autistic people have different sensitivities and preferences and it is important to ask what works and for whom.

The temporal setting

Time is an abstract concept that can be difficult to cope with. In addition, uncertainty about what the future holds (whether it is the next task or the next day) is distressing. Schedules in the form of appointment diaries and timetables are an everyday tool that can offset these difficulties. They help people to understand what will be happening and when; by bringing predictability, they allow people to anticipate events and plan constructively. They can also be used to show that time is passing and where someone is as they progress through their daily programme. In autism, they are always visual, using physical objects, pictures,

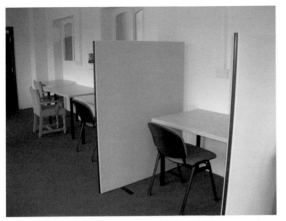

Figure. 15.3 Dividers at a desk where activities are being taught allowing individuals to focus on new and unfamiliar tasks

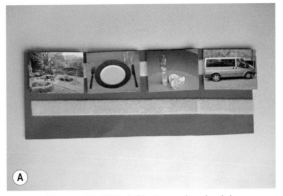

Figure. 15.4(A) A Photograph schedule

text, or symbols and covering anything from part of a day to several days or months. For some they start as simply as 'now this, then that'. The individual should be encouraged to use the schedule as a support, forewarning them of upcoming changes and helping them in negotiating a programme. Examples of these are in Figures 15.4A-C)

Work systems

Using all of these principles, TEACCH developed a system that allows autistic people to make the most of their ability to function independently. Their 'work systems' guide the individual across a wide range of activities and settings that might include, for example, their work area, bedroom, bathroom, kitchen, and dining room. For example, they may be set out as a sequence of cards (the autistic person exchanging or collecting the card as they go through the tasks) or a list, coloured or tabulated for clarity (see Figure 15.5).

Task organisation

TEACCH uses 'task organisation' to help autistic people where they have limited organisation and sequencing skills and difficulty in combining and integrating ideas. Tasks are presented visually, broken down to show their different components in order. People differ in the amount of structure they need, ranging from simple reminders (Figure 15.6) to a very structured 'shoebox task' (in which the component is presented as a single unit, with clear start and finish points, for the individual to focus on).

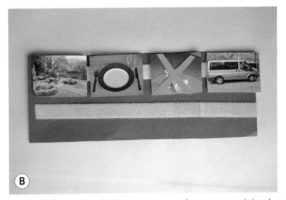

Figure. 15.4(B) A change system where an activity has been cancelled

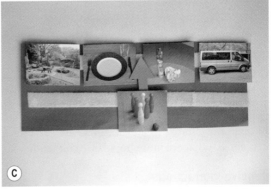

Figure. 15.4(C) A change system where an activity has been added

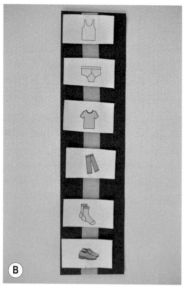

Figure. **15.5** A work system used by an adult to get dressed in the morning. He has organisational and sequencing problems

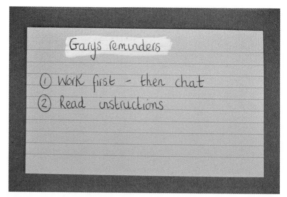

Figure. **15.6** A cue card used by an autistic person who also has mild intellectual disability and who panics when faced with written instructions. These take him through his day as well as preventing him from becoming distracted from his work

---

READER ACTIVITY 15.4

Samuel is a 26-year-old autistic man who has recently moved into a small residential home. Staff report that he asks constantly what is happening and when. He finds even small changes in his timetable difficult to cope with.

The house is very homely but a little cluttered. The dining room is such a lovely large sunny room that it is used for many different activities, although there are two other rooms that they could use as well.

- Reflect on what might help Samuel to understand what is happening.
- Consider the range of systems you might put in place.
- Consider what environmental changes might need to occur.

SPECIFIC INTERVENTIONS

Although not limited to autism, these are some of the interventions that are more popular in this field.

Intensive Interaction

Contrasting with behavioural approaches that aim to teach, train or direct the autistic person are those that are based on following the individual's lead, seeking to enter their world on their terms. The worker copies and follows the actions of the individual in order to build a relationship, treating all their actions as communicative. Used with people who have little functional communication, often having severe intellectual disabilities and autism, it focuses on the quality of the interaction itself rather than on a task or outcome (see also Chapter 5) and was developed in the UK as Intensive Interaction (Zeedyk et al, 2009). Paediatric Autism Communication Therapy (Pact Training, 2021) and Floortime in the USA are also intensive interaction methods (Interdisciplinary Council on Development and Learning, 2021) whilst it is also a central theme of the Options or Son-Rise Program (Autism Treatment Center of America, 2008). Links to these organisations can be found in the online Useful resources.

An underpinning element of such approaches is that they affect both parties and the relationship between them, rather than just doing something to the autistic person. There is substantial evidence of the effectiveness of PACT (Carruthers et al, 2020) and it shows promise in its adaptation in countries with scant resources (Divan et al, 2019).

Social stories

People accept ideas more readily when they come in the form of a story and this is used to promote social behaviour using Social Stories (Gray and Garand, 1993).

The story is simple, non-judgemental, very concrete and tailored to the person to give them a model of how to approach a specific experience. Written from the listener's viewpoint, it consists of clear, concise and accurate statements about that social situation, what is happening and why, and what the typical response might be. It requires the author to make a close study of the behaviour that is to be reinforced or changed and, while there is clear guidance and tuition on how to compose Social Stories, they also need practise and experience. A start might be to complete Reader activity 15.5.

READER ACTIVITY 15.5

Jane is in her late teens and has autism and a mild intellectual disability. Her dentist has become concerned that she rarely brushes her teeth. Jane does not want to take on the burden of routine brushing in a life that she sees as already cluttered with routines and she has avoided visiting the dentist for the last decade.

- Read the advice and guidance on Social stories at the National Autistic Society (England, Wales and Scotland) website https://www.autism.org.uk/advice-and-guidance/topics/communication/communication-tools/social-stories-and-comic-strip-conversations
- Think about how you might start to change Jane's view about caring for her teeth.

Although there are many accounts of its effectiveness at all ages, the evidence is more equivocal on closer scrutiny and shows the methodological difficulties of autism research although a shift towards visual story-telling may be more effective (Hanrahan et al, 2020).

Sensory Integration Therapy

This focuses on the unusual sensory awareness frequently present in autism (see also Chapter 13). A systematic assessment to provide a *sensory profile* leads into a *sensory diet,* a plan that may combine avoiding or neutralising adverse stimuli with promoting more positive ones. They may include adaptations to the environment (removing flickering lights), personal strategies (wearing earphones) and the use of comforting stimuli. Known as *stimming* the last can include a wide variety of repetitive behaviours, including fidgeting, rocking and doodling. A variant is the **Low Arousal Approach** which, besides sensory approaches, uses techniques which include

relaxation and physical exercise. The approach is wide-ranging, encompassing not just the individual but also the people and objects around them (see Box 15.5).

Medication

The British Association for Psychopharmacology has published guidelines on the use of medication in autism (Howes et al, 2018). While it has no place in the routine treatment of the autism's core characteristics at present, their severity will increase with malaise and improve with its treatment, whether antibiotics for tonsillitis, antihistamines for hay-fever or a drug to treat anxiety or depression. Anxiety appears to be helped particularly by those drugs that improve serotonin transmission, both the newer antidepressants and the atypical neuroleptics such as risperidone. The risk is that medication may be overused to control disruptive and violent behaviour, assuming that it stems from anxiety. Autism may be a marker for an unpredictable and individual response to psychotropic drugs, altered sensitivity and more frequent adverse effects. This is effectively illustrated in the tragic case of UK teenager, Oliver McGowan, who developed neuroleptic malignant syndrome (BBC, 2020). More frequent, and often unrecognised, are sedation, obesity and abnormal movements, both immediate and in the longer term. Whatever is prescribed, there must be someone who constantly asks whether it is still necessary or, at least, whether a lower dose might work as well. While it is important to identify and treat additional medical difficulties such as epilepsy, depression and attention deficit, this should be only one part of a wider coordinated approach that includes psychological therapies, education and environmental change (Erickson et al, 2007; Myers et al, 2007).

Many biological treatments are strongly sold by evangelical advocates to families who feel that in the absence of anything else there is little to be lost and much to be gained. The sheer variety of remedies testifies to the lack of any all-round winner. In their time, there was strong evidence of the effectiveness of both fenfluramine and secretin only for it to evaporate in the heat of more rigorous research methodology. What did emerge from the secretin trials (where saline was as effective as secretin) was the power of a placebo (which presumably altered the way the family behaved towards the individual) as well as the methodological difficulties of researching this field (Sandler and Bodfish, 2000).

📄 BOX 15.5   The use of a sensory programme

A seventeen-year-old with ASC, a severe intellectual disability and no useful speech lives in residential care. The staff, struggling to manage his bouts of extreme overactivity and self-injury, referred him to an occupational therapist for a sensory assessment.

This suggested that he had hyporeactive vestibular and proprioceptive systems; the sensations he was registering were insufficient and, through his disturbed behaviour, he was seeking to increase this input. The staff, concerned that he would become over aroused, blocked this sensory seeking leaving him unable to obtain the stimulus he required to self-regulate and calm himself. This, in turn, led him to try harder, becoming disorganised and over-aroused. He appeared to shift abruptly from under- to over-arousal. His environment was often unstructured and unpredictable.

The remedy included staff education, the introduction of a sensory diet and modifications to his environment.

- Staff training focused on the ability of motor activities to alter arousal levels as well as the effect of deep pressure and proprioceptive activities on the central nervous system (CNS); the basis of self-regulation.
- The sensory diet used a rocking chair, fidget toys, and vibrating pillows as well as activities such as tug of war, walking carrying a backpack, sucking thick liquid through straws or from sports bottles, and swimming. As he flipped easily from under to over arousal, activities that were more likely to alert him, such as spinning and arrhythmic movements were avoided.
- Environmental modification provided more predictability together with a structured visual timetable. Central were structured sessions within a separate classroom and elimination of long periods of time in the kitchen where much of his self-injurious and overactive behaviour occurred. Classroom activities were structured in a clear and visual way using shoebox tasks. Proprioceptive activities were scheduled prior to work activities to help him organise and calm himself.

Within a month there was less self-injury and he was measurably more able to attend and to engage in tabletop activities.

CONCLUSION

While autism is frequent in the general population, it is even more so in those with intellectual disabilities. Here it adds an extra layer of disability to be recognised and managed in its own right. If missed, it blocks the more standard approaches to the management of intellectual disability and psychiatric disorder, leaving not just the individual but also their family and professionals thwarted and disheartened. However, with the development of new insights, strategies, attitudes and services, this is an exciting time for all involved.

REFERENCES

American Psychiatric Association. (2013). *Diagnostic and statistical manual of mental disorders (DSM-5)*. Arlington, VA: American Psychiatric Publishing.

Baird, G., Simonoff, E., Pickles, A., et al. (2006). Prevalence of disorders of the autistic spectrum in a population cohort of children in South Thames: the Special Needs and Autism Project (SNAP). *Lancet, 368*, 210–215.

Balfe, M., & Tantam, D. (2010). A descriptive social and health profile of a community sample of adults and adolescents with Asperger syndrome. *BMC Research Notes, 3*, 300.

BBC. (2020). *Autistic Bristol teenager Oliver McGowan's death was 'avoidable'*. Available at: https://www.bbc.co.uk/news/uk-england-bristol-54602417. [Accessed 13 January 2021].

Brede, J., Babb, C., Jones, C., et al. (2020). 'For me, the anorexia is just a symptom, and the cause is the autism': investigating restrictive eating disorders in autistic women. *Journal of Autism and Developmental Disorders*.

Brugha, T. S., Spiers, N., Bankart, J., et al. (2016). Epidemiology of autism in adults across age groups and ability levels. *British Journal of Psychiatry, 209*, 498–503.

Bryson, S. E., Bradley, E. A., Thompson, A., et al. (2008). Prevalence of autism among adolescents with intellectual disabilities. *The Canadian Journal of Psychiatry, 53*, 449–459.

Carruthers, S., Pickle, A., Slonims, V., et al. (2020). Beyond intervention into daily life: a systematic review of generalisation following social communication interventions for young children with autism. *Autism Research, 13*, 506–522.

Charman, T., Baird, G., Simonoff, E., et al. (2018). Efficacy of three screening instruments in the identification of autistic-spectrum disorders. *British Journal of Psychiatry*, *191*, 554–559.

Croen, L. A., Zerbo, O., Qian, Y., et al. (2015). The health status of adults on the autism spectrum. *Autism, 19*, 814–823.

Crompton, C. J., Hallett, S., Ropar, D., et al. (2020). 'I never realised everybody felt as happy as I do when I am around autistic people': a thematic analysis of autistic adults' relationships with autistic and neurotypical friends and family. *Autism*.

Daniels, J. L., Forssen, U., Hultman, C. M., et al. (2008). Parental psychiatric disorders associated with autism spectrum disorders in the offspring. *Pediatrics, 121*, E1357–E1362.

De Bildt, A., Sytema, S., Ketelaars, C., et al. (2003). Measuring pervasive developmental disorders in children and adolescents with mental retardation: a comparison of two screening instruments used in a study of the total mentally retarded population for a designated area. *Journal of Autism and Developmental Disorders, 33*, 595–605.

Divan, G., Vajaratkar, V., Cardozo, P., et al. (2019). The feasibility and effectiveness of PASS Plus, a lay health worker delivered comprehensive intervention for autism spectrum disorders: pilot RCT in a rural low and middle income country setting. *Autism Research, 12*, 328–339.

Erickson, C. A., Posey, D. J., Stigler, K. A., et al. (2007). Pharmacotherapy of autism and related disorders. *Psychiatric Annals, 37*, 490–500.

Fletcher-Watson, S., & Bird, G. (2020). Autism and empathy: what are the real links? *Autism, 24*, 3–6.

Grandin, T. (2006). *Thinking in pictures: and other reports from my life with autism*. London: Bloomsbury Books.

Gray, C. A., & Garand, J. D. (1993). Social stories: improving responses of students with autism with accurate social information. *Focus on Autistic Behavior, 8*, 1–10.

Green, J., Absoud, M., Grahame, V., et al. (2018). Pathological demand avoidance: symptoms but not a syndrome. *The Lancet Child & Adolescent Health, 2*, 455–464.

Haelle, T. (2019). *Identity-first vs. person-first language is an important distinction*. Available at: https://healthjournalism.org/blog/2019/07/identity-first-vs-person-first-language-is-an-important-distinction/. [Accessed 25 February 2021].

Hannant, P., Cassidy, S., Van De Weyer, R., et al. (2018). Sensory and motor differences in autism spectrum conditions and developmental coordination disorder in children: a cross-syndrome study. *Human Movement Science, 58*, 108–118.

Hanrahan, R., Smith, E., Johnson, H., et al. (2020). A pilot randomised control trial of digitally-mediated social stories for children on the autism spectrum. *Journal of Autism and Developmental Disorders*, 1–15.

Happé, F., & Frith, U. (2006). The weak coherence account: detail-focused cognitive style in autism spectrum disorders. *Journal of Autism and Developmental Disorders, 36*, 5–25.

Happé, F., & Frith, U. (2020). Annual research review: looking back to look forward – changes in the concept of autism and implications for future research. *Journal of Child Psychology and Psychiatry, 61*, 218–232.

Hirvikoski, T., Mittendorfer-Rutz, E., Boman, M., et al. (2016). Premature mortality in autism spectrum disorder. *The British Journal of Psychiatry, 208*, 232–238.

Howes, O. D., Rogdaki, M., Findon, J. L., et al. (2018). Autism spectrum disorder: consensus guidelines on assessment, treatment and research from the British Association for Psychopharmacology. *Journal of Psychopharmacology, 32*, 3–29.

Jackson, L. (2002). *Freaks, geeks and Asperger syndrome: a user guide to adolescence*. London: Jessica Kingsley.

Jones, C. R. G., Simonoff, E., Baird, G., et al. (2018). The association between theory of mind, executive function, and the symptoms of autism spectrum disorder. *Autism Research, 11*, 95–109.

Kamp-Becker, I., Albertowski, K., Becker, J., et al. (2018). Diagnostic accuracy of the ADOS and ADOS-2 in clinical practice. *European Child & Adolescent Psychiatry, 27*, 1193–1207.

Kraijer, D., & De Bildt, A. (2005). The PDD-MRS: an instrument for identification of autism spectrum disorders in persons with mental retardation. *Journal of Autism and Developmental Disorders, 35*, 499–513.

Krug, D. A., Arick, J. R., & Almond, P. J. (1988). *The Autism Behavior Checklist*. Portland, OR: ASIEP Education Company.

Lewis, L. F. (2017). A mixed methods study of barriers to formal diagnosis of autism spectrum disorder in adults. *Journal of Autism and Developmental Disorders, 47*, 2410–2424.

Lord, C., Brugha, T. S., Charman, T., et al. (2020). Autism spectrum disorder. *Nature Reviews Disease Primers, 6*, 1–23.

Lord, C., Rutter, M., & Le-Couteur, A. (1994). Autism diagnostic interview – a revised version of a diagnostic interview for caregivers of individuals with possible pervasive developmental disorders. *Journal of Autism and Developmental Disorders, 24*, 659–685.

Maenner, M. J., Shaw, K. A., & Baio, J. (2020). Prevalence of autism spectrum disorder among children aged 8 years

– Autism and Developmental Disabilities Monitoring Network, 11 sites, United States, 2016. *MMWR Surveillance Summaries*, *69*, 1.

Mandy, W. P. L., & Skuse, D. H. (2008). Research review: what is the association between the social-communication element of autism and repetitive interests, behaviours and activities? *Journal of Child Psychology and Psychiatry*, *49*, 795–808.

Milton, D. E. M. (2012). On the ontological status of autism: the 'double empathy problem'. *Disability & Society*, *27*, 883–887.

Myers, S. M., Johnson, C. P., & Council on Children with Disabilities. (2007). Management of children with autism spectrum disorders. *Pediatrics*, *120*, 1162–1182.

Packham, C. (2016). *Fingers in the sparkle jar. A memoir.* Random House.

Parihar, R., & Ganesh, S. (2016). Autism genes: the continuum that connects us all. *Journal of genetics*, *95*, 481–483.

Piven, J., & Palmer, P. (1999). Psychiatric disorder and the broad autism phenotype: evidence from a family study of multiple-incidence autism families. *American Journal of Psychiatry*, *156*, 557–563.

Polderman, T. J. C., Hoekstra, R. A., Posthuma, D., et al. (2014). The co-occurrence of autistic and ADHD dimensions in adults: an etiological study in 17 770 twins. *Translational Psychiatry*, *4*, e435.

Povey, C. (2015). What should services for people with autism look like? *Advances in Autism*, *1*, 41–46.

Rapoport, J., Chavez, A., Greenstein, D., et al. (2009). Autism spectrum disorders and childhood-onset schizophrenia: clinical and biological contributions to a relation revisited. *Journal of the American Academy of Child and Adolescent Psychiatry*, *48*, 10–18.

Rodgers, H., & Mccluney, J. (2020). *Prevalence of autism (including Asperger syndrome) in school age children in Northern Ireland: annual report 2020.* Belfast: Information & Analysis Directorate, Department of Health.

Rutter, M., Kreppner, J., Croft, C., et al. (2007). Early adolescent outcomes of institutionally deprived and non-deprived adoptees. III. Quasi–autism. *Journal of Child Psychology and Psychiatry*, *48*, 1200–1207.

Rydzewska, E., Hughes-Mccormack, L. A., Gillberg, C., et al. (2019). General health of adults with autism spectrum disorders – a whole country population cross-sectional study. *Research in Autism Spectrum Disorders*, *60*, 59–66.

Sandler, A. D., & Bodfish, J. W. (2000). Placebo effects in autism: lessons from secretin. *Journal of Developmental and Behavioral Pediatrics*, *21*, 347–350.

Schopler, E., Reichler, R. J., & Renner, B. R. (1988). *The Childhood Autism Rating Scale (CARS)*. Los Angeles: Western Psychological Services.

Shields, K., & Beversdorf, D. (2020). A dilemma For neurodiversity. *Neuroethics*.

Simonoff, E., Kent, R., Stringer, D., et al. (2019). Trajectories in symptoms of autism and cognitive ability in. *Journal of the American Academy of Child & Adolescent Psychiatry*.

Siu, A. M. H., Lin, Z., & Chung, J. (2019). An evaluation of the TEACCH approach for teaching functional skills to adults with autism spectrum disorders and intellectual disabilities. *Research in Developmental Disabilities*, *90*, 14–21.

Skuse, D., Warrington, R., Bishop, D., et al. (2004). The developmental, dimensional and diagnostic interview (3di): a novel computerized assessment for autism spectrum disorders. *Journal of the American Academy of Child and Adolescent Psychiatry*, *43*, 548–558.

Westwood, H., & Tchanturia, K. (2017). Autism spectrum disorder in anorexia nervosa: an updated literature review. *Current Psychiatry Reports*, *19*, 41.

Whitney, D., & Stansfield, A. J. (2019). Should we be accepting self-referrals for autism assessments? *Advances in Autism*, *6*, 121–127.

Wing, L. (2005). Personal communication.

Wing, L., Leekam, S. R., Libby, S. J., et al. (2002). The Diagnostic Interview for Social and Communication Disorders: background, inter-rater reliability and clinical use. *Journal of Child Psychology and Psychiatry and Allied Disciplines*, *43*, 307–325.

World Health Organisation. (2018). *The ICD-11 classification of disease for morbidity and mortality statistics.* Geneva: World Health Organisation.

Zeedyk, S. M., Davies, C., Parry, S., et al. (2009). Fostering social engagement in Romanian children with communicative impairments: the experiences of newly trained practitioners of Intensive Interaction. *British Journal of Learning Disabilities*, *37*, 186–196.

16

Mental health in people with intellectual disabilities

Laurence Taggart and Peter Langdon

KEY ISSUES

- Contrary to some historical perspectives there is clear evidence across many countries that people with intellectual disabilities can develop mental health problems / psychiatric disorders and in some cases the prevalence is higher than the general population.
- A range of inter-related factors contribute towards mental health problems amongst people with intellectual disabilities and these can be best understood using the bio-psycho-social model of health.
- A systematic and structured approach to gathering information about the typical and atypical signs and symptoms of mental health problems is important for ensuring effective treatment.
- Multi-professional team working is essential for ensuring a person-centred response to the assessment and treatment of mental health problems.
- A range of evidence-based bio-psycho-social interventions exist to treat mental health problems in people with intellectual disabilities.
- Mental health promotion throughout the lifespan of people with intellectual disabilities is vital for promoting mental wellbeing.

INTRODUCTION

The World Health Organization (WHO, 2001, p. 1) has defined mental health as, "…a state of well-being in which the individual realizes his or her own abilities, can cope with the normal stresses of life, can work productively and fruitfully, and is able to make a contribution to his or her community". Mental health is seen as a subjective state which can vary according to external events/ stressors/demands and an individual's ability to cope or manage these demands. It is a core part of general health and is not simply the absence of psychiatric disorder (World Health Organization [WHO], 2004), or merely the presence of happy emotions. People who do not have mental health problems can be unhappy, anxious or irritated. Generally, mental health is comprised of emotional, psychological and social well-being, all incorporating a sense of self-realisation, mastery and autonomy.

For some individuals, emotional, psychological and social functioning may be affected, and this may present as changes in emotions, thoughts, perceptions, memory or behaviours for an extended period of time affecting activities of daily living. These changes are sometimes referred to as signs and symptoms when they begin to take a form represented by a psychiatric disorder and are reported to a mental health care professional. In some circumstances, a person may be diagnosed with a psychiatric disorder.

Contrary to some historical perspectives there is clear evidence across many countries that people with intellectual disabilities can develop mental health problems / psychiatric disorders and in some cases the prevalence is higher than the general population. Within this chapter, the advancements and achievements that have occurred in the care of people with intellectual disabilities who have mental health problems over the last two decades will be discussed. We begin by asking you to read and reflect on Joan's story in Box 16.1 as you will be asked to answer a number of questions throughout this chapter regarding her mental health problem.

📄 BOX 16.1   Joan's story

Joan is a 19-year-old woman with a mild intellectual disability. She lives with her mother and father and has three sisters; all are now married, have children and live locally. At the strong request of Joan's parents, she attended a mainstream primary school and was supported to attend a mainstream secondary school. Her parents found it difficult to accept Joan had an intellectual disability and was different from her three sisters although were contented with her progression through school. However, Joan recalls numerous accounts of being bullied and having no friends.

It was not until Joan's late teens that her behaviour changed. Joan became uncommunicative, isolating herself from her family, wanting to remain in her bedroom and not wanting to go out of the house. Joan's weight was increasing. Her parents would describe some of her behaviours as bizarre; she tended to vocalise unintelligibly while pacing in her bedroom, had cut her own hair, and had removed wires from various electrical items in her bedroom.

As a result of these behaviours she was referred to mainstream psychiatry, whereupon identification that she had an intellectual disability she was transferred to the care of the local intellectual disability community team. This multi-disciplinary team initially gathered information about Joan from a wide range of sources. Joan was assessed by a medical practitioner who discovered that there was an under-secretion of her thyroid gland. The nurses also discovered that around the time of Joan's menstrual cycle her behaviours intensified. Within the interview with both parents, it was identified that there was a history of mental illness in the mother's family. Both parents were not accepting that their daughter could have a mental health problem as well as an intellectual disability.

Joan was also approached and asked about her behaviours. An intellectual disability nurse undertook an unstructured interview with Joan using the Mini PAS-ADD Interview. From careful interviewing with Joan, she reported to the psychiatrist that she heard a man and woman's voice talking to each other about Joan, and sometimes directly to her, telling her what to do; she did not know either person, but they strongly influenced her behaviours.

From this information, she was diagnosed with first episode schizophrenia. Working in partnership with Joan and her parents, members of the multi-disciplinary team developed a bio-psycho-social package of care. Joan was prescribed Depo-Provera to regulate her menstrual cycle, levothyroxine for hypothyroidism, and olanzapine to manage her auditory hallucinations. By using flash cards, headphones, word searches and other diversional activities initiated by Joan, her community intellectual disability nurse was able to work with her to manage but also live with her auditory hallucinations. Socially, Joan's week was structured; she attended a local drop-in centre for people with intellectual disabilities for 2 days and participated with a college of further education programme 1 day. Joan also now has a befriender; they go out every Saturday into her local town.

WHAT DO WE MEAN BY THE TERM 'MENTAL HEALTH PROBLEMS'?

The terms 'mental health problems', 'mental illness' and 'psychiatric disorders' have been used within society interchangeably to cover a wide range of feelings and behaviours which represent a recognisable pattern that causes significant and enduring distress or disability, interfering with functioning. These feelings and behaviours should not be consistent with what would be expected when encountering a common stressor (e.g. bereavement).

Recognising when people with intellectual disabilities have mental health problems is sometimes problematic because many have difficulties with cognitive and communication skills. This means that it can be hard for them to communicate their internal states (i.e. emotions, perceptions, reasoning and memories) and behaviours, making it more difficult for others to understand what it is happening. Consequently, some people with intellectual disabilities may not receive a clinical diagnosis. People with intellectual disabilities who do not receive a psychiatric diagnosis may still have 'mental health problems'.

 READER ACTIVITY 16.1

Identify a person with an intellectual disability who has a psychiatric disorder and list their signs and symptoms.
You can find out more about mental health and intellectual disabilities by visiting the online and free training resources available from MindEd, available without setting up an account: https://www.minded.org.uk/LearningContent/LaunchForGuestAccess/543727

Types of mental health problems/psychiatric disorders

Like non-disabled people, people with intellectual disabilities can also develop an array of mental health problems or psychiatric disorders. Each of these groups of disorders are made up of a number of core signs/symptoms contained within two classification systems. These are the *International Classification of Diseases-11 (ICD-11)* (World Health Organization [WHO], 2018), developed for practitioners with the previous version adopted for use within Europe, Canada, South America, Russia, Australia and Asian countries including China.

Diagnostic and Statistical Manual of Mental Disorders (DSM-5) (American Psychiatric Association [APA], 2018) developed for practitioners in the United States.

The following are some of the main psychiatric conditions.

Mood disorders

This group contains disorders in which the main sign is a marked change in mood. The mood change is usually associated with a change in the overall level of emotion, perception and activity. Most affective disorders tend to be recurrent and the onset of individual episodes can often be related to stressful events or situations. Disorders within this group include bipolar disorder, depressive disorder, recurrent depressive disorder, and dysthymia disorder.

Anxiety, Obsessive Compulsive, and disorders specifically associated with stress

A group of disorders in which anxiety-related symptoms are the core sign, and for some people this can occur in certain well-defined situations. As a result, these situations are avoided or endured with dread. Physical or somatic symptoms like palpitations, feeling faint, trembling and muscular tension are often associated with secondary fears of dying, losing control or going mad. The symptoms have a negative impact upon people's ability to take part in areas of functioning like education, work and relationships with others. Other disorders in this group include agoraphobia, social anxiety disorder, specific phobias (characterised by extreme and persistent fear of specific objects or situations that present little or no real threat) such as panic disorder, generalised anxiety disorder, obsessive-compulsive disorder, adjustment disorders and post-traumatic stress disorder.

Schizophrenia or other primary psychotic disorders

This group brings together a range of psychotic disorders with schizophrenia being the most common condition. Schizophrenia is characterised by disorganised thinking and speech, hallucinations, delusions, disorganised behaviour and blunted affect. Other disorders include schizoaffective disorder, acute and transient psychotic disorder, and delusional disorder. An example of this condition is illustrated in the case of Joan.

Neurocognitive disorders

This group of disorders comprises a range of conditions that are grouped together on the basis of their having in common a demonstrable aetiology in brain injury/disease. Dementia is a syndrome due to disease of the brain in which there is disturbance of memory, thinking, orientation, comprehension, language and judgement. Other disorders in this group include dementia in Alzheimer's disease with early and late onset, vascular dementia and dementia due to Lewy body disease.

Personality disorders

These are a group of mental disorders that are characterised by unhelpful behavioural patterns, impulsivity, affective states, and thoughts which occur consistently across contexts and depart substantially from what is culturally expected, or in other words, social norms. They include borderline, or emotionally unstable, personality disorder, antisocial personality disorder as well as obsessive-compulsive, avoidant, schizotypal and narcissistic personality disorder, as well as others. They are grouped into three clusters.

The first cluster of disorders are the odd or eccentric personality disorders and include paranoid, schizoid and schizotypal personality disorders. They are characterised by withdrawal and social awkwardness and tend to be characterised by unhelpful cognition and avoidance of social situations (e.g. thoughts that others are going to cause you harm, emotional detachment and social isolation, and odd or unusual beliefs).

The next cluster of disorders are characterised by behavioural problems including difficulties with impulsivity and the ability to regulate affective states. The personality disorders that fall into this cluster are borderline, narcissistic, histrionic and antisocial personality disorder. For those with antisocial personality disorder, they will have a history of harming or hurting other people and animals, they may damage property, engage in deceit and act with impulse rather than consider the consequences of their actions. They may have difficulties with experiencing guilt or taking responsibility for their actions and may have been diagnosed with conduct disorder during adolescence. Those with borderline personality disorder often experience intense affect which is often unstable and may lead to behavioural outbursts and related behavioural problems including risk taking and self-harming behaviours. Those with histrionic personality disorder also present with extremes of affect along with excessive attention-seeking, while those with narcissistic personality disorder have a marked sense of entitlement and see themselves as special or talented, demanding special treatment from others.

The final cluster of personality disorders include avoidant, dependent and obsessive-compulsive personality disorder. The key defining feature of this cluster is anxiety, where those with avoidant personality disorder will avoid others because they view themselves as inadequate or likely to be subjected to criticism, while those with dependent personality disorder will experience anxiety associated with fears of being alone, and will demonstrate behaviours which encourage others to take care of them. Those with obsessive-compulsive personality disorder will effortfully work to make sure that things are orderly and perfect within most life domains including exerting control within social relationships in order to neutralise or reduce anxiety.

There are issues associated with making a diagnosis of personality disorder when someone also has an intellectual disability. For example, many people with intellectual disabilities are inherently dependent upon others and behaviours, for example, self-injurious and other challenging behaviours, may be exhibited by some people with intellectual disabilities because they are associated with a communicative function rather than a personality disorder. However, it is possible that some of the behaviours exhibited by people with personality disorder also serve a communicative function (i.e. attempting to communicate psychological distress to others) and some have suggested that deliberate self-harm, often seen in personality disorder, and self-injurious behaviour seen amongst people with intellectual disabilities, have a shared aetiology (Ernst et al, 2010). This situation can often present as markedly complex and skilful assessment by experienced clinicians is required. For a discussion of some of these issues see Moreland et al (2008).

Prevalence of mental health problems

Mental health problems can occur across the lifespan of the person, whether they have a disability or not. Young people, adults and older people with intellectual disabilities can and do experience the same range of mental health problems as people without. Not only does this population experience the same types of clinical conditions but there is an increasing body of evidence highlighting that people with intellectual disabilities have been found to have higher rates of certain mental health problems than the general population (Cooper et al, 2007a, 2018). However, prevalence rates of mental health problems amongst this group do tend to vary, one reason being differences in the severity of the intellectual disability as a result of the level of cognitive impairment and limited communication skills thereby making diagnosis more complex (Hove and Havik, 2010). Other inter-related reasons as to why prevalence rates vary include the following:

- According to Allen (2009) diagnostic overshadowing, behavioural overshadowing (i.e. presence of challenging behaviour) and psychiatric overshadowing (i.e. the person using psychotropic medication) may make obtaining an accurate diagnosis more difficult. For example, behaviours that are associated with having an intellectual disability may be mistaken as symptoms of a mental health problem such as unusual speech, poor social skills, or difficulties regulating affect. These 'atypical' behaviours could lead to 'diagnostic confusion' and difficulties identifying whether a person has a mental health problem (Jamieson and Mason, 2019).
- Many people with mild intellectual disabilities may be able to verbally report how they feel regarding their subjective internal mental health (i.e. emotions, perceptions, cognition) and their behaviours with minimal assistance however this will be difficult for those with limited communication and moderate to severe/profound intellectual disabilities. Consequently, how this group of people express themselves may be through behaviours that are not identified as typical signs/symptoms of a specific mental health condition such as an affective disorder like depression. This manifestation or expression

can be described as 'atypical symptomology' or 'behaviours that challenge' (Hemmings, 2007) and is often referred to as *diagnostic overshadowing*.

- Different screening instruments also reflect variation in prevalence rates. For example, information can be collected based upon screening tools developed for adults without disabilities who can self-report such as Beck's Depression Inventory (Beck et al, 1961) and Hamilton Anxiety Scale (Hamilton, 1959). Such instruments can be used with adults with mild intellectual disabilities but are less reliable for adults with moderate to profound intellectual disabilities. For those with moderate to profound intellectual disabilities, there are instruments that are completed with someone who knows the person well like a carer, parent or staff member. These are referred to as proxy-rated instruments and include the:
- Developmental Behaviour Checklist – 2 (Gray et al, 2018)
- PAS-ADD Schedules (Moss, 2002)
- Reiss Scale (Reiss, 1988)
- Psychopathology Instrument for Mentally Retarded Adults (PIMRA) (Matson, 1988).

Prevalence rates of mental health problems in young people

Meltzer et al (2000) in a large national survey in England, Scotland and Wales found that 13% of boys and 10% of girls aged between 11 and 15 years without intellectual disabilities had mental health problems. Emerson (2003), using secondary analysis of the Meltzer et al (2000) sample, found that children and adolescents with intellectual disabilities were four times more likely to have a mental health problem compared with their non-disabled peers. In an international systematic review of nine studies that compared the mental health of children with and without intellectual disabilities, those with disabilities were more likely to have a mental health problem. Taggart et al (2007), in a study that examined the mental health status of children and adolescents with intellectual disabilities living in state care (i.e. children's home, foster care) in Northern Ireland, found over three-quarters of these young people had a mental health problem.

Prevalence rates of mental health problems in adults

Affective disorders have been reported to be more common in people with intellectual disabilities than the general population; rates of depression and bipolar disorders have been reported to be higher compared to adults without disabilities (Cooper et al, 2007a, 2018; Hassiotis et al, 2014). Likewise, people with intellectual disabilities are more likely to develop anxiety disorders (Hassiotis et al, 2014), and post-traumatic stress disorder as a result of major life event(s) or trauma compared to their non-disabled peers (Mason-Roberts et al, 2018).

Studies also report higher prevalence rates of psychosis and personality disorders. Several studies have examined schizophrenia in people with mild/moderate intellectual disabilities and have reported that prevalence rates are four to six times higher than reported in the non-disabled population (Cooper et al, 2007b, 2015; Hemmings, 2014). Higher rates of schizophrenia have also been reported for adults with mild/moderate intellectual disabilities (Cooper et al, 2018).

Eating disorders such as binge eating, pica, anorexia nervosa, bulimia nervosa, food refusal and psychogenic vomiting (i.e. patients vomit in the absence of any physical cause) have been found to exist in adults with intellectual disabilities, again at a higher prevalence. However, unlike the non-disabled population, no differences have been found in the extent to which this affects males and females (Hove, 2004). In relation to substance misuse in people with intellectual disabilities, Van Duijvenbode and Vandernagel (2019), in a systematic review of 138 studies from 2000-2018, reported that adults with borderline to mild intellectual disabilities were more likely to be at a higher risk of developing a substance use disorder compared to the non-disabled population. Loneliness, bereavement, trauma and mental health problems have been cited as some of the reasons for adults with intellectual disabilities using substances (Taggart et al, 2008). Papagavriel et al (2020) found that loneliness is more prevalent in people with borderline intellectual disability.

Prevalence rates of mental health problems in older people

Older people with intellectual disabilities also develop mental health problems in addition to the recognised dementias. Several studies have reported higher rates of affective disorders, anxiety disorders, bipolar disorder and schizophrenia (Cooper et al, 2015). Prevalence rates of these clinical conditions have again been reported to be higher compared with older people without intellectual disabilities. Nevertheless, it is the dementias that

have been reported to be significantly higher, particularly amongst people with Down syndrome, when compared to this population's non-disabled peers (Strydom and Sinai, 2014). A more detailed exploration of this issue can be found in Chapter 26.

USING A BIO-PSYCHO-SOCIAL MODEL TO UNDERSTAND MENTAL HEALTH

In attempting to understand why people with intellectual disabilities are more likely to develop mental health problems as compared to the non-disabled population, the International Association for the Scientific Study of Intellectual & Developmental Disabilities (IASSIDD, 2001), in a report to the World Health Organization (WHO), proposed adopting a functional framework that examined the whole person. This was in comparison to the opposing medical model that had been traditionally employed across medicine, psychiatry and nursing where the mental health problem was viewed as organic and based within the person. This model, taken from the International Classification of Functioning Disability and Health (ICF) (World Health Organization [WHO], 2007), provided a holistic, proactive approach to understanding how mental health problems develop, but also how such problems can be prevented, if possible (see Figure 16.1). The model identifies the key risk factors for developing mental health problems in four inter-related segments: biological, developmental, psychological and social (Emerson and Hatton, 2014). For the purposes of application to practice, this model will be applied to understanding the specific risk factors for the development of mental health problems in three client groups: young people, women, and people from Black And Minority Ethnic (BAME) groups, all with intellectual disabilities.

Young people with intellectual disabilities

Researchers have identified several risk factors for why young people with intellectual disabilities, including children with autism, are more likely to develop mental health problems compared to their non-disabled peers. These may include:

Biological

Having a specific genetic condition (e.g. Fragile X, foetal alcohol syndrome, Prader–Willi syndrome) or autism, having a severe/profound intellectual disability, having sensory and communication problems, sex (i.e. males are more likely to develop Attention Deficit

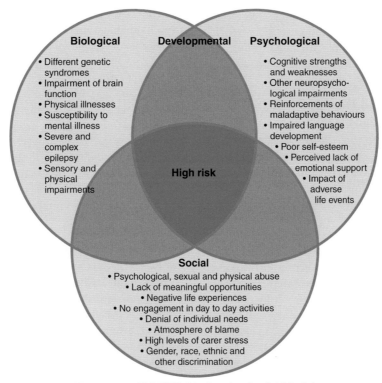

Figure 16.1 IASSIDD Bio-Psycho-Social Model

Hyperactivity Disorder (ADHD) and conduct disorders whereas females are more likely to develop affective and anxiety disorders) (Tsakanikos and McCarthy, 2013).

Developmental and Psychological

The primary caregiver(s) having a mental health problem(s), family history of mental health problems and/or substance abuse, presence of negative role model(s) and the employment of punitive child management practices within the family home (Taggart et al, 2010a).

Social

High levels of social deprivation, poverty, family composition (i.e. single parent), little opportunities for education and recreation, excessive amounts of free time, limited friends, lack of meaning in life, social exclusion (Emerson and Hatton, 2014; Ratcliffe et al, 2015; Munir, 2016; Allington-Smith, 2019).

Women with intellectual disabilities

Women without intellectual disabilities are more likely to develop specific mental health problems compared to

men that include affective disorders, bipolar disorder, anxiety disorders, eating disorders, borderline personality disorder and pre-/peri-menstrual disorders and therefore it could be argued that women with intellectual disabilities are more likely to develop mental health problems (Taggart et al, 2008, 2009a, 2010b). Commonly identified risk factors for this group include the following:

Biological

Physical issues related to hormonal changes, reproduction, sexual health including contraception, and use of psychotropic medication associated with weight gain.

Developmental and Psychological

Juggling multiple roles (i.e. caring for children, caring for family members, looking after the household), negative life events, sexual abuse, domestic violence, how having an intellectual disability affects the woman and her identity, relationships, loss of children and loneliness.

Social

Poverty, inequality, social isolation, restricted social support networks, lack of employment, education and recreation (O'Hara, 2008; Taggart et al, 2008, 2009a,b, 2010a).

People from Black And Minority Ethnic (BAME) groups with intellectual disabilities

Research shows that people with intellectual disabilities from ethnic backgrounds are more likely to have poorer physical and mental health (Magaña et al, 2016). The Healthcare Commission (2007) in the UK found that people from different ethnic groups were more likely to be admitted to hospital and community psychiatric clinics compared to their white counterparts: the majority of admissions were found to be for underlying mental health issues. There is growing evidence that people from ethnic communities are more likely to live in poverty, be unemployed, live in poor social housing, be socially isolated and are more likely to be exposed to more negative life events. In addition, people from ethnic communities may not have health information in a format that they can access/understand and may not utilise health services (Raghavan and Waseem, 2007).

RECOGNISING THE SIGNS/SYMPTOMS OF MENTAL ILL HEALTH

In order for health care professionals to recognise the signs/symptoms of mental ill health in the general population, the ICD-11 (WHO, 2018) and the DSM 5 (APA, 2018) classification systems are used.

Both classification systems undertake a similar task, that is to define the clinical picture of the person in order to provide an accurate diagnosis. These two systems provide a clinical psychiatric diagnosis based upon a range of signs/symptoms, or a cluster of these, often generated during a clinical interview and from other supportive sources which can be direct observation or a review of historical records (e.g. medical or educational records). Furthermore, verbally reporting these signs/symptoms will aid the health care professional in attempting to understand the nature of the mental illness, the potential causes of the illness and to develop an effective treatment package. Joan's story in Box 16.1 highlights the importance of the person's verbal reports. When Joan was interviewed, she disclosed that she

sometimes heard the voice of a man and woman talking to each other about her.

Another development has been the publication of the DC-LD: Diagnostic Criteria for Psychiatric Disorders for Use with Adults with Intellectual Disabilities/Mental Retardation, by the Royal College of Psychiatrists (RCP, 2001). The aim of this classification system is "to improve upon existing general population psychiatric diagnostic classificatory systems" for people with intellectual disabilities (RCP, 2001). There is also the Diagnostic Manual – Intellectual Disability – 2 (DM-ID-2) which is an adapted version of the DSM-5 for use with people who have intellectual disabilities (Fletcher et al, 2016).

Typical clusters of signs/symptoms of mental ill health

Current standardised mental health classification systems as described above attempt to identify the symptoms the person describes and presents with, within clusters or groups of typical signs/symptoms using six main categories. Devine and Taggart (2008) grouped these typical signs/symptoms into six core clusters:

1. Somatic (or physical symptoms)
2. Emotional
3. Behavioural
4. Thought/cognition/perception
5. Attention or motivation
6. Activities of Daily Living (ADLs).

Based on these signs/symptoms, a health care professional also needs to know the length of time the person has been experiencing these signs/symptoms (i.e. 2 weeks, 1 month, 6 months). In order to identify a correct diagnosis, the person must display several identified signs/symptoms for these clusters for a specified period of time.

Atypical clusters or behaviours that challenge

People with mild intellectual disabilities will probably display many of the typical signs/symptoms of mental ill health as detailed within the ICD-11 (APA, 2018) or DSM-5 (WHO, 2018). Some of these signs/symptoms may be more marked such as agitation, crying, short-temperedness, loss of skills or needing more prompting to use skills, social withdrawal, irritability, avoidance, agitation and loss of interest in activities they usually enjoy. Other signs/symptoms may not be directly observable to family carers or front-line staff (i.e. loss of confidence or low self-esteem) and are more difficult to identify.

For people with moderate to severe/profound intellectual disabilities and additional problems (i.e. limited communication skills, sensory disabilities and autism) they may display signs/symptoms that can be described as 'atypical' or 'behaviours that challenge', that is they are not normally recognised as characteristic for a specific mental health problem (Hemmings, 2007). These are displayed in Box 16.2. This evidence is based upon a very similar structured approach a psychiatrist or clinical psychologist would employ within the DSM-5 (APA, 2018), ICD-11 (WHO, 2018), DC-LD (RCP, 2001), DM-ID-2 (Fletcher et al, 2016) as described above.

 READER ACTIVITY 16.2

Focus on an individual with intellectual disabilities and possible mental health problems.

Think about the signs and symptoms that they are displaying.

Use the list in Box 16.2 to identify if the person is displaying any or all of these signs/symptoms.

ASSESSING MENTAL HEALTH PROBLEMS

When undertaking a comprehensive mental health assessment of a person with intellectual disability, care must be undertaken to collate various information from multiple informants in order to ensure the accuracy of the data collected (Simpson, 2009; Moss and Hurley, 2014). The sharing and testing of this information will help health care professionals to develop a working hypothesis of the possible underlying mental health problem or other underlying conditions. Based on this information, a clinical diagnosis can be made, and/or a formulation developed incorporating bio-psycho-social models of mental illness. The two together are used to develop and implement a bio-psycho-social intervention package which is directly informed by theory and research about what interventions work best. The National Institute for Health and Care Excellence (NICE) (2016) recommended several steps for assessing the mental health needs of people with intellectual

 BOX 16.2 **Possible signs and symptoms of mental health problems**

- **Somatic** (or physical symptoms): palpitations, feeling faint, trembling, muscular tension, dizziness, dry mouth, gastric problems, sickness and vomiting.
- **Emotional:** feeling down, sad, weepy, elevated mood, mood swings, short-tempered, frustrated, low self-esteem, lack of confidence, incongruent affect.
- **Behavioural:** idleness, increases or decreases in appetite and subsequent weight change, increases or decreases in sleeping, self-harm, suicidal ideation (i.e. thoughts about planning the suicide act but not actually carrying it out), lethargy, listlessness, disinterest.
- **Thought/cognition/perception:** worried, anxious, apprehensive and nervous, thought disturbance, ideas of self-harm, concentration, orientation, feelings of guilt, remorse, worthlessness, hopeless, disorganised speech, speech that wanders off track or is obliquely related, using made-up words.
- **Attention or motivation:** lethargy, withdrawal, loss of interest in life, negativity, lack of interest in normal routines, inattention.
- **Activities of daily living (ADL):** changes in routine, loss of self-care skills and appearance, loss of social skills, disinterested in work, family, life or hobbies.
- **Atypical or behaviours that challenge:** changes in facial expression, biting (self and others), grinding teeth, increase in repetitive hand movements, increase in sexual behaviour, changes in posture, lack of responsiveness, increase or decrease in vocalisation, disruptive behaviour, thumb-biting, self-injurious behaviour, increased agitation, screaming, spontaneous crying, stereotypical behaviours, non-compliance, seeking greater reassurances and increase in seizure activity, pica, skin-picking, aggression, destruction of property.

disabilities. Box 16.3 identifies the key sources of information that can be gathered about the factors that may predispose, precipitate and/or maintain the person's behaviours.

BOX 16.3 Recommendations for assessment of mental health problems in people with intellectual disabilities based on NICE (2016)

A professional with expertise in mental health problems in people with intellectual disabilities should coordinate the mental health assessment and conduct it with the person with an intellectual disability, their carers and other professionals (if needed)

Speak to the person on their own to find out if they have any concerns (including safeguarding concerns) that they don't want to talk about in front of their carers

When conducting mental health assessments, be aware that an underlying physical health condition may be causing the problem; and a sensory or cognitive impairment may mask an underlying mental health problem; and that mental health problems can present differently in people with more severe intellectual disabilities

When conducting mental health assessments, consider the person's level of distress, understanding of the problem, living arrangements and settings where they receive care, strengths and needs

Assess and review all areas of the person's bio-psycho-social being including
- cultural, ethnic and religious world
- genetic aetiology of the intellectual disability
- the nature, duration and severity of the presenting mental health problem / behaviours
- physical and psychiatric health, medications, past treatments and responses

- assess the person's family, social circumstances, environment and recent life events
- the level of drug or alcohol use as a potential problem in itself and as a factor contributing to other mental health problems
- recent changes in behaviour using information from family members, carers, staff or others involved in the assessment as well as information from relevant records and previous assessments

Develop a formulation of the mental health problem covering
- an understanding of the nature of the problem and its development
- precipitating and maintaining factors; any protective factors
- the potential benefits, side effects and harms of any interventions
- the potential difficulties with delivering interventions
- the adjustments needed to deliver interventions
- the impact of the mental health problem and associated risk factors on providing care and treatment

Provide the person, their family members and other carers, all relevant professionals with a summary of the assessment in an agreed format and accessible language that sets out the implications for care and treatment

Consider use of standardised rating scales

Use of standardised rating scales

Using standardised rating scales to obtain a baseline profile of the person with an intellectual disability, and changes from the baseline, will provide further objective evidence and also support the family carer, front-line staff and clinicians in identifying that there is a problem(s) by collecting evidence via a structured framework. These scales should be part of a holistic comprehensive assessment process involving information from other sources as outlined in Box 16.3. Rating scales should be used to collect data on the person's baseline behaviours in four core areas and can identify the interplay between the risk factors as demonstrated

within the bio-psycho-social model above. Examples include:

1. Physical health (for example the OK Health Checklist, Matthews and Hegarty, 1997).
2. Functioning ability (for example the Adaptive Behaviour Scale, Nihra et al, 1993).
3. Challenging behaviours (for example the Aberrant Behaviour Checklist, Aman and Singh, 1986).
4. Mental health (for example the PAS-ADD Checklist or Interview, Moss, 2002).

These are examples of some standardised rating scales that could help to build an established record of the person's physical health, inventory of functioning skills, levels of challenging behaviour and mental health status. In addition, the tools can be used to monitor changes in the person's treatment and evaluate the impact of the intervention package, thereby ensuring the person returns to their optimal level of physical health and functional ability. Given the bio-psycho-social factors in the aetiology of the person's mental health problem, utilising such standardised rating scales can help 'unscramble' the various other potential causes that lead to the signs/symptoms and behaviours.

Assessing young people with intellectual disabilities

Assessing children and young people with intellectual disabilities should be based upon the risk factors identified for young people with intellectual disabilities discussed earlier in this chapter. Complete Reader activity 16.3 in the online resource to further develop your understanding.

A number of mental health standardised rating scales have been developed for recognising potential problems in young people without intellectual disabilities; conversely some of these tools have been used with young people with intellectual disabilities and have been found to be reliable. One example is the Strengths and Difficulties Questionnaire (SDQ) (Goodman, 1999). The SDQ has been successfully employed with young people with mild intellectual disabilities to assess their emotions, behaviours and functional impairment. The SDQ consists of five subscales (emotions, conduct, inattention–hyperactivity, peer problems and pro-social (positive) behaviour). The SDQ has been reported to have moderate to strong reliability and validity when used with parents, teachers and as a self-rating tool. Emerson (2005) reported that the extended SDQ was a simple and robust tool to also measure the mental health of young people with intellectual disabilities. This scale is freely available to download and use (see Useful resources online).

A specific screening tool that has been developed for young people with intellectual disabilities is the Cha-PAS (Moss et al, 2007) which is part of the PAS-ADD Schedules identified above. The Cha-PAS is a 97-item screening instrument that assesses mental health. This tool examines depression, anxiety, ADHD, compulsions, conduct issues, psychotic disorders and the autistic spectrum. Specific training is required to use this tool.

Assessing women with intellectual disabilities

In assessing the mental health of women with intellectual disabilities, again the bio-psycho-social model (see Figure 16.1) should be an underpinning guide. In addition, a gender-sensitive approach to assessment and intervention should also be undertaken, recognising the specific risk factors that women face regarding the development of mental health problems as illustrated by Joan's story (see Box 16.1) and Vidusha, an Asian woman, in Reader activity 16.4 online. This assessment should include a greater recognition of the obstetric (i.e. pregnancy) and gynaecological issues (i.e. hormonal, peri-and post-menstrual health, contraception, sexual health care issues) and issues related to unequal power within society that many women experience and its link with behavioural and mental health problems (Eogan and Wingfield, 2010).

INTERVENTIONS FOR MENTAL HEALTH PROBLEMS

In keeping with a focus on the bio-psycho-social model, there is no one singular cause for the development of mental ill health in people with or without intellectual disabilities, but a cumulative number of risk factors that must be examined in greater detail. To fully understand the predisposing, precipitating and/or maintaining factors, a bio-psycho-social assessment must therefore be undertaken. Likewise, in treating the person's underlying mental health problem, a bio-psycho-social approach should be employed in order to develop an effective range of interventions. The need for individualised assessments and person-centred planning of interventions also needs to be core to any multi-element intervention package that may include any of the following, singularly or in combination.

Psychopharmacology

Psychotropic medications such as antipsychotics, antidepressants, mood stabilisers, including anti-epileptic medications and lithium, anti-anxiety medications including benzodiazepines, psychostimulants, beta-adrenergic blockers, opioid antagonists are used widely among people with intellectual disabilities. Sheehan et al (2015) highlighted that psychotropic medication remains the first line of defence in managing both mental ill health and challenging behaviours in approximately 50%–63% of this population. The authors purported *"that the proportion of people with intellectual disability who have been treated with psychotropic drugs far exceeds the proportion with recorded mental illness. Antipsychotics are often prescribed to people without recorded severe mental illness but who have a record of challenging behaviour"* Sheehan et al, 2015, p. 1

Indeed Sheehan and Hassiotis (2017) in a systematic review of the use of antipsychotics to manage challenging behaviour in this population found that antipsychotics can be reduced or discontinued in a substantial proportion of adults who use them for challenging behaviour. Because of these concerns, NHS England has embarked on a major campaign called "STopping Over Medication of People with intellectual disability, autism or both (STOMP)" (NHS England, 2020).

Chyka (2000) claims that many of the antipsychotic medications used to manage mental ill health and challenging behaviour in people with intellectual disabilities score highly in the league tables of deaths caused by their side effects, including:

- a range of somatic or physical symptoms
- cholinergic effects (i.e. dry mouth, increase in heart rate, increase in blood pressure, blurred vision, memory problems, loss of coordination, sensitivity to heat), dyskinetic movement disorders (i.e. involuntary repetitive writhing or jerking movements)
- neuroleptic malignant syndrome (i.e. fever, severe muscle rigidity, altered consciousness, automatic arousal and can lead to death)
- memory impairment
- pseudo-parkinsonian symptoms (i.e. unsteady gait, bent posture, expressionless face and tremors).

Despite these serious side-effects, medication prescribed within strict guidelines can serve a clinical purpose. Deb (2018) provided detailed guidelines on the use and management of psychotropic medication for this population. The use of medication must be a therapeutic treatment component that is part of a larger package and not a tool to create a convenient short-term respite for medical personnel or for caregivers. Antipsychotic medication used for behaviour should be reviewed regularly and a person-centred approach taken to treatment. Joan's story (Box 16.1) shows that, whilst diagnosed with paranoid schizophrenia, part of her treatment package was medication but there was a psycho-social intervention package as well. Medication was not the only treatment employed to manage her auditory hallucinations; in addition, medication was also used to regulate her menstrual cycle. You can read more about the use of medication in the management of challenging behaviour in the next chapter.

Cognitive Behavioural Therapy

Cognitive Behavioural Therapy (CBT) aims to augment unhelpful thoughts, or cognitions, that an individual may have about themselves, their past, and their future, as well as unhelpful patterns of behaviour. CBT has been found to successfully treat the following conditions in people with intellectual disabilities (see Vereenooghe and Langdon, 2013):

- Anxiety management (Dagnan and Jahoda, 2006; Douglass et al, 2007).
- Anger management (Rose et al, 2008).
- Bereavement (Summers, 2003).
- Depression (Jahoda et al, 2006).
- Low self-esteem (Whelan et al, 2007).
- Management of auditory hallucinations in psychosis (Kirkland, 2005).
- Obsessive compulsive disorder (Willner and Goodey, 2006).
- Sex offenders (Keeling and Rose, 2006).

CBT is not suitable for all people with intellectual disabilities, and everyone should be assessed to determine their suitability. Dagnan et al (2000) outline several components that will determine suitability, which include an assessment of general language, level of intellectual ability, ability to recognise and understand emotions, and ability to link events to emotion. However, there is some evidence that people with moderate to mild intellectual disabilities can be taught some of these skills (Bruce et al, 2010; Vereenooghe et al, 2016; Vereenooghe et al, 2015).

While some individuals with intellectual disabilities may have difficulty taking part in structured psychological therapy, over 20-years ago Hurley et al (1998) suggested that therapy could be adapted to improve accessibility. Some of the suggested changes included simplifying interventions and sessions, making sessions shorter, using drawings and pictorial aids, simplifying language use, increasing flexibility, tailoring content to developmental level, and including carers, staff, or family members within therapy.

Joan's story (Box 16.1) clearly illustrates the success of a number of strategies to manage her auditory hallucinations: flash cards, headphones, word searches and other diversional activities such as brisk walks, activities that both Joan and her parents were trained in, thereby supporting Joan to continue to live within her family and remain in her local community.

Psychodynamic psychotherapy

Psychodynamic psychotherapy is focused heavily upon the development of a trusting relationship between the client and the therapist which becomes the mechanism by which change occurs (Beail et al, 2005). There is growing evidence in the literature of psychotherapeutic approaches being used successfully to address emotional difficulties, such as poor self-esteem, psychotic behaviour, anxiety and sexually inappropriate behaviour among people with intellectual disabilities (RCP, 2001). However, Shepherd and Beail (2017) concluded that while the associated literature suggests that this psychotherapy may be effective, there are currently no controlled trials and concerns have been expressed about methodological quality of existing studies suggesting that the evidence base is not yet conclusive.

Eye Movement Desensitisation and Reprocessing

Eye Movement Desensitisation and Reprocessing (EMDR) is an intervention that has been highly recommended by NICE to treat those who suffer from Post-Traumatic Stress Disorder (PTSD). Until recently, there has only been a small number of individual case studies that have used EMDR with adults with intellectual disabilities (see Mevissen et al, 2011; Barrowcliff and Evans, 2015, for two examples of single case studies). There have been several recent studies that have explored using EMDR with adults with intellectual disabilities with larger samples including those who may have communication problems meaning that reporting the traumatic memory is difficult. For example Karatzias et al (2019) in the UK undertook a randomised feasibility study of 29 adults with intellectual disabilities who had experienced trauma; half the sample received EMDR and the other half received routine clinical care. As this was a feasibility study, this study showed that the adults with intellectual disabilities could be recruited, consented, baseline and follow-up data collected and the participants randomised to the EDMR intervention could engage in the 8–12 sessions. The results demonstrate improvements in anxiety although the sample size is too small to show clinical effectiveness; a full definitive trial is needed. The EMDR protocol may need to be adapted for use with people who have intellectual disabilities which may include using others to tell the trauma story in the presence of the person with an intellectual disability and the therapist (Lovett, 1999).

Family therapy

Considering the central and key role that good family life plays in maintaining positive mental health (see Health promotion, below), it is surprising how little family therapy appears to be used in the field of intellectual disabilities. The most likely constant in the individual's life is the family, while professional personnel and systems of care delivery are likely to frequently change. Therefore, alongside individual therapeutic work, it makes sense that more targeted intervention is directed at working with families. It is also important to recognise that many people with intellectual disabilities live in 'family' groups and can be supported by staff teams. Family therapy can be successfully applied to help address emotional issues such as loss, isolation, anxieties about sexuality and concerns about failure, whereby the issues can be fully explored with all members of the family participating and helping each other (Baum, 2007).

Solution-Focused Brief Therapy

While Solution-Focused Brief Therapy (SFBT) has become a widely used form of psychotherapy in the UK, there is little published on its use in services for people with intellectual disabilities. Smith (2005) discusses SFBT's potential uses with people with intellectual disabilities and provides a case illustration of its application with a man with a mild intellectual disability referred to clinical psychology services for 'anger management'. The author reports the effectiveness of SFBT in diminishing this man's anger issues. In a series of case studies, Roeden et al (2011) investigated the utility of SFBT with ten adults with intellectual disabilities. They reported improvements in psychological functioning and reductions in maladaptive behaviours following treatment. Similarly, SFBT has been delivered to families who have a child with intellectual disability (Lloyd and Dallos, 2006).

Psychoeducational interventions

One of the first key elements considered necessary for early intervention in mental health has been engagement and psychoeducation, either in groups or individually (as in Joan's story at Box 16.1) with people with intellectual disabilities. Group programmes usually include education about the mental illness, medication and the role of biological, psychological and social risk factors linked to parental stress. Some examples include a psychoeducational group for men who have sex with men (Withers et al, 2001), adults with borderline to mild intellectual disabilities who have psychosis (Crowley et al, 2008) and parents of children with intellectual disabilities (Schultz et al, 1993).

The aims and objectives of these groups have varied from trying to improve members' self-esteem, empowerment, medication adherence to increasing understanding about their illness, improving levels of managing their positive and negative symptoms, and empowering the individual to develop and maintain self-management and access to services (Crowley et al, 2008).

Social interventions

It is important to remember that for many individuals with intellectual disabilities:

> "... it is the specific handicaps they experience in housing, employment, income, social networks, leisure opportunities, and so on, which gives them their greatest frustrations, and their greatest sense of alienation."
> Fryers, 1997, p. 112.

In addition to those shown in Figure 16.1, other factors that enhance susceptibility to mental illness amongst people with intellectual disabilities include their experiences of stigma (Scior and Werner, 2016). Consequently, following assessment, it may be determined that one or any number of social factors might have contributed significantly to the development of mental ill health. In such circumstances, it is important to intervene through manipulating or changing the environment and/or situation (Dagnan, 2007).

Social interventions can address issues such as mental ill health as well as poverty, communication skills, access to leisure, employment, family relationships and education (Emerson and Hatton, 2014). They are focused on providing for the individual or groups the opportunity to have a meaningful life, to make choices, to have adequate leisure opportunities and to be free from the constraints of social exclusion. Social interventions require adopting a more proactive, public health-based approach which focuses on prevention.

READER ACTIVITY 16.5

In what activities do you engage that keep you emotionally well?

Keep a record of your answers.

Think of someone with an intellectual disability who you know or support.

How accessible might these activities be to this person?

What might be the barriers?

What might be needed to help facilitate access?

HEALTH PROMOTION

The Department of Health (2001) in the UK highlighted a two-stage model of promoting mental health:

1. **Reducing risk factors:** poverty, deprived communities, high unemployment, financial difficulties, poor educational opportunities, high crime rates, emotional/physical/sexual abuse, high stress levels, social exclusion, bereavement, family break up, long-term caring, gender.
2. **Increasing protective factors:** quality environments, increasing self-esteem and empowerment, self-management skills, social participation.

There are numerous health promotion programmes for people with intellectual disabilities, many of which have been reviewed by Scott and Havercamp (2016). Black and Devine (2008) developed a mental health promotion booklet for parents, teachers and front-line staff who care for children and young people with intellectual disabilities, entitled Head Start (see Useful resources online). The booklet targets those factors that make young people resilient or protect against them developing mental ill health, as well as highlighting potential risk factors. Below is a list of key factors to help build resilience; although each factor is important, they all overlap, interact and reinforce each other:

- Good physical health.
- Exercise and activity.
- Success and achievement.
- Self-awareness.
- Positive family connections.
- Friendships and relationships.
- Meaningful social activity.
- Support during changes and transitions.
- Involvement in making choices and decisions.
- Care and support.

In Head Start (Black and Devine, 2008) each one of these 10 factors are discussed individually, and practical tips are offered to help carers supporting people with intellectual disabilities to have good mental health. For example, young people with intellectual disabilities who have some understanding and awareness of themselves and the challenges they face are more likely to have stronger emotional resilience. It is important that from an early age children and young people are helped to see and regard their intellectual disabilities as being only one aspect of themselves. This is about helping to build confidence and enabling them to recognise their strengths as much as their limitations. Examples include the following:

- Children and young people should be given opportunities to talk about the limitations imposed by their disabilities
- It is important to be open and honest about the disabilities and to help them understand more about their condition. Many organisations provide useful resources to explain conditions and the likely effects on living and lifestyle
- Group work with peers is one way of helping children and young people with intellectual disabilities understand that everyone is unique and that everyone has their own limitations
- Involve the young person in activities and pursuits that provide the best match with their ability. Focus on activities where participation is not going to draw attention to their disability
- Emphasise and focus your energy on their talents.

INTERPROFESSIONAL WORKING

Throughout this chapter, clear evidence has been shown that to obtain an accurate clinical picture of a person with an intellectual disability, information must be gathered from a range of sources. Such sources of information include family carers, teachers, day-care staff, residential staff, nurses, social workers, psychiatrists and speech and language therapists.

Costello et al (2007) reported that front-line care staff play a key role helping to recognise people with intellectual disabilities who may have difficulties with their mental health. Yet few staff have received training in mental health and evidence about the effectiveness of training is scant. Using a pre–post study design, significant improvements in staff knowledge, attitudes and referral decisions were observed. Costello et al (2007) concluded that brief training interventions may improve awareness of mental health problems.

CONCLUSION

In order to address mental health problems amongst people with intellectual disabilities, readers need to have a clear understanding of the typical and atypical signs/symptoms of the presenting problem as well as the risk factors. Collating this information together can be fraught with difficulty in the population of people with intellectual disabilities and even more complicated with people who have limited or no communication. Multiple informants are required to gather this information so an accurate diagnosis and/or formulation can be made, and a multi-modal intervention package of care developed. Utilising the bio-psycho-social framework as proposed within this chapter will offer readers a more holistic approach to addressing the person's mental health problem, providing a more effective, efficient, and evidence-based intervention. Although the chapter has emphasised the importance of recognising the signs/symptoms of mental ill health and developing an intervention package, this chapter has also highlighted the importance of mental health promotion and prevention in attempting, where possible, to avoid such problems from developing, starting with people with intellectual disabilities themselves.

REFERENCES

Allen, D. (2009). The relationship between challenging behaviour and mental ill-health in people with intellectual disabilities: a review of current theories and evidence. *Journal of Intellectual Disabilities, 12*, 267–294.

Allington-Smith, P. (2019). Children with intellectual disabilities and psychiatric problems. In M. Scheepers & M. Kerr (Eds.), *Seminars in the psychiatry of intellectual disability* (3rd ed.). University Cambridge Press.

Aman, M. G., & Singh, N. N. (1986). *Aberrant Behaviour Checklist manual.* New York: Slosson.

American Psychiatric Association (APA). (2018). *Diagnostic and statistical manual of mental disorders (DSM-5)* Arlington, VA: APA.

Baum, S. (2007). The use of family therapy for people with learning disabilities. *Advances in Mental Health and Learning Disabilities, 1*(2), 8–13.

Barrowcliff, A. L., & Evans, G. A. L. (2015). EMDR treatment for PTSD and intellectual disability: a case study. *Advances in Mental Health and Intellectual Disabilities, 9*(2), 90–98.

Beail, N., Warden, S., Morsley, K., et al. (2005). Naturalistic evaluation of the effectiveness of psychodynamic psychotherapy with adults with intellectual disabilities. *Journal of Applied Research in Intellectual Disabilities, 18*(3), 245–252.

Beck, A. T., Ward, C., & Mendelson, M. (1961). Beck Depression Inventory (BDI). *Archives of General Psychiatry, 4*, 561–571.

Black, L. A., & Devine, M. (2008). *Head Start: promoting positive mental health for children and young people with a learning disability*. Northern Ireland: South Eastern Health and Social Care Trust.

Bruce, M., Collins, S., Langdon, P., et al. (2010). Does training improve understanding of core concepts in cognitive behaviour therapy by people with intellectual disabilities? A randomized experiment. *British Journal of Clinical Psychology, 49*, 1–13.

Chyka, C. (2000). How many deaths occur annually from adverse drug reactions in the United States? *American Journal of Medicine, 109*(2), 122–130.

Cooper, S. A., Smiley, E., Finlayson, J., et al. (2007a). The prevalence, incidence, and factors predictive of mental ill-health in adults with profound intellectual disabilities. *Journal of Applied Research in Intellectual Disabilities, 20*(6), 493–501.

Cooper, S. A., Smiley, E., Morrison, J., et al. (2007b). Psychosis and adults with intellectual disabilities. *Social Psychiatry and Psychiatric Epidemiology, 42*, 530.

Cooper, S., Smiley, E., Allan, L., et al. (2018). Incidence of unipolar and bipolar depression, and mania in adults with intellectual disabilities: prospective cohort study. *British Journal of Psychiatry, 212*(5), 295–300.

Cooper, S., McLean, G., Guthrie, B., et al. (2015). Multiple physical and mental health comorbidity in adults with intellectual disabilities: population-based cross-sectional analysis. *BMC Family Practice, 16*, 110.

Costello, H., Bouras, N., & Davis, H. (2007). The role of staff training in improving community care staff awareness of mental health problems in people with intellectual disabilities. *Journal of Applied Research in Intellectual Disabilities, 20*, 228–235.

Crowley, V., Rose, J., Smith, J., et al. (2008). Psycho-educational groups for people with a dual diagnosis of psychosis and mild intellectual disability. *Journal of Intellectual Disabilities, 12*(1), 25–39.

Dagnan, D. (2007). Psychosocial interventions for people with intellectual disabilities and mental ill health. *Current Opinion in Psychiatry, 20*(5), 456–460.

Dagnan, D., & Jahoda, A. (2006). Cognitive-behavioural intervention for people with intellectual disability and anxiety disorders. *Journal of Applied Research in Intellectual Disabilities, 19*(1), 91–98.

Dagnan, D., Chadwick, D., & Proudlove, P. (2000). Toward an assessment of suitability of people with mental retardation for cognitive therapy. *Cognitive Therapy and Research, 24*, 627–636.

Deb, S. (2018). The use of medication for the management of problem (challenging) behaviour in adults who have intellectual disabilities. Available at: http://www.intellectualdisability.info/mental-health/articles/the-use-of-medications-for-the-management-of-problem-behaviours-in-adults-who-have-intellectual-disabilities. [Accessed 8 December 2020].

Department of Health. (2001). *Valuing people: a new strategy for learning disability for the 21st century*. London: The Stationery Office.

Devine, M., & Taggart, L. (2008). Improving practice in the care of people with learning disabilities and mental health problems. *Nursing Standard, 22*(45), 40–48.

Douglass, S., Palmer, K., & O'Connor, C. (2007). Experiences of running an anxiety management group for people with a learning disability using a cognitive behavioural intervention. *British Journal of Learning Disabilities, 35*, 245–252.

Emerson, E. (2003). The prevalence of psychiatric disorders in children and adolescents with and without intellectual disabilities. *Journal of Intellectual Disability Research, 47*, 51–58.

Emerson, E. (2005). Use of the Strengths and Difficulties Questionnaire to assess the mental health needs of children and adolescents with intellectual disabilities. *Journal of Intellectual and Developmental Disability, 30*(1), 1–10.

Emerson, E., & Hatton, C. (2014). *Health inequalities and people with intellectual disabilities*. Cambridge: Cambridge University Press.

Eogan, M., & Wingfield, M. (2010). Obstetric and gynaecological disorders. In J. O'Hara, J. McCarthy, & N. Bouras (Eds.), *Intellectual disability and ill health*. Cambridge: Cambridge University Press.

Ernst, C., Morton, C. C., & Gusella, J. F. (2010). Self-injurious behaviours in people with and without intellectual delay: implications for the genetics of suicide. *The International Journal of Neuropsychopharmacology, 13*, 527–528.

Fletcher, R. J., Barnhill, J., & Cooper, S. A. (2016). *Diagnostic manual – intellectual disability: a textbook of diagnosis of mental disorders in persons with intellectual disability*. National Association for the Dually Diagnosed.

Fryers, T. (1997). Impairment, disability, and handicap: categories and classifications. In O. Russell (Ed.), *Seminars in the psychiatry of learning disabilities* (pp. 16–30). London: Royal College of Psychiatrists.

Goodman, R. (1999). The extended version of the Strengths and Difficulties Questionnaire as a guide to child psychiatric cases and consequent burden. *Journal of Child Psychology and Psychiatry*, 40, 791–799.

Gray, K., Tonge, B., Einfeld, S., et al. (2018). *Developmental Behaviour Checklist 2*. WPB.

Hamilton, M. (1959). The assessment of anxiety states by rating. *British Journal of Medical Psychology*, 32, 50–55.

Hassiotis, A., Stueber, K., Thomas, B., et al. (2014). Mood and anxiety disorders. In E. Tsakanikos & J. McCarthy (Eds.), *Handbook of psychopathology in intellectual disability. Autism and child psychopathology series*. New York: Springer.

Healthcare Commission. (2007). *A life like no other: a national audit of specialist inpatient healthcare services for people with learning difficulties in England*. London: Healthcare Commission.

Hemmings, C. P. (2007). The relationship between challenging behaviours and psychiatric disorder in people with severe intellectual disabilities. In N. Bouras & G. Holt (Eds.), *Psychiatric and behavioural disorders in development disorders in development disabilities and mental retardation 2007*. Cambridge: Cambridge University Press.

Hemmings, C. P. (2014). Schizophrenia spectrum disorders. In E. Tsakanikos & J. McCarthy (Eds.), *Handbook of psychopathology in intellectual disability. Autism and child psychopathology series*. New York: Springer.

Hove, O. (2004). Prevalence of eating disorders in adults with mental retardation living in the community. *American Journal of Mental Retardation*, 109, 501–506.

Hove, O., & Havik, O. E. (2010). Developmental level and other factors associated with symptoms of mental disorders and problem behaviour in adults with intellectual disabilities living in the community. *Social Psychiatry and Psychiatric Epidemiology*, 45, 105–113.

Hurley, A. D., Tomasulo, D. J., & Pfadt, A. G. (1998). Individual and group psychotherapy approaches for persons with mental retardation and developmental disabilities. *Journal of Developmental and Physical Disabilities*, 10, 365–386.

International Association for the Scientific Study of Intellectual & Developmental Disability. (2001). *Mental health and intellectual disabilities: addressing the mental health needs of people with intellectual disabilities*.

Jahoda, A., Dagnan, D., Jarvie, P., et al. (2006). Depression, social context and cognitive behavioural therapy for people who have intellectual disabilities. *Journal of Applied Research in Intellectual Disability*, 19(1), 81–90.

Jamieson, D., & Mason, J. (2019). Investigating the existence of the diagnostic overshadowing bias in Australia. *Journal of Mental Health Research in Intellectual Disabilities*, 12(1–2), 58–70.

Karatzias, T., Brown, M., Taggart, L., et al. (2019). Results of a randomised-feasibility trial of Eye Movement Desensitisation and Reprocessing (EMDR) for DSM-5 posttraumatic stress disorder in adults with intellectual disabilities. *Journal of Applied Research in Intellectual Disability Research* https://doi.org/10.1111/jar.12570.

Keeling, J. A., & Rose, J. L. (2006). The adaptation of a cognitive-behavioural treatment programme for special needs sex offenders. *British Journal of Learning Disabilities*, 34(2), 110–116.

Kirkland, J. (2005). Cognitive-behaviour formulation for three men with learning disabilities who experience psychosis: how do we make it make sense? *British Journal of Learning Disabilities*, 33(4), 160–165.

Lloyd, H., & Dallos, R. (2006). Solution-focused brief therapy with families who have a child with intellectual disabilities: a description of the content of initial sessions and the processes. *Clinical Child Psychology and Psychiatry*, 11(3), 367–386.

Lovett, J. (1999). *Small wonders. Healing childhood trauma with EMDR*. New York: The Free Press.

Magaña, S., Parish, S., Morales, M. A., et al. (2016). Racial and ethnic health disparities among people with intellectual and developmental disabilities. *Intellectual and Developmental Disabilities*, 54(3), 161–172.

Mason-Roberts, S., Bradley, A., Karatzias, T., et al. (2018). Multiple traumatization and risk of harm in people with intellectual disabilities and DSM-5 PTSD: a preliminary study. *Journal of Intellectual Disability Research*, 62(8), 730–736.

Matson, J. L. (1988). *The PIMRA manual*. Orland Park, IL: International Diagnostic Systems.

Matthews, D. R., & Hegarty, J. (1997). The 'OK' Health Check: a health assessment checklist for people with learning disabilities. *British Journal of Learning Disabilities*, 25(4), 138–143.

Meltzer, G., Gatward, R., Goodman, R., & Ford, T. (2000). *The mental health of children and adolescents in Great Britain*. London: Office for National Statistics.

Mevissen, L., Lievegoed, R., Seubert, R., et al. (2011). Do persons with intellectual disability and limited verbal capacities respond to trauma treatment? *Journal of Intellectual & Developmental Disability*, 36(4), 278–283.

Moreland, J., Hendy, S., & Brown, F. (2008). The validity of a personality disorder diagnosis for people with an intellectual disability. *Journal of Applied Research in Intellectual Disabilities*, 21(3), 219–226.

Moss, S. (2002). *PAS-ADD schedules*. Brighton: Pavilion.

Moss, S., Friedlander, R., & Lee, P. (2007). *The Cha-PAS Interview*. Brighton: Pavilion.

Munir, K. M. (2016). The co-occurrence of mental disorders in children and adolescents with intellectual disability/intellectual developmental disorder. *Current opinion in psychiatry*, 29(2), 95–102.

Moss, S., & Hurley, A. D. (2014). Classification and diagnostic systems. In E. Tsakanikos & J. McCarthy (Eds.), *Handbook of psychopathology in intellectual disability. Autism and child psychopathology series*. New York, NY: Springer.

National Institute for Health and Care Excellence. (2016). *Mental Health problems in people with learning disabilities: prevention, assessment and management*. NICE guideline [NG54]. Available at: https://www.nice.org.uk/guidance/ng54/chapter/Recommendations#assessment. [Accessed 8 December 2020].

Nihra, K., Leland, H., & Lambert, N. (1993). *AAMR Adaptive Behaviour Scale* (2nd ed.). New York: Harcourt Brace.

NHS England. (2020). *Stopping over-medication of people with a learning disability (STOMPLD)*. Available at: https://www.england.nhs.uk/learning-disabilities/improving-health/stomp/. [Accessed 8 December 2020].

O'Hara, J. (2008). Why should I care about gender. *Advances in Mental Health and Learning Disabilities*, 2, 9–18.

Papagavriel, K., Jones, R., Sheehan, R., et al. (2020). The association between loneliness and common mental disorders in adults with borderline intellectual impairment. *Journal of Affective Disorders*, 277, 954–961.

Raghavan, R., & Waseem, F. (2007). Services for young people with learning disabilities and mental health needs from South Asian communities. *Advances in Mental Health in Learning Disabilities*, 1(3), 27–31.

Ratcliffe, B., Wong, M., Dossetor, D., et al. (2015). The association between social skills and mental health in school-aged children with autism spectrum disorder, with and without intellectual disability. *Journal of Autism and Developmental Disorders*, 45, 2487.

Reiss, S. (1988). *Reiss Screen for maladaptive behaviours*. Worthington, OH: IDS.

Roeden, J. M., Maaskant, M. A., Bannink, F. P., et al. (2011). Solution-focused brief therapy with people with mild intellectual disabilities: a case series. *Journal of Policy and Practice in Intellectual Disabilities*, 8(4), 247–255.

Rose, J., Dodd, L., & Rose, N. (2008). Individual cognitive behaviour intervention for anger. *Journal of Mental Health Research in Intellectual Disabilities*, 1(2), 97–108.

Royal College of Psychiatrists. (2001). *Diagnostic criterion for people with learning disabilities (DC-LD)*. London: Royal College of Psychiatrists.

Schultz, C. L., Schultz, N. C., Bruce, E. J., et al. (1993). Psychoeducational support for parents of children with intellectual disability: an outcome study. *International Journal of Disability, Development and Education*, 40(3), 205–216.

Scior, K., & Werner, S. (Eds.). (2016). *Intellectual disability and stigma: stepping out from the margins*. Basingstoke: Palgrave Macmillan.

Scott, H. M., & Havercamp, S. M. (2016). Systematic review of health promotion programs focused on behavioral changes for people with intellectual disability. *Intellectual and Developmental Disability*, 54(1), 63–76.

Sheehan, R., & Hassiotis, A. (2017). Reduction or discontinuation of antipsychotics for challenging behaviour in adults with intellectual disability: a systematic review. *Lancet Psychiatry*, 4, 238–256.

Sheehan, R., Hassiotis, A., Walters, K., et al. (2015). Mental illness, challenging behaviour, and psychotropic drug prescribing in people with intellectual disability: UK population-based cohort study. *British Medical Journal (Clinical Research Edition)*, 351, h4326.

Shepherd, C., & Beail, N. (2017). A systematic review of the effectiveness of psychoanalysis, psychoanalytic and psychodynamic psychotherapy with adults with intellectual and developmental disabilities: progress and challenges. *Psychoanalytic Psychotherapy*, 31(1), 1–24.

Simpson, N. (2009). Clinical assessment. In A. Hassiotis, D. A. Barron, & I. Hall (Eds.), *Intellectual disability psychiatry: a practical handbook*. Chichester: Wiley-Blackwell.

Smith, I. C. (2005). Solution-focused brief therapy with people with learning disabilities: a case study. *British Journal of Learning Disabilities*, 33(3), 102–105.

Strydom, A., & Sinai, A. (2014). Dementia. In E. Tsakanikos & J. McCarthy (Eds.), *Handbook of psychopathology in intellectual disability. Autism and child psychopathology series*. New York: Springer.

Summers, S. J. (2003). Psychological intervention for people with learning disabilities who have experienced bereavement: a case illustration. *British Journal of Learning Disabilities*, 31, 37–41.

Taggart, L., Cousins, W., & Milner, S. (2007). Young people with learning disabilities living in state care: their emotional, behavioural and mental health status. *Child Care in Practice*, 13(4), 401–416.

Taggart, L., Huxley, A., & Baker, G. (2008). Alcohol and illicit drug misuse in people with learning disabilities: implications for research and service development. *Advances in Mental Health in Learning Disabilities*, 2(1), 11–21.

Taggart, L., McMillan, R., & Lawson, A. (2009a). Women with intellectual disabilities: risk and protective factors for psychiatric disorders. *Journal of Intellectual Disabilities*, 13(4), 321–340.

Taggart, L., McMillan, R., & Lawson, A. (2009b). An exploration of the characteristics of women with learning disabilities and psychiatric disorders admitted into a specialist hospital. *Advances in Mental Health in People with Learning Disabilities*, 3(1), 30–41.

Taggart, L., McMillan, R., & Lawson, A. (2010b). Staffs' knowledge and perceptions of working with women with intellectual disabilities and psychiatric disorders. *Journal of Intellectual Disability Research*, 54(1), 90–100.

Taggart, L., Taylor, D., & McCrum-Gardner, E. (2010a). Individual, life events, family and socio-economic factors associated with young people with intellectual disability with and without behavioural/emotional problems. *Journal of Intellectual Disabilities*, 14(4), 267–288.

Tsakanikos, E., & McCarthy, J. (2013). *Handbook of psychopathology in intellectual disability: research, practice, and policy (Autism and child psychopathology series).* Springer.

Van Duijvenbode, N., & Vandernagel, J. E. L. (2019). A systematic review of substance use (disorder) in individuals with mild to borderline intellectual disability. *European Addiction Research*, 25(6), 263–282.

Vereenooghe, L., Gega, L., Reynolds, S., & Langdon, P. E. (2016). Using computers to teach people with intellectual disabilities to perform some of the tasks used within cognitive behavioural therapy: a randomised experiment. *Behaviour Research and Therapy*, 76, 13–23.

Vereenooghe, L., & Langdon, P. E. (2013). Psychological therapies for people with intellectual disabilities: a systematic review and meta-analysis. *Research in Developmental Disabilities*, 34, 4085–4102.

Vereenooghe, L., Reynolds, S., Gega, L., & Langdon, P. E. (2015). Can a computerised training paradigm assist people with intellectual disabilities to learn cognitive mediation skills? A randomised experiment. *Behaviour Research and Therapy*, 71, 10–19.

Whelan, P., Haywood, S., & Galloway, P. (2007). Low self-esteem: group cognitive behaviour therapy. *British Journal of Learning Disabilities*, 35(2), 125–130.

Willner, P., & Goodey, R. (2006). Interaction of cognitive distortions and cognitive deficits in the formulation and treatment of obsessive-compulsive behaviours in a woman with intellectual disability. *Journal of Applied Research in Intellectual Disabilities*, 19(1), 67–74.

Withers, P., Ensum, I., Howarth, D., et al. (2001). A psychoeducational group for men with intellectual disabilities who have sex with men. *Journal of Applied Research in Intellectual Disabilities*, 14(4), 327–339.

World Health Organization. (2018). *ICD-11: international statistical classification of diseases and related health problems* (10th Rev.). Geneva: WHO.

World Health Organization. (2007). *International classification of functioning.* Geneva: WHO. Available at: https://www.who.int/classifications/icf/en/. [Accessed 11 December 2020].

World Health Organization. (2004). *Promoting mental health: concepts, emerging evidence, practice (summary report).* Geneva: WHO.

World Health Organization. (2001). *Strengthening mental health promotion.* Factsheet No. 220. Geneva: WHO.

17

Understanding and responding to behaviour

James Ridley and Petri Embregts

KEY ISSUES

- There are many different ways of understanding the concept of challenging behaviour and interpretations may vary across the life span.
- Prevalence and types of behaviours, including self-injury, will vary between individuals, the cause of which may be multifaceted.
- Comprehensive and holistic assessment of the individual is necessary to establish the underlying cause and function of behaviour and should include physical and mental health checks.

- Prescribed intervention and management approaches must be person centred, with interventions adapted to meet individual need. Their ultimate aim should be to improve the quality of life of the person with an intellectual disability.
- Whilst national/international legislation and ethical practices may vary, the assessment, management and support of an individual with behaviour that challenges should reflect a human rights approach.

CHAPTER OUTLINE

INTRODUCTION

Challenging behaviour is something that reflects a significant range of experiences, outcomes and presentations which can be challenging to the individual, their family or carers, and the providers of services who may be commissioned to offer support. The term should never be considered as a diagnostic label where the focus is likely to be only on the behaviour presented, but rather it should be seen as offering the opportunity to explore the functions of these behaviour(s), to utilise assessments and interventions which are holistic and person centred. The focus of behavioural support should be the development of opportunities which improve overall quality of life and respect the rights of the individual, by offering proportionate responses which should also support the evolution of services. This chapter will explore the concept of challenging behaviour from a variety of different perspectives and outline positive measures that can be employed to minimise the effect on self and others whilst maximising quality of life.

DEFINITIONS AND ASSOCIATED ISSUES

The term 'challenging behaviour' continues to be the most recognised label linked to people with intellectual disabilities who present with behaviours deemed to be challenging or problematic, and shows an evolution from terms being used such as abnormal, aberrant, disordered, disturbed, dysfunctional and maladaptive behaviours (Wolkorte et al, 2019). The term has become generally used and accepted across services within education, health and social care, however its interpretation and associated approaches may be impacted by their service-based expectations; because of this there are known to be several definitions which seek to explain and explore the term challenging behaviour (Wolverson, 2003). An early definition by Blunden and Allen (1987, p. 14) provides an interesting beginning to the exploration of challenging behaviour,

> "We have decided to adopt the term challenging behaviour rather than problem behaviour or severe problem behaviour since it emphasises that such behaviours represent challenges to services rather than problems which individuals with learning difficulties [intellectual disabilities] in some way carry around with them. If services could rise to the 'challenge' of dealing with these behaviours they would cease to be problems."

Recognising that services have a responsibility for challenging themselves in relation to how they support an individual should be considered positive and evolutionary, with clearer links to establishing personalised support; this is in contrast to the past when challenging behaviour was considered a problem inherent only in the individual. Where the focus remains on the individual and "their" behaviour then there is more likelihood for consideration to be aligned to the person receiving treatments or "cures", where the behaviours are seen as requiring care, control and the direction of professionals (Nunkoosing and Haydon-Laurelt, 2011).

Possibly the most often used definition of challenging behaviour is that given by Emerson (1995, p. 3),

> "Culturally abnormal behaviour(s) of such an intensity, frequency or duration that the physical safety of the person or others is likely to be placed in serious jeopardy, or behaviour which is likely to seriously limit use of or result in the person being denied access to ordinary community facilities."

This definition highlights the potential impact of challenging behaviour, identifying that a person's behaviour may place them or others in jeopardy and therefore limit or lead to the denial of access to ordinary facilities, restricting social inclusion, engagement and participation which may impact on their rights. A more contemporary consideration of Emerson's (1995) definition given by the collaboration of the Royal College of Psychiatry (RCPsych), British Psychological Society (BPS) and Royal College of Speech and Language Therapists (RCSLT) (Banks et al, 2007) includes how behaviour may be responded to, with the inclusion of responses which may be restrictive, aversive or lead to exclusion,

> "Behaviour can be described as challenging when it is of such an intensity, frequency or duration as to threaten the quality of life and/or the physical safety of the individual or others and is likely to lead to responses that are restrictive, aversive or result in exclusion."
>
> Banks et al, 2007, p. 10

Wolverson (2003) highlighted that the use of definitions related to challenging behaviour may also influence the interventions which are designed in response such as the use of restraint and restrictive practice. Although these definitions do not highlight legislation they do offer the potential to recognise how approaches can be influenced by frameworks such as human rights-based legislation, (e.g. the UK Human Rights Act, 1998), and associated international conventions for example the European Union Charter of Human Rights (European Union, 2012), United Nations Convention on the Rights of the Child (UNCRC) (UN General Assembly, 1989), and the United Nations Convention on the Rights of People with Disabilities (UNCRPD) (UN General Assembly, 2007).

As people with intellectual disabilities are experiencing greater longevity then they also experience increased risk of developing dementia, and although challenging behaviour should not be seen as an inevitable consequence for people with intellectual disabilities living with dementia (Kerr, 2007), it is recognised that behavioural changes may be the first signs of the onset of the condition (British Psychological Society (BPS) and Royal College of Psychiatry (RCPsych), 2015). Within literature about people living with dementia the description "Behaviours that Challenge" (BtC) appears and, according to the BPS (BPS, 2019, p. 1), can be defined as:

"An expression of distress by the person living with dementia (or others in the environment) that arises from unmet health or psychosocial need(s). The behaviours often reflect attempts by the person living with dementia to maintain a sense of control, dignity and wellbeing, and/or to ease discomfort or distress."

Although this definition is not specifically written or designed to consider the needs of people with intellectual disabilities it does suggest that behaviour is about unmet needs and its function relates to a person's attempts to maintain control, dignity and wellbeing.

The diversity of the lived experiences of people with intellectual disabilities, for instance those who experience mental health difficulties or come into contact with the criminal justice system, cannot be ignored (Department of Health (DH), 2007). The use of broad definitions and checklists can lose sight of the individual and lead to challenging behaviour being viewed as typical for people with intellectual disabilities which increases the risk of labelling or diagnostic/behavioural overshadowing (Disability Rights Commission (DRC), 2006). A view that this is typical presentation for a population group could in turn lead to a reluctance on the part of service providers to undertake further analysis to establish other causes for an individual's behaviour. Blunden and Allen (1987) stated that challenging behaviour is about the challenge to services, therefore when supporting individuals with challenging behaviour the responsibility to establish a clear understanding of the function of the behaviour is on the service. If services recognise their responsibilities to explore the challenges that they are presented with, then this can support service development and lead to the design of effective approaches and services for individuals.

PREVALENCE AND DEMOGRAPHY

Current UK guidance produced by the National Institute for Health and Care Excellence (NICE) (2015) indicates that the prevalence of challenging behaviour for people with intellectual disabilities ranges between 5%–15%. However, there are known variations with a number of studies showing prevalence as low as 4% or as high as 80% (Chung et al, 1996; Emerson et al, 2001; Bowring et al, 2019). Emerson et al (2001) indicates that variations in prevalence rates can relate to a number of factors such as: whether the research has focused only on a specific form of challenging behaviour such as self-injury; the environment where the sample population is situated

> ### BOX 17.1 Key facts
>
> - Prevalence of challenging behaviour in people with intellectual disabilities within the UK who are in contact with education, health or social care services is between 10–15% (NICE, 2015)
> - Age is a contributing factor to prevalence with more demanding behaviours being seen in those between the age of 10–20yrs, the highest prevalence being recorded between the age of 20–40yrs, with much lower recorded prevalence in those over the age of 60yrs (Holden and Gitlesen, 2006)
> - Behaviour which involves aggression, destruction of property and self-injury is positively correlated to the severity of intellectual disability (Moss et al, 2000; Poppes et al, 2010)
> - Males are more likely than females to display challenging behaviour (Moss et al, 2000; Emerson et al, 2001)
> - Challenging behaviour is increased for individuals who experience additional needs, such as visual impairment 12–15%, hearing impairment 8–20%, and communication difficulties 45% (DH, 2007)
> - Challenging behaviour is more prevalent if there is the coexistence of intellectual disability and mental ill health and is estimated to affect between 10 and 46% (Priest and Gibbs, 2004; DH, 2007).
> - Challenging behaviour has a greater prevalence in hospital or institutional/residential services (NICE, 2015; Dworschak et al, 2016).

such as within the community, hospital-based care or within education; how the study defines what is challenging behaviour such as *demanding* or *less demanding* challenging behaviour (Emerson et al, 2001). Some of the additional variations in prevalence can also be attributed to the ways in which the demographic profile of people with intellectual disabilities can influence the data. An example of this can be seen in the study completed by Holden and Gitlesen (2006) who identified that challenging behaviour was more common in younger people and rare in those over the age of 60. Box 17.1 provides an overview of the relationship between key demographics and the prevalence and manifestation of challenging behaviour amongst people with intellectual disabilities.

The prevalence and demographics of self-injurious behaviour

Borthwick-Duffy (1994) reported that as many as 10–50% of people with intellectual disabilities may at some point display self-injurious behaviour. According to Cooper et al (2009), examples of self-injurious behaviour include head punching, hitting or banging self against hard objects and biting self, however the eating of inedible items known as *pica* is also referred to as an additional serious and life-threatening form of self-injury (Call et al, 2015). Huisman et al (2018) identified the prevalence of self-injurious behaviour as up to 30% for those who were not supported within institutional or residential settings, and up to 41% of those who were, thus demonstrating linkage between an individual's living environment and the perceived complexity of their needs. Further exploration of the environment shows continued variations in prevalence where lower rates are seen in day services (3–10%), those with special educational needs (3–12%) and even greater reductions for those living at home (1–4%) (Gates 2007). However, there is also some recognition that the level of a person's intellectual disability is a factor in the display of challenging behaviour with those with severe intellectual disabilities showing a prevalence of 73% in comparison with 19% of those with moderate intellectual disabilities and 17% of those with mild intellectual disabilities (Heslop and Macaulay, 2009). Prevalence may be further affected by the presence of additional sensory needs and impairments, ambulatory difficulties, limited expressive communication skills, and undiagnosed pain or trauma (physical, emotional and psychological) (Heslop and Macaulay, 2009). These are represented below as organic and biological considerations.

CAUSATION

Establishing the potential reason(s) for challenging behaviour and/or self-injurious behaviour requires a comprehensive assessment. The causes of challenging behaviour and self-injurious behaviour are multifaceted but can be broadly categorised into three main areas which are:

- Organic/Biological
- Behavioural/Psychological
- Social/Environmental (Wolverson, 2003; Gates and Mafuba, 2015)

It is important to note, however, that very often an individual may experience more than one of these causes simultaneously. There might also be instances where a single cause influences another, and in some cases creates a situation where the initial behaviour is maintained. This is illustrated in Daniel's story in the accompanying online resource.

Organic and biological considerations

It is often the case that some people consider challenging and/or self-injurious behaviour to be associated with the person having an intellectual disability. This can be referred to as diagnostic or behavioural overshadowing, and the consequences of this can be that the cause of a person's challenging behaviour is not properly assessed or investigated. There are, however, some genetic conditions where challenging behaviour and/or self-injurious behaviour is known to be intrinsically linked. According to Murphy (1994) two conditions which can be biologically defined as presenting a significant increase in the prevalence of specific behavioural difficulties are Lesch-Nyhan and Prader Willi syndromes. Individuals with Lesch-Nyhan syndrome are more likely to engage in self-injurious behaviours including biting their own lips or hands (Wolverson, 2011). Those with Prader–Willi syndrome experience an inability to suppress and manage appetite, which can result in behaviours linked to their demanding and continued attempts to gain access to food; individuals with Prader-Willi syndrome also experience a high prevalence (85%) of self-injurious behaviour (Didden et al, 2007). Huisman et al (2018) found in their review that there was also a notable increased prevalence in those with Smith-Magenis, Cri du Chat, and Cornelia de Lange syndromes. It is important to understand that these syndromes are relatively rare and although there may be an increased prevalence of challenging behaviour and/or self-injurious behaviour amongst affected individuals, it is unlikely that the genetic features of the condition represent its sole cause.

Increased prevalence has also been linked to people with autism (Wolverson, 2011), the presence of epilepsy (Kwok and Cheung, 2007), or those with the beginnings of dementia, a condition that often has an earlier onset amongst people with intellectual disabilities than the general population (BPS and RCPsych, 2015). A more detailed exploration of these conditions can be found within Chapters 15, 14 and 26 respectively.

Endogenous opiates and self-injurious behaviour

According to Roy et al (2015) self-injurious behaviour (e.g. head slapping) has an increased level of prevalence amongst people with intellectual disabilities. One hypothesis is that such behaviour is perpetuated through the consequential release of endogenous opiates that produce a morphine-like effect in the body (Wisely et al, 2002). This effect serves to relieve anxiety, tension, as well as alleviating pain. Murphy (1999) identifies that prolonged exposure to such opiates can create addictive chemical changes. Moreover the pleasurable feelings of euphoria that are experienced is likely to ensure that an individual repeats this behaviour (Gates, 2007; Winchel and Stanley, 1991).

The addictive element of self-injurious behaviour can also be considered where the individual presents with pica behaviour which involves ingesting inedible or non-nutritious objects. Pica is classed as a serious and concerning form of self-injurious behaviour where there is an increased risk for the surgical removal of an indigestible mass (a bezoar) or threat to life (Stiegler, 2005; Matson et al, 2013). The addictive element of pica for people with intellectual disabilities is suggested as being linked to individuals seeking items which offer characteristics that meet their sensory or physiological needs (Call et al, 2015). An example of this is where people who demonstrate pica behaviour seek out cigarette butts to ingest as they become addicted to the nicotine still available in these (Piazza et al, 2002).

Behavioural/Psychological considerations

Bond et al (2019) identified that the lived experiences of people with intellectual disabilities can influence a person's emotional, psychological and behavioural presentation throughout the lifespan. People with intellectual disabilities are more likely to experience a range of adverse life events, in part because of their association with institutional type services and/or the lack of autonomy they may have due to being dependent on care givers (Hatton and Emerson, 2004). This increased exposure to adverse life events can increase the potential for psychological or emotional trauma being a cause of challenging behaviour (Martorell and Tsakanikos, 2008). Significantly, what for many people may be regarded as non-aversive life events such as moving home or changes in routines can have potentially traumatic consequences for someone with an intellectual disability. Wood et al (2018) suggested that where an individual has access to skills and emotional resources such as self-perception and self-regulation, then they are more likely to be able to manage adverse events which occur across the lifespan. Consideration must therefore be given to those who

may not have these skills and psychological resources as this could increase adversity and trauma which is then presented as challenging behaviour.

Social/Environmental considerations

The importance of the social environment on the manifestation of challenging behaviour should be seen as having an equal level of influence to those considerations already highlighted. Hardy and Joyce (2011) indicated that the environment is an influencer on a person's mood, comfort and overall wellbeing. An individual's interaction with the environment and their associated social interactions, which may be over stimulating or under stimulating, will have a profound effect on behaviour, therefore an understanding of a person's sensory needs and daily activities is also key to establishing potential causation (Rattaz et al, 2018). Establishing how an individual experiences their social environment should be explored, as it may be construed as aversive thus creating increased levels of anxiety which can be displayed as challenging behaviour (Perez et al, 2012; Bowring et al, 2019). Contrarily the environment may also be able to offer a level of support for the individual, representing a place of relative safety.

 READER ACTIVITY 17.1

Firstly, think about the environments where people with intellectual disabilities live. Consider how the characteristics of these environments may influence a person's behaviour in a way that may challenge support services.

Secondly, identify from these characteristics which ones could be used to support the individual with behaviour that challenges support services.

Stigma and labelling

Challenging behaviour can be seen as a social construct, that is the product of the interaction between an individual and their environment (Banks et al, 2007). The central principle of social constructionism is that an individual's interpretation of reality is a subjective composite derived from language and cultural perceptions. Foucault (1990) extended this concept to explain how negative labelling in relation to stigmatised groups can lead to them being treated in controlling and other unacceptable ways. That is, people displaying challenging behaviour are often associated with numerous negative assumptions about the individual or group so labelled. Pilgrim and Rogers (1999) introduced the concepts of primary and secondary labelling and the powerful effect this might have on a person's life. Primary labelling is the process of giving a label in the first instance and secondary labelling explains how once a person has been given a negative label they will seem to exhibit the expected symptoms associated with it. This can result in support staff who might expect behaviours to occur as an expected consequence of a given label (Wilner and Smith, 2008). It may also be the case that a person labelled as having challenging behaviour may internalise the label and its negative connotations and 'act out' the behaviours expected as a result of it, therefore creating a sense of behavioural overshadowing where negative perceptions further reduce the ability to see and generate individualised approaches. Although attempts have been made to avoid challenging behaviour from becoming an altogether negative label, it is often associated with a degree of pathology and therapeutic pessimism, some of which is as a consequence of the label, resulting in poor expectations and self-fulfilled prophecies (Bicknell and Conboy-Hill, 1992). As Wolfensberger (1975, p. 2) concluded,

> "It is a well-established fact that a person's behaviour tends to be profoundly affected by the role expectations that are placed upon him. Generally, people will play the roles that they have been assigned. This permits those who define social roles to make self-fulfilling prophecies by predicting that someone cast into a certain role will emit behaviour consistent with that role. Unfortunately, role appropriate behaviour will then often be interpreted to be a person's 'natural' rather than elicited mode of acting."

Worldwide, much legislation and resulting social policy over the past 40 years has been developed in order that the harmful effects of institutionalisation can be eradicated and most large institutions, particularly in Western countries, have now been closed. It was expected that the closure of these large institutions would reduce the levels of challenging behaviour displayed amongst individuals with intellectual disabilities (Lemay, 2009), however this has not happened in all cases and increases may be expected in some instances. The development of specialist contemporary challenging behaviour services has resulted in the re-institutionalisation of many

people with challenging behaviour; it is also the case that newer specialist services may be subdivided by labels, so that within a single service there are units for personality disorder, autistic spectrum conditions, self-injurious behaviour and assessment and treatment thus potentially further pathologising individuals.

With respect to stigma and challenging behaviours, a lack of familiarity with, and knowledge about, people with intellectual disabilities displaying challenging behaviours has been reported by mainstream health professionals (Pelleboer-Gunnink et al, 2017), and this may affect the ongoing challenges regarding inclusion of this group in mainstream healthcare services. To facilitate inclusion in these services, it would be recommended to include contact and collaboration with experts-by-experience in the education programmes of health professionals. Moreover, inclusion would benefit from an understanding of 'equal' treatment that means reasonable adjustments (or accommodations) instead of undifferentiated treatment for people with intellectual disabilities and challenging behaviours. Notably, Pelleboer-Gunnink et al (2019) reported scepticism among care providers towards the feasibility of community inclusion for people with high support needs, including those with challenging behaviours. That is, they tended to be ambivalent about whether people with intellectual disabilities and challenging behaviour should be protected or empowered. This finding is of particular interest as people with intellectual disabilities themselves reported, among others, experiences of over-protection, lack of recognition, and dependence on support as essential expressions of stigmatising treatment (e.g., Giesbers et al, 2019; Jahoda and Markova, 2004; Jahoda et al, 2010). Moreover, stigmatisation seemed to be related to subgroups of people with intellectual disabilities; it seemed to be the strongest for people with more severe or profound intellectual disabilities, and for people with high support needs including those who displayed challenging behaviour.

Parenting and family issues

The perception that children with intellectual disabilities are different from children without can lead to 'faulty' parenting that often results in behaviour that is perceived to be challenging. Rolland (1993) has discussed the concept of centripetal forces (i.e., forces pushing family members together) and centrifugal forces (i.e., forces driving family members apart) in relation to caring for a child with chronic support needs. Centripetal forces might be associated with challenging behaviour as children with intellectual disabilities may be overprotected and thus discouraged from reaching their full potential (McConachie, 1986). In such situations, behaviours associated with early stages of child development are maintained into adulthood when they are viewed as challenging. Moreover, Vetere (1993) has discussed how children with intellectual disabilities can be 'infantilised'. This is a process in which those with intellectual disabilities are treated as 'eternal children' and therefore expected to display some of the often difficult behaviours associated with childhood. Centrifugal forces, on the other hand, can result in the child with an intellectual disability being blamed for family disintegration and dissonance, resulting in problems with attachment such as psychological abuse or emotional abandonment and eventually challenging behaviour (Rolland, 1993).

With respect to family issues, it is imperative to adopt a broad perspective when encouraging family support. In this respect, it is important to not only look at the support people with intellectual disabilities receive from significant others, but also how they can reciprocate, hence, to what extent do they support significant others in return (Giesbers et al, 2019). Support staff should be facilitated to initiate a dialogue with both people with intellectual disabilities and their significant others, to help build mutual relationships and to enhance their social inclusion.

 READER ACTIVITY 17.2

Consider and list possible differences in the early life experiences of children with intellectual disabilities from those without.

Try to explain how these differences can lead to the development of challenging behaviour and the possible effects of this on the lives of people labelled as having challenging behaviour.

Self-injurious behaviour associated with abuse and attachment

People with intellectual disabilities are more at risk of psychological distress and abuse compared to people without, which might manifest as challenging behaviour (Emerson and Einfeld, 2011). That is, challenging behaviour may develop as an attempt to draw attention to the fact that one has been abused. In addition, challenging behaviour may be a manifestation of socially learned behaviour that can develop as a result of consistent exposure to environments in which abuse and aggression are accepted forms of behaviour (Emerson and Einfeld, 2011). These are important factors to consider as it is proposed that self-injurious behaviour may serve several functions that develop as a consequence of these. Examples include how support staff may fulfil a 'pseudo' parental role, and individuals displaying the behaviour may perceive negative responses to self-injury as aberrantly rewarding as any attention is more rewarding than none. Some forms of self-injurious behaviour involve damage to the skin (e.g., scratching, cutting, burning, and picking). Babiker and Arnold (1997) discuss how the skin is used throughout life, particularly by mothers, to communicate attachment, love, to bond and to ease by patting, stroking and kissing. In the case of mothers, fathers and a child with an intellectual disability, the attachment may be dysfunctional, broken or damaged. As such, self-injurious behaviour related to damaging the skin can be a physical representation of the associated emotional distress.

Self-injurious behaviour may also serve a purpose of engendering a particular response that is not usually expected in their relationship with support staff. For example, if support staff are perceived to be indifferent to them, then an individual might display self-injurious behaviour to engender a more caring response. The 'comforting' action and the immediate attention of the first aid and treatment of wounds may demonstrate this. In addition, self-injurious behaviour can also serve the function of being a psychological defence mechanism, such as projection. That is, some people with intellectual disabilities displaying self-injurious behaviours may find their thoughts and feelings too overwhelmingly distressing, unacceptable or inadmissible and may 'project' them onto support staff. Self-injurious behaviour may also serve as a regulatory function within the individual allowing the individual to cope with feelings of distress and anxiety (Babiker and Arnold, 1997). Some individuals may find that the trauma of the abuse they have endured causes them to 'dissociate', and the only way they can return to 'reality' is by injuring themselves in order to feel the sensations which arise. Dissociation is the psychological process associated with experiences of trauma whereby the only way a person can manage the emotional distress is to mentally distance themselves from it by replacing it by inflicting physical pain (Klonsky, 2007).

PRINCIPLES OF ASSESSMENT OF CHALLENGING BEHAVIOUR

The assessment of an individual's behaviour needs to be based on a view that the individual and their behaviour is likely to have developed through a process of experience and learning. Previously, the interpretation of a person's behaviour was founded on the notion that this learning process was primarily based on either positive or negative experiences, which therefore reinforced their behaviour (e.g., Pavlov, 1927; Skinner, 1953), however there is also an assumption that behaviour could be learned vicariously. Bandura (1977) suggested that individuals can learn to behave in certain ways by observation of others, called 'social learning theory'. The outcome of the social learning theory is that an individual may utilise or repeat behaviours that they have observed which can then result in some form of reward or reinforcement (Wolverson, 2011). However, it should be mentioned that whatever the rationale for a person's behaviour, it will always have meaning and it is a result of an unmet need (Pitonyak, 2002). In a sense, difficult behaviours can be considered to be messages that can tell important things about an individual and the quality of their life.

If behaviour has meaning and is used to support an individual to satisfy an unmet need, then assessment must be completed in a way that supports the interpretation of the meaning of their behaviour, and enables the individual to either meet their own needs or be supported by others who understand their needs. As identified by Horner (1994), the role of support staff is not about fixing people, but about their ability to support individuals by facilitating more effective environments. When considering assessment of the environment for an individual, it is important to explicate what that is; an environment could be represented as the person's internal environment (e.g., physical, emotional, psychological) but also as the external environment being related to things that occur around the individual.

Exploring through assessment the reason or causation of challenging behaviour must be completed with a clear understanding that it can be complex and linked to multiple factors. Therefore, the assessment approach and interventions need to reflect the individual and must be based on a clear and specific range of rights-based person-centred approaches and strategies. This section of the chapter will outline the key elements of good practice in relation to the assessment of challenging behaviour and some of the assessment tools utilised to support.

Person-centred assessment

It is imperative that the assessment process is person centred and includes a wide-ranging contextual analysis of a person's challenging behaviour; this is likely to include the involvement of both direct and indirect support providers and families, and is formulated within a multi-disciplinary and multi-agency context (Wolverson, 2011). This process of assessment will require a clear understanding and exploration of current behaviours with a thorough factual description of the behaviour(s) being displayed. Examples of some of the behavioural assessment tools which may be used for this purpose are given in Box 17.2. The individual's past and current experiences also need to be explored as their experience within environmental contexts may have contributed, or is continuing to contribute, to the causation and maintenance of the challenging behaviour. The section on causation explained how challenging behaviour can be caused by organic, environmental and psychological factors, and that it can be also influenced by a complex combination of these.

BOX 17.2   Behavioural assessment tools

- Adaptive Behaviour Scale (Nihira et al, 1993)
- Aberrant Behaviour Checklist (Aman and Singh, 1986)
- Brief Behavioural Assessment Tool (BBAT), (Smith and Nethell, 2014)
- Challenging Behaviour Interview (CBI) (Oliver et al, 2003)
- Functional Analysis Interview (FAI) analysis of problem behaviour (O'Neil et al, 1997)
- Motivation Assessment Scale (MAS) (Durand and Crimmins, 1988)
- Questions About Behavioural Function (QABF) (Paclawskyj et al, 2000)
- Scatterplot (Touchette et al, 1985)

Assessment of organic causation

It is widely known that the health needs of people with intellectual disabilities are likely to exceed those of the general population, with poor physical health also having the potential to impact on the person's mental health and wellbeing (Hardy et al, 2016). An essential part of the assessment process in relation to challenging behaviour is identifying whether the person is experiencing any health-related concerns (Emerson et al, 2012). Not assessing the health needs of the individual increases the potential for diagnostic overshadowing (DRC, 2006). NICE (2015) identifies that a physical health assessment should be completed that includes a review of all current health interventions including medications and associated side effects, and that from this an agreed plan for managing a person's physical health care needs is completed and shared. The assessment may be able to access information from health-related assessments such as the "OK Health Check" (Matthews, 2004), an annual health check, or a person's health action plan which is designed to offer an individualised account of a person's health needs (Howatson, 2005). However, where particular health needs are identified, then more specific assessments may need to be completed which could also support an understanding of the function of the person's behaviour.

Assessment of mental ill health

Similarly to physical health conditions, people with intellectual disabilities will experience greater levels of mental ill health when compared to the general population (Priest and Gibbs, 2004; Cooper et al, 2009). Recognition continues to grow that for some individuals their behaviour may be attributed to undiagnosed psychiatric conditions (Smiley, 2005), with studies demonstrating that a wide range of challenging behaviours displayed by people with intellectual disabilities, including self-injury, can be an atypical feature of mental ill health in this population (Emerson et al, 1999; Taggart and Slevin, 2006). Emerson et al (1999) identified that the display of challenging behaviour in people with intellectual disabilities can cause difficulty in the assessment of mental health, with Raghavan and Patel (2005) indicating that the reason for this difficulty relates to the overlap in presentation between mental illness and challenging behaviour. With this close relationship and presentation, further consideration needs to be given to diagnostic/behavioural overshadowing which may lead to differing interventional approaches. Assessment of mental ill health in the population of people with intellectual disabilities is discussed in more detail in Chapter 16 of this book.

INTERVENTIONS

This section of the chapter will outline a range of interventions to support people with challenging behaviour, with discussion as to how their design and implementation should be both dependent on the individual nature of the person and the reality of practice. As indicated in previous sections, any interventions related to the support and management of challenging behaviour must be person-centred and based on a comprehensive assessment. McBrien and Felce (1995) identify that the purpose of a functional analysis is to establish the potential reasons why a person may be displaying challenging behaviour and what factors serve to reinforce the person's behaviour (thus making it more likely to be repeated). Such an approach is commonly known as ABC – *antecedent* (what was happening before), *behaviour* (what was happening during), and the *consequence* (what happened afterwards) (ABC) (Gates et al, 2002). This is further illustrated in Reader activity 17.3 in the online resource where a breakdown of an ABC approach is given. Therefore, any interventions should be designed in a way which enables the individual to meet their needs, develop new skills, and experience greater opportunities which supports them to experience improved quality of life.

Allen et al (2005) and McCue (2000) identified that interventions need to be based on the following concepts:

- Interventions should be designed to alter systems, not individuals.
- Behavioural approaches should seek to improve the quality of life of individuals, not merely attempt to eradicate challenging behaviour.
- Some behaviours may have more than one function, and they may operate differently in different contexts/environments.
- A detailed functional assessment must be conducted prior to any form of intervention.

Contemporary interventions for people with intellectual disabilities displaying challenging behaviour are increasingly integral parts of a systemic response that offers a global therapeutic approach to challenging behaviour in all aspects of a person's life (Heslop and Macauley, 2009; Kaur et al, 2009). This global approach should be used to develop individualised interventions which recognise the importance of proactive strategies (environmental and antecedent management, skill development, communication support) which focus on potentially problematic issues before the behaviours occur, and reactive strategies (self-protection, supporting distress, managing crises) which identify how support should be offered when a person presents with challenging behaviour (Adams and Allen, 2001). The establishment of proactive and reactive strategies continues to be the recommended best practice approach in services for people with intellectual disabilities and challenging behaviour (DH, 2007; NICE, 2015).

Positive Behavioural Support

Recognition that both proactive and reactive strategies need to be individualised and considered alongside a comprehensive understanding of a person's needs is the foundation of many behavioural and interventional approaches such as Positive Behavioural Support (PBS) (LaVigna and Willis, 2012; Gore et al, 2013). According to Kincaid (2016) the main features of Positive Behavioural Support relate to it being based on a full and ongoing assessment of the individual and their needs, that it respects the person and their rights as well as maintaining their dignity, and that it can be applied not only with individuals but also within larger organisational levels. Gore et al (2013) identified 10 key components linked to Positive Behavioural Support and these are shown in Table 17.1.

PBS is becoming increasingly advocated as a person centred response to the needs of people with intellectual disabilities who display challenging behaviour within both the UK and internationally. There is some recognition that this approach can demonstrate a level of effectiveness in the management of challenging behaviour across a wide range of service settings and across the lifespan (LaVigna and Willis, 2012; Gore et al, 2013; Hassiotis et al, 2018).

Functional Analysis/Behavioural approaches

A functional analysis is conducted to support an understanding of the function of the person's challenging behaviour. This may lead to a hypothesis as to the reason/function of the person's behaviour and how it is being maintained (as in the aforementioned ABC approach). Interventions which are designed in line with this will likely focus on differing aspects of change to support the person, an antecedent approach will look to consider what was happening before a person's behaviour with a view that the stimulus or event that influences the person's behaviour can be controlled or managed. However not all antecedents can be avoided therefore this approach should link with a number of additional interventions and supportive skills development.

TABLE 17.1	Key components of PBS
Values	1. Prevention and reduction of challenging behaviour occurs within the context of increased quality of life, inclusion, participation, and the defence and support of valued social roles
	2. Constructional approaches to intervention design build stakeholder skills and opportunities and eschew aversive and restrictive practices
	3. Stakeholder participation informs, implements and validates assessment and intervention practices
Theory and Evidence Base	4. An understanding that challenging behaviour develops to serve important functions for people
	5. The primary use of applied behaviour analysis to assess and support behaviour change
	6. The secondary use of other complementary, evidence-based approaches to support behaviour change at multiple levels of a system
Process	7. A data-driven approach to decision making at every stage
	8. Functional assessment to inform function-based intervention
	9. Multicomponent interventions to change behaviour (proactively) and manage behaviour (reactively)
	10. Implementation support, monitoring and evaluation of interventions over the long term

Reproduced with from Gore et al (2013)

Behaviour based interventions are concerned with the establishment of alternatives to the behaviour (Gates et al, 2002). Designing interventions based on this approach should therefore enable the person to meet their needs by using other means, however as Emerson (2005) identifies, when using a behaviour based intervention the alternative behaviour needs to have the same level of equivalence or serve the same function as the person's original behaviour. Examples of this could be supporting people through modelling the new behaviours, forward and backward chaining (see Chapter 12), or functional communication training. The final aspect of this is the consequence-based interventions; these, according to Cooper et al (2009), are designed to only influence and affect future behaviours and are unlikely to offer any functional or supportive alternative. As consequence-based interventions are based on what happens after the behaviour has been presented then there is the potential for them to be punishing, with punishment-based approaches being clearly controversial and not supportive of the principles of non-aversive and person centred care which is advocated in many countries (Kearney, 2008).

Active support

People with intellectual disabilities who present with challenging behaviour are more likely to have limited opportunity for activities or experiences and are at risk of exclusion. The philosophy behind active support is that it seeks to enable and promote an individual's access to activities which may support skill development, enable greater engagement, improve quality of life, but also establish activities that are planned with staff/families/carers therefore also supporting their engagement (Flynn et al, 2018). Mansell (1998), stated that "Active Support" has four core components,

- Real activities at home and in the community
- Staff organise the support they offer
- Staff use an "enabling" style of interaction
- Staff improve their practice.

Active support is a person centred interventional approach which can be used as part of planning someone's support in a way that facilitates meaningful engagement, e.g. such as completing household tasks (hoovering, shopping, etc.). It employs the principles of positive behavioural support with the overall aim of improving a person's quality of life (LaVigna and Willis, 2012). Although active support has limited evidence related to its direct effectiveness on the reduction of challenging behaviour (Beadle-Brown et al, 2012), there are studies which have shown a significant decrease in challenging behaviour, for example, disruptive and anti-social behaviours where the principles of active support have been used (Koritsas et al, 2008).

Cognitive Behavioural Therapy (CBT)

Priest and Gibbs (2004) indicated that people with intellectual disabilities have a disproportionate experience of mental illness in comparison to the general population, with Brown et al (2013) suggesting that up to a third of adults have difficulties with emotional regulation which may be associated with increased challenging behaviour. The presentation of challenging behaviour and self-harm may, as some suggest, be a consequence of differences in thinking and cognition (Turnbull, 2007; Wilberforce, 2003). It is also possible to suggest that these often unconscious, negative cognitions are attributable to an individual's life experiences, their environmental experiences and social 'setting' conditions (Wolverson, 2003).

Adapted forms of cognitive behavioural therapy (CBT) and other 'talking therapies' have been used to support people with an intellectual disability across a range of difficulties, including challenging behaviour (BPS, 2015). According to Carr et al (2016) the CBT approach involves supporting the individual to replace problematic/challenging behaviours with more adaptive ways of thinking, feeling and interacting, developing new skills and adaptive approaches which would be supportive of many behavioural interventions where skills development is an interventional factor. Wilberforce (2003) identified additional universal benefits which may help to support the individual and decrease levels of challenging behaviour presented,

- a relationship based on person-centredness, trust, mutual respect and genuineness
- the offer of support and reassurance
- a working alliance in which the individual and therapist work in partnership
- the individual develops insight into their patterns of behaviour
- healthy and positive responses are reinforced by the therapist
- the client feels empowered and listened to.

The process of therapeutic intervention is as important as the content. Some individuals with intellectual disabilities will need an adapted approach with the BPS (2015) indicating that the therapist should consider an individual's level of understanding and strengths, as well as their physical, neurological, cognitive, sensory and communication needs. Examples of this might include developing self-reporting tools that display visual prompts, employing open-ended questions, and recognising that this group may have difficulty in identifying recent events or be acquiescent to the therapist (Priest and Gibbs, 2004; Hassiottis et al, 2012).

Restrictive practice/Restraint

Restrictive practices and restraint are only justifiable where they are based on a full and proportionate understanding of an individual's behaviour. Individualised support must include the identification of non-restrictive approaches such as assisting an individual with their own self-management or using appropriate de-fusion/de-escalation approaches, all of which need to be reflective of a continued individualised approach.

According to the Restraint Reduction Network (Ridley and Leitch, 2019) the use of restrictive interventions and restraint can lead to an infringement of a person's human rights; therefore, their use must be closely monitored, reviewed and be proportionate. People with intellectual disabilities have been identified as a group who are more likely to experience increased levels of restraint and restrictive practice with Emerson (2002) suggesting that in the UK 50–60% regularly experienced some form of physical restraint, with more recent estimates suggesting that total numbers of incidents of physical restraint by one or more members of staff in mental health hospitals in England reported by NHS mental health Trusts in 2011–2012 was over 39,883 (MIND, 2013). For people with intellectual disabilities this focus has also highlighted the increased use of medication which may be prescribed as a chemical restraint; medications such as anti-psychotics being used in the management of challenging behaviours without a psychiatric diagnosis (Glover et al, 2014). Physical and chemical restraint and some other examples of restrictive practices are presented in Box 17.3.

The use of restrictive interventions is not without additional risk and in some circumstances may create an increase in the presentation of an individual's behaviour,

> ### BOX 17.3   Examples of restrictive practices
>
> - Observation (which may include technical surveillance, or other forms of technology)
> - Seclusion (within a specifically designed and mandated environment)
> - Long Term Segregation
> - Physical restraint
> - Mechanical restraint (such as hand cuffs, soft restraints, bed sides)
> - Chemical restraint (such as certain prescribed medication, as and when required medications (PRN) and, depending on the environment, rapid tranquilisation)

which may be related to the individual's overall experience or as a response to trauma which may be physically, emotionally or psychologically linked to the restriction. To help the individual. and those providing support, there must be a commitment to ensuring that there is post-intervention de-brief which can be used to further explore appropriate levels of intervention for an individual (NICE, 2015).

Factors which may contribute to the use of restraint and restrictive practice have included the level of an individual's intellectual disability, their communication ability, and whether they have a psychiatric diagnosis (Emerson, 2002; Allen et al, 2005). It is also recognised that the environment can also be a factor in the use of restraint and restrictive practice with increased prevalence indicated in hospital/institutional services (Lepping et al, 2016).

Other therapeutic approaches

There are a range of additional therapeutic approaches which embrace person-centredness and individual care planning as prerequisites of constructive intervention. These interventions should be considered based on the needs of each individual, and with consideration of the assessed causation related to the challenging behaviour. Readers can explore these interventions by accessing the sources listed after each intervention,

- Family therapy (Wolverson, 2003)
- Structured teaching (Barr et al, 2000)
- The arts therapies (Liebmann, 2000)
- Complementary therapies (Wray and Paton, 2007)
- Intensive interaction (Caldwell, 1999).

Intervention(s) which are designed or identified for use with people with intellectual disabilities should be chosen because they can effectively offer solutions to the causative factors that have led to the challenging behaviour or self-injury being displayed. A one-size fits all approach to intervention is not suitable as it removes the person centred elements of any intervention and may be a breach of the individual's rights. Practitioners must be aware that where there is the potential for an intervention to cause negative, traumatic or increased challenging behaviour, then it must be reviewed with consideration given to the cause or function of the behaviour.

WORKING WITHIN AN ETHICAL AND LEGAL FRAMEWORK

When working with individuals who present with challenging behaviour and those around them, there must be consideration and understanding of the legal and ethical implications related to the assessment, planning and intervention processes. Rights-based approaches to the management of behaviour are becoming more widely acknowledged and accepted; establishing and maintaining them was seen as being progressive and radical (Cornwall and Nyamu-Musembi, 2006). An example of this is the human rights-based approach, offering a robust framework which is supported by national legislation and/or international conventions (Bailey et al, 2010). A human rights-based approach can be used to support a level of assurance, as there is recognition that it can be used to ensure that proportionality and balance is used in the approaches taken as well as offering the facilitation of positive risk management (Whitehead et al, 2009). The inception of the Human Rights Act 1998 within the UK has offered a foundation for practitioners to use when considering the rights of the individual, an example of how this can be translated is shown in Figure 17.1.

International readers will need to observe and refer to their own legislative frameworks where there may be no specific legislation linked to human rights, however most countries offer some recognition of the Universal Declaration of Human Rights (UDHR; UN General Assembly, 1948), the UN Convention on the Rights of the Child (UNCRC; UN General Assembly, 1989), and the UN Convention of the Rights of Persons with Disabilities (UNCRPD; UN General Assembly, 2007).

It is crucial that when considering any assessment or associated interventions related to challenging

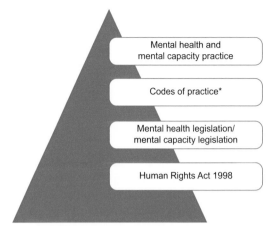

Figure 17.1 The Human Rights Act 1998 as a foundation for other law, guidance and practice * This can be for any codes of practice. The HRA is the foundation, then the next levels up – the law, the codes of practice, the practical decision making and service delivery – sit on top of that foundation. The same process could be applied to any other statute, e.g. Mental Health Act, Care Act, statutory guidance etc. (Reproduced with permission Restraint Reduction Network (RRN) 2019)

behaviour that there is clear recognition and protection of the rights of the person. Legislation should not be considered in isolation as there may be overlapping articles of law which come into play based on a person's age, capacity, or where the intervention considered has its own legislative tool such as a mental health or mental capacity law. Ethical considerations related to the care, support and interventions offered to individuals with challenging behaviour will also require the same level of scrutiny and thought as given to the legislative frameworks. Ethics is referred to as an active process with its applications being linked to a range of ethical theories, ethical approaches, as well as ethical codes of conduct which for some will be linked to their profession such as Nursing and Midwifery Council (NMC, 2018), or those provided by the Behaviour Analyst Certification Board (BACB) (Butts and Rich, 2019; BACB, 2014).

A crucial aspect of supporting a person with intellectual disability who presents with challenging behaviour is that whatever approaches are undertaken clearly protect the individual against a possible infringement of their human rights, and that the approaches advocated from assessment to intervention are proportionate to the behaviour being presented, ensuring that positive risk management is advocated, and that all interventions are focused on improving the person's overall quality of life. To consolidate the learning that has taken place in this chapter access Reader activity 17.4, Daniel's story, in the accompanying online resource.

CONCLUSION

Clearly, understanding the range of factors related to supporting individuals with intellectual disabilities who present with challenging behaviour requires consideration of their overall health, the context and environments in which they live, their life experiences which can impact on the person, and our approaches to practice. Our understanding of the person can be supported using specific assessment tools and practices which enable a clearer exploration of the diversity of influences which can contribute to not only the initial development of challenging behaviour, but also the maintenance of these behaviours such as those which are a response to trauma or biological reinforcers. Recognition needs to be given to how we use this understanding of an individual's needs to support them to develop new and existing skills, open up or renew opportunities that are individualised but also take into consideration their rights, as well as those afforded to those who are around them. We must ensure that the assessment, intervention and long-term opportunities are person centred, valued by the individual and enable a better quality of life.

REFERENCES

Adams, D., & Allen, D. (2001). Assessing the need for reactive behaviour management strategies in children with severe challenging behaviour. *Journal of Intellectual Disability Research*, *45*(4) 335–334.

Allen, D., Evans, J., Hawkins, S., & Jenkins, R. (2005). Positive behavioural support: definition, current status and future directions. *Intellectual disability Review*, *10*(2), 4–11.

Aman, M. G., & Singh, N. N. (1986). *Aberrant Behaviour Checklist manual*. New York: Slosson.

Babiker, G., & Arnold, L. (1997). *The language of injury: comprehending self-mutilation*. Leicester: British Psychological Society.

Bailey, S., Ridley, J., & Greenhill, B. (2010). Challenging behaviour: a human-rights based approach. *Advances in Mental Health and Intellectual Disabilities*, *4*(2), 20–26.

Bandura, A. (1977). *Social learning theory*. NJ: Prentice Hall.

Banks, R., Bush, A., Baker, P., et al. (2007) *Challenging behavior: a unified approach (clinical and service guidelines for supporting people with learning disabilities who are at risk of receiving abusive or restrictive practices)*. College Report CR, 144. London: The Royal College of Psychiatrists, the British Psychological Society and the Royal College of Speech and Language Therapists.

Barr, O., Sines, D., Moore, K., et al. (2000). Structured teaching. In B. Gates, J. Gear, & J. Wray (Eds.), *Behavioural distress: concepts and strategies*. London: Bailliere Tindall.

Beadle-Brown, J., Hutchinson, A., & Whelton, B. (2012). Person-centred active support – increasing choice, promoting independence and reducing challenging behaviour. *Journal of Applied Research in Intellectual Disabilities*, *25*, 291–307.

Behaviour Analyst Certification Board. (2014). *Professional and ethical compliance code for behaviour analysts*. Littleton, CO.

Bicknell, J., & Conboy-Hill, S. (1992). The deviancy career and people with mental handicap. In A. Waitman & S. Conboy Hill (Eds.), *Psychotherapy and mental handicap*. London: Sage.

Blunden, R., & Allen, D. (1987). *Facing the challenge: an ordinary life for people with learning disabilities and challenging behaviour*. London: King's Fund.

Bond, L., Carroll, R., Mulryan, N., et al. (2019). The association of life events and mental ill health in older adults with intellectual disability supplement to the Irish Longitudinal Study on Ageing. *Journal of Intellectual Disability Research*, *63*(5), 454–465.

Borthwick-Duffy, S. A. (1994). Prevalence of destructive behaviours. In T. Thompson & D. B. Gray (Eds.), *Destructive behaviour in developmental disabilities: diagnosis and treatment*. Thousand Oaks, CA: Sage.

Bowring, D. L., Painter, J., & Hastings, R. P. (2019). Prevalence of challenging behaviour in adults with intellectual disability, correlates, and association with mental health. *Current Developmental Disorders Reports*, *6*(4), 173–181.

British Psychological Society (BPS), & Royal College of Psychiatry (RCPsych). (2015). *Dementia and people with intellectual disabilities*. Leicester: BPS.

British Psychological Society (BPS). (2015). *Psychological therapies and people who have learning disabilities*. Leicester: BPS.

British Psychological Society (BPS). (2019) Evidence briefing: "Behaviour that challenges" in dementia. Available at: https://www.bps.org.uk/sites/www.bps.org.uk/files/Policy/Policy%20-%20Files/Evidence%20briefing%20-%20behaviour%20that%20challenges%20in%20dementia.pdf. [Accessed 1 April 2020].

Brown, J. F., Brown, M. Z., & Dibiasio, P. (2013). Treating individuals with intellectual disabilities and challenging behaviors with adapted dialectical behavior therapy. *Journal of Mental Health Research in Intellectual Disabilities*, 6(4), 280–303.

Butts, J. B., & Rich, K. L. (2019). *Nursing ethics: across curriculum and into practice*. Burlington: Jones & Bartlett Learning.

Caldwell, P. (1999). *Person to person: establishing contact and communication with people with profound learning disabilities and extra special needs*. Brighton: Pavilion.

Call, N. A., Simmons, C. A., Lomas Mevers, J. E., et al. (2015). Clinical outcomes of behavioural treatments for pica in children with developmental disabilities. *Journal of Autism, and Developmental Disabilities*, 45, 2105–2114.

Carr, A., Linehan, C., O'Reilly, G., et al. (Eds.). (2016). *The handbook of intellectual disability and clinical psychology practice*. London and New York: Routledge.

Chung, M. C., Cummella, S., Bickerton, W. L., et al. (1996). A preliminary study on the prevalence of challenging behaviours. *Psychological Reports*, 79, 1427–1430.

Cooper, S. A., Smiley, E., Allan, L., et al. (2009). Adults with intellectual disabilities: prevalence, incidence and remission of self-injurious behaviour, and related factors. *Journal of Intellectual Disability Research*, 53(3), 217–232.

Cornwall, A., & Nyamu-Musembi, C. (2004). Putting the 'rights-based approach' to development into perspective. *Third World Quarterly*, 28(8), 1415–1437.

Department of Health. (2007). *Services for people with learning disabilities and challenging behaviour or mental health needs*. Available at: http://www.dh.gov.uk/en/Publicationsandstatistics/Publications/PublicationsPolicyAndGuidance/DH_080129.

Didden, R., Korzilius, H., & Curfs, L. (2007). Skin-picking in individuals with Prader-Willi syndrome: prevalence, functional assessment, and its comorbidity with compulsive and self-injurious behaviours. *Journal of Applied Research in Intellectual Disabilities*, 20(5), 409–419.

Disability Rights Commission (DRC). (2006). *Equal treatment: closing the gap*. Stratford upon Avon: DRC.

Durand, M., & Crimmins, D. (1988). *The MAS administration guide*. Topeka, KS: Monaco.

Dworschak, W., Ratz, C., & Wagner, M. (2016). Prevalence and putative risk markers of challenging behaviour in students with intellectual disabilities. *Research in Developmental Disabilities*, 58, 94–103.

Emerson, E. (1995). *Challenging behaviour: analysis and intervention in people with learning disabilities*. Cambridge: Cambridge University Press.

Emerson, E. (2002). The prevalence of reactive management strategies in community-based services in the UK. In D. Allen (Ed.), *Ethical approaches to physical interventions: responding to challenging behaviour in people with intellectual disabilities* (pp. 15–28). Kidderminster: BILD.

Emerson, E. (2005). Working with people with challenging behaviour. In E. Emerson, C. Hatton, J. Bromley, & A. Caine (Eds.), *Clinical psychology and people with intellectual disabilities* (pp. 127–153). Chichester: Wiley.

Emerson, E., & Einfeld, S. L. (2011). *Challenging behaviour*. Cambridge University Press.

Emerson, E., Hatton, C., Robertson, J., et al. (2012). *People with learning disabilities in England 2011*. Lancaster: Learning Disabilities Observatory, University of Lancaster.

Emerson, E., Kiernan, C., Alborz, A., et al. (2001). The prevalence of challenging behaviours: a total population study. *Research in Developmental Disabilities*, 22(1), 77–93.

Emerson, E., Moss, S., & Kiernan, C. (1999). The relationship between challenging behaviours and psychiatric disorders in people with severe developmental disabilities. In N. Bouras (Ed.), *Psychiatric and behavioural disorders in people with severe developmental disabilities and mental retardation*. Cambridge: Cambridge University Press.

European Union. (2012). *Charter of fundamental rights of the European Union*. 2012/C 326/02. Available at: https://www.refworld.org/docid/3ae6b3b70.html. [Accessed 26 October 2020].

Flynn, S., Totsike, V., Hastings, R. P., et al. (2018). Effectiveness of active support for adults with intellectual disability in residential settings: systematic review and meta-analysis. *Journal of Applied Research in Intellectual Disabilities*, 31, 983–998.

Foucault, M. (1990). *Madness and civilisation: a history of insanity in the age of reason*. London: Routledge.

Gates, B. (2007). Theory and practice of managing self-injurious behaviour in people with learning disabilities. In B. Gates (Ed.), *Learning disabilities: toward inclusion*. Edinburgh: Churchill Livingstone.

Gates, B., Gear, J., & Wray, J. (2002). *Behavioural distress: concepts and strategies*. Edinburgh: Ballière Tindall.

Gates, B., & Mafuba, K. (2015). *Learning disability nursing: modern day practice*. Oxon: CRC Press.

Giesbers, S. A., Hendriks, L., Jahoda, A., et al. (2019). Living with support: experiences of people with mild intellectual disability. *Journal of Applied Research in Intellectual Disabilities*, 32(2), 446–456.

Glover, G., Bernard, S., Branford, D., et al. (2014). Use of medication for challenging behaviour in people with intellectual disability. *The British Journal of Psychiatry*, 205, 6–7.

Gore, N., McGill, P., Toogood, S., et al. (2013). Definition and scope for positive behavioural support. *International Journal of Positive Behavioural Support*, 3(2), 14–23.

Hardy, S., Chaplin, E., & Woodward, P. (2016). *Supporting the physical health needs of people with learning disabilities.* Brighton: Pavilion.

Hardy, S., & Joyce, T. (2011). *Challenging behaviour and people with learning disabilities: a handbook.* Brighton: Pavilion.

Hassiotis, A., Poppe, M., Strydom, A., et al. (2018). Positive behaviour support training for staff for treating challenging behaviour in people with intellectual disabilities: a cluster RCT. *Health Technology Assessment, 22*, 15.

Hassiotis, A., Serfaty, M., Azam, K., et al. (2012). *A manual of cognitive behaviour therapy for people with learning disabilities and common mental disorders: therapist version.* London: Islington NHS Foundation Trust.

Hatton, C., & Emerson, E. (2004). The relationship between life events and psychopathology amongst children with intellectual disabilities. *Journal of Applied Research in Intellectual Disabilities, 17*, 109–117.

Heslop, P., & Macauley, F. (2009). *Hidden pain? Self-injury and people with learning disabilities.* Bristol: Bristol Crisis Services for Women.

Holden, B., & Gitleson, J. P. (2006). A total population study of challenging behaviour in the county of Hedmark, Norway: prevalence, and risk markers. *Research in Developmental Disabilities, 27*, 456–465.

Horner, R. H. (1994). Functional assessment: contributions and future directions. *Journal of Applied Behaviour Analysis, 27*, 401–404.

Howatson, J. (2005). Health action plans for people with learning disabilities. *Nursing Standard, 19*(43), 51–57.

Huisman, S., Mulder, P., Kuijk, J., et al. (2018). Self-injurious behaviour. *Neuroscience and Biobehavioural Reviews, 84*, 483–491.

Human Rights Act. (1998). Available at: http://www. dh.gov.uk/en/Publicationsandstatistics/Publications/ PublicationsLegislation/DH_4009802.

Jahoda, A., & Markova, I. (2004). Coping with social stigma: people with intellectual disabilities moving from institutions and family home. *Journal of Intellectual Disability Research, 48*(8), 719–729.

Jahoda, A., Wilson, A., Stalker, K., et al. (2010). Living with stigma and the self-perceptions of people with mild intellectual disabilities. *Journal of Social Issues, 66*(3), 521–534.

Kaur, G., Scior, K., & Wilson, S. (2009). Systemic working in intellectual disability services: a UK wide survey. *British Journal of Learning Disabilities, 37*, 213–220.

Kearney, A. J. (2008). *Understanding applied behavior analysis, and introduction to ABA for parents, teachers, and other professionals.* London: Jessica Kingsley.

Kerr, D. (2007). *Understanding learning disability and dementia.* London: Jessica Kingsley.

Kincaid, D. (2016). Staying true to our PBS roots in a changing world. *Journal of Positive Behaviour Interventions, 20*(1), 15–18.

Klonsky, D. (2007). The functions of deliberate self-injury: a review of the evidence. *Clinical Psychology Review, 27*, 226–259.

Koritsas, S., Iacono, T., Hamilton, D., & Leighton, D. (2008). The effect of active support training on engagement and, opportunities for choice, challenging behaviour and support needs. *Journal of Intellectual & Developmental Disability, 33*(3), 247–256.

Kwok, H., & Cheung, P. (2007). Co-morbidity of psychiatric disorder and medical illness in people with intellectual disabilities. *Current Opinion in Psychiatry, 20*(5), 443–449.

LaVigna, G. W., & Willis, T. J. (2012). The efficacy of positive behavioural support with the most challenging behaviour: the evidence and its implications. *Journal of Intellectual and Developmental Disability, 37*(3), 185–195.

Lemay, R. A. (2009). Deinstitutionalization of people with developmental disabilities: a review of the literature. *Canadian Journal of Community Mental Health, 28*(1), 181–194.

Lepping, P., Masood, B., Flammer, E., et al. (2016). Comparison of restraint date from four countries. *Social Psychiatry and Psychiatric Epidemiology, 51*, 1301–1309.

Liebmann, M. (2000). The arts therapies. In B. Gates, J. Gear, & J. Wray (Eds.), *Behavioural distress: concepts and strategies.* London: Bailliere Tindall.

McBrien, J., & Felce, D. (1995). *Working with people who have severe learning difficulty and challenging behaviour: a practical handbook on the behavioural approach.* Kidderminster: BILD.

McConachie, H. (1986). *Parents and young mentally handicapped children: a review of research issues.* Beckenham: Croom Helm.

McCue, M. (2000). Behavioural interventions. In B. Gates, J. Gear, & J. Wray (Eds.), *Behavioural distress, concepts and strategies.* London: Bailliere Tindall.

Mansell, J. (1998). Active support (editorial). *Tizard Learning Disability Review, 3*, 4–6.

Martorell, A., & Tsakanikos, E. (2008). Traumatic experiences and life events in people with intellectual disability. *Current Opinion in Psychiatry, 21*(5), 445–448.

Matson, J. L., Hattier, M. A., Belva, B., & Matson, M. L. (2013). Pica in persons with developmental disabilities: Approaches to treatment. *Research in Developmental Disabilities, 34*, 2564–2571.

Matthews, D. R. (2004). *The 'OK' Health Check: health facilitation and health action planning* (3rd ed.). Fairfield: Preston.

MIND. (2013). *Mental health crisis care: physical restraint in crisis: a report on physical restraint in hospital settings in England.* London: MIND.

Moss, S., Emerson, E., Kiernan, C., et al. (2000). Psychiatric symptoms in adults with intellectual disability and challenging behaviour. *British Journal of Psychiatry*, *177*, 452–456.

Murphy, G. (1994). Understanding challenging behaviour. In E. Emerson, P. McGill, & J. Mansell (Eds.), *Severe learning disabilities and challenging behaviour: designing high quality services*. London: Chapman and Hall.

Murphy, G. (1999). Self-injurious behaviour: what do we know and where are we going? *Tizard Intellectual disability Review*, *4*(1), 5–12.

National Institute for Health and Care Excellence (NICE). (2015). *Challenging behaviour and learning disabilities: prevention and interventions for people with learning disabilities whose behaviour challenges (NG11)*. London: NICE.

Nihira, K., Leland, H., & Lambert, N. (1993). *AAMR adaptive behaviour scale – residential and community examiners manual* (2nd ed.). Austin, TX: Pro-Ed.

Nunkoosing, K., & Haydon-Laurelt, M. (2011). Intellectual disabilities, challenging behaviour and referral texts: a critical discourse analysis. *Disability and Society*, *26*(4), 405–417.

Nursing and Midwifery Council. (2018). *The code: professional standards of practice and behaviour for nurses, midwives and nursing associates*. London: NMC.

Oliver, C., McClintock, K., Hall, S., et al. (2003). Assessing the severity of challenging behaviour: psychometric properties of the Challenging Behaviour Interview. *Journal of Applied Research in Intellectual Disabilities*, *16*, 53–61.

O'Neil, R. F., Horner, R. H., Albin, R. W., et al. (1997). *Functional analysis and programme development for problem behaviour: a practical handbook* (2nd ed.). CA: Brooks Cole.

Paclawskyj, T. R., Matson, J. L., Rush, K. S., et al. (2000). Questions About Behavioural Function (QABF): a behavioural checklist for Functional assessment of aberrant behaviour. *Research in Developmental Disabilities*, *21*, 223–229.

Pavlov, I. P. (1927). *Conditional reflexes*. London: Oxford University Press.

Pelleboer-Gunnink, H. A., Van Oorsouw, W. M. W. J., Van Weeghel, J., et al. (2017). Mainstream health professionals' stigmatising attitudes towards people with intellectual disabilities: a systematic review. *Journal of Intellectual Disability Research*, *61*(5), 411–434.

Pelleboer-Gunnink, H. A., van Weeghel, J., & Embregts, P. J. (2019). Public stigmatisation of people with intellectual disabilities: a mixed-methods population survey into stereotypes and their relationship with familiarity and discrimination. Disability and Rehabilitation. *43*(4), 1–9.

Perez, M., Carlson, G., Ziviani, J., et al. (2012). Contribution of occupational therapists in positive behaviour support. *Australian Occupational Therapy Journal*, *59*, 428–436.

Piazza, C. C., Roane, H. S., Keeney, K. M., et al. (2002). Varying response effort in the treatment of PICA maintained by automatic reinforcement. *Journal of Applied Behaviour Analysis*, *35*, 233–246.

Pilgrim, D., & Rogers, A. (1999). *A sociology of mental health and illness*. Trowbridge: Oxford University Press.

Pitonyak, D. (2002). Opening the door. In J. O'Brien & C. Lyle-O'Brien (Eds.), *Implementing person-centered planning: voices of experience* (pp. 99–120). Toronto: Inclusion Press.

Poppes, P., van der Putten, A. J. J., & Vlaskamp, C. (2010). Frequency and severity of challenging behaviour in people with profound intellectual and multiple disabilities. *Research in Developmental Disabilities*, *31*, 1269–1275.

Priest, H., & Gibbs, M. (2004). *Mental health care for people with learning disabilities*. Edinburgh: Churchill Livingstone.

Raghavan, R., & Patel, P. (2005). *Learning disabilities and mental health: a nursing perspective*. Oxford: Blackwell.

Rattaz, C., Michelon, C., Munir, K., et al. (2018). Challenging behaviours at early adulthood in autism spectrum disorders: topography, risk factors and evolution. *Journal of Intellectual Disability Research*, *62*(7), 637–649.

Ridley, J., & Leitch, S. (2019). *Restraint Reduction Network: training standards*. Birmingham: RRN.

Rolland, J. S. (1993, December). Helping couples live with illness. *Family Therapy News*, 15–26.

Roy, A., Roy, M., Deb, S., et al. (2015). Are opioid antagonists effective in reducing self injury in adults with intellectual disability? A systematic review. *Journal of Intellectual Disability Research*, *59*(1), 55–67.

Skinner, B. F. (1953). *Science and human behaviour*. New York: MacMillan.

Smiley, E. (2005). Epidemiology of mental health problems in adults with a learning disability: an update. *Advances in Psychiatric Treatment*, *11*(3), 214–222.

Smith, M., & Nethell, G. (2014). The Brief Behavioural Assessment Tool – preliminary findings on reliability and validity. *International Journal of Positive Behavioural Support*, *4*(2), 32–40.

Stiegler, L. N. (2005). Understanding pica behaviour: a review for clinical and education professionals. *Focus on Autism and Other Developmental Disabilities*, *20*(1), 27–38.

Taggart, L., & Slevin, E. (2006). Care planning in mental health settings. In B. Gates (Ed.), *Care planning and delivery in intellectual disability nursing*. Oxford: Blackwell.

Touchette, P. E., MacDonlad, R. F., & Langer, S. N. (1985). A scatter plot for identifying stimulus control of problem behaviour. *Journal of Applied Behaviour Analysis*, *18*(4), 343–351.

Turnbull, J. (2007). Psychological approaches. In B. Gates (Ed.), *2007 Learning disabilities: toward inclusion* (5th ed.). Edinburgh: Churchill Livingstone.

UN General Assembly. (2007). *Convention on the Rights of Persons with Disabilities: resolution/adopted by the General Assembly, 24 January.* A/RES/61/106. Available at: https://www.refworld.org/docid/45f973632.html. [Accessed 9 November 2020].

UN General Assembly. (1989). *Convention on the Rights of the Child* (Vol. 1577). United Nations, Treaty Series, 3. Available at: https://www.refworld.org/docid/3ae6b38f0.html. [Accessed 9 November 2020].

UN General Assembly. (1948). *Universal Declaration of Human Rights.* Available at: https://www.refworld.org/docid/3ae6b3712c.html. [Accessed 9 November 2020].

Vetere, A. (1993). Using family therapy in services for people with learning disabilities. In J. Carpenter & A. Treacher (Eds.), *Using family therapy in the 90s.* Oxford: Blackwell.

Whitehead, R., Carney, G., & Greenhill, B. (2009). Encouraging positive risk management; supporting 'a life like any other' using a human rights based approach. In C. Logan & R. Whittington (Eds.), *Self-harm and violence: best practice in managing risk.*

Wilberforce, D. (2003). Psychological approaches. In B. Gates (Ed.), *Learning disabilities: toward inclusion* (4th ed.). London: Baillière Tindall.

Wilner, P., & Smith, M. (2008). Attribution theory applied to helping behaviour towards people with intellectual disabilities who challenge. *Journal of Applied Research in Intellectual Disabilities, 21,* 150–155.

Winchel, R. M., & Stanley, M. (1991). Self-injurious behaviour: a review of the behaviour and biology of self-mutilation. *American Journal of Psychiatry, 148*(3), 306–317.

Wisely, J., Hare, D., & Fernandez-Ford, L. (2002). A study of the topography of self-injurious behaviour in people with learning disabilities. *Journal of Learning Disabilities, 6*(1), 61–71.

Wolfensberger, W. (1975). *The origin and nature of institutional models.* Syracuse: Human Policy Press.

Wolkorte, T., van Houwelingen, I., & Kroezen, M. (2019). Challenging behaviours: views and preferences of people with intellectual disabilities. *Journal of Applied Research in Intellectual Disabilities, 32,* 1421–1427.

Wolverson, M. (2003). Challenging behaviour. In B. Gates (Ed.), *Learning disabilities: toward inclusion* (4th ed.). Edinburgh: Churchill Livingstone.

Wolverson, M. (2011). Challenging behaviour. In H. L. Atherton & D. J. Crickmore (Eds.), *Learning disabilities; towards inclusion* (6th ed.). Edinburgh: Churchill Livingstone.

Wood, D., Campbell, T., Lau, L., et al. (2018). Emerging adulthood as a critical stage in the life course. In N. Halfon, C. Forrest, R. Lerner, & E. Faustman (Eds.), *Handbook of life course health development.* Cham: Springer. https://doi.org/10.1007/978-3-319-47143-3_7.

Wray, J., & Paton, K. (2007). Complementary therapies. In B. Gates (Ed.), *Learning disabilities: toward inclusion* (5th ed.). Edinburgh: Churchill Livingstone.

Working with people with intellectual disabilities suspected of offending

Elizabeth Walsh and Salma Ali

KEY ISSUES

- International estimates suggest that approximately 7–10% of convicted offenders have intellectual disabilities.
- People with intellectual disabilities who come into contact with the criminal justice system are often considered 'vulnerable', more so than the wider criminal justice population.
- They are more likely to find criminal justice processes, including court systems, distressing, confusing and bewildering. This can negatively affect their ability to meaningfully participate in legal proceedings.

- Many people with intellectual disabilities may find it difficult to cope in prison and struggle to access services that aim to meet offence related and healthcare needs.
- Assimilation back into their communities after release can also be problematic.
- Services need to work together to ensure an intellectual disability is identified early in the criminal justice process and ensure that all people with intellectual disabilities who offend are at the forefront of any discussions.

CHAPTER OUTLINE

INTRODUCTION

This chapter explores some of the key issues facing individuals with intellectual disabilities who are involved with the criminal justice system (CJS). The CJS refers to government agencies and institutions whose aim it is to manage accused and convicted criminals throughout the process from pre- arrest to post- release from prison. These may differ between countries but could include police services, the Crown Prosecution Service (CPS, in England and Wales), courts, prisons and probation services.

It is acknowledged that people with intellectual disabilities also come into contact with the CJS as witnesses and victims of crime, however, the focus of this chapter is on those who are in contact with the system because they are suspected or convicted perpetrators of crime. It will cover three main areas.

Firstly, it will discuss prevalence rates of people with intellectual disabilities in the CJS and outline some of the difficulties faced by this group as they are supported to navigate their way through the different stages of the system.

Secondly, an overview of some of the main legal and policy safeguards applicable to this population is provided. This includes consideration of service-level responses and solutions designed to ameliorate the negative impact of the issues faced by people with intellectual disabilities who become involved in the CJS. Whilst it is acknowledged that these will differ between countries, for the purposes of this chapter the UK has been used as an example with which international readers can compare their own local and national systems.

Finally, the chapter walks through the criminal justice pathway, considering the challenges and concerns of people with intellectual disabilities from arrest, through to court, onto prison and then discharge into the community. As internationally focused research that explores the experiences of people with intellectual disabilities who have contact with the CJS is an evolving area, this chapter is based predominately on UK experiences.

People with intellectual disabilities who come into contact with the CJS are often considered 'vulnerable', more so than the wider criminal justice population (McCarthy et al, 2016). Within the CJS, the word 'vulnerable' describes people who are less able to cope with the rigours of, for example, police caution and interview, and who are in need of support. According to Talbot (2008), people with intellectual disabilities in contact with the CJS are discriminated against personally, systemically and routinely throughout. For example, HM Chief Inspector of Prisons for England and Wales (2017) noted that prisoners with intellectual disabilities are frequently excluded from some areas of the prison system which means they are often precluded from therapeutic opportunities to address their offending behaviour.

In general, many people with intellectual disabilities are unlikely to have any distinguishing features that make their condition obvious or easily identifiable. Often there are high rates of overlap and comorbidity between their condition and other mental disorders, which makes identification of this population complex (Hellenbach et al, 2017). Within the CJS, this can have negative implications for an individual's health and well-being not to mention significant effects on legal and criminal justice outcomes.

As noted, people with intellectual disabilities suspected of offending often have difficulties navigating their journey through the CJS, and therefore may be disadvantaged without specialist support (see, for example Gudjonsson and Joyce, 2011; Murphy and Clare, 1995; Søndenaa et al, 2010; Talbot, 2008). Awareness of how mental health-related difficulty may contribute to offending behaviour is relatively well understood, however, the effect of having an intellectual disability is currently less well established.

PREVALENCE OF INTELLECTUAL DISABILITY IN CRIMINAL JUSTICE SERVICES

There are no accurate data concerning the number of people with intellectual disabilities in the CJS, though recent international estimates 'suggest that approximately 7–10% of convicted offenders' are considered to have intellectual disabilities (Hellenbach, 2017). In the UK, there are also no accurate statistics available which identify how many people in contact with the CJS have intellectual disabilities. Average estimates vary widely from 1%–34% (Talbot, 2009; Young et al, 2013; Criminal Justice Joint Inspection, 2014; NHS England, 2016; Prison Reform Trust, 2019), and several studies indicate that individuals with intellectual disabilities are over-represented in the CJS (see Talbot, 2008; Hyun et al, 2013; Hellenbach et al, 2017).

The lack of clarity on prevalence has been attributed to methodological variability including differences in definitions and diagnostic criteria (McKenzie et al, 2012; Royal College of Psychiatrists, 2014), sampling techniques and study designs (Lindsay, 2011; Raina and Lunsky, 2010). The Criminal Justice Joint Inspection (2014) suggest that exact numbers are unknown as there are no accurate records kept nor an agreed definition of what constitutes an intellectual disability.

With regard to specific groups, precise information about prevalence amongst black and minority ethnic offenders also remains sparse, but gender differences have been highlighted. Mottram (2007) reports a higher proportion of women in prison with an IQ below 70 (8%) and between 70–79 (32%) than were found among men.

THE LEGAL AND POLICY FRAMEWORK

Access to justice is a fundamental right, and for people with intellectual disabilities it provides a mechanism to tackle much of the discrimination they face (Beqiraj et al, 2017). For example, they are often denied legal capacity and have difficulty accessing courts and other legal settings. However, individuals with intellectual disabilities are arguably most in need of fair access to justice, but frequently experience barriers to it (Beqiraj et al, 2017).

Different countries have different responses and practices to improving access to justice for people with intellectual disabilities, which are often culture-specific and driven by political decisions. However, international law outlines a set of rights, entitlements and guarantees that are specifically designed to address the needs of people with disabilities.

Article 1 of the United Nations (UN) Convention on the Rights of People with Disabilities (CRPD), (UN, 2006, p. 3) defines persons with disabilities as including

"those who have long-term physical, mental, intellectual or sensory impairments, which in interaction with various barriers may hinder their full and effective participation in society on an equal basis with others."

Article 13 (UN, 2006, p. 9) continues to focus on access to justice and states that

"parties shall ensure effective access to justice for persons with disabilities on an equal basis with others, including through the provision of procedural and age-appropriate accommodations, in order to facilitate their effective role as direct and indirect participants, including as witnesses, in all legal proceedings, including at investigative and other preliminary stages."

Therefore, in order to improve social effects and redress the imbalance that people with intellectual disabilities often face in the CJS, access to justice needs significant improvement.

The UK experience

In the UK there are various legal and policy safeguards aimed at protecting the general welfare of vulnerable people, facilitating their access to treatment and support where appropriate, and subsequently reducing risks of miscarriages of justice that might arise from their vulnerability. Provisions tend to be framed within the language of 'mental disorder' as a broad term encompassing intellectual disabilities alongside mental illness. This is problematic to the extent that it masks the more specific needs of people with intellectual disabilities.

Human Rights Act (1998)

The Human Rights Act (HRA) 1998 came into force throughout the UK in October 2000 and brings the European Convention on Human Rights (ECHR) (1953) into British law. The HRA places an obligation on all public bodies, and on those private bodies that carry out functions previously delivered by the State, to ensure they respect human rights. The most relevant articles of the HRA for the purposes of this chapter are:

- Article 2: the right to life
- Article 3: the right to protection from torture, inhumane or degrading treatment
- Article 5: the right to liberty and security
- Article 6: the right to a fair trial
- Article 8: the right to respect for private and family life
- Article 14: the prohibition of discrimination

An important concept introduced through this Act is that public bodies have a positive obligation to protect rights meaning that they must take active steps to safeguard a person's Convention rights. This is particularly relevant where people are in the care of the State, as are prisoners.

The Police and Criminal Evidence Act (1984)

This statutory framework is largely established by the Police and Criminal Evidence Act (PACE) 1984, and its accompanying Codes of Practice, particularly Code C (Code of Practice for the Detention, Treatment and Questioning of Persons by Police Officers) (Home Office, 2006).

The main policy safeguards for suspects with intellectual disabilities are:

- Diversion away from the CJS.
- An appropriate adult should be called to the police station if a person who is 'mentally disordered or otherwise mentally vulnerable' has been detained.
- A custody officer has a duty to seek clinical attention for a detainee who appears to be suffering from a mental disorder.

There are statutory grounds for excluding confession evidence from a trial, where the confession has been obtained under circumstances in which undue pressure was exerted on a vulnerable suspect in a police interview, or the police failed to ensure that the requisite safeguards were in place.

The Equality Act (2010)

The Equality Act (2010) was created to consolidate previous legislation such as the Disability Discrimination Act (2005) under one broader umbrella in order to prevent discrimination. The Act provides the UK with legislation that prevents the occurrence of discrimination and unfair treatment. Essentially, the Equality Act protects the rights of individuals with all disabilities, compelling agencies to proactively eliminate discrimination as part of their everyday work. Therefore, agencies have a statutory responsibility to ensure that discrimination does not occur, for example, by making reasonable adjustments to existing service provision and ensuring that future provision is accessible to people with disabilities, subsequently promoting inclusion.

The principle of inclusion promotes the legal and human rights of people with disabilities to live full and active lives in society. As well as rights, the concept of inclusion implies that individuals with disabilities have the same duties and obligations as their fellow non-disabled citizens – in this context, the duty to live a law-abiding life (Talbot, 2008). The inclusion agenda thus fosters the presumption that, unless their capacity to participate effectively in the criminal justice process is severely limited, people with intellectual disabilities should be subject to the same due process as anyone else, but with appropriate support.

In criminal justice proceedings, this means that defendants with disabilities should be provided with the practical assistance and facilities they require to participate effectively in proceedings. This helps to ensure two important outcomes. Firstly, that individuals are held to account for alleged offending behaviour, and secondly, they have the same opportunity as anyone else to defend themselves wherever possible.

The Mental Health Act (1983, Am. 2007)

Part III of the Mental Health Act (MHA) 1983, as amended by the Mental Health Act 2007, allows people who are mentally disordered to be diverted from the CJS into compulsory treatment by the healthcare system either before or after conviction. The 2007 Act defines mental disorder as 'any disorder or disability of the mind' (section 1(2)). It is specified, however, that for many of the provisions of the Act, including the Part III provisions discussed here, a person with an intellectual disability should not be considered mentally disordered unless the 'disability is associated with abnormally aggressive or seriously irresponsible conduct on his part' (s. 2(2)). Intellectual disability is defined in the Act as 'a state of arrested or incomplete development of the mind which includes significant impairment of intelligence and social functioning' (s. 2(3)).

Transforming Care

Based on the growing evidence-base, and inception of Liaison and Diversion services (discussed later), the National Health Service's (NHS) Transforming Care (NHS England, 2017) agenda aims to provide better community support to meet the needs of people with intellectual disabilities and other related disorders such as Autistic Spectrum to prevent them from coming into contact with the CJS. Transforming Care acknowledges that people with intellectual disabilities who offend often fall through the gaps of existing services and are likely to be unable to access other services because they are considered to be too able, too high risk or have autism (or another disorder) but not an intellectual disability.

Whilst the Transforming Care agenda recognises that community provision should be preventative in order to reduce the amount of people with intellectual disabilities becoming involved in the CJS, it also recognises the need for a reactive approach which allows services to respond appropriately to those already in contact with CJS. This approach focuses on a collaborative, multidisciplinary and multi-agency approach, where specialist risk assessment is central to the delivery of evidence-based interventions and therapeutic support. Professionals working in this area should be appropriately trained, and where needed, consultancy from other services should be sought to appropriately respond to the needs of this group.

 READER ACTIVITY 18.1

Consider the policy and legislative position in your country.
    How does it compare to what you now know about the UK?

DIFFICULTIES FACED BY PEOPLE WITH INTELLECTUAL DISABILITIES IN THE CRIMINAL JUSTICE SYSTEM

In comparison to their non-disabled counterparts, people with intellectual disabilities are more likely to find criminal justice processes distressing, confusing and bewildering, which can negatively affect their ability to meaningfully participate in and understand legal proceedings. Box 18.1 suggests a range of signs that might suggest a defendant has an intellectual disability. Particular concerns about the ability of this group to

BOX 18.1   Signs that might suggest a defendant has an intellectual disability

Someone with an intellectual disability might:
- respond inappropriately to questions or instructions
- use words inappropriately
- not understand criminal justice and court terminology, e.g. words such as remand, custody and bail
- respond inappropriately to their situation as a defendant in court. For example, falling asleep, gazing around the court room or not paying attention to what is happening
- take longer to answer a question or follow an instruction
- appear unduly anxious, distressed, angry or frustrated
- appear withdrawn and say little in response to questions.

 BOX 18.2   Experiences of people with intellectual disabilities in the CJS

- The judges don't speak English, they say these long words I have never heard of in my life.
- I didn't know what 'remanded' meant. I thought it meant I could come back later.
- I couldn't really hear. I couldn't understand but I said 'yes, whatever' to anything because if I say, 'I don't know' they look at me as if I'm thick. Sometimes they tell you two things at once.
- I was upset; I didn't know why I was there. I really didn't think I had done anything wrong.
- I didn't know what was going on and there's no one there to explain things to you. They tell you to read things and in court you can't just ask for help. The judge thinks you can read and write just because you can speak English (Talbot, 2008)

NB interviewees in this study refer to magistrates as judges

meaningfully participate in legal proceedings include problems understanding the police caution, issues with comprehension and literacy, and making decisions that do not safeguard their wellbeing or protect their rights as suspects or defendants (Parsons and Sherwood, 2016). In addition, they are more likely to be acquiescent and suggestible than those without intellectual disabilities (Clare, 2003) and thus are more vulnerable in police interviews (Gudjonsson, 2003) risking the possibility of wrongful conviction.

In 2008 Talbot, for the Prison Reform Trust, conducted a programme of research with people with intellectual disabilities to explore their experiences of being involved the CJS. A number of difficulties were outlined by this group in relation to their understanding of what was happening and feeling unable to change the situation. The voices of some of the participants in this study are noted in Box 18.2 where they talk about their experiences.

These issues are echoed in a thematic review conducted by Hyun et al (2013) which synthesised findings from research in the UK and USA about the experiences of people with intellectual disabilities who faced arrest and imprisonment. The review reported three common themes: (i) participants did not understand what was happening to them, or why, (ii) they felt alone, and they did not know where to turn, or to whom for support and (iii) they were uncertain about what to say or do.

 BOX 18.3   Practical examples of supporting people with intellectual disabilities in the CJS

- Clocks – The use of a digital clock over an analogue clock
- Easy Read documents – visual/pictorial examples
- Regular breaks – particularly during Court proceedings to aid understanding, prevent cognitive overload, and manage anxiety
- Defendant sits next to their Solicitor and not in the dock
- Removal of wigs and gowns in Crown Court
- Use of an Appropriate Adult in the Police station or an Intermediary in Court
- Use of a toy/stimulus – these may help manage sensory issues
- Considering the timing of the court hearing e.g. in the afternoon following administration of medication

Box 18.3 provides some practical examples that can be considered to support people with intellectual disabilities who are in contact with the CJS along the whole pathway, including in police custody, in court and in prison.

PATHWAY THROUGH THE CRIMINAL JUSTICE SYSTEM

The criminal justice system is comprised of a number of agencies including police, courts, prison and probation services. The offender with intellectual disabilities may pass through just one or all of these agencies. Issues specific to each stage are discussed below.

Police Services

The police have a duty to investigate any criminal offence that is reported to them. This may lead to the arrest of an individual who is suspected of having committed the offence. For people with intellectual disabilities, the fact they have intellectual disabilities is unlikely to have a bearing on *how* any arrest is carried out (Murphy and Mason, 2007) however it might have a bearing on whether the suspect is ultimately arrested.

The police have a degree of discretion when deciding what action to take, including issuing a formal warning, engaging with civil enforcement through anti-social behaviour orders (ASBO), onward referral to social support services and a non-judicial criminal punishment e.g. a fixed penalty notice. Police make decisions about onward action, based on a number of considerations including the nature and seriousness of the offence, the context of the offence e.g. has it taken place in public or in private, and the mental capacity of the offender.

Of particular interest here, is consideration of the mental capacity of the offender. According to Talbot (2011), people with mild intellectual disabilities are more likely to be arrested for an offence than those with more significant intellectual disabilities. This is because people with more significant intellectual disabilities are likely to have limited ability to go out alone and are therefore accompanied in public, making it unlikely that they would be able to engage in illegal activities. The milder the intellectual disability, the more likely that formal action will be taken against a suspect, because the police will be more confident that the suspect can be interviewed and ultimately be held responsible for their actions.

People with intellectual disabilities in police custody face a number of challenges, as do those caring for them. In a joint inspection of the treatment of offenders with intellectual disabilities, HM Inspectorates of Probation, Constabulary, Crown Prosecution and Care Quality Commission inspectors examined four specific stages of the CJS with which an offender with intellectual disabilities could come into contact including police services, the crown prosecution service, the courts and probation (see Criminal Justice Joint Inspection, 2014). When considering the treatment of offenders with intellectual disabilities in police custody, inspectors found that many were not adequately assessed or recorded and nor were police custody suites appropriate environments in which to make assessments of their needs. They noted that *Appropriate Adults* (family members, carers, professionals charged with responsibility to ensure that the rights of a vulnerable person in custody are upheld) were not always called and when they were called, were not trained sufficiently to support people with intellectual disabilities. Of most concern in the literature is the way in which the offender with an intellectual disability experiences police custody and how their condition can impact on their ability to engage fully in the criminal justice process.

In their qualitative study of the needs of people with intellectual disabilities within the Scottish criminal justice system, Mediseni and Brown (2015) note the psychological vulnerabilities faced by people with intellectual disabilities, who can have difficulty understanding questions posed by the police during interviews and who can have 'limited understanding of the potential implications of the responses provided' (p.176). This is supported by Marshall-Tate et al (2019) who note that poor communication skills increase difficulties in terms of ability to obtain, process and understand basic information, give an accurate account of events, and understand and participate in legal proceedings.

In their exploration of the challenges associated with communication for people with intellectual disabilities in police custody, Parsons and Sherwood (2016) note the problems faced by detainees in being able to fully understand their rights and entitlements whilst in custody and highlight the importance of making information more accessible for this group when engaged with the CJS. They provide the perspective of the professional working with people with intellectual disabilities in police custody through qualitative interviews. They note the challenges facing staff that include the existing, thoroughly embedded communication practices in place, as well as the 'volatile environment within which communication takes place' (Parsons and Sherwood, 2016, p. 568), echoing findings from the Criminal Justice Joint Inspection (2014) with regards to the inappropriate environment. Such consideration of initial police contact is not confined to the UK as can be seen in Philip Sabuni's (2020) Zambian account in the accompanying online resource. Whilst it refers to 'a person who appears to be in crisis' (rather than is suspected of offending), similarities in approach at this stage and subsequently can be identified.

Criminal Justice Liaison and Diversion Services

The creation of criminal justice liaison and diversion services in the UK was originally stimulated by the Reed Review (Department of Health/Home Office, 1992) which described the needs of people with mental disorder and intellectual disabilities who offend and called for nationwide provision of properly resourced court assessment and diversion schemes.

Liaison and Diversion services work with the Police and Courts to screen and identify vulnerable suspects and defendants of all ages. One of the most important elements of the work of liaison and diversion schemes is the identification and assessment of an individual's impairments and support needs. Ideally, this would occur prior to the point of charge and inform all subsequent proceedings. Liaison and Diversion practitioners, who are often mental health professionals such as community mental health nurses, provide information to legal professionals about identified support needs during criminal justice processes, make recommendations for reasonable adjustments during Court proceedings and refer people to treatment and support services in the community. Services of this nature encourage better identification of an individual's vulnerability both in relation to mental health and intellectual disability. Subsequently, they enable practitioners to consider appropriate support packages tailored to address individual need.

Originally, the purpose of court diversion services was to identify people whose imprisonment was not in the public interest, was likely to be disproportionately harmful to the offender, and not considered an appropriate setting for the vulnerable offender. For example, James et al (2002) demonstrated that timely diversion from the CJS produced better outcomes both in terms of the person's mental health and in reducing the risk of re-offending.

However, although the Reed Review initiated a service level response, historically services developed in response to this review have been, at best, variable and have largely focused on mental health support rather than for people with intellectual disabilities (Royal College of Psychiatrists, 2014). Services for people with intellectual disabilities in the UK have, in comparison been somewhat left behind.

READER ACTIVITY 18.2

Identify any schemes in your own country that may offer an alternative to custody for people with intellectual disabilities.
What evidence exists as to their effectiveness?

Some years later, the publication of The Bradley Review (Department of Health (DH), 2009) reinvigorated much needed discussion in this area. It aimed to examine the extent to which offenders with mental health problems or intellectual disabilities could be diverted from prison to other services and the barriers to such diversion, in order to make recommendations to government. The review made 82 recommendations, which included greater and more robust screening for offenders with intellectual disabilities at the earliest point in the criminal justice pathway, and adequate training of all criminal justice and healthcare professionals as fundamental to ensuring successful identification, management and resettlement of offenders from this group (Kvarfordt et al, 2005; Talbot and Jacobson, 2010; Talbot, 2012).

It is notable that Bradley (DH, 2009) recognised the many similarities between people with mental health issues and intellectual disabilities, but importantly acknowledged that there are also significant and definitive differences between the two groups such that each group should be considered separately. This underlying principle has improved professional understanding about intellectual disabilities and has driven the development of services and pathways specific for this population.

The National Delivery Plan in 2009 (HM Government, 2009) committed to 'promote and stimulate the development of liaison and diversion services' (paragraphs 3.7–3.12), and importantly, responded to Bradley's recommendations (14 and 28) stating that all police custody suites and all courts "should have access to liaison and diversion services". Since this time considerable progress has been made in the development and implementation of such services. The necessary commissioning has been made available and the need to provide an evaluation of the benefits in terms of cost and reoffending outcomes has been key. Notwithstanding, currently not all areas across the UK have access to Liaison and Diversion services, with approximately 60% reported coverage in 2016. However, the NHS five year forward strategy (NHS England, 2016) planned to have 100% national coverage by 2021.

Whilst the full benefit of Liaison and Diversion services in the UK has yet to be widely reported, there is general consensus of its efficacy (Disley et al, 2016; McKenna et al, 2019) describing an effective delivery model where appropriate identification of intellectual disabilities and mental health problems has taken place. However, this does not mean that there is always agreement between professionals as to the required course of action for an individual i.e. about the appropriateness of taking formal action against some suspects with intellectual disabilities or contrarily diverting them to more appropriate support services. This reflects two conflicting perspectives - on the one hand, the provision of treatment and support for suspects with intellectual disabilities, rather than prosecution may help individuals overcome the problems that led them to (allegedly) offend. On the other hand, failure to arrest and prosecute carries its own risks. For example, the individual who has committed a crime but is not prosecuted may not appreciate the gravity of their actions and may reoffend, and possibly commit more serious offences as a result (McBrien and Murphy, 2006). Another risk is that a suspect may be subjected to compulsory treatment without ever being afforded the opportunity to prove their innocence. In practice, however, diversion from custody may be influenced by the availability of provision for example, paucity of specialist provision towards which a person with intellectual disabilities may be diverted for treatment and/or support, in particular preventative services and low-level support. As an example, in the UK, the recent policy Transforming Care, (NHS England, 2017) has emphasised how people with intellectual disabilities and/or autism often "fall through the gaps" (p. 25) of existing provision, and can often be excluded from intellectual disabilities services because they are either too able, not able enough, too high risk, or have autism but not an intellectual disability. Furthermore, local services are not always willing or able to work with people with offending or challenging behaviour, in many areas there is no intellectual disability forensic service or forensic expertise.

The Criminal Courts

Across many countries there is general recognition that defendants must be able to understand and participate effectively in criminal proceedings. Two aspects that govern how defendants with intellectual disabilities are treated are: the right to a fair trial and fitness to plead. Another relevant component of the legal framework in the UK is that, for a defendant to be convicted, they must not only have committed the criminal act (actus reus) but must also have had a degree of criminal intent or guilty mind (mens rea).

The right to a fair trial

Article 6 of the ECHR sets out the right to a fair trial. It states that everyone charged with a criminal offence should be presumed innocent until proved guilty by law, and establishes five minimum rights for the defendant:

1   to be informed properly, in a language which they understand and in detail, of the nature and cause of the accusation
2   to have adequate time and facilities for the preparation of their defence
3   to defend themselves in person or through legal assistance of their own choosing or, if they do not have sufficient means to pay for legal assistance, to be given it free when the interests of justice so require
4   to examine or to have examined witnesses against them and to obtain the attendance and examination of witnesses on their behalf under the same conditions as witnesses against them
5   to have the free assistance of an interpreter if they cannot understand or speak the language used in court.

These 'minimum rights' are arguably violated where a defendant's intellectual disability significantly inhibits their understanding and involvement in the trial and where the necessary support is not provided. Support for people with intellectual disabilities in court should include, for example, arranging for people to visit the courtroom prior to the trial to become familiar with it, ensuring that clear, simple language is used so the defendant can understand, and allowing the defendant to sit with supporting adults where they can easily communicate with their legal representatives (McConnell and Talbot, 2013).

Fitness to plead

It is a long-standing principle in criminal law in England and Wales that any individual who stands trial must be capable of contributing to the whole process of their trial, starting with entering a plea. The HRA 1998 Article 6 enshrinement of the right to a fair trial reinforces this principle. Where there are concerns about a defendant's mental state or capacity, particularly in serious indictable offences, a 'fitness to plead' hearing can be held in the Crown Court (the court which deals with serious criminal cases, as opposed to the magistrates' court which deals with minor criminal offences). The main criteria used in determining fitness to plead are:

- capacity to enter a plea
- ability to follow the proceedings
- knowing that a juror can be challenged
- ability to question the evidence
- ability to instruct counsel.

The decision is made by the judge, without a jury, on the basis of evidence submitted by two or more appropriately qualified medical practitioners.

If a defendant is found to be fit to plead, the case will continue and support may be made available. If a defendant is found to be unfit to plead, a 'trial of the facts' may be held, at which the jury decides whether or not the defendant committed the act or omission of which they have been accused and three disposals are available to the Court if the jury determines that the accused had committed the act or made the omission:

- a hospital order under the Mental Health Act
- a supervision order which places the individual under the supervision of a social worker or probation officer and may include a treatment requirement
- an absolute discharge.

Concerns have been raised about the broad and somewhat subjective criteria for fitness to plead. The Law Commission has recently launched a review of the current test for determining fitness to plead, noting that the legal principles date back to 1836 when 'the science of psychiatry was in its infancy; and that the application of these antiquated rules is becoming increasingly difficult and artificial' (Law Commission, 2016).

READER ACTIVITY 18.3

With respect to your own country's legal system, determine whether there is a similar process of 'fitness to plead' and against what criteria is it assessed.

Reflect upon the general challenges faced by people with intellectual disabilities that may affect their 'fitness to plead'.

Support in the courtroom

Protection and support for vulnerable witnesses in court has been significantly improved over the past ten years. UK legislation, most notably, Part II of the Youth Justice and Criminal Evidence Act 1999 provides for a range of 'special measures' to assist vulnerable and intimidated witnesses – that is, witnesses who are under 17 or have a mental disorder and/or intellectual disability or have a physical disability or disorder. However, Section 16 of this Act made it explicit that these measures were not designed to cover vulnerable defendants. The fact that vulnerable defendants do not have the same statutory entitlement as vulnerable witnesses to the full range of special measures has been a cause of concern. Hoyano (2001), for example, has argued that this asymmetry of provision could contravene the HRA 1998 Article 6 right to a fair trial especially considering that the vulnerability of a defendant with an intellectual disability can be heightened during court proceedings.

In response to these concerns, steps have been taken towards the extension of special measures to defendants. Section 47 of the Police and Justice Act 2006 amends the special measures provisions to allow a 'vulnerable accused' aged 18 or over to give evidence to the Court by a live television link where certain conditions are met. Under the provisions of the Coroners and Justice Act 2009 the statutory right to support from an Intermediary in court has been extended to vulnerable adult defendants whose ability to give evidence is limited. According to McConnell and Talbot (2013) the role of an intermediary 'is to facilitate two-way communication between the vulnerable individual and other participants in the legal process, and to ensure that their communication is as complete, accurate and coherent as possible' (McConnell and Talbot, 2013, p. 31). However, in the Criminal Justice Joint Inspection (2014) it was reported that in the courts that were reviewed, there was a lack of easy read literature in waiting areas, and that accredited and registered intermediaries were not always available to support defendants with intellectual disabilities.

Sentencing and disposal

In the UK, a vulnerable adult defendant who is convicted of an offence and is not diverted from the CJS at this stage through a Mental Health Act disposal, faces the same range of possible disposals as any other adult offender. These include custody and the community order; the community order can be passed for an offence that is not so serious as to make custody unavoidable, but which merits a more severe disposal than, for example, a fine or discharge.

The sentencing decision is often informed by a pre-sentence report (PSR) prepared by a Probation Officer. The PSR contains information about the offence and the background and circumstances of the offender and includes recommendations for sentence. However, such information is predicated on the Probation Officer being informed or recognising that an individual might have an intellectual disability, and the availability locally of appropriate sentencing options.

Prison

According to Norman (2019) many people with intellectual disabilities may find it difficult to cope in prison and struggle to access services in place to meet support, offence related and healthcare needs. This is echoed in the Criminal Justice Joint Inspection (2015) report where it is reported that in the prisons inspected, prisoners with intellectual disabilities 'are at risk of having a much more difficult time in prison than those who do not,' (p. 4). Inspectors in this report also note their alarm at the extremely poor systems they found in prison for identifying such prisoners. They continue to report that there was no routine screening for intellectual disabilities in prison, only if it was suspected. This is of concern given that they also found prison staff inadequately trained to identify potential intellectual disabilities.

NHS England and Pathways Associates (2019) conducted focus groups with experts by experience who had received or were receiving services in the CJS. Issues specific to prison facing people with intellectual disabilities included a lack of staff with experience in supporting people with intellectual disabilities, a high incidence of physical restraint and being bullied by other prisoners.

How prison staff identify and support prisoners with intellectual disabilities was the subject of a report by the Prison Reform Trust (Talbot and Riley, 2007). A number of important findings emerged from the research, which clearly illustrate the difficulties this group, and those who work with them, face within the prison environment:

> "People with learning disabilities are not routinely identified prior to arriving into prison and once in prison face a number of difficulties. They are more likely to be victimised than other prisoners and are unable to access prison information routinely. They are likely to receive inadequate levels of support of varying quality and, because of their impairments, will be excluded from certain activities and opportunities. Their exclusion from offending behaviour programmes in particular makes it less likely that their offending behaviour will be addressed and more likely that they will return to prison again and again."
>
> *Talbot and Riley, 2007*, p. 45

Talbot (2008) reports that in a Prison Reform Trust study of 173 prisoners' experiences of criminal justice services, over half had trouble making themselves understood in prison whilst two thirds reported verbal comprehension difficulties and were more likely to act out aggressively in frustration. This is also noted by Marshall-Tate et al (2019) who refer to the frustration experienced by people with intellectual disabilities with regards to being unable to understand instructions and subsequently presenting as having challenging behaviour.

Talbot (2008) notes that 'Prisoners were five times as likely as the comparison group to have been subject to control and restraint technique and were three times as likely to have spent time in segregation' (Talbot, 2008, p. vi). Interviewees were asked about their experiences of life in prison and for many it was 'hard', 'stressful', 'scary', 'depressing' and 'lonely'. Some said they felt unsafe; others made of it what they could, taking each day as it came; some were ambivalent. A small number had more positive things to say and some said they preferred being 'inside' than 'out':

> "Sometimes I feel I am better in here than when I'm out. I rely on my family a lot on the outside, so my family aren't under stress when I'm inside."
>
> *Talbot, 2008*, p. 28

In their joint inspection of the treatment of people with intellectual disabilities in prison (see Criminal Justice Joint Inspection, 2015), inspectors reported similar findings to Talbot (2008) although in some areas of prison life, there were examples of good practice including both formal and informal care plans developed in order to alert staff to some of the specific needs of prisoners with intellectual disabilities.

 READER ACTIVITY 18.4

Out of the Shadows: The Untold Story of people with learning disabilities in prison is a 2018 project that used photography to document the personal experiences of people with intellectual disabilities in the UK prison system. Read more about the project here https://www.1854.photography/2018/11/out-of-the-shadows-prison/

Reflect on the importance of people with intellectual disabilities having different mediums through which they can convey their thoughts, feelings and emotions.

Reading and writing

Prisons are largely 'paper based' regimes – that is, information is disseminated in writing, for example displayed on notice boards or contained in booklets, and information for individual prisoners is often 'posted' under cell doors. To get things done, a form or 'application' is completed, for example, accessing health services such as the dentist, choosing meals, and arranging visits from family and friends. Most prisoners with intellectual disabilities who participated in the Talbot (2008) study said they had difficulties reading prison information and filling in prison forms:

> "I know 'a' was sandwiches, so I lived off sandwiches."
>
> *Talbot, 2008*, p. 35

When asked how, if he couldn't read, he knew about prison rules, one prisoner said:

> "That's easy. You know the rules when you break the rules."
>
> *Talbot, 2008*, p. 48

Prisoners with intellectual disabilities who were interviewed in the Criminal Justice Joint Inspection (2015) noted similar issues with navigating prison information and processes. It was noted that Easy Read resources were very limited in most of the five establishments that were inspected. When prisoners were asked about their ability to complete applications, visiting orders and complaints forms, many said they sought help from fellow prisoners:

> "My friend writes it out for me. I find it easy [making an application]. If he wasn't there, I'd ask another prisoner."
>
> *Talbot, 2008*, p. 38

Another stated:

> "I don't really know how to book a visit but opposite me there's a guy who said if I got the VO [visiting order], then he'll help me fill it in."
>
> *Talbot, 2008*, p. 38

Understanding and being understood

Adapting and responding to new situations can cause particular challenges for people with intellectual disabilities. Prisoners with intellectual disabilities who were part of the Criminal Justice Joint Inspection (2015) stated that:

> "the new routine threw me off. It started messing me about. They said the regime was changing but with not much notice. Would have been good to have someone sit with me. I asked questions but they didn't know what was going on."
>
> *Criminal Justice Joint Inspection, 2015*, p. 43

Another said:

> "they have to understand with me that I hate change. I can't stand it."
>
> *Criminal Justice Joint Inspection, 2015*, p. 43

Difficulties such as failure to follow instructions and routines in prison is often viewed as non-compliant or manipulative behaviour and punished accordingly. Prison behaviour deemed disruptive, such as misusing in-cell emergency bells, kicking cell doors and shouting have been linked to prisoners with intellectual disabilities (Loucks, 2007; Bryan et al, 2004). Over two-thirds of interviewees who participated in Talbot's 2008 study experienced difficulties in verbal comprehension skills, including difficulties understanding certain words and in expressing themselves, and over two-thirds said they had difficulties making themselves understood in prison:

> "I muddle up words and that causes problems."
>
> *Talbot, 2008*, p. 38

The Criminal Justice Joint Inspection (2015) explored behaviour management through analysis of the Incentives and Earned Privileges Scheme (IEP) which awards or removes privileges in relation to prisoner behaviour, their commitment to rehabilitation and helping others. Prisoners are placed on one of three tiers: basic, standard or enhanced. Most of the prisons visited as part of the inspection had an IEP policy that specifically referred to the need to support those with an intellectual disability to engage effectively with the scheme in so much as their intellectual disability should not affect their IEP level. Indeed, in one prison that was inspected, it was noted that staff were reluctant to use the basic level for prisoners with intellectual disabilities, showing they were mindful of the potential impact of intellectual disability on behaviour.

Inspectors reported good practice in one of the prisons where punitive measures for poor behaviour were notably different on the unit for more vulnerable prisoners. These included informal, short term sanctions such as the loss of television or exclusion from specific activities for a couple of hours. This enabled staff some flexibility to tie sanctions more flexibly and take into consideration other factors that may influence behaviour. However, given that the IEP scheme not only rewards good behaviour but also prisoners' willingness to help others means that some prisoners interviewed for the inspection were unable to progress in the scheme due to the impact of their intellectual disability.

> "I don't do enough to be enhanced. I just pick up the rubbish on the yard but you have to do more [to be enhanced]. I can't attend the groups [you need to attend to be enhanced, like offending behaviour programmes] or anything as I can't be around lots of people."
>
> p. 41

Being scared and being bullied

Prisons can be intimidating places for the most confident and capable of prisoners and being scared and bullied is not something that happens just to prisoners with intellectual disabilities, with around two-fifths of interviewees in Talbot (2008) saying they had been bullied or that someone had been nasty to them, and slightly less than half said they had been scared:

> "I am a bit scared in the shower; someone got raped by eight lads and then two days later he killed himself and that scared me."
>
> Talbot, 2008, p. 44

According to Talbot (2008), prisoners with intellectual disabilities were more likely to spend time alone in their cell than other prisoners and have fewer things to do. High numbers had clinically significant depression or anxiety. In this study, it was found that they were also the least likely to have a job in prison; to know when their parole or release date was; to be in touch with family and friends; to know what to do if they felt unwell; to know how to make a complaint or to have participated in cognitive behaviour treatment programmes, for example, to address their offending behaviour (Talbot, 2008).

In their report, the Criminal Justice Joint Inspection team stated that 'almost half of all the prisoners we interviewed said they had felt unsafe at the establishment' (Criminal Justice Joint Inspection, 2015, p. 40). One prisoner said:

> "I don't like loud noises or people around me. I can't really explain it. Sometimes I get jumpy, memories come back from other places [I have been to] … the units here are really big and it's really loud on [this wing] because it's a detox wing."
>
> Criminal Justice Joint Inspection, 2015, p. 40

Another stated:

> "some people are bullying but they don't realise they are doing it. It frightens me. I don't really tell officers and you can't really get your point across which is embarrassing. You'll get them into trouble or yourself in trouble, then you'll be called an informant and it puts your life in danger."
>
> Criminal Justice Joint Inspection, 2015, p. 41

There are a wide range of challenges faced by prisoners with intellectual disabilities in both managing their day to day life in prison and subsequently, their ability to progress through their sentence. At the heart of these challenges appears to be difficulties for prisoners with intellectual disabilities to engage with prison processes effectively because of issues with literacy and comprehension and being more vulnerable than other prisoners. The Criminal Justice Joint Inspection (2015) provides a host of recommendations to those responsible for running prison establishments and highlights the need for people with intellectual disabilities to have a support plan in place which clearly identifies how their needs will be met. In addition, they stress the importance of this group having good access to all prison processes, which includes providing written information and forms widely available in an Easy Read format.

Addressing offending behaviour and release from prison

The Criminal Justice Joint Inspection (2015) looked at service provision for people with intellectual disabilities both in prison and in the community after their release. They noted that some positive work was being done in those prisons involved in the inspection, 'to introduce general offending behaviour programmes for offenders with an IQ under 80' (p. 10) but that it does not address the needs of people living with other issues, including those with an autism spectrum disorder or those with Attention Deficit Hyperactivity Disorder. It is reported that people with intellectual disabilities may have difficulty working in groups and as such, require workbooks that can be delivered one to one. Chiu et al (2019) acknowledge that conventional offender rehabilitation programmes may not be appropriate for prisoners with additional needs associated with their intellectual disabilities, which therefore can impact on successful re-entry into the community.

Literature that examines what happens to people with intellectual disabilities after imprisonment is minimal. Two small scale studies from Australia (see Ellem, 2012; Ellem et al, 2012) are cited by Chiu et al (2019) who explore the post- prison life of this group. Some of the key themes reported include the absence of support, limited preparation for life after release and difficulties in finding appropriate accommodation, employment and reconnecting with family and friends, the challenge of staying out of trouble. Ellem (2012) notes that the difficulties identified for people with intellectual disabilities are also seen in their non-disabled peers, however, whilst all groups face the stigma of a criminal conviction, those with intellectual disabilities also face the discriminatory attitudes related to their disability suggesting that they may find life harder on release than other ex-offenders. Some of these difficulties are outlined in Paul's story Reader activity 18.5 in the accompanying online resource.

CONCLUSION

Despite the various legal and policy safeguards described in this chapter, the reality for many people with intellectual disabilities is that the CJS frequently does not recognise or meet their particular needs. This, in a large part, reflects a lack of routine screening for an intellectual disability at an early stage in the criminal justice process. Consequently, suspects with intellectual disabilities receive inadequate support at the police station and may incriminate themselves during police questioning. In court their lack of understanding grows as they struggle to make sense of court proceedings and legal terminology. Once in prison their situation often deteriorates. Their limited numeracy and poor verbal communication skills relegates them to a world of not quite knowing what is going on around them or what is expected of them. They spend more time alone than their peers and have less contact with family and friends. They are more likely to experience high levels of depression and anxiety. They are more vulnerable to ridicule and exploitation. Many will be excluded from programmes to address their offending behaviour, which may mean longer in prison as a result (Talbot, 2008; Chiu et al, 2019).

Since the inception of alternative approaches to custody as illustrated through the UK liaison and diversion services schemes, significant progress has been made to improve the situation of people with intellectual disabilities who offend, although more international research needs to be undertaken to compare and contrast this situation with that of other countries. To maintain the momentum of positive change, services need to work together and the needs of people with intellectual disabilities who offend should be at the forefront of any discussions; all services should ensure future commitment to improving the outcomes of this vulnerable group.

REFERENCES

Beqiraj, J., Lawrence, M., & Wicks, V. (2017). *Access to justice for persons with disabilities: From international principles to practice.* International Bar Association.

Bryan, K., Freer, J., & Furlong, C. (2004). *Speech and Language Therapy for Young People in Prison Project: third project report.* University of Surrey.

Chiu, P., Triantafyllopoulou, P., & Murphy, G. (2019). Life after release from prison: the experience of ex-offenders with intellectual disabilities. *Journal of Applied Research Intellectual Disability, 33,* 686–701.

Clare, I. C. H. (2003). *Psychological vulnerabilities of adults with mild learning disabilities: implications for suspects during police detention and interviewing*. Unpublished PhD thesis, King's College.

Coroners and Justice Act. (2009). Available at: http://www.legislation.gov.uk/ukpga/2009/25/contents.

Criminal Justice Joint Inspection. (2014). *A joint inspection of the treatment of offenders with learning disabilities within the criminal justice system – phase 1 from arrest to sentence*. London: Criminal Justice Joint Inspection.

Criminal Justice Joint Inspection. (2015). *A joint inspection of the treatment of offenders with learning disabilities within the criminal justice system – phase 2 in custody and the community*. London: Criminal Justice Joint Inspection.

Department of Health. (2009). *The Bradley Report: Lord Bradley's review of people with mental health problems or learning disabilities in the criminal justice system*. London: Department of Health.

Department of Health/Home Office. (1992). *Review of health and social services for mentally disordered offenders and those requiring similar services ('The Reed Review')*. London: HMSO.

Disability Discrimination Act. (2005). Available at: http://www.legislation.gov.uk/ukpga/2005/13/contents.

Disley, E., Taylor, C., Kruithof, K., et al. (2016). *Evaluation of the offender liaison and diversion trial schemes*. London: RAND.

Ellem, K. (2012). Experiences of leaving prison for people with intellectual disability. *Journal of Learning Disabilities and Offending Behaviour*, 3(3), 127–138.

Ellem, K., Wilson, J., & Chiu, W. H. (2012). Effective responses to offenders with intellectual disabilities: Generalist and specialist services working together. *Australia Social Work*, 65(3), 398–412.

Equality Act. (2010). Available at: http://www.legislation.gov.uk/ukpga/2010/15/contents.

European Convention on Human Rights (ECHR). (1953). Available at: https://www.echr.coe.int/Documents/Convention_ENG.pdf. [Accessed 18 January 2021].

Gudjonsson, G. H., & Joyce, T. (2011). Interviewing adults with intellectual disabilities. *Advances in Mental Health and Intellectual Disabilities*, 5(2), 16–21.

Gudjonsson, G. H. (2003). *The psychology of interrogations and confessions: a handbook. Wiley series in psychology of crime, policing and law*. Chichester: John Wiley & Sons.

Hellenbach, M. (2017). Supervision of offenders with intellectual disabilities by the probation services: challenges and problems. *Journal of Forensic Psychology*, 2(1), 1–7.

Hellenbach, M., Karatzias, T., & Brown, M. (2017). Intellectual disabilities among prisoners: prevalence and mental and physical health comorbidities. *Journal of Applied Research in Intellectual Disabilities*, 30(2), 230–241.

HM Chief Inspector of Prisons for England and Wales. *Annual report 2016–2017*. London: HM Inspectorate of Prisons

HM Government. (2009). *Improving health, supporting justice: the national delivery plan of the Health and Criminal Justice Programme Board*. London: Department of Health.

Home Office. (2006). *Police and Criminal Evidence Act 1984, (s66(1)), Code C: Code of Practice for the Detention, Treatment and Questioning of Persons by Police Officers*. London: The Stationery Office.

Hoyano, L. (2001). Striking a balance between the rights of defendants and vulnerable witnesses: will special measures directions contravene guarantees of a fair trial? *Criminal Law Review*, 948–969.

Human Rights Act. (1998). Available at: http://www.legislation.gov.uk/ukpga/1998/42/contents.

Hyun, E., Hahn, L., & McConnell, D. (2013). Experiences of people with learning disabilities in the criminal justice system. *British Journal of Learning Disabilities*, 42(4), 308–314.

James, D., Farnham, F., Moorey, H., et al. (2002). *Outcomes of Psychiatric Admissions through the Courts*. RDS Occasional Paper No. 79. London: The Home Office.

Kvarfordt, C. L., Purcell, P., & Shannon, P. (2005). Youth with learning disabilities in the juvenile justice system: a training needs assessment of detention and court services personnel. *Child and Youth Forum* (34), 27–42.

Law Commission. (2016). Unfitness to plead Vol 1: report. Available at: https://s3-eu-west-2.amazonaws.com/lawcom-prod-storage-11jsxou24uy7q/uploads/2016/01/lc364_unfitness_vol-1.pdf. [Accessed 16 January 2021].

Lindsay, W. R. (2011). People with intellectual disability who offend or are involved with the criminal justice system. *Current Opinion in Psychiatry*, 24(5), 377–381.

Loucks, N. (2007). *No one knows: offenders with learning difficulties and learning disabilities – review of prevalence and associated needs*. London: Prison Reform Trust.

Marshall-Tate, K., Chaplin, E., Ali, S., et al. (2019). Learning disabilities: supporting people in the criminal justice system. *Nursing Times*, 115(7), 22–26.

McBrien, J., & Murphy, G. (2006). Police and carers' views on reporting alleged offences by people with intellectual disabilities. *Psychology, Crime & Law*, 12(2), 127–144.

McCarthy, J., Chaplin, E., Underwood, L., et al. (2016). Characteristics of prisoners with neurodevelopmental disorders and difficulties. *Journal of Intellectual Disability Research*, 60(3), 201–206.

McConnell, P., & Talbot, J. (2013). *Mental health and learning disabilities in the criminal courts, information for magistrates, district judges and court staff*. London: Rethink Mental Illness & Prison Reform Trust.

McKenna, D., Murphy, H., Rosenbrier, C., et al. (2019). Referrals to a mental health criminal justice liaison and diversion team in the North East of England. *The Journal of Forensic Psychiatry & Psychology*, 30(2), 301–321.

McKenzie, K., Michie, A., Murray, A., et al. (2012). Screening for offenders with an intellectual disability: the validity of the Learning Disability Screening Questionnaire. *Research in Developmental Disabilities*, *33*, 791–795.

Mediseni, F., & Brown, M. (2015). The needs of people with mild learning disabilities within the Scottish criminal justice system: a qualitative study of healthcare perspectives. *Journal of Intellectual Disabilities and Offending Behaviour*, 6(3/4), 175–186.

Mental Health Act. (1983). Available from: http://www.legislation.gov.uk/ukpga/1983/20/contents.

Mental Health Act. (2007). Available at: https://www.legislation.gov.uk/ukpga/2007/12/contents. [Accessed 18 January 2021].

Mottram, P. G. (2007). *HMP Liverpool, Styal and Hindley study report*. Liverpool: University of Liverpool.

Murphy, G., & Clare, I. C. H. (1995). Capacity to make decisions affecting the person: psychologist's contribution. In R. Bull & D. Carson (Eds.), *Psychology in legal contexts* (pp. 97–128). Chichester, UK: Wiley.

Murphy, G., & Mason, J. (2007). People with intellectual disabilities who are at risk of offending. In N. Bouras & G. Holt (Eds.), *Psychiatric and behavioural disorders in intellectual and developmental disabilities* (2nd ed.). Cambridge: Cambridge University Press.

NHS England. (2014). *Liaison and diversion operating model*. UK: NHS England.

NHS England. (2016). *Strategic direction for health care services in the justice system, 2016–2020*. UK: NHS England.

NHS England. (2017). *Transforming care*. Available at: https://www.england.nhs.uk/wp-content/uploads/2017/02/model-service-spec-2017.pdf.

NHS England, & Pathways Associates. (2019). *Beyond the high fence*. London: NHS England.

Norman, A. (2019). In O. Barr & B. Gates (Eds.), *Oxford handbook of learning and intellectual disability nursing*. Oxford: Oxford Medical Publications.

Office for National Statistics. (2019). Available at: https://www.ons.gov.uk/peoplepopulationandcommunity/populationandmigration/populationestimates/datasets/populationestimatesforukenglandandwalesscotlandandnorthernireland.

Parsons, S., & Sherwood, G. (2016). Vulnerability in custody: perceptions and practices of police officers and criminal justice professionals in meeting the communication needs of offenders with learning disabilities and learning difficulties. *Disability & Society*, *31*(4), 553–572.

Police and Criminal Evidence Act (PACE). (1984). Available at: https://www.legislation.gov.uk/ukpga/1984/60/contents. [Accessed 18 January 2021].

Police and Justice Act. (2006). Available at: https://www.legislation.gov.uk/ukpga/2006/48/contents. [Accessed 18 January 2021].

Prison Reform Trust. (2019). *Bromley briefings*. London: Prison Reform Trust.

Raina, P., & Lunsky, Y. (2010). A comparison study of adults with intellectual disability and psychiatric disorder with and without forensic involvement. *Research in Developmental Disabilities* (31), 218–223.

Royal College of Psychiatrists. (2014). *Forensic care pathways for adults with intellectual disability involved with the criminal justice system*. Faculty Report FR/ID/04). London: Royal College of Psychiatrists' Faculty of Intellectual Disability & Faculty of Forensic Psychiatry.

Søndenaa, E., Palmstierna, T., & Iversen, V. C. (2010). A step-wise approach to identifying intellectual disabilities in the criminal justice system. *European Journal of Psychology Applied to Legal Context*, 2(2), 183–198.

Talbot, J. (2008). *Prisoners voices: experiences of the criminal justice system by prisoners with learning disabilities and difficulties*. London: Prison Reform Trust.

Talbot, J. (2009). No one knows: offenders with learning disabilities and learning difficulties. *International Journal of Prisoner Health*, 5(3), 141–152.

Talbot, J. (2011). Working with offenders. In H. Atherton & D. Crickmore (Eds.), *Learning disabilities: toward inclusion* (6th ed., pp. 339–356). Edinburgh: Elsevier.

Talbot, J. (2012). *Fair access to justice? Support for vulnerable defendants in the criminal courts*. London: Prison Reform Trust.

Talbot, J., & Jacobson, J. (2010). Adult defendants with learning disabilities and the criminal courts. *Journal of Learning Disabilities and Offending Behaviour*, 1(2), 16–26.

Talbot, J., & Riley, C. (2007). No one knows: offenders with learning difficulties and learning disabilities. *British Journal of Learning Disabilities*, 35(3), 154–161.

United Nations Convention on the Rights of People with Disabilities. (2006). Available at: https://www.un.org/development/desa/disabilities/convention-on-the-rights-of-persons-with-disabilities.html.

Young, S., Goodwin, E., Sedgwick, O., et al. (2013). The effectiveness of police custody assessments in identifying suspects with intellectual disabilities and attention deficit hyperactivity disorder. *BioMed Central Medicine*, *11*, 248–259.

Youth Justice and Criminal Evidence Act. (1999). Available at: http://www.legislation.gov.uk/ukpga/1999/23/contents.

Living my best life

'I just want to get the best out of life.

I need people to support me to break down barriers where ever there are barriers stopping me living my best life. Being positive is the only way you'll succeed – if you think negatively, you don't really get anywhere.'

Josh

'I want to become an actor, learn more about cooking and sing in a choir. I'd also like to work with children. I'd need support to find the right training, and help from my family to contact people who might be able to give me some advice. I'd like to explore the world, and I'd need someone to travel with me. There are a lot of wonderful things to think about!'

Charlotte

'I want to make the world more understanding, and open people's eyes to see that difference isn't bad. It should be a more diverse world. I will always stand up for people. I need people to listen and show more compassion to others. I am more tolerant of people now – you need to think about being in someone else's shoes.

Olivia

19

Working with families

Lynne Marsh and Edward McCann

KEY ISSUES

- Family caregivers can be any age or gender, and often have multiple roles and responsibilities related to their caregiving role.
- Across the trajectory of the lives of individuals with intellectual disabilities, the delivery and provision of care is increasingly provided by mothers, fathers, siblings, relatives such as grandparents, aunts, uncles, adoptive and foster parents.

- Caregiving is a continual process that evolves and may change across the life course of the individual's and family's life.
- Caregiving for many becomes a way of life.
- The role of caregiver has evolved requiring professionals to be mindful, respectful and considerate of the many competing roles that mothers, fathers, siblings and grandparents may have in terms of caregiving.

CHAPTER OUTLINE

INTRODUCTION

Almost two thirds of children and adults with intellectual disabilities living in the United Kingdom (UK), Northern Ireland (NI) and the Republic of Ireland (ROI) are now cared for and supported at home. Across the trajectory of the life of a child with an intellectual disability, the delivery and provision of care is increasingly provided by informal caregivers including parents, siblings and relatives such as grandparents, aunts, uncles, adoptive parents and foster parents (Kelly et al, 2019; Leedham et al, 2020; Marsh et al, 2018). Globally, approximately 80% of informal care, also referred to as unpaid or family care, is provided by family caregivers who are likely caring for relatives with disabilities (Heller et al, 2018). The overwhelming majority of caregivers are women (Lafferty et al, 2016; Zigante, 2018) however, more fathers are now sharing caregiving roles and responsibilities for their children with disabilities (Davys et al, 2017; Marsh et al, 2020; Schippers et al, 2020; Seymour et al, 2020).

Historically, care for children and adults with intellectual disabilities in Western countries was largely provided in residential institutions, completely separate from families and local communities (Scott et al, 2008; May et al, 2019). Over the last 50 years, the drive for deinstitutionalisation has dominated social policy changes for people with intellectual disabilities. As a result, care provision in Norway and Sweden (Tøssebro, 2016), Ireland (McCarron et al, 2019), the UK (Department of Health (DOH), 2001), Australia (Wiesel and Bigby, 2015), the United States of America (USA) (Scott et al, 2008) and China (Yang and Tan, 2019) is mainly being provided by informal caregivers. Driven by an ethos of inclusion and normalisation, change in care provision underpinned in legislation and rights based approaches, fully recognises that every individual with an intellectual disability is entitled to have the opportunity to experience a full and equal life with, and not apart from, their family. According to the *United Nations Convention on the Rights of Persons with Disabilities (CRPD)*, these entitlements are founded on the principles that 'promote, protect and ensure the full and equal enjoyment of all human rights by all persons with disabilities' (The United Nations, 2006). However, it should also be acknowledged that some countries still operate different models of residential provision for adults with intellectual disabilities. For example, the majority of Swedish adults with intellectual disabilities still reside and are supported in group homes (Engwall, 2017).

Current estimates suggest that almost 1.5 million people in the United Kingdom have intellectual disabilities, of which 286,000 are children (Foundation for People with Learning Disabilities, 2021). This figure is likely to increase due to the numbers of children surviving with multiple and complex health needs, as well as earlier recognition and detection of children with intellectual and neuro developmental disabilities (Truesdale and Brown, 2017). In Northern Ireland, there are almost 26,500 people registered with intellectual disabilities (Department of Health, Social Services and Public Safety, 2009). Similar numbers have been reported in the Republic of Ireland, with 28,388 people registered with intellectual disabilities of which 10,032 are children under 19 years of age (Hourigan et al, 2018). Such figures illustrate the increasing demands being made on family caregivers.

Globally, another trend emerging is that there are now many adults with intellectual disabilities surviving to middle and older age, living at home in the care of their parents aged 70 years and over (Heller, 2019; Ng et al, 2017). Consequently, family caregivers are ageing in tandem with their adult children whilst remaining as primary caregivers (Baumbusch et al, 2017; Egan and Dalton, 2019; Walker and Hutchinson, 2019). This changing demographic profile needs to be further considered as there are many implications for care provision for both the older adult with an intellectual disability and their ageing caregivers in terms of health, social and future supports. Subsequently, family caregivers are taking more responsibility for the care of their child as they transition through childhood, adulthood and older adulthood, resulting in a growing recognition that caregivers globally are the backbone of care provision, and should be acknowledged, supported and empowered in these competing and often demanding roles (Kelly et al, 2019; Reid and Moritz, 2019; Yang et al, 2016).

Given the increasing and diverse demands being made on family caregivers, there is an urgent need for different types of professionals, including health, educational and social care practitioners, to be fully involved in service provision for children and adults with intellectual disabilities and their family caregivers in order to provide the opportunity and necessary supports for individuals to live full and equal lives.

WHAT IS A FAMILY CAREGIVER?

The composition and presentation of the 'traditional' family has changed and evolved significantly with the recognition that the family unit may comprise single parents (male or female), co-parents and same-sex couples (Carroll, 2018; Goldscheider et al, 2015) all of whom are actively involved in child-caring and child rearing activities. However, in order to fully understand family caregiving and the implications of care provision, it is perhaps useful to define and clarify what caregiving is.

Whilst there are many definitions in existence, there appears to be a general lack of consensus about the definition of "caregiving" in relation to disability (Lee and Burke, 2018). Therefore, it is prudent to review the general literature regarding caregiving to help highlight key issues and enable the conceptualisation and further understanding of this core concept. One such definition from *The Carers (Scotland) Act* 2016, describes a caregiver 'as an individual who provides or intends to provide care for another individual (the "cared-for person")' (Scottish Government, 2016). Another definition drawn from *The Irish National Carers' Strategy 2012* identifies a caregiver as 'someone who is providing an ongoing significant level of care to a person who is in need of that care in the home due to illness or disability or frailty' (Department of Health, 2012). The common thread across both definitions is the provision of care, but perhaps the most accurate available definition that captures the whole gambit of family caregiving is derived from a briefing paper by Betts and Thompson (2016), on legislation, policy and practice of carers in the UK. They define 'caregivers' as

> *"persons who provide care (usually unpaid) to someone with a chronic illness, disability or other long-lasting health or care need, outside a professional or formal employment framework."*
>
> *Betts and Thompson, 2016*, p. 5

This explanation predicates how this type of care is unpaid and almost always informal. The primary reasons why people become caregivers includes having to support an individual who has a physical disability, an intellectual disability, changes in health status (exacerbation of chronic long-term health conditions), age related changes (dementia, anxiety, sensory difficulties, mobility problems) and those experiencing poorer mental health (Care Alliance Ireland, 2015).

The role of becoming a caregiver to a child with an intellectual disability begins from the moment the child is diagnosed with an intellectual disability, and for the majority of caregivers, this role continues across the life of the child and well into adulthood and older adulthood (Brennan et al, 2018; Egan and Dalton, 2019). This means that in many cases, the caregiving role continues for the duration of the caregivers' lifetime and may subsequently fall to siblings, other family relatives or to social care services. Interestingly, a common term now used to refer to informal family caregivers in the context of supporting family members with chronic health problems and disabilities is 'career carers' (Keating et al, 2019) or for those caring for people with complex health conditions, the term 'imposed clinical career' was coined by Carter and Bray (2017). These terms attempt to capture the role of caregivers succinctly as it does, for the majority, become a career. Consequently, caregivers are more likely to have to leave paid employment, giving up on career ambitions and aspirations with *work* taking on a new meaning (Ejiri and Matsuzawa, 2019). Importantly, caregivers can be any age or gender, have multiple almost informal roles and responsibilities and are often faced by uncertainty in these roles across the continuum of caregiving (Arnold and Heller, 2018; Hamedanchi et al, 2016; Lee and Burke, 2018; Pryce et al, 2017).

Over time, changes in economic, social and financial status have changed the demography of caring (Flynn, 2017; Schofield et al, 2019). Many mothers are now returning to paid employment resulting in fathers taking on, through necessity, shared care for their children with and without intellectual disabilities. Much of the available literature has focused on caring through the mothers' lens with less attention on fathers' experiences of caring (McKenzie and McConkey, 2016; Willingham-Storr, 2014). Within the last decade however this research interest has changed and there is a consistent growth of literature from the perspective of fathers (Dunn et al, 2020; Boyd et al, 2019; Marsh et al, 2020), parents with intellectual disabilities (Koolen et al, 2019), siblings (Leedham et al, 2020; Noonan et al, 2018) and grandparents (Miller et al, 2012). This growth is encouraging and indicative of how the role of caregiving has evolved and extended beyond the traditional role of mothers, demanding that professionals be mindful, respectful and considerate of the many competing roles that mothers, fathers, parents with intellectual disabilities, siblings and grandparents may have in terms of caregiving.

In summary, current practice in supporting people with intellectual disabilities demonstrates an increased reliance on informal caregivers who are already stretched and struggling as a consequence of poor government decisions to reduce short break and respite services, reduced financial support often compounded by difficulties accessing appropriate educational, health and social care services in their own local communities (Kelly et al, 2019; Lafferty et al, 2016; Malli et al, 2018; Teo et al, 2018). Unsurprisingly, these increased demands place significant strains on caregivers and consequently impacts on caregiving (Lunsky et al, 2017).

Reader Activity 19.1

We have many different roles within our family and society, such as mother, father, sister, brother, friend, etc. Many more of us will take on additional caregiving roles over the course of our lives.

Make a list of the challenges of taking on an informal caregiving role to a close family relative.

How do you think this role could or would change the relationship?

What do you see as one of the 'biggest successes' of this caregiver role and why?

The relevant issues and concerns will be discussed in the next section of this chapter.

THE IMPACT OF CAREGIVING

The impact of caregiving in the disability research has generally presented an overall picture of negativity through the lens of informal caregivers. Factors include care giver burden, deteriorations in caregivers' own physical and mental health, marital disharmony and financial pressures (Balci et al, 2019; Sit et al, 2020). Fortunately, the last decade in particular, has begun to question this negative narrative and witnessed a global growth of interest in the positive experiences associated with informal caregiving (Beighton and Wills, 2017; Hastings, 2016; Rajan and John, 2017). The inclusion of the positive impact of caregiving is extremely welcome, providing a more balanced view of caregivers' experiences as reported in a systematic review of parents' descriptions of the positive aspects of parenting their child with intellectual disabilities by Beighton and Wills in 2019. Some parents in this review reported a growth in personal strength (increased sense of purpose) and personal development (becoming a better person); enjoying a new outlook on life (seeing life from a different perspective); seeing the child as a source of happiness (joy, happiness and pleasure) and being less judgmental (Beighton and Wills, 2019). This was a consistent finding across international studies with parents from India and Mumbai (Bunga et al, 2020; Mohan and Kulkarni, 2018), siblings from Israel (Zaidman-Zait et al, 2020) and grandparents from the USA (Yang et al, 2018). Building positive working relationships between caregivers and professionals were also noted as a positive aspect of caregiving (Mastebroek et al, 2016). Therefore, caregiving is multifaceted and can be influenced by many factors. It is clearly not one dimensional, rather a complex matter that affects the child and the family across the many life transitions (Brown et al, 2020; Caples et al, 2018; Engwall, 2017; Lee and Burke, 2018; Sit et al, 2020).

Parents

As previously discussed, for many, the role of caregiver commences with the confirmation of a child's intellectual disability (Legg and Tickle, 2019; Marsh et al, 2018) and it is evident across studies, that parents identify themselves and accept early on, that their role is as a caregiver for their child with an intellectual disability (Schippers et al, 2020). Over the years however, much of the research has focused on the impact on families of the younger child (see Chapter 19). This trend appears to be changing and there is a great focus and research interest into the experiences of older parents. This relates to their sons or daughters living longer, and as they age themselves they may have to consider other future caring options available outside of the family unit (Hamedanchi et al, 2016; Pryce et al, 2017; Walker and Hutchinson, 2019).

As a consequence of parental caregiving, recurring themes within the international literature involve challenges such as marital disharmony, caregiver stress and physical and mental health concerns (Dunn et al, 2020). The countries producing the research studies include South Africa (McKenzie and McConkey, 2016), Australia (Sim et al, 2018), UK (Grey et al, 2018; Totsika et al, 2017), Ireland (Dawson et al, 2016) and Norway (Tøssebro and Wendelborg, 2017). It also seems that the impact of poorer health and psychological distress of parents varies considerably and is often associated with distinct factors. These include the level and severity of the child's intellectual disability, the lack of availability of day services, the presence of psychiatric disorders and a lack of information in relation to funding and alternative care options (Dawson et al, 2016; Grey et al, 2018; Pryce et al, 2017; Teo et al, 2018; Totsika et al, 2017). Other concerns identified, that have influenced parental caregiving roles, include the amount of time required for caregiving activities (anything between 8 hours and 100 hours per week) (Lafferty et al, 2016; McKenzie and McConkey, 2016; Sit et al, 2020), the financial consequences of caring, the lack of time for self, partners and other children (Meppelder et al, 2014) and the need for daily life to be constructed around the needs of the child with intellectual disability (Dunn et al, 2020; Engwall, 2017). Parental fears for the future, especially in the event of their death, also feature prominently in parents' narratives of caregiving across studies (Brennan et al, 2018).

Similarly, older caregivers express fears for the future in terms of their own mortality, worries about who will provide care for their child upon their death and the lack of future planning (Brennan et al, 2018; Engwall, 2017; Pryce et al, 2017; Ryan et al, 2014). Older UK caregivers, aged from their mid-sixties to mid-eighties, of adult children with intellectual disabilities, have spoken about 'living one day at a time', and 'living with uncertainty' in these caregiving roles (Pryce et al, 2017).

Some of these older parents (five mothers; three fathers) also concluded that the lack of information, especially in relation to funding and alternative care options and the lack of support from professional services, further compounded their distress and experiences of caregiving (Pryce et al, 2017).

Many of these findings are supported by older adult caregivers in Australia (Walker and Hutchinson, 2019), Canada (Baumbusch et al, 2017), Ireland (Brennan et al, 2018; Egan and Dalton, 2019) and the UK (Dunn et al, 2020). However, it needs to be recognised that many parents, irrespective of their age, enjoy the positive aspects of being a parent of a child with intellectual disability as they appear to gain a sense of personal strength and development as well as attaining a more positive outlook on life through their adult child's intellectual disability (Adithyan et al, 2017; Beighton and Wills, 2019).

Parents with intellectual disabilities

While there are no formal recorded figures in the UK on the number of parents with intellectual disabilities (Tarleton and Turney, 2020), Man et al (2017) recorded that approximately 17,000 parents with intellectual disabilities live in Australia. Emerson and colleagues in 2005 reported that approximately 5,000 parents with intellectual disabilities were living in Scotland, a figure that is over 15 years old (Emerson et al, 2005). This lack of up-to-date and accurate demographic information is concerning given the growth in the numbers of parents with intellectual disabilities (Llewellyn and Hindmarsh, 2015; Tøssebro et al, 2017). Even within the growing population of parents with intellectual disabilities, and since the seminal work of Booth and Booth conducted in the 1990s, (Booth and Booth, 1994, 1996), there has been a distinct lack of research conducted among parents with intellectual disabilities, meaning the experiences of this population are still much less understood (Theodore et al, 2018). Clearly, while people with intellectual disabilities become parents and plan to be parents, the existing research is dominated by the experiences of mothers with intellectual disabilities. There remains a gap in the research literature pertaining to the experiences of fathers with intellectual disabilities (Theodore et al, 2018). As highlighted earlier, this is a similar trend identified in the disability research generally.

In one systematic review, exploring the views and experiences of intimate relationships amongst adults with intellectual disabilities, many adults with intellectual disabilities reported wanting to find a partner, settle down and get married. The findings highlighted that restrictions such as limited privacy and constant monitoring, imposed on them by parents and some healthcare professionals, limited opportunities to meet partners (English and Tickle, 2018). This finding was also mirrored by some of the 11 adults with intellectual disabilities from the UK who were either married or in long term committed relationships (Bates et al, 2017).

When adults with intellectual disabilities have families of their own, they can and do become successful parents when provided with the appropriate and necessary supports (Koolen et al, 2019; Stewart and McIntrye, 2017; Theodore et al, 2018). However, as parents with intellectual disabilities, they face a higher risk of permanent removal of their children by the authorities because of stigma and prejudicial beliefs. They may be viewed by some as unable or incapable of bringing up their children due to their intellectual disabilities (Aunos and Pacheco, 2020; Llewellyn and Hindmarsh, 2015; Meppelder et al, 2014). Another finding emerging from the literature is that a significant majority of parents with intellectual disabilities did not have their children living with them and frequently had to prove their parenting ability to professionals, before they could be permitted to keep their child (Theodore et al, 2018). Some parents find themselves in a position of being unable to access appropriate support from healthcare professionals for fear their parenting will be scrutinised and negatively evaluated resulting in their children being permanently removed from their care (Llewellyn and Hindmarsh, 2015; Meppelder et al, 2014; Schuengel et al., 2017).

Reader Activity 19.2

Time to examine your thoughts and perceptions of parents with intellectual disabilities as caregivers. List at least 3 of your initial thoughts and perceptions about adults with intellectual disabilities as parents.

Now read the following by Kirklees Safeguarding Children Board (2018) *Working with Parental Learning Disability Good Practice Guidance.*

Available at: https://proceduresonline.com/trix-cms1/media/5985/2018-11-02-pld-guidance.pdf

Make a list of at least 3 of your thoughts and perceptions that you would like to change to support parents with intellectual disabilities as caregivers more effectively.

Siblings

As the life expectancy of people with intellectual disabilities increases, the likelihood is that children with intellectual disabilities will outlive their parents. Consequently, many siblings will invariably take on substantive caregiving roles, when their parent can no longer do so (Coyle et al, 2014; Lafferty et al, 2016; Lee et al, 2019). The lack of appropriate residential and support services, or indeed confidence in those that are on offer, can also result in more siblings taking on these caregiving roles (Coyle et al, 2014; Lee and Burke, 2018).

A systematic review of 29 studies examining the caregiving roles of siblings of adults with intellectual disabilities found siblings experienced significant caregiving challenges such as physical, economic, and emotional demands; additional caring responsibilities as family members aged (including parents), and having to navigate disability services (Lee and Burke, 2018). Likewise, Coyle et al (2014) in their USA qualitative study with 15 adult sibling caregivers, all of whom were over 40, reported how, as sibling caregivers, they had to revise and adjust to their caregiving roles over time. This need to adjust related directly to their own ageing, the ageing of their sibling, the changing health and medical needs particularly of their sibling with intellectual disabilities, and additional caregiving responsibilities for their own children and their ageing parents (Coyle et al, 2014). Sibling caregivers referred to how caregiving was a 'balancing-act', and how age related changes such as dementia required them to seek alternative accommodation for their sibling, as they were no longer caring for a sibling with an intellectual disability, but faced with the additional challenges of caring for an ageing sibling with an intellectual disability (Coyle et al, 2014). Also, adequate transition and future planning was found to be largely absent thus adding to the tensions of caregiving evident across sibling narratives (Brennan et al, 2018; Leane, 2020).

The benefits of sibling caregiving have also been reported in some studies and include 'watching the growth of individuals with intellectual disabilities, having close sibling relationships, providing parents with respite, and enjoying their own personal growth' (Lee and Burke, 2018, p. 244). Similarly, positive and negative experiences have been reported in a qualitative study with 18 younger siblings aged 13–16, living with brothers and sisters who had profound intellectual disabilities in the Netherlands (Luijkx et al, 2016), a finding consistent in Leedham et al's (2020) thematic synthesis of 18 studies of siblings' lived experiences of autism of which love and empathy were evident across sibling stories, a welcome and positive aspect of sibling caregiving.

Grandparents

Grandparents often play a significant role in the lives of their grandchildren, especially when their grandchild has an intellectual disability (Yang et al, 2018). For some grandparents, taking on caring roles and responsibilities for their grandchild with intellectual disability was required due to a variety of factors including the death of the biological parent or an inability of the biological parent to care for their child (Crettenden et al, 2018).

For many grandparents there is a dichotomy between initial expectations of being a grandparent and their lived experiences related to their grandchild's intellectual disability (Yang et al, 2018). Yet, many grandparents change their view of what was expected of them in connection to their grandchild's intellectual disability (Prendeville and Kinsella, 2019). They begin to see that their primary caregiving role was one of support to the whole family, i.e. their adult child, their grandchild with an intellectual disability and their other grandchildren (Yang et al, 2018). This altered experience of transitioning from grandparent to being a 'grandparent carer', is evident in a qualitative study with 22 Australian grandparents. These grandparents described how their primary caregiving *"role was to be there to support their child and grandchild, to be positive and to help anyway they could"* (Woodbridge et al, 2011, p. 358). This view is further mirrored by other grandparents who move to live nearer their children and grandchildren and even change jobs and careers to provide the additional caregiving support required to their children and grandchildren (Yang et al, 2018). Many grandparents voice how they have to remain positive for the wider family; self-sacrifice and put the family needs first; work to maintain family relationships; and help to improve quality of life for all the family for as long as they are able (Miller et al, 2012).

These extended caregiving roles for many grandparents are seen as an important resource for the family unit, practically, emotionally, and financially (Miller et al, 2012; Yang et al, 2018). Similarly, to parents caring for their children with intellectual disabilities, grandparents caring for a grandchild with intellectual disability primarily worry about who would look after their grandchild when their own health failed or upon their own death (Crettenden et al, 2018). Yet there are also many positive aspects of caregiving raised across studies related to the love they have for their grandchild and the great joy and satisfaction they derive caring for their grandchildren with and without intellectual disabilities and the wider family.

In summary, the role of caregiving amongst parents, parents with intellectual disabilities, siblings and grandparents, demonstrates similar competing and ongoing challenges. Additionally, an appreciation of the child or adult with intellectual disability and more widely, an understanding of others with intellectual disabilities featured across many family caregivers' experiences. There is also compelling evidence of positive outcomes such as personal growth and development, an increased sense of personal strength, confidence and pride in the achievements of the child with intellectual disability as they increasingly take on these significant caregiving roles (Beighton and Wills, 2017; Sandy et al, 2013; Theodore et al, 2018).

📋 Reader Activity 19.3

Next, time to reflect on the role of informal caregivers and the impact that caregiving responsibilities may have on them. Please make some reflective notes on the key issues and concerns that you feel may impact on their roles.

Then, watch the following YouTube TedX clip on Caring for the Caregivers: https://www.youtube.com/watch?v=duhJHedj82g

When you have viewed the clip, go back to your reflective notes and consider how else you could influence positive change with caregivers as they continue on their caregiving trajectory.

This section of the chapter has considered some of the implications for family caregivers of people with intellectual disabilities. The next section builds upon this by highlighting how best to work effectively with families and build on developing the professional relationship.

WORKING EFFECTIVELY WITH FAMILIES

The provision of person-centred and family-centred care is a crucial role for all professionals supporting individuals with intellectual disabilities and their families, leading to increased satisfaction with support and care and increased well-being for individuals and families (Hakobyan et al, 2020; Ryan and Quinlan, 2018). More recently, co-production has begun to gain momentum in disability research and is considered a useful framework for developing a reciprocal partnership model when working with families (see Figure 19.1). While it has not replaced person-centred or family-centred care, co-production works on the premise that user involvement supports the individual with intellectual disability and their caregiver to be more empowered and in control of their lives rather than decisions being made for them (Murray, 2019). It achieves this through increased involvement in choices, decision making processes and prioritising the needs as perceived by the individual with intellectual disabilities and their caregiver.

The key principle underpinning this framework is that professionals are 'doing with' rather than 'doing for' recipients of services and the partnership is equal and reciprocal. The basis of co-production according to Keenan (2018) and Slay and Penny (2014) are as follows:

- Power is shared between professionals and service users and carers – an equal relationship
- Professionals and service users and carers work in partnership toward agreed goals that will benefit all concerned
- It is about more than participation – service users and carers have a significant role to play
- There is value placed on what service users and carers bring to the table
- Service users and carers are partners in the design, development, review and delivery of services
- All parties in the partnership gain something from their contribution.

By not involving individuals with intellectual disabilities and their family caregivers in their care, the development of a trusting relationship would be impeded, therefore it is imperative that co-production is an integral component of building professional relationships, service planning and delivery (Crettenden et al, 2018).

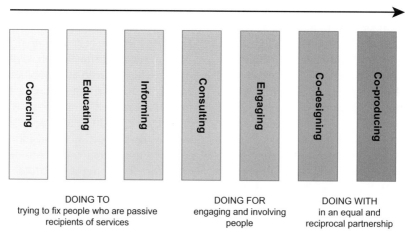

Figure 19.1 **The co-production framework** (Slay and Penny, 2014, in Keenan, 2018)

To conclude this section, and in preparation for the next, Reader activity 19.4 in the accompanying online resource challenges you to reflect upon your current practice.

DEVELOPING PROFESSIONAL RELATIONSHIPS

Professionals play a crucial role in supporting the well-being of people with intellectual disabilities and their family caregivers and while valued overall by caregivers and professionals, it is a relationship that has to be nurtured and developed throughout the caregiving experience (Theodore et al, 2018). Caregivers have reported the need for greater collaboration between themselves and professionals in creating a more flexible person-centred and family centred approach to effective, responsive and appropriate services (Burke et al, 2017; Ryan and Quinlan, 2018). In relation to the professional relationship specifically, a qualitative study with 24 parents (mothers: $n=18$; fathers: $n=6$) highlighted a lack of empathy, and at times dismissive interactions, from professionals thus impacting on their caregiving roles (Ryan and Quinlan, 2018). Other significant external factors reported in the literature affecting professional relationships relate to a lack of professional understanding, limited professional awareness and education of intellectual disability and less positive professional attitudes towards disability (Desroches et al, 2019; Pelleboer-Gunnink et al, 2017).

Additionally, haphazard access to services, administrative delays and bureaucracy, a lack of uniformity and consistency in service provision and poor information sharing have also been identified as recurrent challenges for caregivers in fostering a potential professional relationship (Burke and Heller, 2017; Cohen and Mosek, 2019; Douglas et al, 2017; Ryan and Quinlan, 2018; Whittle et al, 2019). Other issues noted as impeding the professional relationship have been where decisions have been made for caregivers rather than with caregivers (Cohen and Mosek, 2019; Ryan and Quinlan, 2018). Subsequently, caregivers being dismissed by professionals or excluded from health-related decisions have resulted in further power imbalances within the relationship (Brown et al, 2020; Ryan and Quinlan, 2018). These power imbalances feature prominently in a qualitative study, conducted in Israel, by Cohen and Mosek (2019) with 22 mothers of children with intellectual disabilities and 24 professionals (predominately social workers) in which power and the power relationships between these groups were explored. From the findings, four types of power emerged. Firstly, power over; secondly, oppressive power; thirdly, cooperative power and finally collusive power. Power over was when mothers expected emotional support from professionals seeking protection for them and their child. Oppressive power was where mothers expected professionals to value their knowledge and experiences of caring for their child. Cooperative power was the relationship that both groups preferred as there was a genuine and mutual respect of each other's roles. Lastly, collusive power was understood as a shared mutual interest in working in the best interests of the child against a system that both parties thought inadequate (Cohen and Mosek, 2019). The rationale for exploring power and power relationships between professionals and caregivers is that it is an important consideration for collaborative working; collaborative working is often a shared experience and involves prolonged interactions that transcend transitions from childhood to adulthood (Jansen et al, 2017).

Potential solutions proposed by some caregivers to the difficulties of establishing effective working relationships with professionals include developing child-centred rather than system-centred services, the identification of a named and available person to take a family-centred approach to service provision, and more uniformity and consistency in service provision to meet the changing needs of their children (Ryan and Quinlan, 2018). Other solutions proposed by professionals in their experience of supporting sibling caregivers are to nurture and develop positive professional relationships that include professionals encouraging and welcoming sibling involvement, educating siblings on the nature of their relative's disability and assistance with future planning (Burke et al, 2017). A USA survey by Burke et al (2017) of the perceptions of professionals (*n*=290) toward siblings of individuals with intellectual disabilities, highlighted how positive relationships between professionals and siblings were important and helpful as professionals were able to attain accurate and relevant information due to the siblings' in-depth and insightful experiences of their brother or sister.

Likewise, the development of positive professional relationships featured in many of the 15 narratives of Canadian parents (14 mothers) of children with intellectual disabilities (aged 3 to 15). Benefits of these relationships included informational needs being met; the same professional, such as a key worker, being available; the availability of practical tips on supporting and managing the child with intellectual disability from these professionals thus allowing parents to better understand the nature of the child's disability, to develop specific communication and behaviour strategies with their child resulting in a more positive family atmosphere (Sandy et al, 2013; Robert et al, 2015). Likewise, for parents with intellectual disabilities, having professionals who believed in and positively encouraged them as capable parents has been identified as one of the most valued qualities associated with a positive professional relationship (Theodore et al, 2018). Contrarily, however, some

caregivers have reported having needed to source their own specific and relevant information about their child's disability (Douglas et al, 2017; Ryan and Quinlan, 2018) and to navigate through and educate themselves about specific services required for their child which in turn impacted on the professional relationship. Furthermore, when relationships between the professionals and family caregivers break down, potentially as a consequence of unhelpful approaches identified at Box 19.1, experiences of anxiety and frustration for many caregivers supporting relatives with intellectual disabilities have been reported.

Undoubtedly, families want to be involved and expect to be involved in caregiving of their relatives with intellectual disabilities but require emotional, practical and professional support to do so. The end goal therefore is to build family and professional relationships based on reciprocity, mutual respect of each other's roles that seeks solutions in the best interests of the child, the family and the extended family (Ryan and Quinlan, 2018; Theodore et al, 2018). Caregiving is not a static process, but a continual and developing progression, and there is therefore a requirement for caregivers and professionals to build and foster that positive and trusting relationship as caregiving evolves and changes across the life course of the child's and family's life, across the course of the child's disability and across significant periods of transition.

 Box 19.1 Unhelpful approaches to supporting families

- Poor collaborative professional working
- Devaluing or being dismissive of caregivers' expertise and experience
- Not listening or hearing priorities that matter to individuals with intellectual disabilities or their caregivers
- Exclusion from decision making processes
- Service led rather than person-centred and family led services
- Poorly or under resourced services
- Lack of adequate signposting to services, support and entitlements
- Lack of knowledge and awareness of and about disabilities
- Lack of awareness and appreciation for cultural diversity
- Poor engagement and discussion of transition and future planning services and supports.

VALUING THE EXPERT

Family caregivers are usually the people well placed to care for and support their relative therefore should be recognised as experts in their caregiving roles (Leane, 2020). Consistently, in the literature, professionals recognise the importance that collaborative relationships, 'with' rather than 'for', caregivers can result in significant and positive outcomes for the relative with intellectual disability and the wider family (Bunga et al, 2020). A caregiver's unique relationship with their relative that has been developed, maintained and sustained over time, combined with the professional's expertise (knowledge, skills, experience) can result in the care continuum being optimised (Leane, 2020). The caregiver and professional relationship is pivotal across the lifetime of caring and a central part of this relationship are the principles of empowerment, respect, trust, partnership and collaborative working (Sandy et al, 2013).

UNDERSTANDING CHANGING NEEDS

Often caregivers attempt to navigate a diverse range of services such as legal, dental and respite services in order to ensure that their family member's needs are met across the trajectory of caregiving (Burke and Heller, 2017; Lafferty et al, 2016). When the child is initially diagnosed with a specific disability, there are often intense episodes of investigations, speech and language therapies or dietician appointments, as well as linking in with specialist early intervention services. Attendance at these appointments requires additional time and carries financial and travel implications which compete with the day to day management of employment, other caregiving responsibilities and the general running of a household (Brewer, 2018; Brown et al, 2019; Wark et al, 2015). These factors further add to the additional demands associated with caregiving which invariably extend into adulthood when families have to encounter numerous transitions across health, education and social care services (Brown et al, 2020). Often these transitions are perceived by family caregivers as challenging in the absence of effective and clear transition planning and future planning processes (Brown et al, 2019; Garnham et al, 2019).

A more seamless approach to the organising of appointments, accessing financial support and acknowledging the challenges of caregiving is required by all professionals working with families. Therefore, professionals and service providers will be required to work in a more collaborative and synchronous approach now and in the future. Individuals with intellectual disabilities and their caregivers have a wealth of experience and expertise but are content when support from professionals is based on trust, respect and collaboration (Lafferty et al, 2016).

 Reader Activity 19.5

Take some time to view the information on the following link: https://knowhow.ncvo.org.uk/organisation/collaboration/coproduction-and-service-user-involvement

From your reading and engagement with the resources on this website, consider at least 3 ways you would embed this approach in your professional practice when working with people with intellectual disabilities and their family caregivers.

CONCLUSION

Caregiving is a family matter and an evolving process. It is an approach that encourages caregivers to become flexible and adaptable and gain and build on knowledge and experience across their relative's life. Caregivers have entered in to a situation that can often be overwhelming at the beginning and take time to adjust to; many juggle and often struggle to maintain some semblance of what *'normal'* family life should look like. Their 'normality' can become a series of appointments, a life-time full of competing and demanding commitments, and a change in their expectations of their own life trajectory. Caregiving roles and responsibilities are intertwined with professionals and professional services and it is imperative that professionals and services acknowledge the significant impact that caregiving may have on families (Bunga et al, 2020). The breakdown in the professional relationship can be detrimental so the involvement of caregivers in decisions about their child – even when the child is an adult - can foster a more seamless professional dynamic. Whilst the role of caregivers has evolved, so too has the role of professionals who are required to be respectful, considerate and empathetic of the many competing caregiving roles and responsibilities within the family. Therefore, professional support needs to be flexible, sufficient, accessible and supportive so that family caregivers can continue to provide care to their loved ones and achieve with them a quality of life that is rewarding, enriching and fulfilling for their relative (Bunga et al, 2020; Leane, 2020).

REFERENCES

Adithyan, G. S., Sivakami, M., & Jacob, J. (2017). Positive and negative impacts on caregivers of children with intellectual disability in India. *Disability, CBR & Inclusive Development, 28*(2), 74–94.

Arnold, C. K., & Heller, T. (2018). Caregiving experiences and outcomes: wellness of adult siblings of people with intellectual disabilities. *Current Developmental Disorders Reports, 5*(3), 143–149.

Aunos, M., & Pacheco, L. (2020). Able or unable: how do professionals determine the parenting capacity of mothers with intellectual disabilities. *Journal of Public Child Welfare*, 1–27, https://doi.org/10.1080/15548732.2020.1729923.

Balcı, S., Kızıl, H., Savaşer, S., et al. (2019). Determining the burdens and difficulties faced by families with intellectually disabled children. *Journal of Psychiatric Nursing, 10*(2), 124–130.

Bates, C., Terry, L., & Popple, K. (2017). Supporting people with learning disabilities to make and maintain intimate relationships. *Tizard Learning Disability Review, 22*(1), 16–23.

Baumbusch, J., Mayer, S., Phinney, A., et al. (2017). Aging together: caring relations in families of adults with intellectual disabilities. *The Gerontologist, 57*(2), 341–347.

Beighton, C., & Wills, J. (2017). Are parents identifying positive aspects to parenting their child with an intellectual disability or are they just coping? A qualitative exploration. *Journal of Intellectual Disabilities, 21*(4), 325–345.

Beighton, C., & Wills, J. (2019). How parents describe the positive aspects of parenting their child who has intellectual disabilities: a systematic review and narrative synthesis. *Journal of Applied Research in Intellectual Disabilities, 32*(5), 1255–1279.

Betts, J., & Thompson, J. (2016). Carers. *Legislation, Policy and Practice, 24*(17), 1–41. Available at: http://www.niassembly.gov.uk/globalassets/documents/raise/publications/2017-2022/2017/health/2417.pdf. [Accessed 25 August 2020].

Booth, T., & Booth, W. (1994). The use of depth interviewing with vulnerable subjects: lessons from a research study of parents with learning difficulties. *Social Science & Medicine, 39*(3), 415–424.

Booth, T., & Booth, W. (1996). Supported parenting for people with learning difficulties: lessons from Wisconsin. *Representing Children, 9*(2), 99–107.

Boyd, M. J., Iacono, T., & McDonald, R. (2019). The perceptions of fathers about parenting a child with developmental disabilities: a scoping review. *Journal of Policy and Practice in Intellectual Disabilities, 16*(4), 312–324.

Brennan, D., Murphy, R., McCallion, P., et al. (2018). 'What's going to happen when we're gone?' family caregiving capacity for older people with an intellectual disability in Ireland. *Journal of Applied Research in Intellectual Disabilities, 31*(2), 226–235.

Brewer, A. (2018). "We were on our own": Mothers' experiences navigating the fragmented system of professional care for autism. *Social Science & Medicine, 215*, 61–68, https://doi.org/10.1016/j.socscimed.2018.08.039.

Brown, M., Higgins, A., & MacArthur, J. (2020). Transition from child to adult health services: a qualitative study of the views and experiences of families of young adults with intellectual disabilities. *Journal of Clinical Nursing, 29*(1-2), 195–207.

Brown, M., Macarthur, J., Higgins, A., et al. (2019). Transitions from child to adult health care for young people with intellectual disabilities: a systematic review. *Journal of Advanced Nursing, 75*(11), 2418–2434.

Bunga, D., Manchala, H. G., Ravindranath, N., et al. (2020). Children with intellectual disability, impact on caregivers: a cross-sectional study. *Indian Journal of Social Psychiatry, 36*(2), 151.

Burke, M.M., & Heller, T. (2017). "Disparities in unmet service needs among adults with intellectual and other developmental disabilities." *Journal of Applied Research in Intellectual Disabilities, 30*(5), 898–910.

Burke, M. M., Lee, C. E., Arnold, C. K., et al. (2017). The perceptions of professionals toward siblings of individuals with intellectual and developmental disabilities. *Intellectual and Developmental Disabilities, 55*(2), 72–83.

Caples, M., Martin, A. M., Dalton, C., et al. (2018). Adaptation and resilience in families of individuals with Down syndrome living in Ireland. *British Journal of Learning Disabilities, 46*(3), 146–154.

Carer Alliance Ireland. (2015) Family caring in Ireland. Available at: http://www. carealliance. ie/userfiles/file/Family% 20Caring% 20in% 20Ireland% 20Pdf. pdf. [Accessed 23 November 2020].

Carroll, M. (2018). Gay fathers on the margins: race, class, marital status, and pathway to parenthood. *Family Relations, 67*(1), 104–117.

Carter, B., & Bray, L. (2017). Parenting a child with complex health care needs: a stressful and imposed 'clinical career'. *Comprehensive Child and Adolescent Nursing, 40*(4), 219–222.

Cohen, A., & Mosek, A. (2019). 'Power together': professionals and parents of children with disabilities creating productive partnerships. *Child & Family Social Work*, *24*(4), 565–573.

Coyle, C. E., Kramer, J., & Mutchler, J. E. (2014). Aging together: sibling carers of adults with intellectual and developmental disabilities. *Journal of Policy and Practice in Intellectual Disabilities*, *11*(4), 302–312.

Crettenden, A., Lam, J., & Denson, L. (2018). Grandparent support of mothers caring for a child with a disability: impacts for maternal mental health. *Research in Developmental Disabilities*, *76*, 35–45.

Davys, D., Mitchell, D., & Martin, R. (2017). Fathers of adults who have a learning disability: roles, needs and concerns. *British Journal of Learning Disabilities*, *45*(4), 266–273.

Dawson, F., Shanahan, S., Fitzsimons, E., et al. (2016). The impact of caring for an adult with intellectual disability and psychiatric comorbidity on carer stress and psychological distress. *Journal of Intellectual Disability Research*, *60*(6), 553–563.

Department of Health (UK). (2001). *Valuing people: a new strategy for learning disability for the 21st century*. London: Department of Health. Available at: https://assets.publishing.service.gov.uk/government/uploads/system/uploads/attachment_data/file/250877/5086.pdf.

Department of Health, Social Services and Public Safety. (2009). *Delivering the Bamford vision: the response of the Northern Ireland Executive to the Bamford review of mental health and learning disability. Action plan 2009–2011*.

Department of Health (Ireland). (2012). *The Irish national carers' strategy recognized, supported, empowered*. Dublin: Department of Health. Department of Health. Available at: https://assets.gov.ie/10945/d62cf66f0a8f442bb594bbe-0b48ef6ad.pdf.

Desroches, M. L., Sethares, K. A., Curtin, C., et al. (2019). Nurses' attitudes and emotions toward caring for adults with intellectual disabilities: Results of a cross-sectional, correlational–predictive research study. *Journal of Applied Research in Intellectual Disabilities*, *32*(6), 1501–1513.

Douglas, T., Redley, B., & Ottmann, G. (2017). The need to know: the information needs of parents of infants with an intellectual disability a qualitative study. *Journal of Advanced Nursing*, *73*(11), 2600–2608.

Dunn, K., Jahoda, A., & Kinnear, D. (2020). The experience of being a father of a son or daughter with an intellectual disability: older fathers' perspectives. *Journal of Applied Research in Intellectual Disabilities*.

Egan, C., & Dalton, C. T. (2019). An exploration of care–burden experienced by older caregivers of adults with intellectual disabilities in Ireland. *British Journal of Learning Disabilities*, *47*(3), 188–194.

Ejiri, K., & Matsuzawa, A. (2019). Factors associated with employment of mothers caring for children with intellectual disabilities. *International Journal of Developmental Disabilities*, *65*(4), 239–247.

Emerson, E., Malam, S., Davies, I., et al. (2005). *Adults with learning disabilities in England 2003/2004*. Lancaster, PA: Centre for Disability Research.

English, B., & Tickle, A. (2018). Views and experiences of people with intellectual disabilities regarding intimate relationships: a qualitative metasynthesis. *Sexuality and Disability*, *36*(2), 149–173.

Engwall, K. (2017). 'I'm too old to think five years ahead'. Parent carers of adult children with intellectual disabilities in Sweden. *Alter*, *11*(3), 155–167.

Flynn, S. (2017). Perspectives on austerity: the impact of the economic recession on intellectually disabled children. *Disability & Society*, *32*(5), 678–700.

Foundation for People with Learning Disabilities. (2021) Available at: https://www.learningdisabilities.org.uk/learning-disabilities/help-information/learning-disability-statistics-/187687. [Accessed September 22 2021].

Garnham, B., Bryant, L., Ramcharan, P., et al. (2019). Policy, plans and pathways: the 'crisis' transition to postparental care for people ageing with intellectual disabilities in rural Australian carescapes. *Ageing and Society*, *39*(4), 836–850.

Goldscheider, F., Bernhardt, E., & Lappegård, T. (2015). The gender revolution: a framework for understanding changing family and demographic behavior. *Population and Development Review*, *41*(2), 207–239.

Grey, J. M., Totsika, V., & Hastings, R. P. (2018). Physical and psychological health of family carers co-residing with an adult relative with an intellectual disability. *Journal of Applied Research in Intellectual Disabilities*, *31*(Suppl. 2), 191–202.

Hakobyan, L., Nieboer, A.P., Finkenflügel, H. and Cramm, J.M. (2020). The Significance of Person-Centered Care for Satisfaction With Care and Well-Being Among Informal Caregivers of Persons With Severe Intellectual Disability. *Journal of Policy and Practice in Intellectual Disabilities*, *17*(12), 31–42. https://doi.org/10.1111/jppi.12297.

Hamedanchi, A., Khankeh, H. R., Fadayevatan, R., et al. (2016). Bitter experiences of elderly parents of children with intellectual disabilities: a phenomenological study. *Iranian Journal of Nursing and Midwifery Research*, *21*(3), 278–283.

Hastings, R. P. (2016). Do children with intellectual and developmental disabilities have a negative impact on other family members? The case for rejecting a negative narrative. *International Review of Research in Developmental Disabilities*, *50*, 165–194.

Heller, T. (2019). Bridging aging and intellectual/developmental disabilities in research, policy, and practice. *Journal of Policy and Practice in Intellectual Disabilities*, *16*(1), 53–57.

Heller, T., Scott, H. M., Janicki, M. P., et al. (2018). Caregiving, intellectual disability, and dementia: report of the Summit Workgroup on Caregiving and Intellectual and Developmental Disabilities. *Alzheimer's & Dementia: Translational Research & Clinical Interventions*, *4*, 272–282.

Hourigan, S., Fanagan, S., & Kelly, C. (2018). *Annual report of the National Intellectual Disability Database Committee 2017: main findings*. Dublin: Health Research Board. Available at: https://www.hrb.ie/fileadmin/2._Plugin_related_files/Publications/2018_pubs/Disability/NIDD/NIDD_Annual_Report_2017.pdf. [Accessed 20 July 2020].

Jansen, S. L., van der Putten, A. A., & Vlaskamp, C. (2017). Parents' experiences of collaborating with professionals in the support of their child with profound intellectual and multiple disabilities: a multiple case study. *Journal of Intellectual Disabilities*, *21*(1), 53–67.

Keating, N., Eales, J., Funk, L., Fast, J., & Min, J. 2019. 'Life course trajectories of family care', *International Journal of Care and Caring*, *3*(2), 147–163, https://doi.org/10.1332/239788219X15473079319309.

Keenan, P. (2018). *Scoping paper on research evidence and practice relating to co-production*. Available at: http://www.cypsp.hscni.net/wp-content/uploads/2018/06/Co-production-scoping-paper-2018.pdf.

Kelly, C., McConkey, R., & Craig, S. (2019). Family carers of people with intellectual disabilities in Ireland: changes over 10 years. *Journal of Intellectual Disabilities*, 1–9, https://doi.org/10.1177/1744629519866313.

Koolen, J., van Oorsouw, W., Verharen, et al. (2019). Support needs of parents with intellectual disabilities: systematic review on the perceptions of parents and professionals. *Journal of Intellectual Disabilities*, 1–25, https://doi.org/10.1177/1744629519829965.

Lafferty, A., O'Sullivan, D., O'Mahoney, P., et al. (2016). *Family carers' experiences of caring for a person with intellectual disability*. Dublin: University College. Available at: http://nda.ie/nda-files/Family-Carers%E2%80%99-Experiences-of-Caring-for-a-Person-with-Intellectual-Disability.pdf.

Lee, C. E., & Burke, M. M. (2018). Caregiving roles of siblings of adults with intellectual and developmental disabilities: a systematic review. *Journal of Policy and Practice in Intellectual Disabilities*, *15*(3), 237–246.

Lee, C. E., Burke, M., Arnold, C. K., et al. (2019). Correlates of current caregiving among siblings of adults with intellectual and developmental disabilities. *Journal of Applied Research in Intellectual Disabilities*, *32*(6), 1490–1500.

Leane, M. (2020). 'I don't care anymore if she wants to cry through the whole conversation, because it needs to be addressed': adult siblings' experiences of the dynamics of future care planning for brothers and sisters with a developmental disability. *Journal of Applied Research in Intellectual Disabilities*, *33*, 950–961.

Leedham, A. T., Thompson, A. R., & Freeth, M. (2020). A thematic synthesis of siblings' lived experiences of autism: distress, responsibilities, compassion and connection. *Research in Developmental Disabilities*, *97*, 103547.

Legg, H., & Tickle, A. (2019). UK parents' experiences of their child receiving a diagnosis of autism spectrum disorder: a systematic review of the qualitative evidence. *Autism*, *23*(8), 1897–1910.

Llewellyn, G., & Hindmarsh, G. (2015). Parents with intellectual disability in a population context. *Current Developmental Disorders Reports*, *2*(2), 119–126.

Luijkx, J., van der Putten, A. A., & Vlaskamp, C. (2016). 'I love my sister, but sometimes I don't': a qualitative study into the experiences of siblings of a child with profound intellectual and multiple disabilities. *Journal of Intellectual & Developmental Disability*, *41*(4), 279–288.

Lunsky, Y., Robinson, S., Blinkhorn, A., et al. (2017). Parents of adults with intellectual and developmental disabilities (IDD) and compound caregiving responsibilities. *Journal of child and family Studies*, *26*(5), 1374–1379.

Malli, M. A., Sams, L., Forrester-Jones, R., et al. (2018). 'Austerity and the lives of people with learning disabilities'. A thematic synthesis of current literature. *Disability & Society*, *33*(9), 1412–1435.

Man, N. W., Wade, C., & Llewellyn, G. (2017). Prevalence of parents with intellectual disability in Australia. *Journal of Intellectual & Developmental Disability*, *42*(2), 173–179.

Marsh, L., Warren, P. L., & Savage, E. (2018). 'Something was wrong': a narrative inquiry of becoming a father of a child with an intellectual disability in Ireland. *British Journal of Learning Disabilities*, *46*(4), 216–224.

Marsh, L., Brown, M., & McCann, E. (2020). The views and experiences of fathers of children with intellectual disabilities: a systematic review of the international evidence. *Journal of Policy and Practice in Intellectual Disabilities*, *17*(1), 79–90.

Mastebroek M, Naaldenberg J, van den Driessen Mareeuw FA, et al. (2016). Experiences of patients with intellectual disabilities and carers in GP health information exchanges: a qualitative study. *Family Practitioner*, *33*(5), 543–550. https://doi.org/10.1093/fampra/cmw057.

May, P., Vance, R. L., Murphy, E., et al. (2019). Effect of deinstitutionalisation for adults with intellectual disabilities on costs: a systematic review. *BMJ Open*, *9*(9) e025736.

McCarron, M., Lombard-Vance, R., Murphy, E., et al. (2019). Effect of deinstitutionalisation on quality of life for adults with intellectual disabilities: a systematic review. *BMJ Open*, 9(4) e025735.

McKenzie, J., & McConkey, R. (2016). Caring for adults with intellectual disability: the perspectives of family carers in South Africa. *Journal of Applied Research in Intellectual Disabilities*, 29(6), 531–541.

Meppelder, M., Hodes, M., Kef, S., et al. (2014). Parents with intellectual disabilities seeking professional parenting support: the role of working alliance, stress and informal support. *Child Abuse & Neglect*, 38(9), 1478–1486.

Miller, E., Buys, L., & Woodbridge, S. (2012). Impact of disability on families: grandparents' perspectives. *Journal of Intellectual Disability Research*, 56(1), 102–110.

Mohan, R., & Kulkarni, M. (2018). Resilience in parents of children with intellectual disabilities. *Psychology and Developing Societies*, 30(1), 19–43.

Murray, V. (2019). Co-producing knowledge: reflections on research on the residential geographies of learning disability. *Area*, 51(3), 423–432.

Noonan, H., O'Donoghue, I., & Wilson, C. (2018). Engaging with and navigating limbo: lived experiences of siblings of adults with autism spectrum disorders. *Journal of Applied Research in Intellectual Disabilities*, 31(6), 1144–1153.

Ng, N., Wallén, E. F., & Ahlström, G. (2017). Mortality patterns and risk among older men and women with intellectual disability: a Swedish national retrospective cohort study. *BMC Geriatrics*, 17(1), 269.

Pelleboer-Gunnink, H. A., Van Oorsouw, W. M. W. J., Van Weeghel, J., et al. (2017). Mainstream health professionals' stigmatising attitudes towards people with intellectual disabilities: a systematic review. *Journal of Intellectual Disability Research*, 61(5), 411–434.

Prendeville, P., & Kinsella, W. (2019). The role of grandparents in supporting families of children with autism spectrum disorders: a family systems approach. *Journal of Autism and Developmental Disorders*, 49(2), 738–749.

Pryce, L., Tweed, A., Hilton, A., et al. (2017). Tolerating uncertainty: perceptions of the future for ageing parent carers and their adult children with intellectual disabilities. *Journal of Applied Research in Intellectual Disabilities*, 30(1), 84–96.

Rajan, A. M., & John, R. (2017). Resilience and impact of children's intellectual disability on Indian parents. *Journal of Intellectual Disabilities*, 21(4), 315–324.

Reid, N., & Moritz, K. M. (2019). Caregiver and family quality of life for children with fetal alcohol spectrum disorder. *Research in Developmental Disabilities*, 94, 103478.

Robert, M., Leblanc, L., & Boyer, T. (2015). When satisfaction is not directly related to the support services received: understanding parents' varied experiences with specialised services for children with developmental disabilities. *British Journal of Learning Disabilities*, 43(3):168–177.

Ryan, C., & Quinlan, E. (2018). Whoever shouts the loudest: listening to parents of children with disabilities. *Journal of Applied Research in Intellectual Disabilities*, 31, 203–214.

Ryan, A., Taggart, L., Truesdale-Kennedy, M., et al. (2014). Issues in caregiving for older people with intellectual disabilities and their ageing family carers: a review and commentary. *International Journal of Older People Nursing*, 9(3), 217–226.

Sandy, P. T., Kgole, J. C., & Mavundla, T. R. (2013). Support needs of caregivers: case studies in South Africa. *International Nursing Review*, 60(3), 344–350.

Schippers, A., Berkelaar, M., Bakker, M., et al. (2020). The experiences of Dutch fathers on fathering children with disabilities: 'Hey, that is a father and his daughter, that is it'. *Journal of Intellectual Disability Research*, 64(6), 442–454.

Schofield, D., Zeppel, M. J., Tanton, R., et al. (2019). Intellectual disability and autism: socioeconomic impacts of informal caring, projected to 2030. *The British Journal of Psychiatry*, 215(5), 654–660.

Schuengel, C., Kef, S., Hodes, M. W., et al. (2017). Parents with intellectual disability. *Current Opinion in Psychology*, 15, 50–54.

Scotland Government. (2016). Carers (Scotland) Act. Edinburgh: Scottish Government. Available at: https://www.legislation.gov.uk/asp/2016/9/contents/enacted.

Scott, N., Lakin, K. C., & Larson, S. A. (2008). The 40th anniversary of deinstitutionalization in the United States: decreasing state institutional populations, 1967–2007. *Intellectual and Developmental Disabilities*, 46(5), 402–405.

Seymour, M., Giallo, R., & Wood, C. E. (2020). Perceptions of social support: comparisons between fathers of children with autism spectrum disorder and fathers of children without developmental disabilities. *Journal of Intellectual Disability Research*, 64(6), 414–425.

Sim, A., Vaz, S., Cordier, R., et al. (2018). Factors associated with stress in families of children with autism spectrum disorder. *Developmental Neurorehabilitation*, 21(3), 155–165.

Sit, H. F., Huang, L., Chang, K., et al. (2020). Caregiving burden among informal caregivers of people with disability. *British Journal of Health Psychology*. Available at: https://onlinelibrary.wiley.com/doi/epdf/10.1111/bjhp.12434.

Slay, J., & Penny, J. (2014). *Commissioning for outcomes and co-production: a practical guide for local authorities*. London: New Economics Foundation. Available at: http://b. 3cdn. net/nefoundation/974bfd0fd635a9ffcd_j2m6b04bs. pdf.

Stewart, A., & MacIntyre, G. (2017). *Parents with learning disabilities*. Glasgow: Institute for Research and Innovation in Social Services. Available at: https://www.iriss.org.uk/resources/insights/parents-learning-disabilities. [Accessed 23 November 2020].

Tarleton, B., & Turney, D. (2020). Understanding 'successful practice/s' with parents with learning difficulties when there are concerns about child neglect: the contribution of social practice theory. *Child Indicators Research*, 13(2), 387–409.

Teo, C., Kennedy-Behr, A., & Lowe, J. (2018). Contrasting perspectives of parents and service providers on respite care in Queensland, Australia. *Disability & Society*, 33(9), 1503–1527.

The United Nations. (2006). Convention on the Rights of Persons with Disabilities. Available at: https://www.un.org/development/desa/disabilities/convention-on-the-rights-of-persons-with-disabilities.html. [Accessed 23 November 2020].

Theodore, K., Foulds, D., Wilshaw, P., et al. (2018). 'We want to be parents like everybody else': stories of parents with learning disabilities. *International Journal of Developmental Disabilities*, 64(3), 184–194.

Tøssebro, J. (2016). Scandinavian disability policy: from deinstitutionalisation to non-discrimination and beyond. *Alter*, 10(2), 111–123.

Tøssebro, J., Midjo, T., Paulsen, V., et al. (2017). Prevalence, trends and custody among children of parents with intellectual disabilities in Norway. *Journal of Applied Research in Intellectual Disabilities*, 30(3), 533–542.

Tøssebro, J., & Wendelborg, C. (2017). Marriage, separation and beyond: a longitudinal study of families of children with intellectual and developmental disabilities in a Norwegian context. *Journal of Applied Research in Intellectual Disabilities*, 30(1), 121–132.

Totsika, V., Hastings, R. P., & Vagenas, D. (2017). Informal caregivers of people with an intellectual disability in England: health, quality of life and impact of caring. *Health & Social Care in the Community*, 25(3), 951–961.

Truesdale, M., & Brown, M. (2017). *People with learning disabilities in Scotland: 2017 health needs assessment update report*. Edinburgh: NHS Health Scotland. Available at: https://hub.careinspectorate.com/media/1291/people-with-learning-disabilities-in-scotland-2017-health-needs-assessment-update.pdf. [Accessed 23 November 2020].

Walker, R., & Hutchinson, C. (2019). Care-giving dynamics and futures planning among ageing parents of adult offspring with intellectual disability. *Ageing & Society*, 39(7), 1512–1527.

Wark, S., Canon-Vanry, M., Ryan, P., et al. (2015). Ageing–related experiences of adults with learning disability resident in rural areas: one Australian perspective. *British Journal of Learning Disabilities*, 43(4), 293–301.

Whittle, E. L., Fisher, K. R., Reppermund, S., et al. (2019). Access to mental health services: The experiences of people with intellectual disabilities. *Journal of Applied Research in Intellectual Disabilities*, 32(2), 368–379.

Wiesel, I., & Bigby, C. (2015). Movement on shifting sands: deinstitutionalisation and people with intellectual disability in Australia. *Urban Policy and Research*, 33(2), 178–194 1974–2014.

Willingham-Storr, G. L. (2014). Parental experiences of caring for a child with intellectual disabilities: a UK perspective. *Journal of Intellectual Disabilities*, 18(2), 146–158.

Woodbridge, S., Buys, L., & Miller, E. (2011). 'My grandchild has a disability': impact on grand parenting identity, roles and relationships. *Journal of Aging Studies*, 25(4), 355–363.

Yang, X., Artman-Meeker, K., & Roberts, C. A. (2018). Grandparents of children with intellectual and developmental disabilities: navigating roles and relationships. *Intellectual and Developmental Disabilities*, 56(5), 354–373.

Yang, X., Byrne, V., & Chiu, M. Y. (2016). Caregiving experience fo children with intellectual disabilities among parents in a developing area in China. *Journal of Applied Research in Intellectual Disabilities*, 29(1), 46–57.

Yang, W., & Tan, S. Y. (2019). Is informal care sufficient to meet the long-term care needs of older people with disabilities in China? Evidence from the China Health and Retirement Longitudinal Survey. *Ageing & Society*, 1–20, https://doi.org/10.1017/S0144686X1900148X.

Zaidman-Zait, A., Yechezkiely, M., & Regev, D. (2020). The quality of the relationship between typically developing children and their siblings with and without intellectual disability: insights from children's drawings. *Research in Developmental Disabilities*, 96, 103537.

Zigante, V. (2018). *Informal care in Europe. Exploring formalisation, availability and quality*. Available at: http://cite.gov.pt/pt/destaques/complementosDestqs2/Informal_care.pdf.

20

Childhood

Mary Dearing and Maria Pallisera

KEY ISSUES

- Children with intellectual disabilities are children first.
- An intellectual disability may be diagnosed at birth or during childhood, however this diagnosis will have a lifelong impact on the child and their family.
- Although milestones of development may be delayed, some will be achieved.

- Having a child with an intellectual disability may impact upon individual family members, for example, parents, siblings and grandparents.
- Children with intellectual disabilities should be listened to, particularly at life transition as plans are developed to move onto new stages.
- Children with intellectual disabilities have an added risk of harm which should not be underestimated.

CHAPTER OUTLINE

INTRODUCTION

The news of the birth of a baby is usually a jubilant event. Family members and friends often mark this very special experience by buying gifts for both the mother and infant to celebrate the significance of this occasion. When asked during pregnancy about their expectations for the birth of their son or daughter, parents often respond that their greatest desire is for their child to be born healthy. For all parents, the birth of their first baby is an important transition. Whatever mothers and fathers assume parenthood to be, the demands are usually far greater than ever imagined, and the birth of a baby not only brings joy but also additional anxieties, as new parents attempt to work out how they will make

adjustments to their lives. A recent report (Hirsch, 2019) estimates that the overall cost of raising a child until their eighteenth birthday in the UK is approximately £150,000 for a couple, rising to £185,000 for a lone parent. In comparison, a study by Emerson et al (2010) acknowledged that families who support a child with an intellectual disability were considerably more likely to experience poverty and adversity. This may be because there are additional indirect costs to families of children with intellectual disabilities, for example, the ability of a mother to remain in full time employment (Stabile and Allin, 2012). Internationally, research studies suggest that the extra cost of living with a disability may range from 9% of average weekly income in Vietnam

(Braithwaite and Mont, 2009) to 17% in Australia (Saunders, 2006) and in Ireland (Cullinan et al, 2010).

Despite recognised financial restraints, what is more difficult to estimate is the social and emotional price that parents pay for the happiness and pleasure of having a child. When it becomes apparent that a child has been born with, or is later diagnosed as having, an intellectual disability, this price may be set even higher, as this generally unexpected and therefore unplanned event may thrust families into a completely new world of professionals and services of which they have no previous knowledge or awareness. Children with intellectual disabilities may be required to attend a range of health and therapeutic appointments in comparison to a typically developing child (Genereaux et al, 2016). This therefore affects the time that carers have to spend on social activities, and can have both an emotional and financial impact on their well-being. All parents need to adapt to their new situation and may begin to adopt a new set of values, beliefs and expectations. Recent research suggests that younger care givers of children with intellectual disabilities are more likely to experience a mild to moderate burden of care (Egan and Dalton, 2019), however parents also experience personal growth and perceive the parenting of their child with a disability as a source of empowerment leading to feelings of greater personal strength (Waizbard-Bartov et al, 2019).

Intellectual disability (describing a significant impairment in intellectual functioning and significant impairment in adaptive behaviour, relating to the ability to function socially), can be diagnosed at any time in childhood or adolescence provided it occurred before adulthood. However, in general, the more severe the intellectual disability, the earlier it becomes apparent and therefore the earlier it is diagnosed (Stojanovic et al, 2019). With the advancement of medical technology and ultrasound scans, some parents may already know their child could have a disabling condition prior to birth, and through adjustment and acceptance may have already begun to re-model their lives (Carlsson et al, 2017).

For other families the news that their son or daughter has an intellectual disability may imminently follow the birth, whilst for others it may be months or years before they are formally told that their child is developmentally delayed or has a specific condition which results in them having an intellectual disability. However, research from Denmark confirms what is common for families

is that they engage in a wide range of coping strategies, particularly when a diagnosis of an intellectual disability is confirmed. It is at this stage, some parents begin to see their child as an individual with possibilities rather than disabilities (Graungaard et al, 2011).

Although it can be difficult to determine a precise prevalence rate for children with intellectual disabilities, an estimate by Maulik et al (2011) suggests it to be 10.4 per 1000 worldwide. This study affirms that the prevalence of intellectual disabilities can be almost twice as high in low and middle-income countries than in countries with higher incomes. However, recent statistics produced in the UK provide an estimated prevalence of children with intellectual disabilities at 2.5% (Public Health England, 2016). An explanation for the variance in statistics may be accounted for by the diverse assessment and criteria used to determine intellectual disability internationally. Additionally, the construct of intellectual disability varies across cultures, and a stigma still exists which may result in children with intellectual disabilities being a hidden population (Aldersey, 2012). Despite this variance in figures, there is universal agreement that the number of people with intellectual disabilities is set to increase with the advancement of medical technology, and that people with intellectual disabilities are generally living longer (Walker, 2015). It is important therefore that professionals who work with children with intellectual disabilities and their families not only have sufficient knowledge and skill to meet the changing needs of this group, but also consider their own values and attitudes so that positive outcomes can be achieved and effective parent partnerships established. This chapter concentrates on the needs of children with intellectual disabilities and their families, exploring evidence and best practice to support them to live the most rewarding lives possible. To achieve this, the reader will follow the journey a family may take following the diagnosis of an intellectual disability and the effect this may have on the child, their parents, siblings and other family members.

Defining Child

For the purpose of this chapter, the definition of a child has been explored from various perspectives. From a biological perspective, a child can be defined as a human between the stages of birth and puberty. However, when national and international legislation is reviewed there are various definitions of 'child' proposed that are dependent on a range of differential factors; these consequently lead to confusion, particularly in transition to adult services when young people can transfer to different services at different ages. The most widely accepted international definition of child is from the UN Convention on the Rights of the Child (1989). This states that child "means every human being below the age of 18 years unless, under the law applicable to the child, majority is attained earlier" (United Nations [UN], 1989, Article 1). This definition is generally accepted legally across most of the world and there appears to be international agreement that childhood is a stage for children to be in education and be able to play in order to develop into strong and confident individuals (United Nations Children's Fund (UNICEF), 2005).

CHILDREN FIRST

In Europe and some other parts of the world, there has been a positive shift in how children with intellectual disabilities are perceived. Barnes (2012) suggests that the origin of this change is an amalgamation of political activism and scholarship which collectively has generated a shift in perception. This change appears to stem from the move from segregated models of living for some people with intellectual disabilities to more inclusive, community-based provision (World Health Organisation (WHO), 2010). This welcomed shift fosters the belief that children with intellectual disabilities are full and active members of society and are equal to their peers. However adverse opinions continue to exist in some cultures which result in a lack of opportunity for meaningful contribution to community events and inadequate access to healthcare and education (Hervie, 2013). All children should have the opportunity to have the best possible start in life, and the support they need from their families and professionals to encourage them to fulfil their potential.

When children with intellectual disabilities are considered, it is critical that those supporting them remember that above all they are children first; this standpoint was one of the central principles of the UK Children Act (1989). Children with complex health and social care needs have the same wishes and ambitions as other children. They want to live at home, go to school and spend time with their friends and family participating in leisure and community activities (Browne and Millar,

2016). The challenge is to empower children and their families as well as to increase their involvement and inclusion in their communities, so that those communities benefit from the contribution they can make. In circumstances where children are unable to live with their families, then the WHO (2010) promotes that children should live in small family groups with carers acting as surrogate parents with an emphasis on child centred approaches to care.

It is vital that all children have the opportunity to experience childhood; to play, have fun and develop friendships and be encouraged to reach their full potential. From a policy maker's perspective it is well established that to make lasting change, resources should be prioritised between conception and three years (Caceres et al, 2016). Therefore, governments should invest in supporting early cognitive, linguistic and socio-emotional maturity to enable children to flourish in education. In some countries, for example Scotland, a special commission exists to deliver on strategy and policy in this area (Scottish Commission for Intellectual Disability, 2019).

The legislative and policy context

The United Nations Convention on the Rights of Persons with Disabilities (UNCRPD) adopted in 2006, advocates inclusive and equitable education for all children. In some parts of the world children with disabilities are too frequently denied access to any education; according to WHO and the World Bank (2011) children with intellectual disabilities in developing countries have the lowest school enrolment rate. Several reasons underpin this that include limited student interaction because of large class sizes; basic wages for teachers and lack of appropriate resources also contribute to poor engagement with children with intellectual disabilities (Masino and Niño-Zarazúa, 2016). In the western world the medical model of disability, which supported the segregation of children with intellectual disabilities into special education has slowly been eroded with the support of the United Nations Educational, Scientific and Cultural Organisation (UNESCO) Salamanca Statement on Principles, Policy and Practice in Special Needs Education (UNESCO, 1994). This statement promotes that ordinary schools accommodate all children and that educational policies enable children with disabilities to attend neighbourhood schools (UNESCO, 2015). However, even when included in ordinary services, children with intellectual disabilities continue to require dedicated services to address their individual needs.

When the United Nations Convention on the Rights of the Child (UN, 1989) was adopted by the UN General Assembly, it became the most widely ratified and complete statement on the international human rights of children ever produced. The Convention protects specific child rights in international law, defining universal principles relating to the status and treatment of children worldwide. In addition, it is the only international human rights treaty which includes civil, political, economic, social and cultural rights, and it sets out in detail what every child needs for a safe, happy and fulfilled childhood. The Convention identifies that human rights are founded on respect for the dignity and worth of each individual, regardless of race, gender, language, religion, opinions, wealth or ability. It sets minimum standards, stating that every child has the right to survival; the right to the development of their full physical and mental potential; the right to protection from influences that are harmful to their development; and the right to participation in family, cultural and social life (UN, 1989). The existence of separate legislation in some countries pertaining to all children, for example, the UK Children Act (2004), acknowledges both their vulnerability and rights as individuals as well as a group with needs discrete from those of adults.

EARLY IDENTIFICATION AND DIAGNOSIS

As all children are individuals they develop and learn at different rates, and in diverse ways, but some will develop and learn at a much slower pace than their peers. The diagnosis of an intellectual disability is most often made by a Paediatrician (a doctor specialising in the care of children), however for this to happen, it first has to be recognised that a developmental delay is present. This is often referred to as 'global developmental delay', defined as a significant delay in at least two developmental domains. This can include motor skills (gross or fine), speech and language, cognitive skills and activities of daily living often leading to an eventual diagnosis of an intellectual disability (Shevell et al, 2003). Developmental screening can be undertaken by a range of professionals but generally includes assessment of the environment, genetic, biological, social and demographic influences that may positively or negatively have an impact on a child's development (Khan,

2019). In the UK, for example, the Special Education Needs and Disability Code of Practice (Department of Health, 2015) recognises the importance of identifying children with intellectual disabilities early to ensure that these infants and young children are given maximum support. In terms of professional services, early involvement of specialist services may not only improve health outcomes by mitigating the effects of the disability, but also improve the overall wellbeing of the child and, as recognised by Pratt and Patel (2007), the wellbeing of their family.

It is important for all who work with infants and young children to understand child development, to enable them to recognise when a child is not developing as expected. Although every child is unique, and no two children will reach their developmental milestones at the same time, for children with intellectual disabilities detection enables early intervention programmes to commence. Khan (2019) suggests these are vital to improve health care and have a positive impact on individual children and their families; in many cases, the receipt of appropriate services can change the child's developmental trajectory.

In some circumstances, an intellectual disability can be associated with a number of genetic or inherited conditions such as Down syndrome; a specific diagnosis such as this can provide some idea of the difficulties the child may encounter across their lifespan. For parents whose child has a formal diagnosis, and are therefore aware already that their development will be delayed, there will be moments of pride as their child reaches each new milestone. Other parents who have not had a formal diagnosis, or in cases where the origins of the condition are unknown, may experience growing concern if their child does not appear to be developing at the same rate as others of a similar age; in addition they may face difficulties and frustration in having professionals acknowledge this and feel they are treated as over anxious parents (Lundeby and Tøssebro, 2008). Recent technological advances such as genomic hybridization have allowed diagnosis of chromosomal imbalances that cause intellectual disabilities (Zahir and Friedman, 2007). Despite this many parents still experience a long and exhausting diagnostic process as it is often not possible to state a definitive diagnosis as research states only 17% to 50% of conditions are attributed to genetic cause (Kaufman et al, 2010). For those parents whose children do not have a formal diagnosis they may struggle to navigate healthcare systems, and find it harder to obtain financial and educational support (Jewitt et al, 2017).

For parents, the recognition that their child has an intellectual disability can be stressful, and it has been established that initial experiences with health professionals have a major, lasting influence on the parents' ability to cope with their child's condition (Jewitt et al, 2017). Parents require assistance to provide effective care for their child in the first year of life and additionally require emotional support to adjust to their new role. Also, they need assistance finding appropriate information and to establish support networks (Douglas et al, 2016). Professionals should therefore remain acutely aware of how their responses to parental concerns might be interpreted and the manner in which they convey information.

READER ACTIVITY 20.1

Consider where you live, are there support groups for parents to access whose child has received a diagnosis of an intellectual disability?

How accessible are these groups?

What are the strengths and challenges of bringing families together to support each other?

A multitude of terms are used both nationally and internationally that are intended to clarify for parents their child's difficulties but often just add further confusion. Adoption of the term 'delay' rather than 'disability' may be more acceptable as some children may match the achievement of their peers once a specific difficulty has been identified and addressed, for example a hearing or visual impairment. However, for other children, if a significant learning delay persists as the child gets older, and this delay impinges on a number of areas of the child's development, professionals may begin to consider an intellectual disability. This implies they assume that the child will continue to learn at a slower pace than other children of the same age into adulthood. It is therefore essential for professionals to undertake a holistic assessment before diagnosing an intellectual disability. Development is an intricate concept that involves the sequencing of physical and psychological changes which start at conception and follow a defined process, for example, crawling, walking then running. However, development is dependent on a child's life experiences and circumstances that will be individual and unique

(Lindon and Brodie, 2016). Physical processes refer to the changes which happen to a child's body; psychological processes relate to the child's thought, intelligence and language development; and socioemotional processes relate to a child's relationship with other people which may emerge as changes that occur in a child's emotions and personality. The development of an infant is usually measured in terms of what is normal and expected at any given age, but is influenced by both individual maturation rates and experiences (Lindon and Brodie, 2016). Simpson and Weiner (1989) offer the definition of the word development as 'a new stage in a changing situation'. This is relevant in developing countries and from a global perspective, it has been identified that inadequate cognitive stimulation, iodine deficiency and iron deficiency anaemia are visible risks that prevent millions of children from achieving their full potential (Walker and Ward, 2013).

Achieving optimal physical and mental wellbeing

The World Report on Disability (WHO and World Bank, 2011) affirms that people with disabilities experience poorer levels of health than the general population. This is reinforced by the UK report on the Confidential Inquiry into Premature Deaths of People with Learning [Intellectual] Disabilities (Heslop et al, 2013) into the health disparities that exist between people with and without intellectual disabilities (see also Chapter 9). All children should have the right to access primary and mainstream services provided by front line health services for example, family doctors and nursing services. Globally there has been a significant rise in diet related chronic disease; these include conditions such as obesity, cardiovascular disease, cancers and type 2 diabetes (Mozaffarian et al, 2018). Healthy eating initiatives are now at the forefront of many government's agendas internationally, with some countries developing healthy eating recommendations which are consistent with contemporary nutritional science, whilst at the same time take into account the cultural and consumption habits of a particular country (Davis et al, 2019). Research suggests that an increase in a child's weight velocity in preschool years is a strong indicator of obesity in adult life (Birch and Ventura, 2009). Health promoting initiatives are just as important, if not more so, for children with intellectual disabilities who may run increased risks in adulthood of developing potentially life limiting conditions such as diabetes linked to obesity and coronary heart disease. Maïano (2011) concluded that a high number of children and young people with intellectual disabilities are overweight and obese compared to typically developed peers, and are therefore at a higher risk of developing secondary health problems. In an attempt to address this increasing problem, and set the future scene more positively, it is important that health promoting information and education is available in easy read versions, and that screening and preventative measures are routinely offered at an early age for all children with intellectual disabilities.

It is also vital that the mental health of children and young people is not overlooked. Glasper et al (2015) suggest that mental health problems in childhood are rarely a simple single diagnosis and can often be attributed to a symptom of a conflicting social dilemma, for example, bullying or low self-esteem, or may be linked to a genetic condition, e.g. Prader Willi syndrome. Unique challenges exist when attempting to identify and diagnose a mental health problem in a child with an intellectual disability as often symptoms can be falsely attributed to the disability rather than an accompanying mental illness, despite the existence of comprehensive questionnaires to diagnose individuals with dual presentation, for example, the Developmental Behaviour Checklist (Einfield and Tonge, 2002). What is important is how to improve well-being and mental health of individuals across the lifespan, laying the foundations for good mental health in childhood. Children with intellectual disabilities have, for a long period, experienced gaps in services. This is clearly evident where they have been excluded from accessing child and adolescent mental health services because of their primary diagnosis (Toms et al, 2015). This disparity exists despite international research showing there is a much higher prevalence of psychiatric disorders (between 30%–50%) amongst people with intellectual disabilities including children and adolescents (Enfield et al, 2011) (see also Chapter 16).

FAMILY EXPERIENCE

Expectant mothers and fathers are often enthusiastic about their imminent role as parents but for many new parents those early weeks following the birth of their child are tense as they face a unique set of challenges including sleep deprivation, learning new skills in caring for their infant and extensive lifestyle changes. The seminal work of LeMasters (1957) originally recognised

that the transition to parenthood is one of the family's most difficult stages of adjustment. A host of individual factors will influence how parents adjust including the support they receive from family and friends.

In preparation for the birth of a child parents, siblings, grandparents and members of the extended family will consider how the arrival of this new family member will impact on each of them personally. However, when a child is born or is later diagnosed with an intellectual disability, a different process of adaptation may occur. Those parents who can maintain or improve a positive attitude and optimism for their child's future are more likely to be able to mediate the effects of stress and provide effective care for their child (Peer and Hillman, 2012). The reaction of families will vary but it is not unusual for them to grieve the 'loss' of their 'normal' child. Parents report feeling a range of emotions from sadness and disbelief to heartache and anger (Sheehan and Guerin, 2018). However, simultaneously, they also frequently report feeling alarmed by the strength and complexity of the level of protection they feel for their son or daughter (Sheehan and Guerin, 2018). For some parents of children with intellectual disabilities, who initially have difficulties in adjusting, it may be that they are just at the initial stage of a developmental process of coping and adaptation, and have not yet reached a stage at which point they can accept the child, the disability and themselves. Emerging from the literature is recognition of the positive effects and contributions a child with an intellectual disability makes to their parents and families (Miersschaut et al, 2010). Parents of children diagnosed with intellectual disabilities often discuss the impact the birth of their child has had on them personally. For example, the Irish actor Colin Farrell spoke of his experiences of caring for his son with Angelman syndrome

"The struggle of a child with special needs can be so brutal that they tear at the very fabric of your heart, but the love shared and the pure strength and heroism observed is the needle and thread that mends all tears."

Poletto, 2017

 READER ACTIVITY 20.2

Read the following blog
http://www.hopefulparents.org/
Think about your hopes and aspirations for children with intellectual disabilities.

Internationally, the WHO (2010) emphasises the importance of early psychological support to parents when their child first receives a diagnosis of an intellectual disability. Research suggests that early identification and referral to appropriate services can improve lifelong outcomes for these children (King and Glascoe, 2003). However, the emerging science of *epigenetics* (the study of how DNA expression can be changed without altering the structure of DNA itself) reveals that one of the most valuable assets in promoting child development are the interactions between a baby and their caregiver (Winston and Chicot, 2016). The repeated interactions and communication that occurs between the infant and their caregiver help promote pathways for learning and logic to develop; it also provides infants with a secure bond that will help them in later life to maintain healthy relationships.

Mothers

The majority of children with intellectual disabilities continue to reside with, and be brought up by, their birth family even into adulthood (Walker and Ward, 2013). Services available to support parents of children with intellectual disabilities are generally aimed at mothers as they continue to be the parent likeliest to be the primary care giver (Sato et al, 2015). There have been numerous studies undertaken which relate to the effect that having a child with an intellectual disability will have on a mother (see Chapter 19) but most emphasis has been placed on the emotional, financial and physical costs (Mukherjee and Shignapure, 2016).

Fathers

The contribution that fathers of children with intellectual disabilities make has increased, and currently fathers are more engaged with their child and with family life than previous generations (Bostrom and Broberg, 2014). As such, professionals need to engage with fathers as well as mothers to promote their involvement in care of the child (Lamb, 2010). The adjustment that fathers of children with intellectual disabilities are required to make often goes unrecognised, but research suggests that they are more likely to participate in play, nurturing and discipline but less likely to pursue emotional or social support (Dabrowska and Pisula, 2010). Fathers of children with intellectual disabilities experience social isolation and other difficulties adjusting to their new role and feel there is a lack of support from employers (Ly and

Goldberg, 2014). Therefore it is imperative that professionals working with the family should make all efforts to listen to both parents, assist them to adapt to their new situation, and where possible make adjustments to allow fathers to attend meetings.

Siblings

The relationship between children and young people with intellectual disabilities and their siblings has been studied from different perspectives including the model of stress and confrontation which focuses on the emotional experience when faced with having a sibling with an intellectual disability (Meltzer and Kramer, 2016). The relatively recent advancement of inclusive research approaches has allowed new perspectives to emerge that include the viewpoint of children with intellectual disabilities themselves. This approach seeks to understand the nature of the sibling relationship at different stages of development and how these relationships change throughout life (Meltzer and Kramer, 2016). Research has found that siblings can be effective sources of support and company for their disabled brother or sister throughout their lives. Floyd et al (2016) point out that strong relationships between siblings predict a good adjustment to school for children with intellectual disabilities, and that the period of adolescence is a critical moment in the development of relationships between siblings. Informing siblings about the conditions of the disability, and promoting common spaces where the family can share activities, can help strengthen the relationships between siblings.

Grandparents

Recent research (Griggs et al, 2009) demonstrated that approximately a third of maternal grandmothers provided regular child care for their grandchildren, with 40 per cent providing occasional help with childcare. Although there remains little research on the role grandparents play with children with intellectual disabilities, there is some evidence to suggest they too have a similar initial emotional response to the birth of a child with an intellectual disability as parents, experiencing both a period of mourning for the loss of the grandchild they expected, and one of adjustment to the revised situation (Lee and Gardner, 2010).

The role that grandparents of children with intellectual disabilities play is similar to the role of any grandparent; they advise and guide their grandchildren and offer practical, emotional and sometimes financial support to the child's parents. However, research has shown that grandparents of children with intellectual disabilities feel a greater need to protect and support their adult children recognising that they are dealing with challenging circumstances (Findler, 2014). When working with families it is therefore vital to recognise and consider the support that grandparents both provide and may require.

TRANSITION THROUGH CHILDHOOD

Transition points are often thought of as being stressful periods of loss. Indeed, the changes force the search for new personal and community resources and supports. Timely planning that includes the individual with an intellectual disability as the main agent from the very beginning can reduce the tension that is usually related to transitions. Parents, children and young people have to become involved and take a central role in the processes linked to the transition; the planning, training and the necessary collaboration between different agencies (for example, health services, educational services, vocational centres, community and local agencies) (Davis et al, 2015). This section of the chapter explores the different transitions that may take place in the life of a child with an intellectual disability and best practice in meeting the requirements of them.

Children experience different periods of transition throughout their development; particular moments of different duration in which significant changes are often linked to the environment in which they develop, and which generate new situations and challenges. Any transition can lead to challenges but also positive changes, improvements and advances; as such they need to be carefully planned to ensure adequate distribution of support to facilitate the transformation of challenges into progress.

The most significant transitions experienced by most children and young people, whether or not they have intellectual disabilities, are from home to school, from primary school to secondary school, and from secondary school to post-school life. Along with these, there are other specific transitions experienced by some children, such as children with chronic health conditions (CHCs). The transition from hospital to home is one of these, in which the collaboration between parents, healthcare staff and schools is of vital importance. The

development of self-determination and self-care skills are areas of work in which the coordinated efforts of professionals and families are required; any interventions and support must focus on stimulating strengths and abilities (Strnadová and Cumming, 2016). In addition, children and adolescents with CHCs must learn to manage their health conditions outside the home, at school and in the community; the process that takes them from family-focused management to self-care in adolescent and young adult life is another specific transition that is relevant for children and young people. In order to enhance autonomy in the management of their health, it is essential to include school-age children in discussions about their conditions, and families must also be helped to support the child in this process (Beacham and Deatrick, 2015). Beacham and Deatrick indicate the need to support young people to anticipate changes linked to their condition that may appear with puberty, and to incorporate the skills that can help them manage these conditions. Health professionals, who will monitor the children and young people over the years, have a major responsibility in designing, monitoring and evaluating the plan aimed at promoting the autonomy of the child or young person with CHCs. The transition from paediatric (children's) to adult care services is closely linked to this process of gaining a child's autonomy, and also requires close coordination and continuity of health care. It needs a written plan that guides the transition process. It should begin in their early teens and involve parents / primary carers, paediatric health care providers, and the receiving adult health care providers, in addition to the child. It is also very important to ensure accurate tracking mechanisms are established by health care services to monitor the plan to improve post-transition achievements (Zhou et al, 2016).

Home to school

Transition from home to school includes a series of changes experienced by children and their families at stages (depending on the educational provision of each country). Incorporation into preschool settings probably generates the child's first inclusive experience outside of their family. For the first time, it is necessary to build the supports that will help the child to establish social relationships and develop in a context of formal learning, and this requires specific efforts from both the child and their parents, who will have to learn to negotiate with service providers. A transdisciplinary approach including healthcare professionals is recommended. They provide the child's health history, as well as information on their development, and the planning of the supports and abilities that the child should develop at least one year in advance (Strnadová and Cumming, 2016). Among these are those linked to self-determination, essential to the building of foundations for future autonomy. Palmer et al (2013) insist on the need to enhance opportunities to develop choice-making and problem-solving abilities, self-regulation and engagement skills, as they are necessary to facilitate future independence. Collaboration between families and professionals to develop coordinated actions at school and at home is essential, as well as professionals recognising and respecting family beliefs and cultural values.

Primary to secondary school

This transition occurs at around the age of 11 and focuses on formal school experiences, but it entails significant changes for students, their families and teachers. Cultural discrepancies including organisation of school time and teaching spaces, teachers and personal resources, academic requirements that are clearly increasing in the secondary stage and new composition of peer groups, generate insecurities, challenges and opportunities.

Planning the transition in a collaborative way including parents or carers, professionals from both primary and secondary schools, and the young person with disabilities, is essential to encourage integration into secondary school. It is necessary for teachers and other school staff to really listen and recognise the concerns of children and parents before the transition occurs. Since each child is different, so are their needs and demands, and so it is necessary to design individual supports for each child. Listening to young people before the transition can help this process, and supporting them to express their concerns through materials such as photographs, diaries and narratives may be useful (Hughes et al, 2013). This planning should carefully review both the level of self-determination of the young person and the academic, social and behavioural demands that will be required in the different subjects and spaces of the secondary school. This includes taking into account both academic subjects, as well as the routines necessary to make use of the cafeteria and other communal spaces. This preparation will allow for appropriate support

planning to prepare the young person and help in the incorporation of new routines.

The relational challenges linked to this transition deserve a special mention. This is the stage in which the friendships that will accompany the early adolescents throughout their youth are built. Making new friends is a challenge for every teenager when changing to secondary school, and a necessary element for a sense of belonging in the new school. However, literature shows that early adolescents with intellectual disabilities often lose friends in the transition from primary to secondary education. This can be related to the progressive decrease in the presence and participation in ordinary classrooms of young people with intellectual disabilities throughout their trajectory in secondary education (Webster and Blatchford, 2013; Wendelborg and Tøssebro, 2010), and also with the lack of opportunities to participate in structured leisure activities in the community (Callus and Farrugia, 2016) (see also Chapter 21). This restricts the possibility of participating in decisions about how to spend free time and with whom, as well as establishing friendships outside the family circle, so that young people with disabilities cannot exercise their rights to participate on equal terms with others. In this context, school and community play a relevant role by offering extracurricular activities that will help strengthen both the sense of belonging, and establish and strengthen new relationships that can become supportive (Coffey, 2013).

Secondary school to adult life

This section is supported by **Reader activity 20.3, Martha's story** (Part A) in the accompanying online resource.

The process of transition from secondary school to adult life is a temporary situation in which issues related to education, vocational training, independent life and community participation are addressed, and young people make key decisions to guide their personal path according to their own goals. Continuing with post-compulsory education, whether vocational or academic, is one of those decisions; a decision which every young person, whether they have an intellectual disability or not, has to make. Also at this stage, actions are taken that affect areas such as the emancipation from the family, the beginning of the work career path, and social inclusion through the development of social support networks. From this perspective, in the process of the transition of young people with intellectual disabilities to adulthood, several aspects of the Convention on the Rights of Persons with Disabilities (CRPD) (United Nations, 2006) are brought into play: the right to education (Article (art.)24), to work (art.27), to culture and leisure (art. 30) and to independent life in the community (art.19).

The CRPD (UN, 2006) shows that horizons for people with disabilities have widened, that personal itineraries can be absolutely diverse, and that they can take directions that have traditionally been vetoed for people with intellectual disabilities; higher academic education, for example, or the creation of a family. However, in spite of having their rights taken into account, young people with intellectual disabilities experience numerous barriers to continuing their training, to working or to advance in their independent life (European Agency for Fundamental Rights (FRA), 2013). Their transition processes are usually longer and with fewer opportunities. In most countries, when they finish secondary school, their job opportunities are reduced to a sheltered workshop or to day centres (Midjo and Aune, 2018). Young people generally experience difficulties in continuing post compulsory education, and this situation can affect their job recruitment later.

The challenges of the transition process, as well as the actions and tools that can contribute to its improvement, can be distributed in 4 interrelated dimensions represented in Figure 20.1: individual-family; relational; organisational and community.

Individual-family dimension

The processes of transition to adult life constitute unique paths, of which each young person takes centre stage. However, young people and their families complain that they do not have sufficient information about post-secondary alternatives, and ask for opportunities to spend time in potential new settings before making post-school decisions; in addition, young people want to have a say in decisions affecting their lives (Pallisera et al, 2016; Rome et al, 2015). That is why it is crucial for the young person to participate fully in the planning of this process, and to make decisions in the different phases. Professionals from different fields (for example, education, health, work) and family members have a supporting role in helping them answer the question, "What would I like to do in the future?" helping to achieve their goals. In spite of not having been

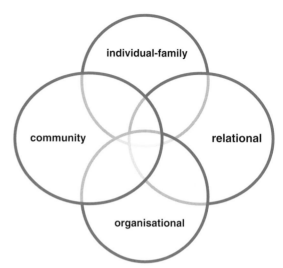

Figure 20.1 Dimensions of transition

able to develop investigations that confirm it, there is professional consensus that Person-Centred Planning (PCP) is a tool that can help increase the participation of young people in the planning of their transition, to give support in the formulation of post-school objectives, and to articulate clear support strategies, involving family, professionals, friends and community agents (Cobb and Alwell, 2009; Kaehne and Beyer, 2014). One of the specific styles of PCP, PATH (Planning Alternatives Tomorrow with Hope), can be a particularly useful resource to organise support for young people in the transition process to help them achieve their desired future goals, as illustrated in Figure 20.2. This process is put into play and centred on the self-determination of the young person, which is why these skills are ratified as a necessary area for work, both in the family context and in the educational centres, during the process of development of the young person (see Chapter 4 for more on person-centred assessment).

Relational dimension

Research shows that young people with intellectual disabilities have less leisure and free time opportunities than their peers without disabilities (Pallisera et al, 2016; Shelden and Storey, 2014; Small et al, 2013). This situation involves difficulties in establishing friendships that can be key to combating social isolation and exclusion. Having a social network composed of peers of the same age constitutes an element of support for the transition to adulthood. This is why it is important to foster the construction of social networks from childhood onwards in providing young people with intellectual disabilities with more resources to meet the challenges of transition (Leonard et al, 2016). Specifically, schools must promote adequate and appropriate opportunities for social interaction and development of communicative skills of adolescents and young people with intellectual disabilities, both in the more academic contexts and in the leisure and recreation areas. Guiding families on the need for children and young people with intellectual disabilities to experience desired leisure, cultural and / or sports experiences that can be shared with other friends of similar ages is another necessary action to be undertaken by school staff. This is reinforced in Chapters 21 and 22.

Organisational dimension

The process of transition to adult life may yield different scenarios (school and post-school) with the involvement of a diversity of centres, projects and services that can provide support, all with different organisational cultures and work practices. Coordination amongst professionals and services is a key element in the improvement of the transition process (Foley et al, 2012; Pallisera et al, 2014). Ensuring transition plans that facilitate the decision-making of the young person and their families by informing them and orienting them appropriately can only be guaranteed by a planning process that begins at the secondary school stage. Its main players and the agents involved must be included, with a clear leadership that ensures the distribution of responsibilities between the different agents and the coordination of the process. The secondary school professionals play a major role in leading planning during the transition process. Regarding curricular practices, it is important to enhance the teaching and learning of competences related to daily life, workplace-related experiences and self-determination (see also Chapter 22).

Community dimension

Linking personal trajectories with training, work and independent life objectives needs support from the community. The local environment is the territorial context where different services and spaces of different kinds (for example, cultural, work, leisure, training) exist that can become places for learning or development of supports. Community agents from different sectors (for example, health, vocational education and training, and work) need to be involved in transition planning, considering the general needs of young people as a group, but also taking into account the particular specific demands of individuals, in order to be able to design personalised processes. Coordination between educational centres, and community associations and services, will enhance the development of volunteer work and work placements that can be very useful for gaining work experience and gaining social competencies that enhance future inclusion.

At this point, pause and return to **Reader activity 20.3,** Martha's story (Part B) in the accompanying online resource.

Research shows that children and young people with intellectual disabilities can make a valuable contribution to the design and provision of services that can help them advance their personal itineraries (Rome et al, 2015). It is the responsibility of adults to find the ways to incorporate the perspectives of young people, by listening to their voices and supporting, if necessary, their decisions on how the transition process should take place.

KEEPING CHILDREN SAFE

Staying safe

Providing care for any child is challenging. Increasingly, the media are highlighting the pitfalls of parenthood as changes in societies occur and the subsequent restrictions these place on children. The United Nations Convention on the Rights of the Child (1989) acknowledges that play is every child's right. However, thirty years ago children had more freedom to express their independence. In 1970 the average nine-year-old girl would have been free to wander 840 metres from her front door. By 2015 this distance has shortened to 500 metres (Schoeppe et al, 2015). Children were permitted to play near their home, and one of the few distractions was television aimed at children aired after school. Today the picture is very different; parents may now feel they need to supervise their adolescent's activities as globally concerns are raised regarding harmful drinking, interpersonal violence and preventable death. The WHO (2019) report that road traffic accidents are now the leading cause of

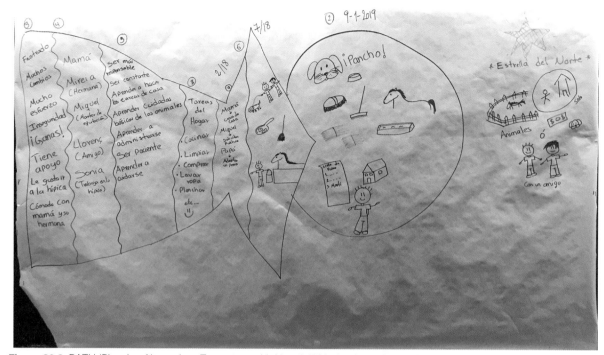

Figure 20.2 PATH (Planning Alternatives Tomorrow with Hope). With thanks to the students of the Master's degree in Inclusive Education: Addressing Diversity, academic year 2017/18, University of Girona

death amongst adolescents. Play is becoming 'endangered' and 'extinct' (Hyndman, 2019), as parents attempt to protect their children from traffic, strangers and pollution. Concern over these potential dangers coupled with acquisition of technological 'must haves' such as personal computers and games consoles have resulted in children spending more time at home in sedentary activities, and less time engaged in social interaction with their peers with one report suggesting that children spend twice as long looking at screens as they do playing outside (Jenkins, 2018).

Increased vulnerability to abuse

Recent research suggests that children with intellectual disabilities are exceptionally vulnerable and they are more likely to experience abuse and neglect than any other children (Helton et al, 2018). Moreover, the presence of multiple impairments appears to increase this risk (Wissink et al, 2015). They also have a decreased knowledge about sexual health and an increased dependency on care givers. Additionally, Franklin et al (2019) cite several concerns expressed by parents, as shown in Table 20.1.

Helping children protect themselves

Although safeguards exist (for example in the UK, the Disclosure and Barring Service which assists employers to make decisions regarding recruitment and prevention of people that may be unsuitable to work with children), families and organisations should not become complacent. Where possible, and appropriate, families should make children aware of risks and promote children keeping themselves safe; in particular, they must educate and stress to their children that people that they already know may harm them, although this is an area that is often overlooked. Efforts into abuse prevention need to be sustained, and programmes should include modelling, discussion and role play and where possible involve caregivers (Pulido et al, 2015).

All children, wherever they are educated, should have the right to teaching to understand the function of their bodies and understand their sexuality. Appropriate and timely education on sexual matters is fundamental for children to protect and understand themselves (Travers et al, 2014). However, there are several barriers identified to sexual health education for children with

TABLE 20.1 Concerns expressed by parents

Their child may
* receive intimate personal care, possibly from a number of carers, which may increase the risk of exposure to abusive behaviour
* have an impaired capacity to resist or avoid abuse
* have communication difficulties or lack of access to an appropriate vocabulary which may make it difficult to tell others what is happening
* not have someone to turn to, may lack the privacy they need to do this, or the person they turn to may not be receptive to the issues being communicated
* be inhibited about complaining because of a fear of losing services
* be especially vulnerable to bullying and intimidation and possibly at risk of being targeted, groomed and exploited by gangs
* be more vulnerable than other children to abuse by their peers.

intellectual disabilities which include that both parents and teachers may lack knowledge and confidence in teaching this subject resulting in anxiety, fear and concern. Additionally, sexual health resources may be limited or may not be reliable and valid and therefore impede teaching (Treacy et al, 2018). Children with intellectual disabilities should be made aware of topics such as self-harm, bullying, drug awareness, sex education and personal safety (see Chapters 22 and 25 for more on sex education).

All individuals who come into contact with children should be familiar with and follow their organisation's procedures for promoting and safeguarding the welfare of children, and know who to contact to express their concerns that a child may be at risk of harm (International Service, 2019). Concerns should be acted upon in the same way as with any other child. They should always listen to what a child is trying to tell them, either verbally or through their presentation, and allow them the time and opportunity to do so; in particular, people who work with children with intellectual disabilities need to consider the communication method of the child. In addition, they should remain alert to non-verbal messages, for example, reluctance to leave with a particular person which may be an indication that they are at risk of harm from that individual (see Chapter 8 for more guidance on safeguarding against abuse and harm).

Displaced children

It is estimated that on any given day 23,000 people are displaced either within their country of origin or in other countries (United Nations High Commissioner for Refugees (UNHCR), 2013). If we accept that an estimated 15% of any population has a disability (WHO, 2010) then a number of these will be children. This specific population of children with disabilities, including those with intellectual disabilities, in any displaced or conflict affected community are vulnerable to discrimination, exploitation and violence but with reduced ability to access services and support (UNHCR and Handicap International, 2011). This is compounded further by limited access to disability-specific health care (Pearce, 2015). Although this group of children with disabilities experience emotional symptoms (Khan et al, 2019) there is little preventative or targeted psychosocial intervention available to support them. In these circumstances, it is vital that children with disabilities are given the right to express their views, and more importantly contribute to decisions affecting their lives. In 2018, UNICEF published guidance which focuses on children with disabilities in humanitarian action which recommends targeted programmes to ensure they receive rehabilitation and assistive devices, in addition to education, protection, health and nutrition, water sanitation and hygiene.

CONCLUSION

The principal message readers should take from this chapter is that children with intellectual disabilities are, above all, children first. Each child will receive a diagnosis at a different time and they, and their families, will experience a process of adaptation. A pervading theme for all children will be transition; how each child (and importantly, their family and carer givers) will adapt to new stages in their life will largely depend upon those who support them and the services available. In many countries, policy exists to guide the development of services and to provide a framework for all professionals to respond to specific health, social and educational needs. It has been established that all children are vulnerable but children with intellectual disabilities may be particularly so. The value placed on providing the best possible start in life for a child with an intellectual disability and their family cannot be overestimated, only then can they begin to achieve their potential and be accepted as a full, contributing member of the society in which they live.

REFERENCES

Aldersey, H. M. (2012). Family perceptions of intellectual disability: understanding and support in Dar es Salaam. *African Journal of Disability*, 1(32).

Barnes, C. (2012). Understanding the social model of disability: past, present and future. In N. Watson, A. Roulstone, & C. Thomas (Eds.), *Routledge handbook of disability studies*. Abingdon: Routledge.

Beacham, B. L., & Deatrick, J. A. (2015). dhildren with chronic conditions: perspectives on conditions management. *Journal of Pediatric Nursing*, 30(1), 25–35.

Birch, L. L., & Ventura, A. K. (2009). Preventing childhood obesity: what works? *International Journal of Obesity*, 33(1), 74–81.

Bostrom, P. K., & Broberg, M. (2014). Openness and avoidance – a longitudinal study of fathers of children with intellectual disability. *Journal of Intellectual Disability Research*, 58(9), 810–821.

Braithwaite, J., & Mont, D. (2009). Disability and poverty: a survey of World Bank poverty assessments and implications. *ALTER – European Journal of Disability Research / Revue Européenne de Recherche sur le Handicap*, 3(3), 219–232.

Browne, M., & Millar, M. (2016). A rights-based conceptual framework for the social inclusion of children and young persons with an intellectual disability. *Disability & Society*, 31(8), 1064–1080.

Caceres, S., Tanner, J., & Williams, S. (2016). Maximizing child development: three principles for policymakers. *Journal of Human Development and Capabilities*, 17(4), 583–589.

Callus, A. M., & Farrugia, R. (2016). *The disabled child's participation rights*. London: Routledge.

Carlsson, T., Starke, V., & Mattsson, E. (2017). The emotional process from diagnosis to birth following a prenatal diagnosis anomaly: a qualitative study of messages in online discussion. *Midwifery*, 48, 53–59.

Children Act. (1989). London: HMSO.

Children Act. (2004). London: HMSO.

Cobb, R. B., & Alwell, M. (2009). Transition planning. Coordinating interventions for youth with disabilities. *Career Development for Exceptional Individuals*, 32(2), 70–81.

Coffey, A. (2013). Relationships: the key to successful transition from primary to secondary school? *Improving Schools*, 16(3), 261–271.

Cullinan, J., Gannon, B., & Lyons, S. (2010). Estimating the extra cost of living for people with disabilities. *Health Economics*. Available at: http://www.interscience.wiley.com.

Dabrowska, A., & Pisula, E. (2010). Parent stress and coping styles in mothers and fathers of pre-school children with autism and Down syndrome. *Journal of Intellectual Disability Research*, 54, 266–280.

Davis, J., Ravenscroft, J., & Bizas, N. (2015). Transition, inclusion and partnership: child, parent and professional led approaches in a European research project. *Child Care in Practice*, 21(1), 3–49.

Davis, K., Esslinger, K., Elvidge Munene, L. A., et al. (2019). International approaches to developing healthy eating patterns for national dietary guidelines. *Nutrition Reviews*, 77(6), 388–403.

Department of Health. (2015). *Special education needs and disability code of practice: 0 to 25 years*. Available at: https://www.gov.uk/government/publications/send-code-of-practice-0-to-25. [Accessed 18 December 2019].

Douglas, T., Redley, B., & Ottmann, G. (2016). The first year: the support needs of parents caring for a child with intellectual disability. *Journal of Advanced Nursing*, 72(11), 2738–2749.

Egan, C., & Dalton, C. T. (2019). An exploration of care–burden experienced by older caregivers of adults with intellectual disabilities in Ireland. *British Journal of Learning Disabilities*, 47(3), 188–194.

Einfeld, S. L., Ellis, L. A., & Emerson, E. (2011). Comorbidity of intellectual disability and mental disorder in children and adolescents: a systematic review. *Journal of Intellectual & Developmental Disability*, 36, 137–143.

Einfeld, S. L., & Tonge, B. J. (2002). *Manual for the Developmental Behaviour Checklist: primary carer version (DBC-P) & teacher version. (DBC-T)*.

Emerson, E., Shahtahmasebi, S., Lancaster, G., et al. (2010). Poverty transitions among families supporting a child with intellectual disability. *Journal of Intellectual & Developmental Disability*, 35, 224–234.

European Agency for Fundamental Rights. (2013). *Choice and control: the right to independent living experiences of persons with intellectual disabilities*.

Findler, L. (2014). The experience of stress and personal growth among grandparents of children with and without intellectual disability. *Intellectual and Developmental Disabilities*, 52(1), 32–48.

Floyd, F. J., Costigan, C. L., & Richardson, S. S. (2016). Sibling relationships in adolescence and early adulthood with people who have intellectual disability. *American Journal on Intellectual and Developmental Disabilities*, 121(5), 383–397.

Foley, K. R., Dyke, P., Girdler, S., et al. (2012). Young adults with intellectual disability transitioning from school to post-school: a literature review framed within the ICF. *Disability & Rehabilitation, 34*(20), 1747–1764.

Franklin, A., Toft, A., & Goff, S. (2019). Parents' and carers' views on how we can work together to prevent the sexual abuse of disabled children. *NSPCC Learning Future of Children, 22*(1), 65–96.

Genereaux, D., Bansback, N., & Birch, P. (2016). Development and pilot testing of a tool to calculate parental and societal costs of raising a child with intellectual disability. *Journal of Intellectual & Developmental Disability, 41*(1), 11–20.

Glasper, E. A., Coad, J., & Richardson, J. (2015). *Children and young people's nursing at a glance.* Chichester: Wiley-Blackwell.

Graungaard, A. H., Andersen, J. S., & Skov, L. (2011). When resources get sparse: a longitudinal qualitative study of emotions, coping and resource creation when parenting a young child with severe disabilities. *Health, 15*(2), 115–136.

Griggs, J., Tan, J. P., Ann Buchanan, A., et al. (2009). 'They've always been there for me': grandparental involvement and child well-being. *Children & Society, 24*(3), 200–214.

Helton, J. J., Gochez-Kerr, T., & Gruber, E. (2018). Sexual abuse of children with learning disabilities. *Child Maltreatment, 23*(2), 157–165.

Hervie, V. M. (2013). *Shut up! Social inclusion of children with intellectual disabilities in Ghana: an empirical study of how parents and teachers experience social inclusion of children with intellectual disabilities.* Master's thesis, University of Nordland.

Heslop, P., Blair, P., Fleming, P., et al. & Russ, L. (2013). *Confidential inquiry into premature deaths of people with learning disabilities (CIPOLD), Final report.*

Hirsch, D. (2019). *The cost of a child in 2019.* London: Poverty Action Group. Available at: https://www.un.org/development/desa/publications/world-population-prospects-2019-highlights.html. [Accessed 25 October 2019].

Hughes, L. A., Banks, P., & Terras, M. M. (2013). Secondary school transition for children with special educational needs: a literature review. *Support for Learning, 28*(1), 24–34.

Hyndman, B. (2019). *Let them play. Kids need freedom from play restrictions to develop.* Available at: http://theconversation.com/let-them-play-kids-need-freedom-from-play-restrictions-to-develop-117586. [Accessed 20 December 2019].

International Service. (2019). *Safeguarding children, young people and vulnerable adult's policy.* Available at: https://www.internationalservice.org.uk/our-safeguarding-policy. [Accessed 19 December 2019].

Jenkins, R. (2018). *Children spend twice as long looking at screen than playing outside.* Available at: https://www.independent.co.uk/life-style/children-screens-play-outside-computer-phone-time-healthy-games-a8603411.html. [Accessed 19 December 2019].

Jewitt, A., Rosser, E., Clement, E., et al. (2017). The role of the Roald Dahl swan (syndromes without a name) clinical nurse specialist; the 12 months experience. *Archives of Diseases in Childhood, 102*(3), A19.

Kaehne, A., & Beyer, S. (2014). Person-centred reviews as a mechanism for planning the post-school transition of young people with intellectual disability. *Journal of Intellectual Disability Research, 58*(7), 603–613.

Kaufman, L., Ayub, M., & Vicent, J. B. (2010). The genetic basis of non-syndromic intellectual disability: a review. *Journal of Neurodevelopmental Disorder, 2*, 182–209.

Khan, L. (2019). Detecting early developmental delays in children. *Pediatric Annals, 48*(10), e381–e384.

Khan, N. Z., Shilpi, A. B., Sultana, R., et al. (2019). Displaced Rohingya children at high risk for mental health problems: findings from refugee camps within Bangladesh. *Child: Care, Health and Development, 45*(1), 28–35.

King, T. M., & Glascoe, F. P. (2003). Developmental surveillance of infants and young children in pediatric primary care. *Current Opinion in Pediatrics, 15*, 624–629.

Lamb, M. E. (Ed.). (2010). *The role of the father in child development* (5th ed.). Hoboken, NJ: John Wiley & Sons.

Lee, M., & Gardner, J. E. (2010). Grandparents' involvement and support in families with children with disabilities. *Educational Gerontology, 36*, 467–499.

LeMasters, E. E. (1957). Parenthood as crisis. *Marriage and Family Living, 19*, 352–355.

Leonard, H., Foley, K. R., Pikora, T., et al. (2016). Transition to adulthood for young people with intellectual disability: the experiences of their families. *European Child & Adolescent Psychiatry,* 1369–1381.

Lindon, J., & Brodie, K. (2016). *Understanding child development: 0-8 years* (4th ed.). London: Hodder Education.

Lundeby, H., & Tøssebro, J. (2008). Exploring the experiences of 'not being listened to' from the perspective of parents with disabled children. *Scandinavian Journal of Disability Research, 10*(4), 258–274.

Ly, A. R., & Goldberg, W. A. (2014). New measures of fathers of children with developmental challenges. *Journal of Intellectual Disability Research, 58*(5), 471–484.

Maïano, C. (2011). Prevalence and risk factors of overweight and obesity among children and adolescents with intellectual disabilities. *Obesity Reviews, 12*, 189–197.

Masino, S., & Niño-Zarazúa, M. (2016). What works to improve the quality of student learning in developing countries? *International Journal of Educational Development, 48*, 53–65.

Maulik, P., Mascarenhas, M., Mathers, C., et al. (2011). Prevalence of intellectual disability: a meta-analysis of population-based studies. *Research in Developmental Disabilities, 32*(2), 419–436.

Meltzer, A., & Kramer, J. (2016). Siblinghood through disability studies perspectives: diversifying discourse and knowledge about siblings with and without disabilities. *Disability and Society, 31*(1), 17–32.

Midjo, T., & Aune, K. E. (2018). Identity constructions and transition to adulthood for young people with mild intellectual disabilities. *Journal of Intellectual Disabilities, 22*(1), 33–48.

Miersschaut, M., Roeyers, H., & Warreyn, P. (2010). Parenting in families with a child with autism spectrum disorders and a typically developing child: mothers' experiences and cognitions. *Research in Autism Spectrum Disorders, 4*, 661–669.

Mozaffarian, D., Angell, S., Lang, T., et al. (2018). Role of government policy in nutrition – barriers to and opportunities for healthier eating. *British Medical Journal, 361*, k2426.

Mukherjee, M., & Shignapure, V. (2016). Challenges faced by parent due to the presence of mentally handicapped person in the family. *The International Journal of Indian Psychology, 3*(3), 61–77.

Pallisera, M., Fullana, J., Puyaltó, C., et al. (2016). Changes and challenges in the transition to adulthood: views and experiences of young people with learning disabilities and their families. *European Journal of Special Needs Education, 31*(3).

Pallisera, M., Vilà, M., & Fullana, J. (2014). Transition to adulthood for young people with intellectual disability: exploring transition partnerships from the point of view of professionals in school and postschool services. *Journal of Intellectual and Developmental Disability, 39*(4), 333–341.

Palmer, S. B., Summers, J. A., Brotherson, M. J., et al. (2013). Foundations for self-determination in early childhood: an inclusive model for children with disabilities. *Topics in Early Childhood Special Education, 33*(1), 38–47.

Pearce, E. (2015). 'Ask us what we need': operationalizing guidance on disability inclusion in refugee and displaced persons programs. *Disability and the Global South, 2*, 460–478.

Peer, J. W., & Hillman, S. B. (2012). The mediating impact of coping style on stress perception for parents of individuals with intellectual disabilities. *Journal of Intellectual Disabilities, 16*(1), 45–59.

Poletto, C. (2017). *Colin Farrell to parents of children with special needs: you are not alone.* Available at: https://www.today.com/parents/colin-farrell-parents-special-needs-kids-you-are-not-alone-t120277. [Accessed 17 January 2021].

Pratt, H., & Patel, D. (2007). Learning disorders in children and adolescents. *Primary Care: Clinics in Office Practice, 34*(2), 361–374.

Public Health England. (2016). *People with learning disabilities in England.* London: GOV.UK.

Pulido, M. L., Dauber, S., Tully, B. A., et al. (2015). Knowledge gains following a child sexual abuse prevention program among urban students: A cluster-randomized evaluation. *American Journal of Public Health, 105*, 1344–1350.

Rome, A., Hardy, J., Richardson, J., et al. (2015). Exploring transitions with disabled young people: our experiences, our rights and our views. *Child Care in Practice, 21*(3), 287–294.

Sato, N., Araki, A., Ito, R., et al. (2015). Exploring the beliefs of Japanese mothers caring for a child with disabilities. *Journal of Family Nursing, 21*(2), 232–260.

Saunders, P. (2006). *The costs of disability and incidence of poverty.* Sydney: Social Policy Research Centre, University of New South Wales.

Scottish Commission for Learning Disability. (2019) Available at: https://www.scld.org.uk/. [Accessed 4 December 2019].

Schoeppe, S., Duncan, M. J., Badland, H. M., et al. (2015). Too far from home? Adult attitudes on children's independent mobility range. *Children's Geographies, 14*, 482–489.

Sheehan, P., & Guerin, S. (2018). Exploring the range of emotional response experienced when parenting a child with an intellectual disability: the role of dual process. *British Journal of Learning Disabilities, 46*(2), 109–117.

Shelden, D. L., & Storey, K. (2014). Social life. In K. Storey & D. Hunger (Eds.), *The road ahead* (pp. 233–254).

Shevell M., Ashwal, S., Donley, D., et al. (2003). Practice parameter: evaluation of the child with global developmental delay: report of the Quality Standards Subcommittee of the American Academy of Neurology and the Practice Committee of the Child Neurology Society. *Neurology, 11*(3), 367–380.

Simpson, J. A., & Weiner, E. S. C. (Eds.). (1989). *Oxford English dictionary* (2nd ed.). Oxford: Clarendon Press.

Small, N., Raghavan, R., & Pawson, N. (2013). An ecological approach to seeking and utilising the views of young people with intellectual disabilities in transition planning. *Journal of Intellectual Disabilities, 17*(4), 283–300.

Stabile, M., & Allin, S. (2012). The economic costs of childhood disability. *Future Child, 22*(1), 65–69.

Stojanovic, J. R., Miletic, A., Peterlin, B., et al. (2019). Diagnostic and clinical utility of clinical exome sequencing in children with moderate and severe global developmental delay/intellectual disability. *Journal of Child Neurology* 8830738 1987983.

Strnadová, I., & Cumming, ThM. (2016). *Lifespan transitions and disability. A holistic perspective.* UK: Routledge.

Toms, G., Totsika, V., Hastings, R., et al. (2015). Access to services by children with intellectual disability and mental health problems: population-based evidence from the UK. *Journal of Intellectual & Developmental Disability, 40*(3), 239–247.

Travers, J., Tincani, M., Whitby, P., et al. (2014). Alignment of sexuality education with self-determination for people with significant disabilities: a review of research and future directions. *Education and Training in Autism and Developmental Disabilities, 49*(2), 232–247.

Treacy, A. C., Taylor, S. S., & Abernathy, T. V. (2018). Sexual health education for individuals with disabilities. A call to action. *American Journal of Sexuality Education, 13*(1), 65–93.

United Nations Educational Scientific and Cultural Organisation (UNESCO). (1994). The Salamanca Statement and Framework for Action on Special Needs Education. Available at: http://www.unesco.org/education/information/nfsunesco/pdf/SALAMA_E.PDF. [Accessed 4 December 2019].

United Nations High Commissioner for Refugees (UNHCR) & Handicap International. (2011). *Need to know guidance: Working with persons with disabilities in forced displacement.* Geneva: UNHCR. Available at: http://www.unhcr.org/4ec3c81c9.pdf. [Accessed 17 January 2021].

United Nations High Commissioner for Refugees (UNHCR). (2013). *Displacement: the new 21st century challenge. UNHCR global trends 2012.* Geneva: UNHCR.

United Nations Children's Fund (UNICEF). (2005). The state of the world's children. Available at: https://www.unicef.org/sowc05/english/childhooddefined.html. [Accessed 12 November 2019].

United Nations Children's Fund (UNICEF). (2018). *Children with disabilities in situations of armed conflict: discussion paper.* UNICEF.

United Nations. (2006). *Convention on the Rights of Persons with Disabilities.* Available at: https://www.un.org/disabilities/documents/convention/convoptprot-e.pdf. [Accessed 29 January 2017].

United Nations. (1989). *Convention on the Rights of the Child.* London: UNICEF UK.

Waizbard-Bartov, E., Yehonatan-Schori, M., & Golan, O. (2019). Personal growth experiences of parents to children with autism spectrum disorder. *Journal of Autism and Developmental Disorders, 49*(4), 1330–1341.

Walker, C. (2015). Ageing and people with learning disabilities: in search of evidence. *British Journal of Learning Disabilities, 43*(4), 246–253.

Walker, C., & Ward, C. (2013). Growing older together: ageing and people with learning disabilities and their family carers. *Tizard Learning Disability Review, 18*(3), 112–119.

Webster, R., & Blatchford, P. (2013). The educational experiences of pupils with a statement for special educational needs in mainstream primary schools: results from a systematic observation study. *European Journal of Special Needs Education, 28*(4), 463–479.

Wendelborg, C., & Tøssebro, J. (2010). Marginalisation processes in inclusive education in Norway: a longitudinal study of classroom participation. *Disability & Society, 25*(6), 701–714.

Winston, R., & Chicot, R. (2016). The importance of early bonding on the long-term mental health and resilience of children. *London Journal of Primary Care, 8*(1), 12–14.

Wissink, I. B., an Vugt, E., Moonen, X., Stams, G. J. J., & Hendriks, J. (2015). Sexual abuse involving children with an intellectual disability (ID): a narrative review. *Research in Developmental Disabilities, 36*, 20–35.

World Health Organisation (WHO). (2010). *Better health, better lives: children and young people with intellectual disabilities and their families.* Geneva: WHO.

World Health Organisation (WHO) and World Bank. (2011). *World report on disability.* Geneva: WHO.

Zahir, F., & Friedman, J. M. (2007). The impact of array genomic hybridization on mental retardation research: a review of current technologies and their clinical utility. *Clinical Genetics, 72*, 271–287.

Zhou, H., Roberts, P., Dhaliwal, S., et al. (2016). Transitioning adolescent and young adults with chronic disease and/or disabilities from paediatric to adult care services – an integrative review. *Journal of Clinical Nursing, 25*(21–22), 3113–3130.

21

Leisure and friendships

Roy McConkey and Theresa Lorenzo

KEY ISSUES

- Friendships, free-time and leisure pursuits add to everyone's quality of life, yet around the world many people with intellectual disabilities lead lonely and unfulfilled lives.
- Our current models of support services may inhibit people from developing a rich social and leisure life.
- A new type of relationship is required between paid staff and the people they support, one that actively promotes the social status of people with intellectual disabilities, creates opportunities for their active participation in community activities, and supports the development of social networks and friendships.
- A primary aim of modern support services should be to link people into the network of community facilities and services in their locality rather than trying to meet their needs within specialist, segregated provision.

CHAPTER OUTLINE

INTRODUCTION

"People with learning (intellectual) disabilities want to lead ordinary lives and do the things that most people take for granted. They want to study at college, get a job, have relationships and friendships, and enjoy leisure and social activities. Many people need support to do these things; and some will need high levels of support on an ongoing basis as well as multi-agency investment to have any kind of meaningful life."

Department of Health (DH), 2009, p. 83

This chapter is primarily aimed at all staff working in services to assist people with intellectual disabilities. As you will read, it is within their gift to promote an active social and leisure life for the people they support rather than inhibiting or indeed denying them this opportunity, albeit unintentionally. Staff must be active partners with self-advocates, family carers and the wider community in the creation of inclusive leisure activities.

Just as leisure and friendships add to the quality of all our lives, so it should be for people with intellectual disabilities, yet many of them lead lonely, unfulfilled lives. In many countries this loneliness is due to the stigma and shame still associated with this disability that forces families to keep their child hidden from others. But this lifestyle persists even when people receive modern support services which ostensibly offer much better opportunities than the institutionalised provision of yesteryear. Hence promoting a richer social life for people with intellectual disabilities has to go beyond the limitations inherent in much of our current service practices and priorities with their focus on disabilities rather than abilities. Rather as Martin Seligman (2011) noted: "removing disabling conditions is not remotely the same as building the enabling conditions of life" (p. 53).

Fundamental to this new approach, is promoting the social status of people with intellectual disabilities. Engagement in community leisure activities can be an ideal means for doing this and in this respect these activities are a means to an end and not just an end in themselves. This theme is examined in the opening section of the chapter. Here too, the contribution of friendships and active leisure activities to the quality of people's lives is summarised as is the impact on their emotional well-being, increased self-reliance and the promotion of positive self-images. Moreover these outcomes can be realised in even the most impoverished settings.

The second section of the chapter describes the solitary and passive nature of the leisure activities of children and adults with intellectual disabilities and outlines the main barriers that inhibit the formation and maintenance of friendships and their participation in more active leisure pursuits. This section challenges the priorities and presumptions that underlie service provision based on a 'deficit' or 'care' model. An alternative approach based around *creating opportunities* is proposed.

The third section of the chapter describes the supports (both personal and contextual) that encourage the formation of social networks out of which leisure pursuits and friendships can emerge. A particular feature is the mediating role that paid support staff can play in supporting friendships and the qualities required to achieve this goal. But the contribution made by befrienders is arguably especially more valuable in low resource countries. The goal, nonetheless, is the same; individuals are empowered to experience mutual relationships within expanded social networks.

Throughout the chapter two questions reoccur on which readers need to ponder. Might our current models of support services in health and social care actually inhibit people from developing a rich social and leisure life? Is a new type of relationship required between professional staff and the people they support?

THE SOCIAL STATUS OF PEOPLE WITH INTELLECTUAL DISABILITIES

People with intellectual disabilities don't have a high status within society. In part it's because most people across the world have little contact with this group. Second, the public's image of them, admittedly perceived through the media, remains one of helplessness. Third, people in local communities are reluctant to have personal contact; fearing that they would not know what to say or how to react (McConkey, 2019).

We also have to admit that the special services for this group have done them no favours in raising their status. The era of long-stay institutions may be drawing to a close in more affluent countries but the memory lingers on. *'Putting people away'* implied worthlessness; even a threat to the well-being of others in the family or community.

Yet the community services that have replaced them – be they special schools, group homes or day centres – also have a glass wall around them that keeps people with intellectual disabilities apart from society. And while the public commonly applaud the patience and dedication of staff working in such services, they frequently go on to add: "*I could never do your job*". The implicit message is clear – special people need special staff. In fact the predominant rationale for many of the specialist services for people with intellectual disabilities can reinforce negative stereotypes of them as the following examples illustrate

- The **'social care model'** as found in residential care homes, nursing homes and day centres - creates and reinforces images of people who need looking after. And not just among the general public but also relatives, visitors and even the staff who work there.
- The **'treatment model'** as typified by challenging behaviour teams and therapists admitting people to 'assessment and treatment' units - implies that these are people who need to be 'fixed' because of some underlying abnormality.
- The **'training model'**, as represented by special needs courses at Further Education Colleges and vocational training centres can unwittingly imply people's incompetence; geared as they are to low-level skills and courses that result in no accredited awards.

BOX 21.1 The parable of the fish

If the fish in a stream were dying, we would not assume that we could solve the problem by pulling the fish out of the stream and allowing them to swim in a clean fish tank for 30 minutes each day, and then returning them to the stream for the remainder of the day.

Rather we would begin a systematic search to find out what was causing the fish to die. If the health of the fish were important to us we would do what was necessary to restore the health of the stream so that the fish could thrive. *Mary Taylor.*

Of course these various models of services may be justified on other grounds but what is especially concerning is when the personnel working in them do little to challenge the negative images created and leave to someone else the task of promoting community integration and social inclusion, just like the parable of the fish (see Box 21.1).

However social inclusion will only be achieved when everyone takes responsibility for it, no matter which service they work in or the type of job they do. This chapter is targeted at *all* staff working in services that support people with intellectual disabilities; be they in specialist disability provision, mainstream services or community-based rehabilitation. Promoting leisure opportunities cannot be left to specialists with new titles such as 'befriender co-ordinator' or 'community link workers'. Such people or services may have a contribution to make but we contend that their efforts will be considerably enhanced if they performed their roles as part of a partnership with all the other people of influence in the person's life.

Enhancing the social status of marginalised groups

In the last two decades we have gained a better understanding as to how the social inclusion of marginalised people, such as those with disabilities, can be enhanced. The foundation stone is to actively enhance the social status of the excluded group while being clear about their rights within society (World Health Organisation (WHO) and World Bank, 2011). It's a generation since the United Nations first proclaimed the rights of disabled persons in 1976 but this has been updated by the Convention of Rights of Persons with Disabilities (United Nations, 2006). Article 30 of this convention states:

> *"the right of persons with disabilities to take part on an equal basis with others …. in recreational, leisure and sporting activities."*

These rights-based statements resulted from many years of lobbying by disabled activists, family carers and professionals to ensure that people with disabilities had access to the same opportunities as other citizens and to put an end to discriminatory practices. Even the general public acknowledges the marginalisation and exclusion of people with intellectual disabilities. In a national opinion survey undertaken in Ireland, only 39% agreed that people with intellectual disabilities are able to participate fully in life (McConkey, 2019). So, statements of rights and even specific legislation alone are unlikely to produce changes in people's mind-sets and attitudes.

People with disabilities face the negative consequences of ongoing discrimination. In a national survey in England, about one-third of the nearly 3,000 people interviewed stated that someone had been rude or abusive to them in the past year because of their intellectual disabilities (Emerson et al, 2005). Likewise in developing countries women with intellectual disabilities are the targets for sexual exploitation and abuse (Lorenzo and Kathard, 2018). There are still many miles to go in the pursuit of full acceptance and respect for all citizens in modern societies.

Valued social roles

Wolfensberger (1972), the Canadian sociologist, long championed the need to reduce the devalued status of people whom society views as different. He identified four means for enhancing their social status and their potency has been confirmed in the decades since.

Project positive images of disability

The various talents of people with disabilities need to be promoted and we don't just mean in the media; too often their failings and incompetence are stressed by service staff. This negativity can easily go unnoticed. Perhaps we need to rebalance the wording of our assessment reports, team briefings, service brochures, fundraising appeals, and be more careful of the images we paint through word-of-mouth.

People with intellectual disabilities also need to be given opportunities to prove themselves and have their successes applauded. That is how their self-confidence and self-esteem grows. This growth in turn changes other people's perceptions as well. Ordinary activities of leisure and work provide an ideal context for stimulating this growth globally, such as creative arts and sporting achievements (Darragh et al, 2016).

Use ordinary settings

People who are different have to be seen in the ordinary settings of shops, bars and buses; in schools, colleges and businesses; and in socially valued settings such as on television programmes, in theatres and concerts. Community presence may work best when it involves individuals or pairs of people rather than larger groups of people with intellectual disabilities, and for them to be seen in the company of their peers who are non-disabled, emphasising their equal status.

Create social exchanges

People lose some of the stigma of their disability as they meet and mix with others. The public's reaction is often "*they're not as different as I thought!*" However, for people meeting a person with an intellectual disability for the first time, this interaction needs to happen in a planned and purposeful way, perhaps based around a shared activity in a familiar setting to reduce their apprehensions. There are numerous opportunities for facilitating such interactions in any community from schools to sports, and clubs to pubs (McConkey et al, 2009).

Expect achievement

People with intellectual disabilities may be slow to learn but they can learn as various chapters in this book illustrate. Moreover their initial attempts are often no predictor of ultimate success in learning. So beware of giving up too soon! If we do not expect achievement then we will not persevere in encouraging people to learn, which in turn will impact on their self-confidence and motivation. They may come to feel it is safer not to take on new challenges rather than risk failure.

So what do services need to do in order to ensure that people with intellectual disabilities take on valued social roles within society? Obviously creating new images of this group is a crucial first step but in itself is insufficient to ensure their inclusion in society. We might gain some clues by considering how this occurs for others within society. Children are an example as are other marginalised groups such as immigrants and refugees. Remarkably the same strategies apply in human societies around the world.

PROMOTING SOCIAL INCLUSION THROUGH LEISURE

Alongside schools and workplaces, leisure pursuits are a major means through which we become integrated within our communities not only in childhood but as teenagers, adults and older people. A brief reflection quickly identifies why this integration occurs and the benefits it can bring:

- Leisure pursuits are usually done in the company of others. It is possible to spend all of your free-time alone, but this is the exception. Shared activities provide opportunities for conversations, for working together to achieve a common outcome and for helping each other out when the need arises.
- Leisure embraces a huge diversity of activities which means that individual preferences and talents can be accommodated. Everyone does not need to do the same thing, people can be directed towards the activities that suit them best.
- Leisure offers opportunities for personal growth and development. Admittedly this happens more so in some situations than in others but then people are wise to this and they move on when they have exhausted the possibilities and before boredom sets in.
- Through leisure we can demonstrate our talents, obtain a sense of achievement and gain a more positive self-image. The affirmation of others is especially necessary in creating a sense of being needed.
- Participation in active leisure pursuits brings positive benefits to children and adolescents in terms of their overall feelings of happiness and improved self-concept which does not happen with passive activities such as PlayStations or watching television.
- Friendship, good social relations and strong supportive networks improve people's health at home, at work and in the community. Although well attested with non-disabled persons (Wilkinson and Marmot, 2003), these findings are likely to be just as true, if not more so, for people with intellectual disabilities.

- The availability of communication technology and social media such as mobile phones, Facebook and Skype enables people to maintain contact especially for those with physical, visual and/or hearing impairments albeit accessibility barriers remain to be overcome (Lorenzo et al, 2018).

Processes not products

But people don't just engage in leisure for the sake of the activity; people may train hard at sports, attend choir practices and frequent discos, but it is not just the activity that's important, they value the companionship, the sense of achievement and the opportunity to chat with others. This line of argument gives rise to a variant of the chicken and egg conundrum as to which comes first – do people need the talents and competences before they can start to join in leisure pursuits, or do they acquire these competences through active participation in leisure pursuits? The answer is likely to be a bit of both. You probably take part in certain leisure activities because you have some of the required skills but you persist in the hope that your tennis, photography, dancing or whatever can get better.

Strangely this freedom is often not given to people with intellectual disabilities. Rather the dominant attitude has tended to stress the need to 'prepare' them to take part in community activities and for them to prove themselves competent before they are considered 'ready' for leisure pursuits with others (Gjermestad et al, 2017). A similar attitude kept many people living in institutions for far longer than they needed to, as the more competent persons were selected first. Likewise certain people now living in group homes may not be taken on outings because they may 'create a scene'.

Such attitudes are doubly disadvantaging. People are not given the opportunity to learn in settings that are supportive of their learning and yet they have to meet the same standards of non-disabled people when there. It is rather like saying that a person will never learn to swim and then giving them no opportunity to go to the swimming pool. That's called a self-fulfilling prophecy and people with intellectual disabilities have no need for prophets of doom.

Failure of opportunities

A radical conclusion also emerges from this debate; could it be that people with intellectual disabilities are incompetent not because of their impairments but because they have not been given the same opportunities to learn as their non-disabled peers? This view harmonises with the position of disabled activists who promote a social, rather than medical model of disability (Oliver, 1996). Rather than focusing on a person's deficits, the emphasis is on creating equal opportunities for participation and inclusion. For example, Valuing People Now (DH, 2009) outlined some of the ways service thinking needs to change in England to bring this about but their proposals are applicable internationally:

- work in close partnership with families as well as other services and link into broader community developments ...
- think beyond nine-to-five working days and include evenings and weekends;
- invest in making community-based facilities and settings that are accessible for all; and
- develop a clear de-commissioning strategy that shows how money will be drawn down from traditional services and re-invested in wider opportunities (p. 83).

Likewise the World Health Organization's Guidelines (2010) on community based rehabilitation emphasise the involvement of people with disabilities and their families in decision making and the mobilisation of resources at a local community level to facilitate participation and inclusion. To further illustrate some of the key points made in this section, here is a Reader Activity for you to try.

 READER ACTIVITY 21.1 Keeping a diary

Identify a person with an intellectual disability who you know well.

Keep a diary for one week (7 days) of all the activities they do morning, afternoon and evening.

Note also the people with whom they did the activities or who were present with them.

Once you have the information you can identify how many activities were outside of their home, how many could be classed as active pursuits and how many they did with their friends rather than with staff support.

People's aspirations

Most people with intellectual disabilities aspire to have the same opportunities as their non-disabled peers (Merrells et al, 2018). For example, in Spain, Badia et al (2013) interviewed nearly 240 people and found that they wanted more social and physical activities. Kampert and Gorenczny (2007) found that increased community involvement and more socialisation opportunities were the most common desires expressed by over 250 individuals in Pennsylvania, USA. Likewise, having meaningful activities and spending time socialising and meeting other people, were the dominant themes in interviews undertaken with 87 people from a range of services in England and Scotland (Miller et al, 2008). So too in Northern Ireland, social activities were the most commonly selected goals when over 120 people were invited to identify three things they would like to try in the coming six to nine months; with entertainment and sporting activities the next most popular (McConkey and Collins, 2010a).

But having friends was just as important as the activities. When Murray (2002) sought the views of over 100 young people with a range of disabilities through various participatory methods, she concluded:

"Whilst opportunities to try out a range of leisure activities and pursuits are appreciated, it is the opportunity to be in mutually valued relationships that young disabled people identify as the key to the possibility of their inclusion in mainstream culture."

Murray, 2002, p. 70

The remainder of this chapter examines how these governmental and personal aspirations can be put into practice.

REMOVING BARRIERS TO ACTIVE LEISURE

If the aspiration, motivation and potential competence is there, what is it that stops people with intellectual disabilities from participating in active leisure pursuits? When asked, they are well aware of the barriers they face. Emerson et al (2005) and Lorenzo et al (2018) identified two main ones: limited and/or inaccessible transport and minimal support from friends and carers.

The informants in the focus groups organised by Abbott and McConkey (2006) also noted insufficient or inaccessible community amenities which was compounded by the location of people's living accommodation. But they also highlighted the influence of service staff and management on the options provided for them as did Miller et al (2008). The participants in this study also recounted further barriers arising from staffing of services, namely continuity of staffing in people's lives and the shortage of staffing.

Finally, barriers exist within community amenities. For instance Brodin (2009) found in a survey of Swedish municipalities that the absence of trained staff and financial constraints were the twin barriers in making outdoor education more accessible to adults with intellectual disabilities.

But significant as these barriers are, perhaps there are two more fundamental ones to promoting leisure pursuits for people with intellectual disabilities, particularly in more affluent countries; namely our conceptions of leisure and the role of support staff in services.

DEFINITIONS OF LEISURE

Leisure is often interpreted as activities undertaken in our 'free-time' after work is completed. But how meaningful is this interpretation for people whose lives consist solely of free-time? With them, the term 'pass-time' is probably a more appropriate one in that the goal is to find activities primarily as a means for passing the time for them; hence the dominance of watching television, listening to music or playing computer games in their leisure repertoires. Moreover these pastimes make little demand on support staff or family carers in that when people are occupied in them, they can get on with their own work. Thus it is easy to convince ourselves that people have a life full of leisure – so what more do they want?

If, however, we viewed leisure in terms of active pursuits in which people invest energy, enthusiasm, effort and enjoyment, then we would be more conscious of how bereft of leisure their lives really are. Of course people themselves realise this gap as indeed do the family carers of children and teenagers (Overmars-Marx et al, 2019) but it is rare for support services to acknowledge the lack of active pursuits.

It has been argued that an active leisure life is the main means of providing a better quality of life for those people for whom employment and/or independent living is less likely to be an option (Patterson and Pegg, 2009). Stebbins (2000) coined the phrase 'serious leisure' which he defined as:

"the systematic pursuit of an amateur, hobbyist, or volunteer core activity that is highly substantial, interesting, and fulfilling and where, in the typical case, participants find a career in acquiring and expressing a combination of its special skills, knowledge, and experience."

Stebbins, 2000, p. 3

Enabling people to become leisure activists requires more systematic support strategies around this outcome than happens in services at present. But the realisation of this need only becomes apparent when we reconceptualise the meaning of leisure and why it is important to do so; two themes we will return to in the third section of the chapter.

ROLE OF SERVICES AND SUPPORT STAFF

A second fundamental barrier is the role of staff in support services. This finds expression in different ways: firstly, in terms of personal support. McConkey and Collins (2010b) surveyed 245 staff working in either supported living schemes, shared residential and group homes, or in day centres. Staff were asked to rate, in terms of priority to their job, 16 tasks that were supportive of social inclusion and a further 16 tasks that related to the care of the person they supported. Across all three service settings, staff rated more care tasks as having higher priority than they did the social inclusion tasks. The staff who were most inclined to rate social inclusion tasks as NOT being applicable to their job were those working in day centres; female rather than male staff, those in front-line jobs rather than senior staff, and those in part-time or relief positions rather than full-time posts. Thus there could be sizeable proportions of staff who do little to actively support the social and community engagement of the people in their services. Clement and Bigby (2009) go on to suggest that staff working with individuals who have more severe and profound disabilities see them as so different that terms such as 'inclusion' were not meaningful for them.

Pockney (2006) identified another dilemma for staff. People receiving support are much more inclined to name staff as their friends but not the other way round. Staff may be wary of encouraging an over-friendly relationship with individuals particularly through involving them in their own social networks. Activities done with a group of persons rather than as a 'two-some' provide an additional safeguard for staff even though group outings rarely provide opportunities for people to extend their social networks by meeting and becoming acquainted with others (Lippold and Burns, 2009).

At another level, services may fail to maintain or extend the social connectedness of people they have supported over periods of time. Bigby (2008) examined the informal relationships of a randomly selected group of people who had been resettled from Australian institutions into community-based accommodation. After five years, the residents had not formed any new relationships and the numbers in touch with family members had decreased. Similar findings have been reported in Ireland for people moving to personalised accommodation and support from congregate settings (McConkey et al, 2019).

When the perennial problems of staff turn-over and shortages of staffing are added in, then it is no surprise that there are major failures in supporting people to maintain friendships and preferred activities outside of the home. This is crucial when people move from one service to another, notably young people leaving school or people moving from the family home into supported accommodation. Taken together, these barriers provide formidable obstacles for support services and their staff to create a more active and social lifestyle for people with intellectual disabilities. But they can be overcome.

CREATING ACTIVE AND SOCIAL LIFESTYLES

Figure 21.1 summarises the proposals that people with intellectual disabilities identified for overcoming the four types of barriers they experienced to their social inclusion which were described above (Abbott and McConkey, 2006). Person-centred planning events, team meetings of support staff and periodic reviews of services all provide opportunities for changes to be made in the way individuals are supported to overcome the specific barriers they face.

However, three broad strategies hold particular promise for most individuals (Louw et al, 2019).

- Creating social opportunities so that people meet and mix with others in society.
- Identifying informal supporters or 'befrienders' with mutual interests who can mentor their companions with disabilities in social situations.
- Generating opportunities for people to make useful contributions which other people value, and from which they benefit.

Although these three dimensions are inter-related we will examine each one in turn. As you will read, leisure pursuits – along with having paid work – offer all these opportunities but remember, it is not the product of the activity on which its value is judged but rather what the person gains through participating.

READER ACTIVITY 21.2   Assessing social inclusion

On the list of activities below, tick off those you have done in the past four weeks.

Then talk to, or think about, one or more people with intellectual disabilities whom you know. Tick off the activities they have done in the past four weeks.

Put a circle around those the person did on their own or with their friends (rather than with support staff or when attending day centres).

Are there any differences between the listings? Why is this?

How many different activities did the people with intellectual disabilities do on their own or with friends?

What does this activity tell you about their opportunities to have an active social and leisure life?

Activities	I have done	Person 1 has done	Person 2 has done
Out for a walk with one or two others			
Had an outing by car with others			
Gone on a bus, train journey			
Been in a café/restaurant/pub			
Been to shopping centres/supermarkets			
Visited park/beach/outdoor events and places			
Been to cinema, theatre, concerts, museums			
Been to swimming pool, water parks			
Watched sports events – football, rugby, ice-hockey			
Took part in *outdoor* sports/activities with others e.g. football, cricket, tennis.			
Took part in *indoor* sports/activities with others – gym, karate, bowling, darts, snooker			
Had a holiday/weekend break			
Attended church, religious celebrations			
Been to dance/drama/art classes			
Gone to discos/clubbing			
Had a friend to visit at home.			
Had a friend to sleep-over			
Visited a friend/relative at his/her house			
Slept over at a friend's house			
Had party/celebration at home			
Please list any other leisure activities not covered by the above			

Widening social networks

How might we widen people's social networks? Left to their own devices, people with intellectual disabilities often fail to meet and get on with other people. Many lack the conversational skills and social graces needed to initiate interactions with strangers. They may have even greater difficulties locating opportunities in their neighbourhood for socialising and finding their way to them. What they need is a match-maker! Someone who knows the needs, interests and talents of the person with a disability but also who knows what's going on in the locality or is capable of tracking down possible opportunities, such as social clubs, church groups, yoga classes, educational activities not forgetting more informal opportunities such as visiting friends. It certainly helps if support staff are from the same neighbourhood and have grown up in it. They will then be very familiar with the people and amenities it has to offer. Research on the role of community rehabilitation workers

Personal ability and skills

- Access to appropriate skills training (literacy/numeracy/budgeting/independent travel).
- Getting to know the neighbourhood.
- Encouragement from staff to socialise.
- Information, access and encouragement towards a healthy lifestyle.

Staff and management

- Being listened to by staff and managers.
- Support to make your own plans and go out independently.
- More staff available for one-to-one support or better use of available advocacy and volunteer groups to do this.
- Up-to-date information on community opportunities.
- Enabled to live independently.

The community

- Education of the community – schools etc.
- Accessible information provided on activities/events.
- Make links with community through Open Days in services
- More advocates and volunteers to accompany individuals
- Increased use of existing (mainstream) facilities and activities.

The home/scheme

- Use of a named driver/known local taxi firm.
- Support to access activities available locally.
- Free/affordable/accessible transport options.
- Taught/allowed to use public transport.

Figure 21.1 Suggested solutions to the barriers to social inclusion by people with intellectual disabilities

in Southern Africa found that they were able to foster inclusion, coordinate access to services, act as mentors and supporters to both disabled and non-disabled youth, and provide information to facilitate participation in community development activities, including social activities (van Pletzen et al, 2014). Staff living elsewhere and coming to work in a different area, should make the effort to find out about the community in which their work is based. Sadly, few managers and staff think to do this.

The next step is arguably the more difficult. The matchmaker has to ask if people are prepared to welcome new members. Schwartz (1992) identified this simple task as one of the most crucial weapons in the armoury of social connectors. Equally he notes the reluctance there can be on the part of professional staff and carers to ask favours of others. Why?

- Perhaps because they are afraid of being rejected; people may say no? Yet experience and research suggests that the majority of people are disposed to be of assistance and very few would ever be rude and critical in refusing to participate (Bigby and Wiesel, 2019).
- Or maybe staff and carers feel that no one can quite measure up to the task or that there are too many risks involved? So they continue to shoulder the responsibility.

Again experience shows that professional staff and carers tend to over-estimate risk and they do not consider that the person with an intellectual disability may respond differently to the 'new' person and setting (see Chapter 6 for more on the issue of risk and response to risk).

- Or more worrying, could it be that they feel there is nothing in it for the other person; that there are no benefits to befriending a person with an intellectual disability? Yet family carers and voluntary helpers are so much more adapt at naming these benefits than are professional staff (Ferrer et al, 2016).

Having found people, the next crucial role of the matchmaker is that of introducing them to one another. Like a good host or hostess, the matchmaker needs to put the two sets of people at their ease by facilitating the conversation, modelling interactions, suggesting joint activities for them to do and when the opportunity arises, discretely withdrawing for a time so that they take on the responsibility for maintaining the interaction.

Finally, the matchmaker needs to be supportive of the blooming partnerships by keeping in touch with both parties; checking how things are going; making discrete suggestions and subtly praising them for how well they are coping with the challenge.

Rarely are these connecting tasks written into the job descriptions of professional workers nor are people recruited to these jobs for their 'people-making' skills. Paradoxically though, most of us acquire these skills and utilise them in our personal lives so perhaps their deployment in the service of people with intellectual disabilities could be readily promoted if only the will to do so was there!

Of course certain circumstances can make it easier to create and extend people's social networks (Shelley et al, 2018). Renewing former acquaintances is one strategy that has been used to re-connect people with intellectual disabilities with peers they may have known in years gone by at school, day centres or long-stay hospitals. A similar strategy has proved effective for people to reconnect with family members with whom they may have lost touch (Mihaila et al, 2020). Invitations to visit the person with an intellectual disability in their home can be a useful starting point. Yet it is surprising how few people are encouraged to use their homes in cities or towns as a place for meeting others (Emerson and McVilley, 2004); it happens more easily in villages and rural areas.

Another fruitful strategy can be connecting people with others who have intellectual disabilities, particularly when people have control over the group's activities as happens in advocacy groups (see Chapter 7 for more on self-advocacy groups). Some groups now provide a range of services and supports to their members including educational classes, social events, income generation and holiday breaks. These also provide opportunities for closer and more intimate relationships to develop (see Chapter 25).

Modern technology also offers opportunities for people to keep in touch with their friends. Just as people with intellectual disabilities have learnt to use mobile phones, so too with some tutoring and practice they could master using Skype, email and social networking sites on their tablets or smartphones. As these become cheaper and more portable, they offer new opportunities for people to connect with others, provided they have the support to get started (Den Brok et al, 2015). But as discussed in the previous chapter of this book there can be barriers that need acknowledging and overcoming.

Befriending and mentoring

Getting people involved in active leisure pursuits requires more than support from staff or access to social networks. A promising option is to recruit 'befrienders' or 'buddies' who are of similar age, background and interests to the person needing support and who are willing to share some of their leisure time with a chosen partner (Southby, 2019). Although befriending may start as a contrived relationship, it can grow into more genuine, lasting friendships.

Another approach is the recruitment of peer mentors with the aim of developing the social and communication skills required by people with intellectual disabilities to participate successfully in community life (Wilson et al, 2013). The mentors are often more suited to this task than professional staff as they have more time to spend with the person with an intellectual disability, they can establish more equal relationships and may have greater insights into the issues that youth face in their society.

A variety of strategies can be used to recruit befrienders or mentors, including newspaper and radio adverts, but the most successful has been through word-of-mouth from people who already have some involvement, such as other staff in the services or their network of family and friends. Interested persons need the opportunity to gradually 'opt-in' through a series of meetings so that they become fully aware of all that is involved. Careful vetting procedures also need to be in place. A contact person needs to be nominated whom befrienders and mentors can easily contact at any time if they have queries or if they encounter any problems. They have a vital role in proactively supporting the befrienders and mentors especially in giving them feedback on the importance of their contribution. Other key factors to forming stable relationships include a notably strong orientation process, appropriate matching and a high degree of reciprocity in the experience (Wymer and Starnes, 2001).

Most befrienders and mentors do not receive any payment although their expenses should be re-imbursed. Most are offered a time-limited commitment, say for 12 months, which can be renewed if all is going well. Equally they can honourably withdraw when their commitment has been fulfilled.

Befriending and mentoring can occur as stand-alone schemes to support community inclusion but the ethos of both can often be combined in other activities. Three contrasting examples follow.

Participation in sports

The Special Olympics movement has demonstrated internationally, the latent willingness there can be in communities to befriending and mentoring people with intellectual disabilities. Although the focus is on playing sport – and there are many to choose from – the mentoring provided by coaches extends into wider social skills while the volunteers offer the friendship and encouragement needed to nurture self-confidence and self-esteem (Tint et al, 2017). The Unified Sports initiative, in which combined teams of players with and without disabilities train and compete together, provides opportunities for meaningful peer-to-peer friendships that will further social inclusion beyond the sports field (McConkey et al, 2013). Similar opportunities may be provided through Paralympics, the International Sports Federation for Persons with Intellectual Disability as well as mainstream sporting clubs and national sports bodies.

Family placement

Family placement schemes are another example of befriending and mentoring (Robertson et al, 2011). Here people with disabilities – adults as well as children – are placed with carefully selected families for day-time breaks or overnight stays in their home. Although initially intended to provide a 'respite' break for family carers, these schemes also provide opportunities for the person with an intellectual disability to become part of another social network, and to experience the leisure pursuits that the host families are involved in. Indeed some family carers also comment on the relationship they have built up with the host family and how the schemes have widened their social and support networks. In some countries adults with intellectual disabilities live with the host families fulltime as an alternative to residential placements.

Circles of friends

Another approach attracting much interest recently is that of creating 'circles of support' or 'circles of friends' (Duggan and Linehan, 2013). Reader activity 21.3 in the accompanying online resource encourages you to develop these with the people you support. There is no prescription for the form and format these take as they will be guided very much by the wishes and needs of the person with an intellectual disability as identified in their person-centred plan. That said there are some common strands in such circles They might include family members – siblings, cousins, aunts and uncles; neighbours and acquaintances; co-workers for people in work settings; members of clubs, churches and such

like who know the person. The circle deliberately does NOT have professional workers as members although they can have a key role as facilitators or 'go-betweens' in starting the circles. In developing countries in particular, families have been identified as an anchor and catalyst for the participation of disabled youth in sport, recreation and other free time activities (Lorenzo et al, 2018). Likewise occupational therapy students who are required to do service learning as part of their training, have worked with Community Rehabilitation Workers to help communities support disabled youth to take action that promotes their active citizenship and their participation in sport, recreation and cultural activities and events in their communities (Lorenzo et al, 2015).

The depth of friendship will vary across the members of the circle. Some may be prepared to be intimately involved; others will continue as acquaintances but they will be better informed than previously. The circle can seek out social, educational, employment as well as leisure opportunities and support people within them (Mental Health Foundation, 2020).

The idea of circles of support can find expression in other ways. For example, Key Ring (n.d.) is a housing provider for people with intellectual disabilities that works by building up mutually supportive networks among the tenants living within a geographical area as well as linking them into the communities where they live. Likewise new forms of day provision often operate on the basis of creating social networks for their clients by slotting them into educational, employment and recreational opportunities in the community (Towell, 1988). As yet, there have been few formal evaluations of these networks as to whether or not they fulfil their promise but informal feedback from members is very positive.

Likewise in less affluent countries, community rehabilitation workers are well placed to build support systems in local communities for mothers and caregivers of children with disabilities who have expressed the need for respite. They have created safe social spaces for youth with disabilities to socialise with others, for example, watching sport at stadiums or on television together in a club (Lorenzo et al, 2018).

Potential drawbacks

The success of befriending and mentoring schemes is not guaranteed. Steps must be taken to overcome some of their potential drawbacks.

- The matching of 'friends' is often done by a professional worker or scheme coordinator, which means that the person with an intellectual disability has very limited scope for choosing and developing their own friendships.
- The 'friendship' that develops runs the risk of being artificial in the sense that the non-disabled person is invariably cast in the role of helper and supervisor. Through time these expectations can place quite a strain on the relationship.
- If the non-disabled person is no longer able or willing to continue, there is the added problem of finding a replacement while dealing with possible feelings of disappointment and loss in the person left behind.
- The befriender approach is an example of adopting a specialist solution to a disability issue but therein lies the major risk of all; a befriender absolves everyone else – busy support staff and social workers for example – from their responsibilities of nurturing friendships and leisure opportunities for the people with whom they work.

Creating opportunities for contributions

Notions of helplessness pervade many people's perceptions of adults with intellectual disabilities. Many appeals for donations are based on this premise but this approach further alienates them from society as people in need of charity. In reality, many more people with intellectual disabilities could be active contributors to society if given the opportunities, preparation and support. We highlight two areas in particular; household tasks and voluntary work.

Household tasks

One area that is easily overlooked in helping people to become contributors is that of household tasks. Skills such as vacuuming and cleaning floors are a necessary part of housekeeping but they can also be deployed in various kinds of employment. Window cleaning, gardening, cooking, ironing and car washing can be a hobby for some and an additional source of income for others. It also equips them for entertaining visitors in their home and relieves support staff from extra chores that otherwise might fall on them. But perhaps the biggest gain is that when people are seen to be competent in one area such as housekeeping, then more comes to be expected of them. Maybe they could go alone to the shop …. stay over with friends … cut the neighbour's grass.

Front-line staff working in services are 'expert' in household chores and in their own families. Many will have taught and encouraged their partners and children to acquire these skills. Why then do so many staff (and parents, it has to be said) do the housework for people with intellectual disabilities rather than supporting them to learn to do it for themselves? We suspect it is a systems failure. The social care model is so pervasive that people come to see their jobs as looking after people; who like the elderly or the chronically ill, cannot be expected to do things for themselves. Other services which espouse person-centredness and following clients' choices, are reluctant to force the issue of housework if clients opt not to learn. Indeed some advocates will proclaim that it is what staff are paid to do, so why should they do the housework? Both of these explanations bring us back to the central ethos of our support services and the vision we hold for the lives of people with intellectual disabilities. In the words of the United Nations Rights statement, is it to give them: *"full participation and inclusion"*?

Voluntary work

Another undeveloped area is the potential for people to undertake voluntary work that benefits others. This work can be a substitute for paid employment when job opportunities are scarce or people are unable to fully meet the demands of an employer (see Chapter 23). But voluntary work provides positive benefits such as opportunities to meet and to work alongside other people and even to pursue particular interests and hobbies alongside personal gains, such as increased self-confidence, improved social skills, larger social networks and acquiring practical and work skills (Trembath et al, 2010).

As with other job opportunities, people need preparation and training in order to succeed as volunteers. The issue is: who provides this? Enrolling for classes in further education and vocational training is one possibility, but probably the best way is learning on-the-job with the help of a mentor or a 'job coach' (see Chapter 23). This person could be a specialist worker from a training and employment agency but equally they might get support from a Community Based Rehabilitation worker already assisting the person with an intellectual disability in their home, or another volunteer engaged in the work takes on the job of training the new recruit. Arrangements must be in place too for ongoing monitoring and support.

Sadly, many mainstream volunteer agencies whose remit covers recruitment and training have been slow to embrace the concept of people with disabilities as volunteers. But maybe they reflect the perceptions held by support staff who don't see volunteering as an opportunity but rather a risk too far.

OPPORTUNITIES AND RISKS

It's appropriate that we end with the most challenging aspect of creating social and leisure opportunities for people with intellectual disabilities: the management of risk. Old definitions of the condition we now call 'intellectual disability' made mention of the person's inability to "*guard against common dangers*". They were also considered not to be responsible for their actions if mishaps occurred. In recent years, Health and Safety Legislation plus policies on the Protection of Vulnerable Adults coupled with the regulation and inspection of services has encouraged service providers to minimise any risks to the people in their care. Although the intentions are laudable, one unfortunate consequence is that service users are very often denied opportunities because of the increased risk they are perceived to pose. People cannot go swimming because there is no trained lifeguard at the pool; tenants in a supported living scheme cannot go to the shops unaccompanied; and teenagers are discouraged from using public transport.

The underlying presumption of their need for constant protection is, however, open to question – people with intellectual disabilities should be supported to take responsibility for their decisions and actions. This will enable them to become more self-reliant and less dependent on others. As yet, remarkably little research has been undertaken in how this can happen. We are equally ignorant of how best to achieve a balance between minimising risks and creating opportunities.

A few pointers are self-evident. First, risk has to be judged for each individual. It cannot be based on a person's membership of a group. In this respect the person's competences and personality have to be considered alongside their previous experience of making decisions and managing risks. But how do they gain these experiences unless given the opportunity to do so?

Second, the nature of risk varies from one context to another. The hazards associated with riding a bicycle to work are different to staying alone in the house overnight. Reduced competence in one should not preclude

the other. Yet staff prohibitions are often based on such generalisations.

Third, people's perceptions of risk vary; most teenagers see fewer dangers than do their parents (McConkey and Smyth, 2003). Similarly staff or family carers tend to be more risk aversive than young adults with intellectual disabilities. Who is to say, their perceptions are invalid?

Chapter 6 explores these issues in greater detail. Suffice to say, that denying people opportunities on the grounds of risk is no longer a valid option. Rather the onus is placed on supporters to find the opportunities in which risk can be successfully managed.

CONCLUSION

Hopefully this chapter has given you a new vision as to how people with intellectual disabilities can lead more fulfilled lives. Some readers will dismiss the ideas as idealistic; citing individuals with certain complex needs as examples as to why change is not possible for everyone or anyone! Others will maintain that the community is not a safe place for vulnerable people and efforts to place them there, will encounter avoidable risks. These viewpoints have some validity but it is question of balance. To date, the numbers of people who have had the opportunities for socialising, contributing and taking responsibility are small. But they are a growing number. People with Down syndrome, for instance, have successfully attained GCSEs, passed their driving test, obtained paid work in McDonalds, live in their own flat and married the love of their life!

These successes, and others like them, did not come about by chance. Three key strategies were employed

1. **Looking beyond special services.** The opportunities provided by the wider society are more adept at creating the types of opportunities outlined in this chapter than are so-called 'specialist' services. Hence a primary aim of modern services should be to link people into the network of ordinary services rather than trying to meet their needs solely within specialist provision

2. **Supporting people to be where they want or need to be.** Services directed at leisure and work should not take place in special buildings, exclusively for people with intellectual disabilities. Rather they should be created around people who share a common activity and purpose, and where people with intellectual disabilities will be supported to take their place within these networks.

3. **Believing that change is possible.** It's easy to think that a person with a disability can never change or have a better life. But that becomes a self-fulfilling prophecy. Rather we need to be adaptive and creative in helping people to become what they could be and in managing the risks encountered along the way

The novelist Chinua Achebe pictures creation as an ongoing process, we might even call it re-creation. He writes,

"It is early on creation day. There is still a lot ahead of us. There is the afternoon up to the evening. And so it's important to understand that the world is very young. There is a lot of work to do. This is our task ... to improve the human world."

Achebe, 2004, p. 35

Thankfully we have the knowledge to make the human world more inclusive of all its members, now all we need is the political, spiritual, mental, physical and emotional will to do so.

REFERENCES

Abbott, S., & McConkey, R. (2006). The barriers to social inclusion as perceived by people with intellectual disabilities. *Journal of Intellectual Disabilities*, 10(3), 275–287.

Achebe, C. (2004). *Hands that shape humanity: little book of wisdom*. Mayfair: Capetown.

Badia, M., Orgaz, M. B., Verdugo, M. A., et al. (2013). Patterns and determinants of leisure participation of youth and adults with developmental disabilities. *Journal of Intellectual Disability Research*, 57(4), 319–332.

Bigby, C. (2008). Known well by no-one: trends in the informal social networks of middle-aged and older people with intellectual disability five years after moving to the community. *Journal of Intellectual & Developmental Disability*, 33(2), 148–157.

Bigby, C., & Wiesel, I. (2019). Using the concept of encounter to further the social inclusion of people with intellectual disabilities: what has been learned? *Research and Practice in Intellectual and Developmental Disabilities*, 6(1), 39–51.

Brodin, J. (2009). Inclusion through access to outdoor education: learning in motion (LIM). *Journal of Adventure Education and Outdoor Learning*, 9(2), 99–113.

Clement, T., & Bigby, C. (2009). Breaking out of a distinct social space: reflections on supporting community participation for people with severe and profound intellectual disability. *Journal of Applied Research in Intellectual Disabilities*, 22, 264–275.

Darragh, J. A., Ellison, C. J., Rillotta, F., et al. (2016). Exploring the impact of an arts-based, day options program for young adults with intellectual disabilities. *Research and Practice in Intellectual and Developmental Disabilities*, 3(1), 22–31.

Department of Health. (2009). *Valuing people now: a new three-year strategy for people with learning disabilities*. London: DH.

Den Brok, W. L. J. E., & Sterkenburg, P. S. (2015). Self-controlled technologies to support skill attainment in persons with an autism spectrum disorder and/or an intellectual disability: a systematic literature review. *Disability and Rehabilitation: Assistive Technology*, 10(1), 1–10.

Duggan, C., & Linehan, C. (2013). The role of 'natural supports' in promoting independent living for people with disabilities; a review of existing literature. *British Journal of Learning Disabilities*, 41(3), 199–207.

Emerson, E., Mallam, S., Davies, I., et al. (2005). *Adults with learning difficulties in England 2003/04*. London: National Statistics and Health and Social Care Information Centre.

Emerson, E., & McVilly, K. (2004). Friendship activities of adults with intellectual disabilities in supported accommodation in northern England. *Journal of Applied Research in Intellectual Disabilities*, 17, 191–197.

Ferrer, F., Vilaseca, R., & Bersabé, R. M. (2016). The impact of demographic characteristics and the positive perceptions of parents on quality of life in families with a member with intellectual disability. *Journal of Developmental and Physical Disabilities*, 28(6), 871–888.

Gjermestad, A., Luteberget, L., Midjo, T., et al. (2017). Everyday life of persons with intellectual disability living in residential settings: a systematic review of qualitative studies. *Disability & Society*, 32(2), 213–232.

Kampert, A. L., & Gorenczny, A. J. (2007). Community involvement and socialization among individuals with mental retardation. *Research in Developmental Disabilities*, 28, 278–286.

KeyRing. (n.d.). Available at: https://www.keyring.org/. [Accessed 26 September 2020].

Lippold, T., & Burns, J. (2009). Social support and intellectual disabilities: a comparison between social networks of adults with intellectual disability and those with physical disability. *Journal of Intellectual Disability Research*, 53(5), 463–473.

Lorenzo, T., & Kathard, H. (2018). Disabled women and violence in South Africa. In S. Shah & C. Bradbury-Jones (Eds.), *Global perspectives on disability, violence and protection over the life-course: an edited collection*. UK: Routledge.

Lorenzo, T., McKinney, V., Bam, A., et al. (2018). Mapping the participation of disabled youth in sport and free time activities to facilitate youth development. *British Journal of Occupational Therapy* December online.

Lorenzo, T., Motau, J., van der Merwe, T., et al. (2015). Community rehabilitation workers as catalysts for disability: inclusive youth development through service learning. *Development in Practice*, 25(1), 19–28.

Louw, J. S., Kirkpatrick, B., & Leader, G. (2019). Enhancing social inclusion of young adults with intellectual disabilities: a systematic review of original empirical studies. *Journal of Applied Research in Intellectual Disabilities*. https://doi.org/10.1111/jar.12678.

McConkey, R. (2019). Public perceptions of the rights of persons with disability: national surveys in the Republic of Ireland. *Alter: European Journal of Disability Research*.

McConkey, R., Bunting, B., Keogh, F., et al. (2019). The impact on social relationships of moving from congregated settings to personalized accommodation. *Journal of Intellectual Disabilities*, 23(2), 149–159.

McConkey, R., & Collins, S. (2010a). Using personal goal-setting to promote the social inclusion of people with intellectual disability living in supported accommodation. *Journal of Intellectual Disability Research*, 54(2), 135–143.

McConkey, R., & Collins, S. (2010b). The role of support staff in promoting the social inclusion of persons with intellectual disabilities. *Journal of Intellectual Disability Research*, 54(8), 691–700.

McConkey, R., Dowling, S., Hassan, D., et al. (2013). Promoting social inclusion through unified sports for youth with intellectual disabilities: a five nation study. *Journal of Intellectual Disability Research*, 57(10), 923–935.

McConkey, R., Dunne, J., & Blitz, N. (2009). *Shared lives: building relationships and community with people who have intellectual disabilities*. Amsterdam: Sense Publishers.

McConkey, R., & Smyth, M. (2003). Parental perceptions of risks with young adults who have severe learning difficulties contrasted with the young people's views and experiences. *Children and Society*, 17, 18–31.

Mental Health Foundation. (2020). *Circles of support and circles of friends*. Available at: https://www.mentalhealth.org.uk/learning-disabilities/a-to-z/c/circles-support-and-circles-friends. [Accessed 6 August 2020].

Merrells, J., Buchanan, A., & Waters, R. (2018). The experience of social inclusion for people with intellectual disability within community recreational programs: a systematic review. *Journal of Intellectual & Developmental Disability*, 43(4), 381–391.

Mihaila, I., Handen, B. L., Christian, B. T., et al. (2020). Leisure activity in middle-aged adults with Down syndrome: initiators, social partners, settings and barriers. *Journal of Applied Research in Intellectual Disabilities*. https://doi.org/10.1111/jar.12706.

Miller, E., Cooper, S. A., Cook, C., et al. (2008). Outcomes important to people with intellectual disabilities. *Journal of Policy and Practice in Intellectual Disabilities*, 5(3), 150–158.

Murray, P. (2002). *Hello! Are you listening? Disabled teenagers' experience of access to inclusive leisure*. York: Joseph Rowntree Foundation.

Oliver, M. (1996). *Understanding disability: from theory to practice*. Basingstoke: Macmillan.

Overmars-Marx, T., Thomése, F., & Meininger, H. (2019). Neighbourhood social inclusion from the perspective of people with intellectual disabilities: relevant themes identified with the use of photovoice. *Journal of Applied Research in Intellectual Disabilities*, 32(1), 82–93.

Patterson, I., & Pegg, S. (2009). Serious leisure and people with intellectual disabilities: benefits and opportunities. *Leisure Studies*, 28(4), 387–402.

Pockney, R. (2006). Friendship or facilitation: people with learning disabilities and their paid carers. *Sociological Research Online*, 11(3), 89–97.

Robertson, J., Hatton, C., Wells, E., et al. (2011). The impacts of short break provision on families with a disabled child: an international literature review. *Health & Social Care in the Community*, 19(4), 337–371.

Schwartz, D. B. (1992). *Crossing the river: creating a conceptual revolution in community and disability*. Cambridge: Brookline Books.

Seligman, M. E. (2011). *Flourish: a visionary new understanding of happiness and well-being*. London: Nicholas Brealey Publishing.

Shelley, K., Donelly, M., Hillman, A., et al. (2018). How the personal support networks of people with intellectual disability promote participation and engagement. *Journal of Social Inclusion*, 9(1), 37–57.

Southby, K. (2019). An exploration and proposed taxonomy of leisure-befriending for adults with learning disabilities. *British Journal of Learning Disabilities*, 47(4), 223–232.

Stebbins, R. (2000). Serious leisure for people with disabilities. In A. Sivan & H. Ruskin (Eds.), *Leisure education, community development and populations with special needs* (pp. 101–108). Oxon: CABI.

Tint, A., Thomson, K., & Weiss, J. A. (2017). A systematic literature review of the physical and psychosocial correlates of Special Olympics participation among individuals with intellectual disability. *Journal of Intellectual Disability Research*, 61(4), 301–324.

Towell, D. (Ed.). (1988). *An ordinary life in practice: Developing community-based services for people with learning disabilities*. London: King's Fund Centre.

Trembath, D., Balandin, S., Stancliffe, R. J., et al. (2010). Employment and volunteering for adults with intellectual disability. *Journal of Policy and Practice in Intellectual Disabilities*, 7(4), 235–238.

United Nations. (2006). Convention on the Rights of Persons with Disabilities. Available at: http://www.un.org/disabilities/.

van Pletzen, E., Booyens, M., & Lorenzo, T. (2014). An exploratory analysis of community-based disability workers' potential to alleviate poverty and promote social inclusion of people with disabilities in three Southern African countries. *Disability & Society*, 29(10), 1524–1539.

Wilkinson, R., & Marmot, M. (Eds.). (2003). *Social determinants of health: the solid facts* (2nd ed.). Denmark: WHO.

Wilson, N. J., Bigby, C., Stancliffe, R. J., et al. (2013). Mentors' experiences of using the active mentoring model to support older adults with intellectual disability to participate in community groups. *Journal of Intellectual & Developmental Disability*, 38(4), 344–355.

Wolfensberger, W. (1972). *The principle of normalisation in human services*. Toronto: National Institute on Mental Retardation.

World Health Organisation. (2010). *Community based rehabilitation guidelines*. Geneva: WHO.

World Health Organisation and World Bank. (2011). *World report on disability*. Geneva: WHO.

Wymer, W. W., Jr., & Starnes, B. J. (2001). Conceptual foundations and practical guidelines for recruiting volunteers to serve in local nonprofit organizations: part I. *Journal of Nonprofit & Public Sector Marketing*, 9(1–2), 63–96.

22

Access to education

David S. Stewart

KEY ISSUES

- Facilitating inclusive education for children and young people with intellectual disabilities has been the focus of both national and international policy and legislation and remains a hotly debated issue.
- Educators need training and support to better understand students with intellectual disabilities, particularly those with accompanying complex needs.
- There needs to be a broad and balanced educational curriculum, preparing children and young people with intellectual disabilities for life ahead with robust planning and preparation to ensure smooth transition when leaving school.

- Planning needs to be holistic and underpinned by clear partnership working between the young person, their family and other relevant carers and professionals.
- Opportunities must be provided to develop the student voice, ensuring students are empowered and their opinions valued.
- National governments need to ensure that there are strategies in place to ensure a workforce able to meet the needs of students.

CHAPTER OUTLINE

INTRODUCTION

Education for children and young people with intellectual disabilities has an interesting history, and it is important at the start of this chapter to review past provision to better understand current practices and situations today. Understanding national policies and codes of practice is vital if sense is to be made of the procedures and practices in schools, and how they affect students and their families. No subject is more hotly debated than inclusion and the constant question, "Does it matter where children are taught?". Further to this are questions about the relevance and appropriateness of what children are taught – does it equip them for life, does it challenge? In short, do current systems ensure entitlement to a full and enriched education? These are some of the issues that will be considered in this chapter.

Moving on from school can be a difficult time for students but for those with intellectual disabilities it can be particularly traumatic; a smooth transition may be affected by the choice of what is available to them after finishing school, and for others after finishing college. In either situation a smooth process of transition depends on schools and colleges working in close partnership with the child, their parents and families to determine their individual needs and explore the best options available to them. The essential elements of this partnership will be discussed in the latter half of this chapter. We begin by placing the education of children with intellectual disabilities within an international context.

WHERE SHOULD CHILDREN AND YOUNG PEOPLE BE TAUGHT?

Inclusion is probably one of the most talked about subjects within the area of special education and the question of whether or not children and young people with intellectual disabilities should be educated alongside their mainstream peers, or in separate provision, continues to be hotly debated. The right to education has been a feature of different international agreements ranging from the United Nations Convention on the Rights of the Child (UN, 1989) through to the United Nations Declaration on the Rights of Persons with Disabilities (UN, 2006) and the most recent Cali commitment to equity and inclusion in education (United Nations Educational, Scientific and Cultural Organisation [UNESCO], 2019).

It is just over 25 years since more than 300 people representing both governments and other international organisations met in Salamanca, Spain to pledge their support for inclusive education for children with disabilities. The outcome of this meeting was the *Salamanca Statement* that re-affirmed their commitment to education for all children, regardless of individual differences, a statement of intent that had previously been outlined in the 1948 Universal Declaration of Human Rights and at the 1990 World Conference of Education for All (UNESCO, 1994). At the heart of the agreement was a number of key principles:

1 every child has a fundamental right to education, and must be given the opportunity to achieve and maintain an acceptable level of learning,
2 every child has unique characteristics, interests, abilities and learning needs,
3 education systems should be designed and educational programmes implemented to take into account the wide diversity of these characteristics and needs,

4 those with special educational needs must have access to regular schools which should accommodate them within a child centred pedagogy capable of meeting these needs,
5 regular schools with this inclusive orientation are the most effective means of combating discriminatory attitudes, creating welcoming communities, building an inclusive society and achieving education for all; moreover, they provide an effective education to the majority of children and improve the efficiency and ultimately the cost-effectiveness of the entire education system (UNESCO, 1994: *Salamanca Statement*).

Principles 4 and 5 illustrate the Statement's commitment to encouraging countries, which were still developing their special education provision, to establish inclusive education from the start, rather than having both mainstream schools and special schools. However there remains a wide variance in terms of the degree to which this has occurred. In 2019 Peter Mittler reflected that 25 years on both UNESCO and governments "have failed to follow up on the Salamanca statement in respect to the number of children with disabilities who remain excluded from primary and pre-primary education" (Ainscow et al, 2019). Indeed, in countries such as the UK, where substantial progress had been made in this area, the number of children with special needs in mainstream secondary schools in England actually fell by 24 per cent between 2012 and 2019 (Milmo and Stanton, 2019).

In 2006 the UK Office for Standards in Education, Children's Services and Skills (OFSTED, 2006) commissioned a report: "Does it matter where pupils are taught?" The report concluded that the best outcomes for students with intellectual and/or other disabilities came not from the type but the quality of provision. However, whilst it was acknowledged that there was effective provision across both mainstream and special schools, there was more good and outstanding provision in resourced mainstream schools than elsewhere.

Many countries now have national legislation to support students with Special Educational Needs and Disabilities (SEND) however there are some issues which are common to all and these include:

1 different interpretations of national legislation by state, regional and local authorities,
2 insufficient finances to enable carrying out the national legislation,
3 difficulty of access to assessment and diagnosis,

READER ACTIVITY 22.1

Find out about the specific legislation in your own country that directs the education of children and young people with special educational needs including those with intellectual disabilities.

To what extent does this legislation reflect the philosophy of inclusion?

4 lack of appropriate training for the workforce (Lewis et al, 2019),
5 conflicting legislation, which counters the initial SEND legislation. In the UK for instance the Government's current programme of Academies has seen a large increase in the number of students with intellectual disabilities being excluded from school and a decline in inclusion.

WHAT SHOULD BE TAUGHT?

Education for people with intellectual disabilities has its origins in the work promoted by French physician and educator Eduard Seguin (1812–1880), the Italian physician and educator, Maria Montessori (1870–1952) and the Belgian educator and physician Ovide Decroly (1871–1932). These early methods of education focused on developing order, co-ordination, concentration and independence. Today there is still much discussion as to what should be taught to children and young people with intellectual disabilities, and whether they should follow the same programmes of study as their non-disabled peers (Lawson et al, 2015). This gives rise to a polarisation of views with tension between providing commonality (inclusiveness, equality) and relevance (differentiation) (Norwich, 2010). There has also been the danger of staff, new to special education and perhaps with little prior training, mistaking assessment tools as the basis of a curriculum, which could lead to a very thin education.

Given the diversity of educational needs of children and young people with intellectual disabilities, a single approach will not suffice, as educational provision needs to be tailored, wherever possible to individual learning needs. The chief guiding principle should be that **all** children and young people are entitled to rich and exciting education which will provide them with the skills, knowledge and experiences to maximise their independence, to participate as fully as possible in their community, and have a happy and fulfilling life.

Within the debate about what to teach is also the issue of *entitlement*. For some this might constitute learners having a right to participate in the full curriculum; for others it may mean the learner having the opportunity to do so. In the Australian Curriculum (Australian Curriculum Assessment and Reporting Authority, 2016) this means offering "all students with a disability the right to the same educational opportunities and choices on the same basis with their peers through rigorous, meaningful and dignified programs." This issue of entitlement must never be lost when considering what is appropriate to students with a wide range of abilities. A good example of this was the introduction of Modern Foreign Languages in UK special schools in the early 1990s; one view was *"What's the point of teaching this to these students?"* yet all the evidence has since pointed to the fact that students enjoy the subject and the challenge of learning something new.

The challenge is therefore not how we limit the curriculum for children and young people with intellectual disabilities but how we make entitlement a reality in an appropriate way. Programmes of study need to incorporate a wide range of approaches to ensure that they have access to education that is akin to their particular needs, and at a point when they need it most. As a young person moves toward independence, the requirement to manage money, including budgeting, becomes more of an essential task, therefore a specific focus on the development of basic mathematical skills would be considered a priority at this point in time. As an example, the Australian Curriculum provides for financial literacy education for youth with disabilities (Hordacre, 2016). This is especially important if an individual is the recipient of a personal budget that enables them to have choice and control over the support services they need. This chapter will now move on to consider the subject of numeracy in a little more detail alongside other essential subject areas.

Numeracy

In addition to the benefit of having some basic mathematical competence for facilitating the development of skills required for independent living, maths (or numeracy as it is often referred to) also includes the basics of spatial awareness – how a person's body relates to their environment. This is why physical education is so important in the learning of maths. Children with intellectual disabilities will also need opportunities to explore the shape and size, as well as the properties of objects. More able students may learn to count and sort, and practical and relevant tasks must be encouraged to support this education. However, other concepts such as time and money can be far more difficult for children to grasp. For example, road crossing requires real skills in the assessment of time, distance as well as understanding one's own speed of walking. Even harder are the concepts of estimation which we generally use all the time in our lives. Educators need to employ activities, which will motivate a student to learn numeracy skills. For example, a student may not wish to count out numbers of bricks but can quickly articulate scores on an Xbox game. For younger students, singing rhymes, which reinforce counting, and numbers can be very useful. The thing to remember is that whichever teaching method is employed, it must be meaningful to the individual.

Literacy

An overriding principle in the teaching of reading to people with intellectual disabilities is to have high expectations. There is a real risk that assumptions can be made about a person's capabilities that if untested, can lead to opportunities being lost. *"I never knew he could read!"* is an alarming statement when considered in relation to a 15-year-old. What crucial learning might have been missed because of people presuming certain things about the capability of the child, further evidence of the damage that labelling can cause (see Chapter 2).

We are surrounded by print so how does a young person with an intellectual disability make sense of this world without support to engage with different types of literature? Reading requires an ability to decode letters, words and/or symbols culminating in the comprehension of what is being conveyed. Teachers will be aware of the challenges which hearing and speech difficulties (common in children and adults with intellectual disabilities) bring to the process of teaching reading. Sometimes there has been sole emphasis on social sight vocabulary (words a learner recognises on sight without having to decode them or work them out e.g. EXIT, Bus stop) and whilst this is an important aspect of education there is a danger that other abilities to read text can be missed.

Children and young people can read for pleasure or information, but it has to be acknowledged that some children with intellectual disabilities will never grasp the skills of reading words. This does not mean, however,

that they cannot, like everyone else, enjoy the pleasure of books. Their engagement can be facilitated through reading to them or following a sequence of a story through the illustrations. Every school should have a good library, which is accessible to all. Bag Books (2020), a form of sensory storytelling, is also a good way of facilitating children of all abilities to engage with stories.

Sport and physical education

Physical activity encourages general fitness with benefits in terms of obesity and mental development. We know from statistics that obesity in adults with intellectual disabilities is a concerning issue with higher levels amongst this population than their non-disabled peers (Gawlik et al, 2018) and lower levels of physical activity (Collins and Staples, 2017; see also Chapters 9 and 10). In the latter study this was a particular concern for children with Down syndrome or Autistic Spectrum Disorder (ASD) not achieving the recommended 60 minutes of daily moderate to vigorous physical activity (MVPA). Such knowledge thus reinforces the importance of introducing exercise into the daily lives of children from an early age.

Schools must ensure that students have access to a full range of physical education. Physical education can also develop cross-curricular skills such as expressive and receptive language, mathematics and literacy; the challenge however is how to make sport and physical education accessible to all. Good practice suggests sharing ownership for curriculum design and learning with the students, whilst considering what constitutes physical education is demonstrated by research in New Zealand (Petrie et al, 2018). In terms of exercise, there needs to be a focus on what physical activities a young person can continue to do into adulthood. If school sports have all been about team sports, the reality is that few young people with and without disabilities continue in team sports once they have left school. As students leave school, they and their families need to be signposted to leisure and sports services which will be able to support them. These are particularly important as an acceptance of an inactive lifestyle by carers, resource limitations, paid carer preferences or communication issues between family carers and paid carers have all been found to be barriers to leisure opportunities for people with intellectual disabilities (Cartwright et al, 2016) so the earlier this dialogue takes place at school the better.

Rebound therapy

Rebound therapy using trampolines is increasingly popular in schools. Through the effects of vibration, it can reduce high muscle tone and stimulate those with low muscle tone. It has been shown to benefit airway management, ensuring lungs are kept in good condition, and improve co-ordination (Haghigh et al, 2019) although more research is still needed to fully assess its benefits. It is important that rebound therapy is carried out by accredited trainers who can develop appropriate programmes to develop the skills of the young person.

In addition to physical education, a healthy lifestyle might also be promoted in schools through engagement with food preparation activities,

Movement and dance

The benefits of dance for children and young people with intellectual disabilities range from developing an awareness of movement possibilities, to sensitivity of movement and expression, to choreographing their own dance. It allows them to follow sequence and promotes co-ordination and poise. There is a range of approaches that teachers can employ to teach skills in this area including Margaret Morris Movement, Robins Educational Rhythmics, Wolfgang Stange's therapeutic calisthenics or more popularly, Sherborne Development Movement. Sherborne's methodology is based on the work of Rudolf Laban (1879–1958), an Austro-Hungarian dancer, choreographer and dancer/movement theoretician, and encourages body awareness, spatial awareness and positive self-image (see Useful resources online); it also promotes relationships with a partner, and trust and confidence in self and others. The partner work is a particular strength of this approach (Weston, 2012).

Assistive technologies to support learning and communication

> *"Communication, and the interaction between staff and learners and among learners themselves, is fundamental to education and acknowledged to lie at the centre of the curriculum for this group."*
> *Goldbart and Ware 2015*, p. 258

Whilst this statement was made in relation to people with profound and multiple needs, the same can be said for all students with intellectual disabilities. Teachers need to provide appropriate learning environments and support for children to develop their communication abilities. Students must have the opportunity to listen as well as to express themselves. Individual students will communicate in different ways, and staff need to be sensitive to their individual methods of communication. Many of the individual methods of communication that can be employed by schools have been discussed in Chapter 5. This section therefore focuses specifically on the use of assistive technologies in education.

The last twenty years has seen a revolution in the development of assistive technologies in schools to support the communication needs of children and young people with intellectual disabilities. This includes the use of switches such as BIGmack (a large button device that enables the user to send a single message) that give students a voice, empowering them to take control of their environment. Eyegaze technologies have also enabled children with little mobility to communicate, read and create their own writing. The use of robots has also been successful particularly in motivating students (Hedgecock et al, 2014). The "No Isolation" robot from Norway has been created to support students whose health might mean long periods in hospital (see Useful resources online).

Assistive technologies have been used to support students to explore the relationship between cause and effect, and to promote language development or improve a student's sense of direction (Boot et al, 2018). Interactive whiteboards, iPads or other tablets, and visual collaboration systems, have enhanced the learning of students. Schools have engaged with colleagues in higher education to develop, and importantly to evaluate, the use of assistive technology. The training and support of staff is critical if students are to get the full benefit.

The Arts

Whilst the Arts may be used therapeutically it is important to remember all students have an entitlement to arts education as well. New technologies are enabling greater access for students with intellectual disabilities to participate and engage in music and art. Projects such as 'Able Orchestra' (Orchestras Live, 2020) have demonstrated how even students with the most severe physical disability can create and enjoy music. However, barriers do exist and may include opportunity and access restrictions in addition to negative attitudes (Dance4, 2013). Opportunities

READER ACTIVITY 22.2

Think about a child or adult with an intellectual disability that you support.

Reflect upon how different assistive technologies might be employed to enhance their communication skills.

Consider what might be the strengths and/or barriers to their use.

How could these be overcome?

to work with outside providers should be an essential part of the Arts programme. Visits to the theatre, galleries, concerts and exhibitions enhance the learning experience of young people. Local and national arts organisations are generally keen to work with schools. The internationally renowned Matthew Bourne Dance Company runs a project, *In Our Shoes*, which is very accessible to a wide range of students with different disabilities (see Useful resources online). Particularly important is the training it provides for school staff to find accessible ways to introduce, develop and teach dance in schools settings (see Useful resources online). Encouraging parents and families to value the arts for their child is important to ensure that this education continues at school, and once the young person enters adult life.

Friendships and relationships

To ensure students spend time with their friends outside of school and college, schools need to work with families and other agencies to facilitate opportunities. After school clubs and school residentials can help foster such friendships, for students who are not invited to the same parties or sleepovers as their peers without disabilities; families with a child with a disability may also feel unable to entertain another child with a disability at home. School trips, including residentials where students spend a few days away from their family can also facilitate opportunities for children with intellectual disabilities to do fun things with friends in the evenings and at weekends. They also get the opportunity to be away from their parents, thus developing their independence. Summer schools can be vital in giving young people a chance to meet their friends in the holidays to counter the loneliness they might experience (Clark and Nwokah, 2011). Students with complex needs will find access to these opportunities even more difficult,

and schools need to carefully consider how this can be facilitated.

Supporting students to sustain friendships and relationships once they have left school is crucial as without this support these could be lost. Alumni Associations, which keep people in touch, can be invaluable. In terms of facilitating the maintenance of friendships the school can be a catalyst and support social activities and clubs. Schools, which organise activities for its alumni, can also evaluate the impact of the education it has provided. Simple things like making sure every former student receives a birthday or Christmas card are greatly valued. When a person no longer has family left, this small gesture shows that people still care. Providing extra-curricular activities are an excellent way for students to develop and sustain their friendships (Brooks et al, 2014).

Sexual education

"Although we can shape (and mis-shape) sexual experiences, sexuality is not an optional extra, which we in our wisdom can choose to bestow or withhold according to whether or not some kind of intelligence test is passed."
Craft 1987, p. 19

For young people with intellectual disabilities, sex and relationship education is a vital area of the curriculum, yet its delivery in schools, whether mainstream or special, is still very varied. Sometimes political inertia in giving guidance to schools has meant very diverse access to this education. Such education is important for it cannot be assumed that students have acquired information, knowledge, beliefs and appropriate behaviours as other young people might do. It will be important to remind colleagues that students have a right to an education to help them understand themselves, their sexual development, the choices open to them, and their right to protection from sexual abuse and exploitation.

Young people need to be aware of their own sexual health and safety. They need to value themselves. Without education there is the danger that students might find themselves in difficulty because of inappropriate sexualised behaviour, or because of a lack of assertiveness training making them liable to abuse.

Research would indicate that parents and families are very keen that schools deliver content in this area (Güven, 2015) so schools should be prepared to work closely with them to devise a mutually agreed approach. For instance, if talking about masturbation being a private activity, the school will need to talk with the family about the child's bedroom being the private place. Many students are not generalist learners so each situation needs to be explained. If talking about safer sex in relation to using a condom, then this needs to be explained that this is with whomever they are having sex, whether it be a male and female or two men. To not do so can leave students vulnerable to unsafe practices.

Students will often have difficulties understanding the nature of friendships and relationships. Someone being friendly is not the same as a "friend" and these are lessons, which need to be taught. Students will require help understanding their own emotions and those of others. As they approach adolescence, some students may find the experience very difficult; prophylactic education is important, preparing young girls for periods or boys for wet dreams. Some students may become distressed as they begin to have hair on their body or face and will need to be supported in coming to terms with growing up. *Sexual expression: A Relationships and Sex Education (RSE) resource for people with learning difficulties and disabilities* (Brook, 2020) can be a useful educational resource.

As previously stated, support for the development of friendships is also important. There is a real danger that young people may be friendless and therefore potentially vulnerable. Issues of same sex relationships may also occur and schools should ensure they are in a good position to advise and support young people and their families in such cases. Guidance on such issues is becoming more common as recognised by its inclusion in key pieces of policy and guidance (see Department of Education, 2019, as a UK example). Educators will need to be mindful of a range of views within society and need to have good dialogue with parents and families to explain the purpose of the education is to ensure their child leads a happy, fulfilled and safe life.

With the increasing use of technology, students will need sound education to support them in the appropriate use of the internet. They need to be aware of the dangers of on-line dating and chat rooms and sexting. For those who may be friendless it is all too easy to be manipulated online (see also Chapter 8).

Schools may feel vulnerable about facilitating sex education for children and young people with intellectual disabilities; as such an example of good practice is for a school to establish a monitoring group consisting of staff, governors, parents and others from the wider community to monitor what happens in school, advise and support staff and work with parents and families, providing training and advice. It can also create and advise on appropriate resources.

Community and global awareness

Students will wish to have access to their community where they can feel safe and confident. Schools can give opportunities for students to take part in community activities such as fund raising for good causes. This might be collecting for those who are disadvantaged in the community or raising money for people who are homeless. It is important that they learn they can play their part in their local community. Engaging in school festivals and working with young people from other schools encourages confidence. The more opportunity students in mainstream education have to meet children with intellectual disabilities, the more it is hoped that some of the stereotypes such as those outlined in Chapter 2 will be challenged and an atmosphere of tolerance and support engendered. Global networks allow young people to learn about others in the world. Modern technology allows them to contact other young people across the world, learning about differences and similarities. eTwinning as part of the Erasmus programme has seen over 80,000 eTwinning projects take place since its inception. It is an excellent way for students to learn about each other's cultures (see Useful resources online).

There are, of course, practicalities when facilitating access to the community. For those with complex needs this may require preparation. A class of 10 students with profound and multiple intellectual disabilities (PMID) may need 4 minibuses to get to an event. Booking theatres and other venues needs forward planning to ensure success. Schools need to work closely with other agencies such as sports, arts and cultural venues to ensure inclusion into the community. If a student has a less than positive experience this may affect their feelings of confidence and safety.

PROFOUND AND MULTIPLE INTELLECTUAL DISABILITIES (PMID)

Amongst children with intellectual disabilities are some whose educational needs are worthy of further consideration; students with Profound and Multiple Intellectual Disabilities (PMID). This group poses real challenges for schools in ensuring that the content of their education, and its mode of delivery, meets their individual needs. Children in this group tend to need education that very much focuses on the self and how things and ideas relate to their most immediate needs.

Over the last ten to fifteen years, advances in medical science and care have meant that children who historically may have died before school age are now within the education system. This has led to many challenges for school staff who may have had no previous experience of working with children with such complex needs. Children and young people with PMID have health conditions that co-exist. These conditions overlap and interlock creating a complex profile. The co-occurring and compounding nature of this complexity requires a personalised learning pathway that recognises children and young people's unique and changing learning patterns.

Children and young people with PMID present with significant difficulties, e.g. physical disabilities, sensory impairments, communication needs and serious medical conditions. They need specific support and strategies, which may include transdisciplinary input, to engage effectively in the learning process, and to participate actively in classroom activities and the wider community. Teachers must also take the possibility of mental ill health into consideration when assessing and planning for education. Schools need to adopt a supportive culture, engaging with other agencies. The provision of trained counsellors is becoming more common in schools (Buckley and Mahdavi, 2018); this is important as certain behaviours may incorrectly be attributed to the disability rather than appreciating that the young person has significant issues affecting their mental well-being (see also Chapter 16). Staff need to think of strategies, which can support the mental health needs of students, such as enabling them to develop skills to understand and express their emotions, using pictures, signs and other communication aids. The use of art, music and movement can encourage children to express and release their emotions in ways they feel secure.

Carpenter (2011) has stated that

"Sustainable learning can occur only when there is meaningful engagement. The process of engagement is a journey, which connects a child and their environment (including people, ideas, materials and concepts) to enable learning and achievement."

The Engagement Profile and Scale is a classroom tool (Specialist Schools and Academies Trust, 2011) which allows educators to focus on the child's engagement as a learner and create personalised learning pathways for students with complex needs. Further useful information and resources to support teaching and learning for students with complex intellectual disabilities can be found in the PMLD Link website (2020), which highlights standards of practice for school staff, and The Complex Needs website (2012). Links to both of these websites can be found in the Useful resources online.

TRANSITIONS AND PREPARING FOR ADULTHOOD

In the school life of a young person with an intellectual disability there can be several transitions; this could be between different types of schools or from one age group to another. All such transitions need to be planned so that a student feels confident and safe. The most challenging transition however is that of leaving school and moving to adult provision such as day centres or further education colleges.

Preparing for Adulthood is a UK government programme that prepares young people with intellectual disabilities for when they leave school, focussing on education, training and employment, independent living, health and participation in society (see Useful resources online). Right from the early years, education staff need to be thinking about skills and knowledge which will equip students with intellectual disabilities for their future life. There will be some students with complex needs for whom life expectancy may be limited but one must always have an eye to the future. For families this can be a most distressing time not least because they are generally moving from statutory services to permissive ones, and they may not know what is available for their adult child. Moreover, funding issues mean that some services may have limited availability and/or capacity, so advanced planning is required to ensure that needs and wishes of a young person are addressed.

Students should be at the forefront of any transition process, being actively involved in the planning and preparation. The student and family may begin to meet a new range of professionals who should help with the process yet some of the input comes far too late and many students and their families become very anxious. In research with parents in the USA, there was concern about inefficient and siloed systems with a disconnect between school and community (Franklin et al, 2019). For those with additional health needs there needs to be a detailed consultation with health professionals. Within a school environment access to health staff may be everyday but will generally be far less in adult provision. If a young person is going to require health support at college or in adult provision, a transitions professional may be able to give support.

One option for students leaving school may be some form of further education. During their last few years at school students may have had tasters of further education courses so that they will have some ability to choose what they wish to study at college. However not all further education is inclusive or may be less tolerant of certain behaviours. Progression routes may limit the time a student spends at a college and there might not always be clear routes post-college. Parents may find themselves in another transition process only two years after their child has left school. Options of courses may also be limited. Tracking of young people once they have left school is inconsistent and there needs to be greater longitudinal studies to evaluate outcomes.

In preparing young people, schools need to be mindful of the skills required for independent living. Some students may always need some level of support, but they also need to be encouraged to do as much for themselves as possible. For those who are able, support in understanding budgets and the value of money is required. Experience of household expenses such as food items and utility bills are an important aspect of life. This can begin with their access to mobile phones, which will be one of the first utility bills they encounter. Food budgeting needs to be done in conjunction with healthy food options and further emphasises the need for basic numeracy skills.

Students will need support in thinking of where they will live in the future. Schools and colleges need to have a particular focus on future housing options and provide young people and their families with information and resources so that they can fully understand what is available (see also Chapter 24). For those who have been taught out of area and are returning to their home this is of immediate concern (more about transition planning can be found in Chapter 20).

It is important that students have access to courses that are for recreation and pleasure as well as those for life skills. Provision of leisure activities can be a difficulty in more rural areas. Research in Canada (Roult et al, 2017) found access and financial considerations could present a challenge but there are clearly benefits for the person with an intellectual disability, their relationship with their environment and for the family. This is echoed in experiences in the UK where evening classes for poetry, dance and drama give opportunities for people to engage with their friends in meaningful and enjoyable activities.

The world of work is still the dream of many young people and for some there is the offer of work experience similar to school schemes, but gaining employment is far less a reality. Education and training for students with intellectual disabilities post-school is generally vocational however evidence would suggest that few obtain employment following engagement with these programmes (Rooney, 2016; Agarwal et al, 2020). The emphasis tends to be on basic numeracy, literacy and Information Technology (IT) and can often seem to be a repetition of what the young person had at school. Furthermore, where a young person has the possibility of work, the courses that they have followed tend not to be relevant to the type of employment offered. Whilst much will depend on the individual college, it is important that all partners strive to support an individual with an intellectual disability to access education and training that will be relevant and useful to them in the next stage of their life (Zainal and Hashim, 2019).

Doing voluntary work or working in co-operatives is a much more likely option. National programmes, which support the employment of people with disabilities, may have less of a success record with people with intellectual disabilities. For instance, in the USA, with less access to benefits there is a greater impetus to find employment whilst in the UK the provision of financial support through welfare may actually hinder access to paid employment.

Whilst the issue of employment is specifically discussed in the next chapter of this book, it is worth mentioning the importance of preparatory work. A useful programme developed by Nottingham Trent University (2019) called *Being on time: My Appearance* gives training in preparing for work or school. This encourages students to estimate the time needed to get ready in the morning before work or school.

RECORDING AND ASSESSMENT OF PROGRESS

It is important that students have individual education plans with targets to be met. Measurement of achievement towards meeting these targets requires good assessment and recording processes. Accurate assessment is essential to securing and measuring student progress. Age and prior attainment are the starting point for developing expectations of student progress. Getting good comparative data, particularly for students with PMID and other complex needs can be difficult, but teachers, learners and their parents and carers need to know whether they are making good progress. Schools need to be challenged where learners are not making good progress. Better use of data can raise expectations even for students working at lower levels throughout their school career.

One of the most important purposes of assessment is to inform teaching and learning. Every learner needs to know how he or she is doing, what he or she needs to do to improve, and how to get there. Particularly for those at the early stages of learning it is more challenging to make accurate and reliable judgements. Reliability is often based on moderation. Can a child perform the same task at a different time and for a different teacher? To support rigorous teacher assessment, effective procedures for moderation are needed to ensure assessments are sound and consistent across class teams and teaching groups within a school and between clusters of schools.

In terms of assessment and targets students should be involved as much as possible. This takes planning and preparation but can be very effective for the young person taking some control over their lives. Where possible they should be involved in their individual education plan. The use of pictures, symbols, and video recordings can assist the young person in becoming involved. Creating visual pathways in which the young person's hopes and dreams are recorded as well as how this is to be achieved creates a very useful resource, which also holds individual providers and professionals to account (see Haringey's Guide in the Useful resources online). Young people should be supported to manage their own health, ensuring they have regular health checks and health plans are in place to support their access to health. The transition from services, which may have been automatic whilst they were children, will need to be re-established as adults (see also Chapter 20).

Developing the student voice

The United Nations Convention on the Rights of the Child 1989 states "children who are capable of forming views, have a right to receive information, to express an opinion and to have that opinion taken into account in any matters affecting them." The challenge is to ensure that children and young people with intellectual disabilities are afforded this right. Giving students a voice must start in the early years. Work on self-esteem is crucial for a child or young person for them to appreciate that they are important, and that people will listen to them. Young people need to be given confidence whatever form of communication they might use.

Where possible they should take part in all decision-making processes in education. This includes setting targets, choosing a school, contributing to the assessment of their needs, annual reviews and the transition process. All children, regardless of whether they attend a special or mainstream school, should be given the same chance to take part in discussions about their education. There will need to be different levels of support provided for individual students. Some may need greater time to express their views. A young person may have a different view to the parent and that view should be listened to.

Involving a student in the education process can demand some creative thinking and much preparation and planning, but the results and the richness of the engagement are always well worth the effort. For instance, pictorial recording during the meeting is an effective way of ensuring the student has understood what is being discussed. A permanent image of this acts as a powerful reminder when being reviewed. Making the young person the centre of that picture is crucial in identifying what needs to happen and who will make it happen; this is important for all concerned. Preparing the young person beforehand is critical so that he or she is aware of what is going to happen in any discussion. They need time to consider what they want to say. Practical considerations such as the following need to be made:

- Where does the young person feel comfortable?
- How long does the young person need to be in the meeting?
- Who needs to be there? Expecting the voice from a young person in a room full of professionals is often unrealistic. Are there other opportunities for the professionals to meet?

- How do we learn the views of people with PMID and other complex needs? What work has been done with them and their families prior to the meeting?

Involving students at the earliest opportunity is highly beneficial. Supporting them to develop the confidence to convey their views and opinions, hopes and fears might be established through ventures such as School Councils and Youth Parliaments. Students may also join advocacy groups organised by other agencies (see also Chapter 7).

In School Councils students are given opportunities to speak for themselves or on behalf of their fellows. Some students may need to have an advocate to support them. These supported groups can be very useful to develop skills and confidence. Often the Councils will report on issues, which are of concern to students who are seeking solutions. They may be given a budget to begin the process of having responsibility and this is another way that numeracy skills can be developed.

It has also been found that students who attend drama and theatre groups develop a confidence that enables them to take part in debate and discussions. Students learn to speak up, project themselves and articulate their thoughts (Kempe and Tissot, 2012). Posture is also improved as they are taught to raise their head when speaking and direct their voice to the listeners. This may seem very obvious, but these are skills that need to be learnt if the young person is to become an effective contributor. Ferguson (2019) demonstrates how a multisensory theatre performance can use facial expressions, gestures, intonation of voice and objects to enhance the engagement of those with PMID.

For students with PMID it is important to ensure that they too have a voice. As already discussed there are many simple switches and devices available that can make a significant difference to young people in simple everyday choice making. Being able to ask for a drink or being able to turn on the radio when the young person wants to listen is wonderfully empowering. Staff need to persevere and explore all technologies, which are now available. Many schools will be working with local colleges and universities to develop improved access for students with disabilities. Portable eye-controlled communication devices can be very liberating for some students.

Where advocates are used to support students it is important to ensure that this is not just the view of one person, with research in Canada (Bennett et al, 2017)

cautioning against the subjective interpretation by professionals. Sometimes it has been useful to have a small group for an individual. In one example a young man clearly became distressed in shops. In his advocacy group the female staff tried to think of ways to help. The sole male worker remarked that he hated shopping and that perhaps the young man was no different, and this should be taken into account. This led to a much more satisfactory conclusion.

When supporting young people it may be useful to include a young person without intellectual disabilities, as they are able to bring a broader context. A young person with a disability may feel that they are being disadvantaged by something their parent does not allow them to do. It may be nothing to do with their disability but their age or safety and this would equally apply to their non-disabled peers. In an inclusive drama group discussion about boundaries placed by parents, students with intellectual disabilities were surprised that their non-disabled fellows had limits placed on how much time they could use the computer.

Citizenship education provides an opportunity to inform young people of their rights and responsibilities. While people with intellectual disabilities have rights, they may not know about them, or if they do, they may not be able to exercise them. The sooner such rights and responsibilities are discussed in school the more likely that this information will support future learning and behaviours. In both mainstream and special schools, staff need to ensure that students with intellectual disabilities have access to this information and knowledge. Those who have responsibility for timetabling must ensure that there is time for this information to be repeated and reinforced.

As part of social cohesion, schools might consider the global dimension as part of the wider curriculum, and this is just as relevant for students with special educational needs. Schools will be working with partner schools across the globe. To support this work there is a variety of schemes such as the International School Award (British Council, 2020). This encourages schools to audit what they are doing in relation to the Global Dimension and to plan for further action. As part of Citizenship education, students need to have the sense that not only are they local citizens, but they are also world citizens. What goes on elsewhere does affect their lives. If wars are being fought there is less money for disability services. Children like themselves in other countries may not have the same entitlements. This is all part of the greater disability agenda.

Some schools may have links through their local twinning associations or their national agencies. This enables staff to visit schools in other countries and promotes students learning about young people from diverse backgrounds. For schools finding a similar school can be an interesting experience. Supported by the European Union (EU), an eTwinning project between six special schools adopted a toy owl who spent time in each school. Students took pictures of their school and community with the owl and shared this with the other schools, enjoying learning about each other's cultures. Using technology is a way for schools to make contact. This is useful for short projects when a visit would not be possible. The teaching of a modern foreign language in school is also relevant here – it can be a positive experience for students acquiring a new skill and enjoying putting the simple phrases they learn to good use when abroad or entertaining foreign visitors.

There is much to be learnt and shared by such international co-operation. Students with intellectual disabilities enjoy visits to schools in other countries. They have also been supported at international conferences, speaking to and learning from others from around the world.

WORKING WITH OTHERS

To ensure that students, whether in mainstream or special provision, receive the most appropriate education, due attention needs to be made to ensuring a highly skilled workforce. Whilst there is already a lot of excellent skill expertise within education systems, which needs to be celebrated, there is still inconsistency in the effectiveness of the support provided to learners. Box 22.1 identifies some of the issues, which need to be addressed to ensure a workforce confident in its ability to deliver high quality education.

Multi-agency working

Students who are identified with intellectual disabilities will usually have a number of other needs, be they medical, emotional or social. From an early age many will have contact with a wide range of professionals, and this will continue into school life. In special schools, in particular, there may be several health professionals on site, and in other schools there will be many peripatetic staff visiting.

> ### BOX 22.1   Ensuring a workforce competent to deliver high quality education
>
> - Special educational needs awareness for teachers needs to be prioritised by organisations in charge of teacher teaching.
> - Mainstream and special schools need to be encouraged to work together to share best practice and expertise. Rather than working in competition, collaboration should drive forward the sharing of ideas and knowledge.
> - Schools should audit training needs in relation to special educational needs.

Colleagues from different agencies will have received a variety of training and education. On some professional training courses there may be little in the way of input on children and young people with intellectual disabilities. Often professionals have little idea of the training of others. This can get in the way of working together and there needs to be more cross-sector training.

The relationship between professionals may be dependent on the service level agreements organised by agencies and this will vary greatly. For many there will be involvement of social care, whether for respite care or for other social needs. Psychologists, mentors, doctors, transition workers will also engage with the students and their families. With so many people working on behalf of students it is important that there is good multi-agency working. People need to understand the roles of others and what they can contribute to the lives of the young people.

Working with parents and families

It is clear that for schools, "families in all their shapes, sizes and guises should be at the heart of everything they do. It is important, that their interactions empower families rather than de-skill them" (Carpenter and Rawson, 2015, p. 87). It is recognised that decisions made about provision for students in school are strengthened by embedding an expectation that parents are, where possible, fully engaged in and part of the process of reviewing and implementing strategies to support learning. To ensure this engagement, parents may need guidance on how to support their child's learning and school staff are alive to the part parents can and should play. To enable schools to ensure engagement rather than mere involvement by parents they need to consider issues including those at Box 22.2.

Early intervention is clearly vital and once a child is identified as having a special educational need, some countries might provide early years advisers such as Portage workers who work with families and their children. In some areas voluntary organisations may run schools for parents, as indeed will some schools. The whole process of special education can be very complex. Parents will be generally completely unaware of what needs to happen. They may still be coming to terms with the child's disability, yet parents should be used as a fountain of knowledge for they know their child better than anyone else.

Parents need to feel they can be active in the life of the school. Where possible a parent room provides possibilities for training, listening and support. A home/school liaison officer within a school can provide a real support to parents and families. Parents are encouraged to become parent governors and become involved in the life of the school. For special schools there is always the issue of distance from the child's home and also the fact that their child cannot communicate about what they have done during the day. Home school diaries and telephone calls help in keeping families in touch. Parent evenings, other meetings and social events are important to ensure parents feel part of their child's education.

There may be particular issues for siblings. In a mainstream setting there may be bullying because the student has a brother with a disability and if the child attends a special school, the siblings may have no idea what it looks like. Activities where families can attend with their child are much to be encouraged. Families should be signposted to seek support from independent agencies. These may be organisations for particular disabilities for example Down Syndrome South Africa, the Fragile X Association of Australia or those for rare disabilities such as Unique in the UK and NORD in the USA (see Useful resources online). They can make sure that parents' views are heard and understood, and they are active ensuring these views impact on local policy and practice. They can play a critical role in informing parents about processes and rights. Professionals should never underestimate how difficult it can be for a parent trying to negotiate the minefield of bureaucracy.

Increasingly services in schools have been responsive to the differences across and within ethnic minorities when delivering culturally appropriate services. These include interpretation services, dietary needs and care needs. Croot (2012) reminds us, however, that families from ethnic minorities are similar to the rest of the community in wanting their concerns addressed, trusting relationships with professionals, and better outcomes for their children. She warns that services based on assumption of ethnicity can lead to professionals prejudging familial needs. Meeting needs with reduced resources can bring additional pressures for schools, thus it is ever more important to make creative use of available use of human resources within school and the local neighbourhood.

Modern technologies can provide convenient and instant methods of sharing information with parents. For those working with families who use a second language the Seesaw app (see Useful resources online) has proved very positive for both families and schools. Yet new technologies are not for everyone and schools need to establish a family's preferred method of communication. Many parents still prefer the home-school diary. Some schools find Home-School Agreements very useful for establishing an expectation on families to contribute to plans of action.

📄 BOX 22.2   Promoting parental engagement

- Ideally there should be a senior member of school staff who champions the review process and develops the engagement of parents and families.
- Develop accessible jargon-free formats of communication. A good example for working with parents who may use a second language is the Seesaw (2020) communication app.
- Be aware of barriers, which may hinder engagement such as costs, childcare, transport, and need for interpreters.
- Survey parents about the type of support that they need.
- Develop opportunities to engage parents in the school curriculum so that they can support their child at home.
- Provide training for school staff so that they have better understanding of how to engage parents.
- Encourage those parents who may be able to support other families.

READER ACTIVITY 22.3

Consolidate your knowledge and understanding of the key issues covered in this chapter by reading Jo's story in the online resource and answering the accompanying questions.

CONCLUSION

Education for children and young people with intellectual disabilities has come a long way and there is much to celebrate. The rights of children and young people with special educational needs and disabilities have been enshrined in legislation, with education and equality a statutory duty on schools and state authorities. However, unless there is greater and more consistent funding to support this legislation, opportunities to access an appropriate education will be diminished. Research needs to focus on the disparity between national legislation and its interpretations by authorities at a local or state level. There is a real need to focus on the multi-disciplinary working, with a holistic approach, which supports the student with intellectual disabilities wherever they happen to be educated.

REFERENCES

Agarwal, R., Heron, L., & Burke, S. L. (2020). Evaluating a postsecondary education program for students with intellectual disabilities: leveraging the parent perspective. *Journal of Autism and Developmental Disorders*.

Ainscow, M., Slee, R., & Best, M. (2019). Editorial: the Salamanca Statement: 25 years on. *International Journal of Inclusive Education*, *23*(7–8), 671–676.

Australian Curriculum Assessment and Reporting Authority. (2016). Sydney: Acara.

Bag Books. (2020). Multi-sensory stories for people with learning disabilities Available at: http://www.bagbooks.org/. [Accessed 22 November 2020].

Bennett, S., Gallagher, T., Shuttleworth, M., et al. (2017). Teen dreams: voices of students with intellectual disabilities. *Journal on Developmental Disabilities*, *23*(1), 64–75.

Boot, F. H., et al. (2018). Access to assistive technology for people with intellectual disabilities: a systematic review to identify barriers and facilitators. *Journal of Learning Disability Research*, *62*(10), 9000–9921.

British Council. (2020). International School Award. Available at: https://www.britishcouncil.org/school-resources/accreditation/international-school-award. 900– 921 [Accessed 30 December 2020].

Brook. (2020). Sexual expression: a relationship and sex education (RSE) resource for people with learning difficulties and disabilities. Available at: https://www.brook.org.uk/resources/. [Accessed 18 January 2021].

Brooks, B. A., Floyd, F., Robins, D. L., et al. (2014). Extracurricular activities and the development of social skills in children with learning and specific intellectual disabilities. *Journal of Learning Disability Research*, *59*(7), 678–687.

Buckley, M., & Mahdavi, J. N. (2018). Bringing children from the margins to the page: counselors supporting students with learning disabilities. *Journal of School Counseling*, *16*(23).

Carpenter, B., Egerton, J., Brooks, T., Cockbill, B., et al. (2011). *The Complex Learning Difficulties and Disabilities Research Project: developing pathways to personalised learning*. London: Specialist Schools and Academies Trust.

Carpenter, B., & Rawson, H. (2015). Working with families: partnerships in practice. In P. Lacey, R. Ashdown, P. Jones, et al. (Eds.), *The Routledge companion to severe profound and multiple learning difficulties* (pp. 80–89). London: Routledge.

Cartwright, L., Reid, M., Hammersley, R., et al. (2016). Barriers to increasing the physical activity of people with learning disabilities. *British Journal of Learning Disabilities*, *45*(1).

Clark, K., & Nwokah, E. (2011). Play and Learning in Summer Camps for Children with Special Needs. *American Journal of Play*, *3*(2).

Collins, K., & Staples, K. (2017). The role of physical activity in improving physical fitness in children with learning and developmental disabilities. *Research in Developmental Disabilities*, *69*, 49–60.

Complex Needs. (2012). Training materials for teachers of learners with severe, profound and complex learning difficulties. Available at: http://www.complexneeds.org.uk/. [Accessed 22 November 2020].

Craft, A. (1987). *Mental handicap and sexuality – issues and perceptions*. Tunbridge Wells: Costello.

Croot, E. J. (2012). The care needs of Pakistani families caring for disabled children: how relevant is cultural competence? *Physiotherapy*, *98*(4), 351–356.

Dance4. (2013). *Changing perceptions*. Nottingham: Dance4.

Department of Education. (2019). Relationships education, relationships and sex education (RSE) and health education Available at: https://assets.publishing.service.gov.uk/government/uploads/system/uploads/attachment_data/file/908013/Relationships_Education__Relationships_and_Sex_Education__RSE__and_Health_Education.pdf. [Accessed 30 December 2020].

Ferguson, A. (2019). Raising the bar through inclusive theatre. Available at: http://frozenlighttheatre.com.

Franklin, M. S., Beyer, L. N., Brotkin, S. M., et al. (2019). Health care transition and young adults with intellectual disability: views from parents. *Journal of Pediatric Nursing, 47*, 148–158.

Gawlik, K., Zwierzchowska, A., & Celebańska, D. (2018). Impact of physical activity on obesity and lipid profile of adults with learning disability. *Journal of Applied Research of Intellectual Disability, 31*, 308–311.

Goldbart, J., & Ware, J. (2015). Communication. In P. Lacy (Ed.), *Routledge companion to severe, profound and multiple intellectual disabilities* (pp. 258–270). London: Routledge.

Güven, S. T. (2015). Sex education and its importance in children with learning disabilities. *Journal of Psychiatric Nursing, 6*(3), 143–148.

Haghigh, A., Mohammadtaghipoor, F., Hamedinia, M., et al. (2019). Effect of a combined exercise program (aerobic and rebound therapy) with two different ratios on some physical and motor fitness indices in intellectually disabled girls. *Baltic Journal of Health and Physical Activity, 11*(1), 24–33.

Hedgecock, J., Standen, P. J., Beer, C., et al. (2014). Evaluating the role of a humanoid robot to support intellectual in children with profound and multiple disabilities. *Journal of Assistive Technologies, 8*(3), 111–123.

Hordacre, A. L. (2016). *Understanding everyday money skills for young people with disabilities.* Adelaide: Australian Industrial Transformation Institute, Flinders University of South Australia.

Kempe, A., & Tissot, C. (2012). The use of drama to teach social skills in a special school setting for students with autism. *Support for Learning, 27*(3), 97–102.

Lawson, H., Byers, R., with Rayner, M., et al. (2015). Curriculum models, issues and tensions. In P. Lacey, R. Ashdown, P. Jones, et al. (Eds.), *The Routledge companion to severe, profound, and multiple learning difficulties* (pp. 233–245). London: Routledge.

Lewis, I., Corcoran, S. L., Juma, S., et al. (2019). Time to stop polishing the brass on the Titanic: moving beyond 'quick-and-dirty' teacher education for inclusion, towards sustainable theories of change. *International Journal of Inclusive Education, 23*(209), 722–739.

Milmo, C., & Stanton, A. (2019). Campaigners warn that special needs children have been forced out of mainstream schools. Available at: https://inews.co.uk/news/education/government-segregation-special-needs-children-mainstream-schools-328706. [Accessed 18 January 2021].

Norwich, B. (2010). Dilemmas of difference, curriculum and disability: international perspectives. *Comparative Education, 46*(2), 113–135.

Nottingham Trent University. (2019) Being on time: my appearance. Available at: https://isrg.org.uk/software/my-appearance/. [Accessed 18 January 2021].

OFSTED. (2006). *Inclusion: does it matter where pupils are taught?* London: OFSTED.

Orchestras Live. (2020). *Able Orchestra.* Available at: https://www.orchestraslive.org.uk/projects/able-orchestra. [Accessed 22 November 2020].

Petrie, K., Devich, J., & Fitzgerald, H. (2018). Working towards inclusive physical education in a primary school: 'some days I just don't get it right'. *Physical Education and Sport Pedagogy, 23*(4), 345–357.

PMLD Link. (2020). Available at: https://www.pmldlink.org.uk/. [Accessed 22 November 2020].

Rooney, N. M. (2016). *Transition-age youth with learning disabilities: providers perspectives on improving post-school outcomes* (Master's dissertation). St Catherine University.

Roult, R., Carbonneau, H., Belley-Ranger, É., et al. (2017). Leisure for people with disabilities in rural Quebec. *Societies, 7*(3), 22.

Seesaw. (2020). Available at: https://web.seesaw.me/platforms. [Accessed 22 November 2020].

Specialist Schools and Academies Trust (SSAT). (2011). *The Complex Intellectual Difficulties and Disabilities Research Project – Engagement Profile and Scale.* Wolverhampton: SSAT.

United Nations. (1989). The United Nations Convention on the Rights of the Child. Available at: https://downloads.unicef.org.uk/wp-content/uploads/2010/05/UNCRC_PRESS200910web.pdf?_ga=2.78590034.795419542.1582474737-1972578648.1582474737. [Accessed 15 January 2021].

United Nations. (2006). Convention on the Rights of Persons with Disabilities (CRPD). Available at: https://www.un.org/development/desa/disabilities/convention-on-the-rights-of-persons-with-disabilities.html. [Accessed 15 January 2021].

United Nations Educational, Scientific and Cultural Organisation [UNESCO]. (2019). *International forum on inclusion and equity in education.* Cali, Colombia.

UNESCO. (1994). *The Salamanca Statement and framework for action on special needs education.* Paris: UNESCO.

Ware, J. (2015). *Engaging learners with complex learning difficulties and disabilities.* London: Routledge.

Weston, C. (2012). Becoming bonded through developmental movement play: review of a parent and child movement group incorporating the theory, practice and philosophy of Sherborne Developmental Movement. *Body Movement and Dance in Psychotherapy, 7*(4), 1–18.

Zainal, M. S., & Hashim, H. (2019). The Implementation of Transition Programme for students with learning disabilities in Malaysia. *Creative Education, 10*(8), 1802–1812.

23

Realising employment: Unfulfilled aspirations?

Julie Ridley, Susan Hunter and Grete Johanne Wangen

KEY ISSUES

- A substantial body of research shows that given the choice, many people with intellectual disabilities would prefer a real job to attending segregated day centres.
- People with intellectual disabilities who seek employment are not always given the encouragement or support they need to find and stay in jobs.
- Despite promising developments in support over the past two decades and a raft of policy, only a small percentage of people with intellectual disabilities are in employment, including in the UK and Norway.
- With the right kind of support and challenging the misconceptions people have about employing people with intellectual disabilities, most can achieve paid jobs in ordinary workplaces.
- An approach known as the 'supported employment model' has been highly effective in making participation in real jobs in their communities a reality for many people with intellectual disabilities.
- Implementing personalised and creative practices in working with people with intellectual disabilities requires health and social care professionals to recognise people's aspirations to be in real jobs; to understand the barriers that sometimes get in the way; and to be knowledgeable about employment outcomes and what effective support looks like.

CHAPTER OUTLINE

INTRODUCTION

Since the early 1980s, being in mainstream employment has become a reality for a growing number of people with intellectual disabilities across the world. The right of all disabled people to participate in the workforce is recognised internationally in policy encapsulated in Article 27 on work and employment of the Convention on the Rights of Persons with Disabilities (United Nations, [UN], 2008), and in practice (European Union of Supported Employment [EUSE], 2010). Policy statements increasingly underline the necessity to increase the range of opportunities disabled people have to be socially integrated, including supporting access to paid jobs in ordinary workplaces (Department for Work and

Pensions [DWP], 2017). The supported employment model, developed in the United States in the 1980s, has been successfully used for decades enabling thousands of people with intellectual disabilities worldwide to enter the labour market, and as a result to contribute to their communities as valued employees and taxpayers. The model uses a partnership strategy to enable disabled people to get and keep employment and supports businesses to employ valuable workers (see website of British Association for Supported Employment [BASE] in online Useful Resources). A convincing body of research and evaluation now exists to show that when people with intellectual disabilities have the right employment support, there is potential to significantly improve people's quality of life, and to increase their participation in local communities, even in the face of welfare cuts (Bates et al, 2017a). Furthermore, as a recent systematic review of the literature found (Beyer and Beyer, 2017), there is also a compelling economic case for employing people with intellectual disabilities.

Despite a body of evidence showing what works, statistics continue to show that the majority of people with intellectual disabilities are far from the workforce, many still attending segregated centres or special provision, with only a minority of people able to fulfil their aspiration to be in a real job (EUSE, 2018; NHS Digital, 2020; Scottish Commission for Learning Disabilities [SCLD], 2018). While this chapter draws extensively on literature from across Europe as well as the USA, it reflects especially on the experience of the authors' own countries, the UK and Norway.

While several empirical studies have indicated overall improvements in quality of life for people in smaller community homes than in large scale institutionalised hospitals (Chowdhury and Benson, 2011; European Union Agency for Fundamental Rights [FRA], 2018), corresponding efforts to promote the inclusion of people with intellectual disabilities in the workforce have been far less impressive. Indeed, for most people with intellectual disabilities a real job continues to be an elusive goal: in the UK, for example, statistics for England for 2019–20 show employment rates for people with intellectual disabilities of only 5.6%, a downward trend year on year after a brief upturn in 2017–18 (NHS Digital, 2020; Hatton, 2018). In Norway, people with intellectual disabilities have even less chance of accessing job opportunities in the open labour market: only

3% of people with intellectual disabilities aged 18 to 25 years and 7% of those aged 26 to 55 years are registered as employed, which means virtually all people with intellectual disabilities are excluded from employment (Wendelborg et al, 2017; Wangen, 2019).

The historic service solution of bringing people together in protected environments, in places such as occupational centres, adult resource centres and sheltered workshops has proven resilient. In these segregated places, people with intellectual disabilities have engaged in industrial contract work and work placements, but such settings have been limited in helping people move onto ordinary jobs in the community. At the same time, some families and carers have expressed reservations about the reconfiguration of day services (Department of Health [DH], 2009a), which can be a powerful barrier to seeking alternatives.

In Western society paid work not only represents an important source of income to satisfy basic needs, but also provides other benefits such as status, occupation, purpose, and the focus of social relationships, the loss of which can result in poor mental and physical health (Bambra and Eikemo, 2009; Bambra, 2010). As such, paid work is a central component in adult identity and people often define themselves, and others, by their occupation. As Roy McConkey (2007) stated in an earlier edition of this handbook, in many cultures people are defined by the nature of their job and many societies value people according to their contribution. Practitioners in health and social care may find themselves at the interface between the wishes of people with intellectual disabilities, the anxieties of their families, changing policy expectations and the legacy of traditional services. Those supporting people with intellectual disabilities have a pivotal role to play in helping them achieve employment if that is a desired goal.

Professionals may be involved in assessment, person centred or lifestyle planning, helping people with intellectual disabilities to identify their needs, aspirations and support requirements (Roulstone et al, 2014; Bates et al, 2017b). The promotion of employment as an option cannot be left solely to employment specialists. It is important that all those involved with people with intellectual disabilities understand the key concepts surrounding employment, the barriers facing individuals who want a real job, and what support is available to achieve this goal.

This chapter adopts a position that perceives disability as a product of social organisation rather than of individual impairment or personal limitation. In the literature this is known as the 'social model of disability' (Oliver, 1990, 1996). In terms of debates regarding employment, this recognises the importance of examining structural as well as individual barriers to employment, and of adopting a broader approach when identifying where the responsibility for change lies and the kinds of solutions that are effective. We begin by examining what is meant by employment.

WHAT IS 'EMPLOYMENT'?

In the literature, the term 'employment' has been used as a rather loose concept that has been variously interpreted and is often synonymous with the term 'work' and includes unpaid and voluntary work as well as paid work (Ridley et al, 2005). While work could be defined as an activity involving the exercise of skills and judgement within set limits prescribed by others, Beyer et al (2004) helpfully clarifies 'employment' as work that someone is paid for at least at the national minimum wage for working a certain number of hours and completing specified tasks. Employment support also covers a wide range of diverse provision, not all of which is focused on supporting people in real paid jobs (European Union [EU], 2012). This is illustrated in Mary's account in Box 23.1 in describing her experience of both unpaid and paid jobs.

Research mapping what employment support is available to people with intellectual disabilities and/or autistic spectrum conditions has often found that the types of support can range from helping people gain and keep jobs in the competitive market, supporting people to run self-employed businesses, through to supporting people in work experience placements and unpaid work (Ridley et al, 2005; EU, 2012; McTier et al, 2016).

BRIEF POLICY CONTEXT

As is widely acknowledged, the issue of employment for people with intellectual disabilities is neither a new idea nor a newcomer to the policy context (DWP, 2017; EUSE, 2018; Parkin et al, 2020). Arguably the Industrial Revolution and its impact on working patterns demanding an organised, skilled and ultimately, literate workforce, propelled the question onto the policy agenda, where it has remained ever since, though with varying degrees of prominence. In the heyday of institutional provision for people with intellectual disabilities, institutions themselves provided often heavy work associated with self-sufficiency in maintaining buildings, growing food and domestic chores - labour in the true sense (Ingham, 2002; Dale, 2004; Reaume, 2004). Community based institutions such as day centres developed patterns of contract work, often repetitive, boring jobs that went unremunerated beyond 'pocket money'. Although contract working has survived in the shape of 'sheltered' workshops, more 'enlightened' welfare policies towards the end of the twentieth century began to promote personal development and social inclusion within day services. This led to the emergence of work experience or placements, usually unpaid, and volunteering as a means of achieving these objectives. Stalker (2001) provides a detailed account of these historical trends.

As the broad rights, equalities and citizenship agendas have gathered momentum in society in general, so has the concept of an 'ordinary life' for people with intellectual disabilities. In other words, services should support individuals to have their own homes in the community and indeed to pursue 'real jobs for real pay' (Wertheimer and Real Jobs Initiative, 1992). Whether in housing, leisure or employment, this has a basis in the 'support' model as opposed to the traditional 'readiness' model of service delivery, where people pass through a range of preparatory stages before graduating into the 'real world'. One criticism of the readiness model in relation to employment was that individuals rarely

> 📄 **BOX 23.1 Mary's story**
>
> Before this job I helped with the lunches at the sheltered housing complex. I used to set the tables for the older people, get the plates ready, serve their lunches, and clear all the tables. It was my job to get their food orders from the menus for the week. I worked 9 hours a week. It was only voluntary work. I was there for 3 years getting £20 a week because that's what you're allowed to earn when you're on benefits. I moved from there onto being in full time employment and came off my benefits.
>
> (Authors' unpublished research)

moved onto paid employment, instead they remained perpetual trainees (Beyer et al, 2004). Originally developed in the USA and now widely implemented across Europe to support people with profound disabilities in employment (Gold, 1980), the supported employment model represents a major shift from readiness thinking to an approach focused on 'place, train and maintain' people in jobs tailored to their individual strengths and interests, whilst providing on-site support through job coaches in a manner that promotes integration into ordinary workforces.

In terms of policy, supporting individuals with intellectual disabilities to get jobs is high on the political agenda. Typical of such policies is the government strategy document, *Valuing Employment Now* (DH, 2009b) applicable to England, which set ambitious goals of placing more people in paid jobs of 16 hours a week or more; tackling barriers to employment; and increasing provision of specialist supported employment personnel and organisations. Later, Scotland's Learning Disability Strategy *The Keys to Life* launched in 2013 identified promoting employment opportunities as a national priority (McTier et al, 2016). More recently, NHS England and NHS Employers launched *NHS Learning Disability Employment* in 2015 to increase opportunities for people with intellectual disabilities employed within the health service through an enhanced support offer. Further, up until May 2019, the DWP ran a 'Proof of Concept' initiative involving nine local authorities offering people with intellectual disabilities and/or autism supported employment to increase their chances of being in real jobs. In a European context, the Vienna Declaration (EUSE, 2018), recently called for urgent action to ensure that the right to employment for all disabled people is implemented. Such policy directives recognise both the moral and economic case, as well as the potential of employment opportunities to increase social inclusion.

Placing the success of UK policies alongside those of comparator countries in Europe and the USA, Beyer and Robinson (2009) concluded that despite a policy trend away from segregated to community-based provision across Europe, the balance of investment remained in favour of specialist workshop provision with limited development of supported employment. Similarly, a mapping exercise involving 30 European countries (EU, 2012) found differential development of supported employment despite strong evidence for its effectiveness. Various weaknesses are identified in the planning and commissioning processes including a loss of capacity in commissioners who understand the importance of real jobs, or the business case for expanding the market for employment support, as well as a failure to link employment supports to the growth of personal and individual budgets (Davies et al, 2012). Critics suggest that too much time and resources are being spent on work preparation and job readiness. Subsequently, the importance of understanding 'what works' and applying this to commissioning supported employment to achieve positive employment outcomes is emphasised (National Development Team for Inclusion [NDTi], 2011; EU, 2012).

In 2006, EUSE drew attention to a range of factors within various countries that impacted differentially on the extent to which supported employment has developed. These included lack of a rights-based approach to disability issues; the absence of a national policy framework for supported employment within an individual country; the lack of dedicated funds to support the implementation of the policy framework; complicated and rigid welfare benefit systems which act as disincentives for people considering full status employment; and a lack of leadership regarding mainstreaming supported employment at national level. A later EU (2012) study of supported employment in 30 European countries found some of these same issues asserting that supported employment should be available to all, and that disabled people should be regarded as jobseekers belonging to countries' mainstream systems. A two-year study on employment support for disabled people in the UK investigating the relationship between investment and outcomes (Greig et al, 2014) concluded that commissioning evidence-based models in the future could radically change the finding that significant sums of money are being spent on service models that do not evidence real job outcomes. Online Reader activity 23.1 encourages further reflection on supported employment policy.

KEY CONCEPTS

In any discussion of employment, it is important to understand the radical shift that occurred during the 1970s-80s from a focus on getting people 'ready' to consider the 'support' they need to achieve individual goals. What is known as the 'support model' (Bradley et al, 1994) evolved from progressive movements in the field of disability and have been highly influential in shaping the goals of human services including how employment support is conceptualised. Traditionally, moving into one's own home and/or getting a job involved progression through various stages and the acquisition of skills until an individual reached a point where services or those in authority felt they were *ready* to take on a specific activity or responsibility. In contrast, the support model places people directly in their own home or job and provides *support* to them where they are; this may be temporary or longer term. In relation to work, it translates into a 'presumption of employability for everyone' (Hagner and DiLeo, 1993, p. 7).

This change was in no small part shaped by the concepts of community participation and inclusion expressed most succinctly in John O'Brien's five accomplishments (O'Brien and Tyne, 1981). These translated the theory and principles of normalisation developed by Wolfensberger (1972, 1983) in North America for practical application. Early ideas of implementing 'normalisation' emerged from Scandinavia arguing that people with intellectual disabilities were entitled to the same patterns of life as those enjoyed in mainstream society with options for work, leisure and accommodation (Nirje, 1980). The writings of Wolfensberger expanded these ideas to consider how historical devaluation of people with intellectual disabilities in Western society and associated stigma could be counteracted by the creation of positive images and socially valued roles – for example, from service recipient to worker, employee or taxpayer. The 'ordinary life' initiative in the UK including an 'ordinary working life' (Kings Fund Centre, 1984), is arguably a direct descendant of normalisation theory. Online Reader activity 23.2 invites further reflection on the nature of employment for people with intellectual disabilities pre-1980.

Whilst these ideas have been instrumental in the transformation of service delivery from large, isolated institutions with their eugenic associations into community-based resources that aspire to promote an inclusive and participatory society, they have not been without their critics in terms of social 'conservatism' in the lifestyles being promoted (Brown and Smith, 1992; Johnson et al, 2010). In theory, as social norms change so do concepts of what is a 'valued lifestyle', but the achievement of what Wolfensberger called 'social role valorisation' has been a more elusive goal. Indeed, research has pointed to less than perfect social

integration outcomes when jobs are for few hours and job quality is poor (Ridley, 2001; Jahoda et al, 2007 McTier et al, 2016). Others have found little evidence of the holistic and strategic approaches that are needed to tackle the social exclusion of people with intellectual disabilities so that they can take advantage of, and benefit from, opportunities such as jobs in ordinary workplaces (Gosling and Cotterill, 2000).

The spread of the above ideas has generated many challenges for practitioners and services from the 1990s onwards, demanding new approaches that emphasise individual choice and self-determination, support and guidance, facilitation rather than direction (Bradley et al, 1994). The degree of choice exercised by an individual in their daily life is affected by the opportunities and the support available. Despite its lesser impact in the field of intellectual disabilities, the social model of disability focuses attention on the responsibility of society to ensure that disabled people are not excluded from the workforce for structural reasons. The implied shift in the power balance in a new type of partnership between disabled people, their families and professionals, is captured in the contemporary term, 'co-production' (Hunter and Ritchie, 2007). This defines quality as conformity with customer requirements and the extent to which they achieve quality of life outcomes, empowerment and choice. The relevance of these concepts to employment are further expanded below. Online Reader activity 23.3 invites further reflection on the meaning of a co-productive approach.

WHY REAL JOBS ARE IMPORTANT

A review of Britain's working age population (Dame Carol Black, 2008) stated that for most people, their job is not only a key determinant of material progress but also a key source of self-worth, family esteem, identity and standing within the community, and a means of social participation and fulfilment. Paid work can be good for health, reversing the harmful effects of long-term unemployment and prolonged sickness absence. Some writers make a direct link between employment and happiness (Bauman, 2008), and with quality of life. Indeed, some have argued that work itself can be used as a single indicator of quality of life (Kiuranor, 1980). From the 1980s onwards, advocates of the 'ordinary life' movement (Kings Fund Centre, 1984; Gathercole and Porterfield, 1985) argued that real jobs offer the following positive benefits for people with intellectual disabilities:

- Meaningful and valued life options
- An income
- A purpose and structure to daily life
- Social links with the community
- Meaningful choices and opportunities
- A sense of personal future

These benefits are clearly highlighted in Edith's story in Box 23.2.

Staggeringly low employment rates for people with intellectual disabilities do not reflect in any way the desire of people with intellectual disabilities to have a job and be part of ordinary workplaces. The consistent message across a number of studies exploring the aspirations of people with intellectual disabilities is that as well as wanting to have friends, to live in an ordinary house, to marry or have a partner, and in some cases to have children, many people want paid jobs (Stalker, 2001; DH, 2009b). This is however sometimes at odds with the views and aspirations of some families and carers (DH, 2009a). Given the choice, people with intellectual disabilities choose paid jobs over attendance at day centres (Racino and Whittico, 1998; Sayce, 2011; McTier et al, 2016). More recently, research with people with intellectual disabilities has found that people want to be in employment, and those that are in very part-time work want jobs that are more hours (Sayce, 2011; Beyer et al, 2004; McTier et al, 2016). In Beyer et al's (2004) research, just under half of those who had been in work in the past or had never worked, wanted a paid job. Similarly, around a third (35%) of people with intellectual disabilities interviewed in a Scottish study (Curtice, 2006) wanted a job.

One study found that people with intellectual disabilities who were in paid work identified money, social interaction, making a contribution to society, and having something to do as the main benefits (Beyer et al, 2004). Other UK studies have found people with intellectual disabilities are more satisfied in supported employment than in their previous day service and reported making new friends at work (Bass, 2000). European research finds clear links between supported employment and better quality of life for people with intellectual disabilities, especially when they are in real jobs in ordinary workplaces, and when there is sufficient support (Verdugo et al, 2006).

 BOX 23.2   Edith's story

Edith works as an events organiser in a nursing home. She plays dominoes and bingo with the residents and makes them cups of tea. Sometimes she goes out with residents. She works 4 afternoons a week for a total of 16 hours per week. She's been in her job for 8 months. This is her first paid job. She is in her 40s and lives with some other people in accommodation with support. Edith really likes her job because she gets to meet new people and because she gets paid. If she didn't have her job, she would really miss meeting people: the residents, the staff and the visitors: "without this, I'd be left out – no family, no friends." Edith's pay helps her to manage her bills better (e.g. her telephone bill). She can also go on holiday, which she's never been able to do before: she's going to Spain. She's also doing more line dancing and buying more clothes. She said that the best thing about the job is "I'm happy. Happiness."

(Ridley et al, 2005, p. 69)

Informants in a Norwegian study highlighted benefits for people with intellectual disabilities in supported employment; these included the importance of being able to make individual choices, and feeling valued and included in society (Wangen, 2019). Alongside such positive claims, is a parallel argument that questions the promotion of employment opportunities and an 'ordinary life', favouring instead the concept of quality of life (Redley, 2009). This line of argument suggests that the danger of adopting employment as the main source of identity and self-esteem is that it reinforces social exclusion and lack of self-worth associated with unemployment (Mayo, 1996; Johnson et al, 2010). Nevertheless, while ideas about the place of employment in current times may seem to be in a state of flux, for most people with intellectual disabilities, paid work is an important determinant of quality of life and economic status. Online Reader activity 23.4 encourages further reflection on the relevance and benefits of participating in the workforce.

SUPPORTED EMPLOYMENT MODEL

The supported employment model emerged from the USA in the mid-1980s and has become a well-established approach across Europe demonstrating success in finding jobs with a range of disabled people and maintaining them in these jobs (Schneider et al, 2002; EU, 2012). In contrast to the readiness model, the supported employment model, evolving from progressive movements in the field of disability, sought to place people directly into jobs and provide the support they need for as long as needed, commonly referred to as 'place, train and maintain' (Leach, 2002). Supported employment developed out of dissatisfaction with the poor employment outcomes of sheltered workshops in the USA (Mank, 1994), and built on the ground breaking research of Marc Gold into the learning capacity of people with severe disabilities to learn skills once considered far too difficult or complex (Gold, 1973, 1980). The concept of 'Try Another Way', both as an ideological and educational principle, evolved from his observations of how people with intellectual disabilities learnt new skills (Gold, 1980). He argued that finding the desired job for the person and then providing the necessary training and support on site in the workplace was both effective and functional from a learning perspective. In line with the early ideas and values of normalisation and social role appreciation (Kristiansen, 1996), jobs should be found in regular workplaces and without prior training or insistence that people were job ready.

In the UK, the growth of agencies offering supported employment since the 1980s has been associated with the failure of traditional Adult Training Centres and Adult Resource Centres to deliver good employment outcomes, and a drive to shift from segregated, group-based services to community-based, individualised solutions. One survey (Beyer et al, 1996) evidenced the expansion from just five agencies offering supported employment in the UK in 1986, increasing to over 200 by 1995, and an estimated 5,000 people nationally, predominantly people with intellectual disabilities, were employed with local employers. This growth was most significant in England and Wales, and somewhat slower in Scotland and other parts of Europe (Sutton, 1999). In Norway, developments started with a two-year pilot project conducted in Oslo supporting 20 people with intellectual disabilities to get and keep jobs in the open labour market (Wangen, 2019). Promising results led to the implementation of a nationwide project during 1992–1995 supporting a range of disabled people, young people who have dropped out of school, people with drug and alcohol problems and people with mental health problems. Three quarters of job seekers in the national project attained jobs or came closer to the labour market including 83% of those with intellectual disabilities (Spjelkavik et al, 2003).

In the USA, supported employment is defined in legislation and supported by a system of federal and state funding. Under the US Rehabilitation Amendments Act 1968, providers are required to target individuals with severe disabilities who require ongoing support in order to perform their work, and jobs must be for a minimum of 20 hours per week. No such stipulation exists in the UK and European versions of supported employment. Nonetheless, a broad definition of supported employment operationalised across Europe is that it means:

Providing support to people with disabilities or other disadvantaged groups to secure and maintain paid employment in the open labour market (EUSE, 2010).

Despite a lack of consensus of definition in the UK and Europe, there is agreement internationally across research and policy commentators that three elements are consistent and are considered fundamental to supported employment (EUSE, 2010):

1. Paid work - individuals should receive commensurate pay for work carried out – if a country operates a national minimum wage then the individual must be paid at least this rate or the going rate for the job;

2. Open labour market – supported employees should be regular employees with the same wages, terms and conditions as other employees who are employed in businesses/organisations within the public, private or voluntary sectors;

3. Ongoing support – referring to job support in its widest sense whilst in paid employment. Support is individualised and meets the needs of both employee and employer.

Initially the model embraced four alternatives thought necessary to adapt to local employment situations and individual service requirements. Three were group-based models, although it is the 'individual placement model' or 'job coach model' (Tannen, 1993) that is generally what is commonly referred to as supported employment in Europe. In relation to supporting people with mental health problems, this is often referred to as the 'Individual Placement and Support' or IPS model, and additional emphasis is placed on the co-location of specialist employment staff, such as job coaches and clinical staff.

A five-stage process for supported employment is identified in an experience-based *Toolkit for Supported Employment* developed by a European partnership of practitioners as a model of good practice (EUSE, 2010). The Toolkit serves to reinforce a consistent methodology for the delivery of specialist supported employment services across Europe, and aims to reinforce the values, standards, principles and process of supported employment. Box 23.3 summarises the five-stage process, which should be considered dynamic and adapted to individual job seeker's needs.

At the heart of this 'place and train' approach is the assumption that employment outcomes are maximised when the training of individuals is implemented on site rather than through pre-vocational methods. A key element is the provision of flexible support to an individual, which it is assumed will vary between individuals and may be required at different stages in the process (EU, 2012). However, it will typically involve training on-the-job, usually involving Training in Systematic Instruction (TSI) methods (Leach, 2002), presence at the workplace for a period after which support may be faded, and regular monitoring visits and/or telephone calls to the individual and/or the employer. The model presumes that there are some individuals who will require support indefinitely and for whom reduction of support would not be appropriate. The important role of support is illustrated in the following case example (see Box 23.4).

 BOX 23.3 Five core processes of Supported Employment

1. **Engagement** – Underpinned by the core values of accessibility to ensure informed choices are made
2. **Vocational Profiling** – Ensuring empowerment to the individual throughout the process
3. **Job Finding** – Self-determination and informed choice are key values in Supported Employment
4. **Employer Engagement** – Accessibility, flexibility and confidentiality are key values to be nurtured through this process
5. **On/Off Job Support** – Flexibility, confidentiality and respect are the key components to successful support measures in paid employment delivered through an Employment Support Worker/Job Coach (EUSE, 2010)

BOX 23.4 Support to get a real job

"The supported employment team helped me get the job. I wouldn't have moved onto the job without them. It would be kind of difficult to do on your own because not everyone is as nice to you. You can phone anytime you want and once a year she comes up and sees how I'm doing in work. Before I got this job Sam came into the interview with me and showed me some wee techniques, ways of answering questions and how you ask questions at interviews. If you've never had interviews it can be very hard so it prepared me and I got the job. I felt better with Sam being there. The supported employment team helped me find the job and fill in the forms. Now I've got a supervisor at work to support me. The women that you work with as well who've been there longer they help me as well. They're all nice there, it makes a difference."

BARRIERS TO EMPLOYMENT

Given the now vast body of research demonstrating successful outcomes for supported employment, the barriers to employment for people with intellectual disabilities would appear to reside in the lack of opportunity, low expectations and problems with support. People with intellectual disabilities report they encounter several barriers to finding and keeping jobs (Allen, 2006). A survey of people with intellectual disabilities in Scotland (Curtice, 2006) cited health, disability, not being able to find suitable employment and the benefits trap as common barriers to work. Barriers appear at three levels: personal or individual; structural and attitudinal barriers.

Personal or individual barriers

At an individual or personal level, adults with intellectual disabilities may lack skills or qualifications that can be easily matched with the current job market and have limited experience of workplace culture and the demands of work. They may have difficulties interacting socially with other people and may sometimes challenge others by their behaviour. Some personal barriers people face can arise from slower than average learning of new tasks, memory issues, communication issues which impact on receiving instruction and giving information, impaired motor function performance, and difficulties with changing routines (Beyer and Beyer, 2017, p. 4). In many respects, they share many of the problems faced by other long-term unemployed people, particularly young adults who have no experience of the job market. One response to these individual barriers, is supported internships through *Project Search*, providing the opportunity to learn employability skills in real workplaces and achieve 50% employment outcomes. Project Search, originally developed at Cincinnati children's Hospital Medical Center in 1996, and applied extensively across the UK (see DFN Project Search, 2020), is based on supported employment best practice. Online Reader activity 23.5 invites further reflection on this notion of job aspirations.

Structural barriers

On a structural level, aspects of the UK social security system and other related systems have long been identified as causing major problems for individuals with intellectual disabilities who want real jobs, as well as impacting on the further development of supported employment (O'Bryan et al, 2000). However, evidence supports the view that skilled and knowledgeable professionals who stay well informed of benefit regulations and changes, and introduce the income potential of employment from the start, can effectively work with such barriers (Hunter and Ridley, 2007; McInally, 2008). Financial calculations to find out whether the individual will be worse off in work are therefore a prime consideration for most disabled people contemplating paid employment, and many employment projects consider this fundamental and always include a full welfare benefits check. A good illustration of this is North Lanarkshire Council Scotland which developed a corporate strategy for supported employment that tackled these barriers by maximising benefits, only supporting jobs of 16 hours plus a week to attract tax credits, increasing opportunities for social integration, and offering school leavers employment options as a matter of routine (Joseph Rowntree Foundation [JRF], 2002; McInally, 2008). The initiative not only doubled individual's disposable income on average, but each job cost half the support costs of a day placement (DH, 2009b). Margaret's story in Box 23.5 illustrates the benefits of this approach.

Structural barriers also include the inflexibility of changing and shrinking job markets, particularly in times of recession. Changing patterns of employment

---

BOX 23.5   Margaret's story

Margaret is 19 years old, has intellectual disabilities and suffers with depression. She attended mainstream education and on leaving school attended a local college for two years. When she was referred to North Lanarkshire Council Supported Employment Service her sole income consisted of £15 Child Benefit. An immediate priority for the service was to maximise Margaret's income. With the assistance of the service she was awarded Income Support and Disability Living Allowance (DLA) increasing her benefit from £15 to £96.85 per week. Margaret started working in a local nursing home in March 2004.
(Ridley et al, 2005, p. 106)

---

mean that for a significant proportion of the population job sharing and temporary part-time work, alongside zero-hour contracts, have become the norm. Since the 1980s tele-working or home-based working are also now more acceptable, and in an increasingly high-tech world there is an expectation that workers are multi-skilled and can demonstrate a portfolio of skills and experience (Handy, 1984). In more recent years, these challenges have led to increased interest in developing supported self-employment initiatives for people with intellectual disabilities to provide more personalised employment opportunities (Bates, 2009). While it has been claimed that a major barrier to supported employment is high rates of unemployment, evidence shows that even in areas with traditionally high rates of unemployment, jobs have been secured when people get the right support (McInally, 2008). Equally, Roulstone et al (2014) identify the need for greater personalisation in employment support to address challenging local labour markets and finite funding. Furthermore, Bates et al (2017a) demonstrated that when people with intellectual disabilities are supported in imaginative and novel ways, they can participate successfully in employment at times of budget cuts and austerity.

Attitudinal barriers

Other people's attitudes and perceptions can be a significant barrier to employment for people with intellectual disabilities. There may have been little or no preparation for employment at school; and their experiences will typically be of segregated services, for example

Adult Training Centres (ATCs), and of institutionalisation, which suggests a need to be working with young people with intellectual disabilities to raise their aspirations (Bates et al, 2017b). One woman with intellectual disabilities in a job commented:

"I sometimes think of all the people left at the day centres and feel sad for them. Even if people can't read or write they should be encouraged all the time to get jobs. The problem is that people get used to going to the ATC, don't believe in themselves anymore and lose their confidence. Eventually they don't bother trying and give up."

Demby, 1992, p. 6

For many of us, employment is an expected aspiration fostered from an early age, but this is often not so for people with intellectual disabilities. Families are disempowered by professionals discouraging them from holding the idea that one day their son or daughter will be in a job, perceiving this generally as 'unrealistic'. Accepting what professionals offer, parents have continued to demand a service system that perpetuates low expectations of people with intellectual disabilities (DH, 2009a; McTier et al, 2016). Although easy to generalise about the over protectiveness of parents, and the at times conflicting interests between people with intellectual disabilities and their family carers, it should be remembered that it was parents, and not professionals, who pioneered the Mencap Pathway Scheme in England and Wales. Parents were also instrumental in many of the changes occurring in the USA and Canada in the 1980s, resulting in a more advanced system of vocational services than in Britain, and more recently in the growth of the service brokerage movement. Mencap, formed by Judy Fryd, a mother of a child with intellectual disabilities in 1946, continues to champion the benefits of employing people with intellectual disabilities and to make the business case (Capper, 2017).

It is often assumed that realising the goal of employment for people with intellectual disabilities depends heavily on an attitudinal shift among employers. However, research findings are inconclusive about what determines how sympathetic an employer will be toward employing people with intellectual disabilities (Unger, 2002). What the research does find, however, is that the most positive employers are those who have previously employed people with intellectual disabilities and/or have experience of support from specialist employment agencies. These employers often emphasise the reliability and dependability of employees with intellectual disabilities, as well as the significance to them in helping them fulfil their duty to implement equal opportunities and give individuals a valuable role in life (Beyer and Beyer, 2017; Capper, 2017). Luecking et al (2004) asserted that employers with experience develop more positive views even when these workers have severe disabilities. A UK survey exploring attitudes about people with intellectual disabilities as employees found that a majority considered that integrated work is best for most, and nine out of ten believed that employing people with intellectual disabilities would not adversely affect the workplace. Several respondents identified a lack of work training measures as the major obstacle to greater inclusion (Burge et al, 2007). In a comprehensive survey of Norwegian companies, roughly 10% responded that they would consider hiring people with intellectual disabilities in the future, indicating a more positive predisposition towards employing people with intellectual disabilities than might be expected (Ellingsen, 2011).

REALITIES OF PRACTICE

Research over the past 20 years or so has identified key challenges and issues with supported employment in practice. These have included differences in how supported employment has been operationalised in practice, and that implementation has slowed despite strong evidence about the effectiveness of the model in achieving positive employment outcomes. Not only this, but those with more severe impairments are least likely to benefit from support. In response to the poor implementation outcomes of supported employment, the sector has developed occupational standards that re-establish inclusion competency, emphasise core principles and values, and serve to (re)assure that provision offers quality employment support. Each of these issues will now be considered in more detail.

Variations in supported employment in practice

Employment support covers a vast canvas of international activity, not all of which is supported employment (Ridley and Hunter, 2006; EU, 2012). Also, supported employment takes many different shapes and forms in the different countries affecting individual access. A consequence of this is that comparison and exchange of knowledge and experience across countries become more complicated. Many of the agencies supporting people with intellectual disabilities are involved in pre-vocational or work preparation activities, and are not working towards employment outcomes (McTier et al, 2016). Furthermore, EU (2012) research finds decreasing numbers of dedicated supported employment services across Europe, which is significant because research demonstrates better financial outcomes for employees supported by services that have dedicated job finders and staff with qualifications (Beyer, 2001).

The type and quality of jobs has varied enormously between supported employment agencies, and this affects the quality of individual outcomes. A key issue identified from research over 20 years ago was the similarity of treatment of disabled and non-disabled people in terms of job recruitment, compensation and training, and this has affected, and continues to affect, the potential for integrating supported employees (Mank et al, 1998). Recognising the centrality of these issues can be seen in UK law which has made it illegal for employers to discriminate against disabled people, and has introduced the requirement for employers to make 'reasonable adjustments' in the workplace (Equality Act 2010, Section 20).

Problems with implementation

Many studies conclude that despite the positive outcomes experienced from supported employment, its implementation, not only in the UK but in other European countries such as Spain, as well as the USA, has been somewhat disappointing (Beyer et al, 2002; Pallisera et al, 2003; Hunter and Ridley, 2007; Beyer and Robinson, 2009). The worldwide trend is only a minority of people with intellectual disabilities participate in the labour market. Even in the USA with a longer history of implementing supported employment, percentages of disabled people in ordinary jobs has been falling over time; studies report falls of disabled people in jobs from 34% in 1986 to 21% by 2010 and this trend has continued (Riesen et al, 2015).

Since the 1990s, there has been a decline in work-oriented schemes in Norway and– at least for a period– an increase in care-oriented schemes for people with intellectual disabilities leaving many people marginalised and on the outskirts of both ordinary and sheltered labour markets. Norwegian studies have also shown a marked decrease in people with intellectual disabilities in supported employment in contrast to other European countries such as Spain, Finland and the UK (Beyer et al, 2010). Only 2.9% of people with intellectual disabilities were in employment with support in Norway in the same year (Reinertsen, 2012; Wangen, 2019). Many countries invest more resources in segregated or specialist provision than in community employment; supported employment appears to have become part of a continuum of responses rather than an alternative to segregated services. Online Reader activity 23.6 invites research into employment services that exist in different areas.

Another issue related to implementation is that many people with intellectual disabilities are in unpaid jobs or working in jobs that are for a few hours. For instance, research in Scotland identified the majority of people with intellectual disabilities were supported in work that was unpaid or voluntary, and those who were in paid jobs were in jobs for under 10 hours per week, some for as little as one or two hours (Ridley et al, 2005). Of those in unpaid or voluntary work placements, 14% had been in these placements for more than four years, challenging the argument that such work placements improve people's employment outcomes. In mapping the employability landscape in Scotland 10 years later, McTier et al (2016) found people with intellectual disabilities in jobs that varied between three and 43 hours per week with the average between 10–20 hours per week, pointing out the need to distinguish between real, sustainable employment and part-time, sheltered employment that should not be viewed as sustainable jobs that people can earn a living from.

Similarly, a UK wide survey of supported employment agencies in the mid-90s (Beyer and Kilsby, 1997) found that almost half of people in supported employment were working less than 16 hours per week with 42% having total earnings of £15 or less. In Norway, of people with intellectual disabilities that are in jobs most work part-time, and a fifth are working less than 10 hours per week (Wendelborg et al, 2017; Wangen, 2019). Working part-time and for short hours, therefore, seems to be a common experience, and as some researchers conclude means that supported employment has not significantly increased the incomes of people with intellectual disabilities entering employment from their previous situation (Beyer and Robinson, 2009). Online Reader activity 23.7 encourages reflection on the quality aspects of jobs.

Inequalities of access

There are consistent inequalities in access to supported employment. This despite the model originally being inspired by the needs of people with higher support needs, and a key principle of supported employment is 'no exclusion', that is, people should not be excluded because it is assumed that they are not ready for work or that they have major challenges (Wangen, 2014). In a survey of employment support in Scotland, only 7% of supported employees were people with severe intellectual disabilities (Ridley et al, 2005). Less well served by existing services were people with autistic spectrum conditions, women with intellectual disabilities and those from black and minority ethnic communities. An early review of supported employment outcomes and practice in the USA also noted that outcomes were harder to obtain for people with severe impairments, and there appeared to be gender differences with more men in supported employment than women (Mank et al, 1998).

Recent years have seen the concept of *Customised Employment* develop in the USA to ensure that supported employment continues to be about tailor-made job development for job seekers with complex support needs (Harvey et al, 2013). This arose from a recognition that the focus of job specialists on securing ordinary working conditions and wages has sometimes taken the focus away from developing jobs based on what best suits the individual and his/her assets and support needs (Griffin et al, 2007; Inge et al, 2018). Customised Employment is thus defined as:

> "*Individualizing the employment relationship between employees and employers in ways that meet the needs of both. It is based on an individualized determination of strengths, needs, and interests of the person with a disability, and is also designed to meet the specific needs of the employer.*"

> *Riesen et al., 2015*, p. 184

The concept has been widely researched in the USA and there is now a growth in control studies involving people with intellectual disabilities. So far, the researchers have developed a fidelity scale for the first stage of the process, which is referred to as 'Discovery' (Riesen, et al. 2019). This is illustrated in Sara's story in Box 23.6 with Reader activity 23.8 providing the opportunity to reflect on the process, applying learning from the chapter.

 BOX 23.6   Sara's story: Illustration of the Discovery process

Sara has complex support needs including some issues with losing her temper and some personal hygiene issues. She also has one big dream: to be a shop assistant in a particular interior and gift shop in Oslo. She has been working in a sheltered workshop, assembling electronic devices. Although her manager is keen to keep her - as she is one of their best workers - Sara's wishes are taken seriously and a work trial was arranged at the shop. She started one day a week, and Andrea, the employment specialist, was with her the whole time. It was agreed that the employer should teach Sara how to behave towards customers in the shop. Andrea should assist Sara with the laundry and personal hygiene at home, as well as monitoring Sara's development at work. After two weeks, Sara said *"it has been so nice to get this job. I have become happier and proud of myself"*. Sara is now in her second working year at the shop and works there three days a week. Andrea drops by every fortnight. The employer says *"Sara is amazing in the shop. She knows where every item is and she is always doing her best. Customers ask her for help"*. Sara now manages the cash register and is at times responsible for closing the shop.

 READER ACTIVITY 23.8   Sara's story: Reflection and application of learning

1. What do you notice about this process and how the supported employment project has worked with Sara?
2. Identify the outcome of this approach for a) Sara; and b) her employer.
3. What are the positive and negative aspects of this job in realising Sara's employment aspirations?

Entrepreneurship is widely reflected in global social trends, and promoted by governmental policies including those of the EU, which in 1999 declared the creation of an 'enterprise culture' to be at the top of the public policy agenda (McQuaid, 2000). Supported self-employment is another adaptation of supported employment, which has responded flexibly to the needs of people with more complex support needs and the importance of personalising job outcomes. Interest in supported self-employment opportunities has grown in the USA (Callahan et al, 2002; Griffin and Hammis, 2003), and there are examples of this being used successfully in supporting people with severe intellectual disabilities. So far in the UK, this has been pursued on a limited scale. Arguably, self-employment provides the necessary flexibility and a better adjustment between disability status and working life, and European studies have found that disabled people generally are more likely to be self-employed than non-disabled people (Pagan, 2009). Several organisations, including the Foundation for People with Learning Disabilities in the UK (Bates, 2009) now provide useful guides to help people with intellectual disabilities move into self-employment. Jenny's story in the accompanying online resource illustrates this.

Improving inclusion competency through standards

The fragility of the sector and need for supported employment services to become more widely available and to be of of consistent quality (O'Bryan et al, 2000) has led to the employment sector addressing inclusion competence through development of international (EUSE, 2010) and national occupational standards for supported employment (British Association for Supported Employment [BASE] and the Learning and Skills Improvement Service [LSIS], 2017). The EUSE Toolkit for Supported Employment (EUSE, 2010) aimed to reinforce a consistent methodology for the delivery of specialist supported employment services through increasing the awareness and competencies of the staff responsible for vocational assessment, job finding and on-going employment support for job seekers and employees. Moreover, the Toolkit aimed to reinforce the core values, standards, principles and process of supported employment.

The concept of inclusion competence is relatively new but seems to have become firmly established in the field of job inclusion. It was developed in Norway and the first edited book on the subject published in 2014 by Frøyland and Spjelkavik. It is a common term for a set of attitudes, knowledge and skills necessary to provide job support to people with complex assistance needs so that they receive and retain regular jobs. The competence consists of social, pedagogical and health professional knowledge of the job seeker's support needs in combination with guidance methodology. Furthermore, inclusion expertise consists of knowledge of how to use ordinary workplaces so that job seekers with complex assistance needs can get a job, and experience both mastery and development in and on the job.

PRINCIPLES FOR BEST PRACTICE

A set of clear principles emerge from both the body of international research into supported employment and provider statements about quality standards. Together these offer a defining framework for considering how best to support people with intellectual disabilities to access and sustain real paid jobs. The following principles (see Box 23.7) are derived from research that sought the opinions of people with intellectual disabilities and others about best practice and quality in supported employment (Ridley and Hunter, 2007).

In terms of an overarching framework, the Supported Employment Quality Framework (SEQF) produced by the British Association for Supported Employment (BASE, 2017), together with transnational partners including Supported Employment Norway, and the European Union of Supported Employment, emphasises how managers and job specialists can work together to improve the quality of supported employment. The SEQF links the five basic principles of supported employment (client engagement, vocational profiling, job finding, employer engagement and job support) to one or more of the nine EFQM (European Foundation for Quality Management) areas. It contains a scored self-assessment toolkit for organisations which can be used to prioritise actions to further improve the quality of support offered to jobseekers and employers. Links to the SEQF can be found in the accompanying Useful Resources online.

CONCLUSION

This chapter has focused on the issue of employment for people with intellectual disabilities. Some may dismiss the idea of employment as unrealistic especially for those considered to have severe intellectual disabilities, and at times of high unemployment and austerity. Others, equally point to the moral and rights-based approach upon which supported employment is founded. It needs to be remembered that the supported employment

BOX 23.7   Principles for supporting people with intellectual disabilities in employment Ridley & Hunter 2007

1. **Real jobs/valued roles** – there should be a clear focus from the outset on securing the outcome of real paid jobs, providing valued roles for people with intellectual disabilities in their communities. As an employee, individuals should be paid the going rate for the job and have the same workplace terms and conditions as other employees

2. **A presumption of employability** – everyone who wants to work should be assumed to be employable with the right support. Employment should be actively considered an option for people with intellectual disabilities and/or autistic spectrum conditions (ASC)

3. **Learn about work on the job** – individuals with intellectual disabilities and/or ASC should be trained on the job rather than preparing for future employment

4. **Flexible support** - people with intellectual disabilities and/or ASC should receive flexible, individualised support that is not time limited and is tailored to meet their individual needs. Follow-on support, and support to develop, progress in or move onto other jobs should be a feature

5. **Promote early participation in employment** – access to employment support should be at the earliest stage possible e.g. at school leaving age. If employment is on the curriculum for disabled pupils, progression to employment will increasingly become more of a natural assumption for everyone

6. **Equality of access** – support to access employment should be available for everyone interested in working regardless of label, support need or perceived level of functioning, including those with more severe intellectual disabilities and/or ASC

7. **Personalisation** – people with intellectual disabilities and/or ASC should be treated as individuals and support should be customised for each person. The emphasis should be on finding out what each person wants to do and where his/her skills and aspirations lie and using these in the job finding and development process

8. **Participation and involvement** – individuals with intellectual disabilities and/or ASC should be fully involved in all aspects of the process, and have the information and support necessary to enable them to participate

9. **Self-determination and choice** – people with intellectual disabilities and/or ASC should be asked about the support they need, be encouraged to express individual choice and be involved in deciding what they want. They should be helped to understand their opportunities fully so they can make informed choices

10. **Social inclusion** – people with intellectual disabilities and/or ASC should be offered real jobs with ordinary or mainstream employers and have the opportunity to work alongside non-disabled co-workers.

approach was originally developed to help people with more severe impairments who would not otherwise be able to access the labour market. The fact that they have been failed should not be taken as evidence that employment is unsuitable for them, but as evidence of the limited implementation of this model so far.

There is great unmet potential in the population of people labelled as having intellectual disabilities, yet many who want real jobs are not being supported or encouraged by those working most closely with them and/or their families to realise their vocational aspirations. Presuming that everyone who wants to work is employable with the right support, is a radical shift in thinking. Until it becomes the default position to offer people with intellectual disabilities, regardless of the severity of their impairments or support needs, the support they need to attain real jobs, they will continue to be in segregated services and on the periphery of their communities. The presumption of employment is the most important underpinning principle of best practice identified by research and is in line with international policy.

Dedication

This chapter is dedicated to the late Rose Trustam who was a tireless campaigner for the rights of people with intellectual disabilities.

Acknowledgements

In updating the chapter, we acknowledge the extensive help received from Huw Davies of the British Association for Supported Employment who gave generously of his time, knowledge and networks. Also significant was the support we received from Dr Simon Jarrett, Editor of Community Living magazine who always knew who we should ask to get the facts right.

REFERENCES

Allen, D. (2006). Life better but jobs scarce, say Scottish respondents. *Learning Disability Practice*, 9(6), 6.

Bambra, C. (2010). Yesterday once more? Unemployment and health in the 21st century. *Journal of Epidemiology and Community Health*, 64, 213–215.

Bambra, C., & Eikemo, T. A. (2009). Welfare state regimes, unemployment and health: a comparative study of the relationship between unemployment and self-reported health in 23 European countries. *Journal of Epidemiology and Community Health*, 63, 92–98.

Bass, M. (2000). *Supported employment for people with learning difficulties.* York: Joseph Rowntree Foundation.

Bates, K. (2009). *In business: developing the self-employment option for people with learning disabilities.* London: Foundation for People with Learning Disabilities.

Bates, K., Goodley, D., & Runswick-Cole, K. (2017a). Precarious lives and resistant possibilities: the labour of people with learning disabilities in times of austerity. *Disability & Society*, 32(2), 160–175.

Bates, K., Davies, J., & Burke, C. (2017b). *When I grow up. Raising the aspirations and employment prospects of young people with learning disabilities. Practical support for schools and colleges.* London: Foundation for People with Learning Disabilities.

Bauman, Z. (2008). *The art of life.* Cambridge: Polity Press.

Beyer, S. (2001). *How does agency organisation impact on employment outcomes?* Paper presented at 5th European Union of Supported Employment Conference, March, Edinburgh.

Beyer, S., Goodere, L., & Kilsby, M. (1996). *The costs and benefits of supported employment agencies.* London: The Stationery Office.

Beyer, S., & Kilsby, M. (1997). Supported employment in Britain. *Tizard Learning Disability Review*, 2(2), 6–14.

Beyer, S., Hedeboux, G., Morgan, C., et al. (2002). *International reflections: an interim report on effective approaches to vocational training and employment for people with learning disabilities from the Labor Project.*

Beyer, S., Grove, B., Schneider, J., et al. (2004). *Working lives: the role of day centers in supporting people with learning disabilities into employment.* Leeds: Department of Work & Pensions.

Beyer, S., & Robinson, C. (2009). *A review of the research literature on supported employment: a report for the Cross-Government Learning Disability Employment Strategy Team.* London: Department of Health.

Beyer, S., Jordán de Urríes, F., & Verdugo, M. (2010). A comparative study of the situation of supported employment in Europe. *Journal of Policy and Practice in Intellectual Disabilities*, 7, 130–136.

Beyer, S., & Beyer, A. (2017). *A systematic review of the literature on the benefits for employers of employing people with learning disabilities.* London: Mencap.

Bradley, V. J., Ashbaugh, J. W., & Blaney, B. C. (1994). *Creating individual supports for people with developmental disabilities – a mandate for change at many levels.* Baltimore: Paul H Brookes.

British Association for Supported Employment (BASE). (2017). Supported employment quality framework. Available at: https://www.base-uk.org/knowledge/supported-employment-quality-framework. [Accessed 15 February 2021].

British Association for Supported Employment (BASE) and the Learning and Skills Improvement Service (LSIS). (2017). *National occupations standards for supported employment.* Available at: https://www.base-uk.org/sites/default/files/pdfs/NOS%20Job%20Coaching%202017.pdf. [Accessed 30 November 2020].

Brown, H., & Smith, H. (1992). *Normalisation. A reader for the nineties.* London: Routledge.

Burge, P., Ouellette-Kuntz, H., & Lysaght, R. (2007). Public views on employment of people with intellectual disabilities. *Journal of Vocational Rehabilitation*, 26(1), 29–37.

Callahan, M., Shumpert, N., & Mast, M. (2002). Self-employment, choice and self-determination. *Journal-of-Vocational-Rehabilitation*, 17(2), 75–85.

Capper, M. (2017). *Good for business. The benefits of employing people with a learning disability.* London: Mencap.

Chowdhury, M., & Benson, B. A. (2011). Deinstitutionalization and quality of life of individuals with intellectual disability: a review of the international literature. *Journal of Policy and Practice in Intellectual Disabilities*, 8(4), 256–265.

Curtice, L. (2006). *How is it going? A survey of what matters most to people with learning disabilities in Scotland today.* Glasgow: Enable.

Dale, P. (2004). Training for work: domestic service as a route out of long-stay institutions before 1959. *Women's History Review*, 13(3), 387–405.

Dame Carol Black. (2008). *Review of the health of Britain's working age population.* London: TSO.

Davies, H., Melling, K., & Wilson, P. (2012). *Personalisation and supported employment. A BILD guide.* British

Association for Supported Employment/British Institute for Learning Disabilities.

Demby, S. (1992). My future is bright. *Community Living*, 6(2), 6.

Department for Work and Pensions (DWP). (2017). *Improving lives: the future of work, health and disability*. London: DWP. White Paper.

Department of Health (DH). (2009a). *Valuing people now: a new three-year strategy for people with learning disabilities. Making it happen for everyone*. London: Department of Health.

Department of Health (DH). (2009b). *Valuing employment now: valuing real jobs for people with learning disabilities*. London: Department of Health.

DFN Project Search. (2020). Available at: https://www.dfn-projectsearch.org/. [Accessed 29 December 2020].

Ellingsen, K. E. (2011). By the far end of the table? On work participation for people with intellectual disability. *Fontene Forskning*, 2(11), 4–19.

Equality Act. (2010). Available at: https://www.legislation.gov.uk/ukpga/2010/15/contents. [Accessed 15 February 2021].

European Union (EU). (2012). *Supported employment for people with disabilities in the EU And EFTA-EEA – Good practices and recommendations in support of a flexicurity approach*. Luxemburg: European Union.

European Union Agency for Fundamental Rights (FRA). (2018). *From institutions to community living for persons with disabilities: perspectives from the ground*. Vienna: European Union Agency for Fundamental Rights.

European Union of Supported Employment (EUSE). (2010). *European Union of Supported Employment toolkit*. Dundee: EUSE/Leonardo Partnership. Available at: http://euse.org/content/supported-employment-toolkit/EUSE-Toolkit-2010.pdf. [Accessed 18 November 2020].

European Union of Supported Employment (EUSE). (2018). Employment for all. Strategies for the implementation of the UN CRPD Vienna Declaration. Available at: http://www.euse.org/images/Vienna_Declaration-EN.pdf [Accessed 18 November 2020].

Frøyland, K., & Spjelkavik, Ø. (Eds.). (2014). *Inclusion skills competence. Ordinary work as an aim and a means*. Oslo: Gyldendal Akademisk.

Gathercole, C., & Porterfield, J. (1985). *The employment of people with mental handicap: progress towards an ordinary working life*. London: Kings Fund Centre.

Gold, M. (1973). Research on the vocational habilitation of the retarded: the present, the future. In N. R. Ellis (Ed.), *International review of research in mental retardation* (Vol. 6). New York: Academic Press.

Gold, M. (1980). *Try another way – training manual*. Champaign, IL: Research Press.

Gosling, V., & Cotterill, L. (2000). An employment project as a route to social inclusion for people with learning difficulties? *Disability & Society*, 15(7), 1001–1018.

Greig, R., Chapman, P., Eley, A., et al. (2014). The cost effectiveness of employment support for people with disabilities. Available at: https://www.ndti.org.uk/resources/the-cost-effectiveness-of-employment-support-for-people-with-disabilities. [Accessed 30 November 2020].

Griffin, C., & Hammis, D. (2003). *Making self employment work for people with disabilities*. Baltimore: Paul Brookes.

Griffin, C., Hammis, D., & Geary, T. (2007). *The job developer's handbook. Practical tactics for customized employment*. Baltimore: Paul Brookes.

Hagner, D. C., & DiLeo, D. (1993). *Working together: workplace culture, supported employment and persons with disabilities*. Cambridge, MA: Brookline Books.

Handy, C. (1984). *The future of work: a guide to a changing society*. London: Blackwell.

Harvey, J., Szoc, R., Dela Rosa, M., et al. (2013). Understanding the competencies needed to customize jobs: a competency model for customized employment. *Journal of Vocational Rehabilitation*, 38, 77–89.

Hatton, C. (2018). Paid employment amongst adults with learning disabilities receiving social care in England: trends over time and geographical variation. *Tizard Learning Disability Review*, 23(2), 117–122.

Hunter, S., & Ridley, J. (2007). Supported employment in Scotland: some issues from research and implications for development. *Tizard Learning Disability Review*, 12(2), 3–13.

Hunter, S., & Ritchie, P. (2007). *Co-production & personalisation in social care: changing relationships in the provision of social care*. London: Jessica Kingsley Publishers.

Inge, K. J., Graham, C. W., Brooks-Lane, N., et al. (2018). Defining customized employment as an evidence-based practice: the results of a focus group study. *Journal of Vocational Rehabilitation*, 48, 155–166.

Ingham, N. (2002). *Gogarburn lives*. Edinburgh: Living Memory Association.

Jahoda, A., Kemp, J., Riddell, S., et al. (2007). Feelings about work: a review of the socio-emotional impact of supported employment on people with intellectual disabilities. *Journal of Applied Research in Intellectual Disabilities*, 21(1), 1–18.

Johnson, K., & Walmsley, J., with Wolfe, M. (2010). *People with intellectual disabilities. Towards a good life?* Bristol: Policy Press.

Joseph Rowntree Foundation. (2002). *Success in supported employment for people with learning difficulties. Findings*. York: Joseph Rowntree Foundation.

Kings Fund Centre. (1984). *An ordinary working life: vocational services for people with mental handicap*. London: Kings Fund Centre.

Kiuranor, C. (1980). An integral indicator of the quality of work and the quality of life. In A. Szalai & Andrews (Eds.), *The quality of life: comparative studies*. London: Sage.

Kristiansen, K. (1996). Normalisation and social role valorisation. Ideological and theoretical foundation for supported employment. In T. Hernes, K. Stiles, & G. Bollingmo (Eds.), *The road to an ordinary job. A new perspective on rehabilitation*. Oslo: Ad Notam.

Leach, S. (2002). *A supported employment workbook*. London: Jessica Kingsley.

Luecking, R., Fabian, E. S., & Tilson, G. P. (2004). *Working relationships. Creating career opportunities for job seekers with disabilities through employer partnerships*. Baltimore: Paul Brookes.

Mank, D. M. (1994). The underachievement of supported employment: a call for reinvestment. *Journal of Disability Policy Studies*, 5(2), 1–24.

Mank, D., Cioffi, A., & Yovanoff, P. (1998). Employment outcomes for people with severe disabilities: opportunities for improvement. *Mental Retardation*, 36(3), 205–216.

Mayo, E. (1996). Dreaming of work. In P. Meadows (Ed.), *Work out – or work in? Contributions to the debate on the future of work*. York: Joseph Rowntree Foundation.

McConkey, R. (2007). Leisure and work. In B. Gates & H. Atherton (Eds.), *Learning disabilities. toward inclusion* (5th ed.). Elsevier.

McInally, G. (2008). Supported employment for people with learning disabilities: the case for full time work. *Tizard Learning Disability Review*, 13(3), 42–46.

McTier, A., Macdougall, L., McGregor, A., et al. (2016). *Mapping the employability landscape for people with learning disabilities in Scotland*. Glasgow: Scottish Consortium for Learning Disabilities.

McQuaid, R. W. (2000). *Defining entrepreneurship – implications for ICT, social enterprise and regional and local development policies*. (Social Science Working Paper No. 33) Edinburgh: Napier University.

National Development Team for Inclusion (NDTi). (2011). *Commissioning employment support*. Available at: https://www.base-uk.org/knowledge/ndti-insights-commissioning-employment-support. [Accessed 20 November 2020].

NHS Digital. (2020). Measures from the Adult Social Care Outcomes Framework: England. Available at: https://files.digital.nhs.uk/6F/78B873/meas-from-asc-of-eng-1920-ASCOF-report.pdf. [Accessed 15 February 2021].

NHS England and NHS Employers. (2015). NHS learning disability and employment: tools and guidance. Available at: www.nhsemployers.org/~/media/Employers/Publications/new%20NHS%20Learning%20Disability%20Employment%20Programme%20Tools%20

and%20Guidance%20Draft%2024%20(2).pdf. [Accessed 15 February 2021].

Nirje, B. (1980). The normalization principle. In R. J. Flynn & K. E. Nitsch (Eds.), *Normalisation, social integration and community service*. Baltimore: University Park Press.

O'Brien, J., & Tyne, A. (1981). *The principle of normalisation: a foundation for effective services*. London: The Campaign for Mentally Handicapped People.

O'Bryan, A., Simons, K., Beyer, S., et al. (2000). *A framework for supported employment*. York: York Publishing Services.

Oliver, M. (1990). *The politics of disablement*. Basingstoke: MacMillan and St Martin's Press.

Oliver, M. (1996). *Understanding disability. From theory to practice*. London: MacMillan.

Pagan, R. (2009). Self-employment among people with disabilities: evidence for Europe. *Disability & Society*, 24(2), 217–229.

Pallisera, M., Vila, M., & Valls, M. J. (2003). The current situation of supported employment in Spain: analysis and perspectives based on the perception of professionals. *Disability & Society*, 18(6), 797–810.

Parkin, E., Kennedy, S., Long, R., et al. (2020). *Support for people with a learning disability*. House of Commons Briefing Paper 07058. Available at: https://researchbriefings.files.parliament.uk/documents/SN07058/SN07058.pdf. [Accessed 20 November 2020].

Racino, J. A., & Whittico, P. (1998). The promise of self advocacy and community employment. In P. Wehman & J. Kregel (Eds.), *More than a job. Security satisfying careers for people with disabilities*. Baltimore: Derek H Brookes.

Reaume, G. (2004). No profits, just a pittance: work, compensation and people defined as mentally disabled in Ontario, 1964–1990. In S. Noll & J. W. Trent (Eds.), *Mental retardation in america: a historical reader*. New York: New York University Press.

Redley, M. (2009). Understanding the social exclusion and stalled welfare of citizens with intellectual disabilities. *Disability & Society*, 24(4), 489–501.

Reinertsen, S. (2012). *National conditions report on the work and activity situation among people with intellectual disability*. Trondheim: National Competence Environment for Intellectual Disability. National Statement on the Conditions.

Riesen, T., Morgan, R. L., & Griffin, G. (2015). Customized employment: a review of the literature. *Journal of Vocational Rehabilitation*, 43, 183–193.

Riesen, T., Hall, S., Keeton, B., et al. (2019). Customized employment discovery fidelity: developing consensus among experts. *Journal of Vocational Rehabilitation*, 50, 23–37.

Ridley, J., & Hunter, S. (2007). *Learning from research about best practice in supporting people with learning disabilities in real jobs: information for commissioners.* Glasgow: Workforce Plus.

Ridley, J., & Hunter, S. (2006). The development of supported employment in Scotland. *Journal of Vocational Rehabilitation, 25*(1), 57–68.

Ridley, J., Hunter, S., & Infusion Co-operative, (2005). *'Go for it!' Supporting people with learning disabilities and/ or autistic spectrum disorder in employment.* Edinburgh: Scottish Executive.

Ridley, J. (2001). Supported employment and learning disability: a life-changing experience? In C. Clark (Ed.), *Adult day services and social inclusion. Better days.* Jessica Kingsley.

Roulstone, A., Harrington, B., & Kwang Hwang, S. (2014). Flexible and personalised? An evaluation of a UK tailored employment support programme for jobseekers with enduring mental health problems and learning difficulties. *Scandinavian Journal of Disability Research, 16*(1), 14–28.

Sayce, L. (2011). Getting in. In *Staying in and getting on: disability employment support for the future.* London: Department for Work and Pensions.

Schneider, J., Heyman, A., & Turton, N. (2002), *Occupational outcomes: from evidence to implementation. An expert topic paper commissioned by the Department of Health.* Durham: Centre for Applied Social Studies, University of Durham.

Scottish Commission for Learning Disability (SCLD). (2018). *Learning disability statistics Scotland, 2018 provisional statistics.* Available at: https://www.scld.org.uk/2018-report/. [Accessed 12 November 2020].

Spjelkavik, Ø., Frøyland, K., & Skardhamar, T. (2003). *Disabled people in ordinary work – inclusion through supported employment.* Oslo: Oslo Met University.

Stalker, K. (2001). Inclusive daytime opportunities for people with learning disabilities. In C. Clark (Ed.), *Adult day services and social inclusion. Better days.* London: Jessica Kingsley.

Sutton, B. (1999). Inclusive employment: international perspectives. In K. Stiles (Ed.), *Beyond borders: global supported employment and people with disabilities.* Training Resource Network.

Tannen, V. (1993). A literature review of supported employment. In A. Pozner & J. Hammond (Eds.), *An evaluation of supported employment initiatives for disabled people.* Sheffield: Employment Department.

Unger, D. D. (2002). Employers attitudes towards persons with disabilities in the workforce: myths or realities? *Focus on Autism and Other Developmental Disabilities, 17*(1), 2–10.

United Nations. (2008). Convention on the Rights of Persons with Disabilities (CRPD). Article 27 Work and Employment. Available at: https://www.un.org/development/desa/disabilities/convention-on-the-rights-of-persons-with-disabilities/article-27-work-and-employment.html. [Accessed 20 December 2020].

Verdugo, M. A., Jordán de Urríes, J. B., Jenaro, C., et al. (2006). Quality of life of workers with an intellectual disability in supported employment. *Journal of Applied Research in Intellectual Disabilities, 19*, 309–316.

Wangen, G. (2014). On work site follow up. In K. Frøyland & Ø. Spjelkavik (Eds.), *Inclusion skills competence. Ordinary work as an aim and a means.* Oslo: Gyldendal Akademisk.

Wangen, G. (2019). *Reaching the target – work inclusion for people with disabilities.* Oslo: Oslo Metropolitan University.

Wendelborg, C., Kittelsaa, A., & Wik, S. E. (2017). *Transition from school to work for pupils with intellectual disability.* NTNU Social Research.

Wertheimer, A. (1992). *Real Jobs Initiative. Changing lives: supported employment and people with learning disabilities.* Manchester: National Development Team.

Wolfensberger, W. (1972). *The principle of normalisation in human services.* Toronto: National Institute on Mental Retardation.

Wolfensberger, W. (1983). Social role valorisation: a proposed new term for the principle of normalisation. *Mental Retardation, 21*(6), 234–239.

24

A home of my own

Pete Richmond and Alice Squire

KEY ISSUES

In this chapter we consider key components of a rights-based approach to housing, with a focus on putting theory into practice. We look at:
- Rights of people with intellectual disabilities
- Non-institutionalised settings

- Being part of community
- Independent living
- Person centred approaches
- Positive relationships between people being supported and supporters.

CHAPTER OUTLINE

INTRODUCTION

Most adults with intellectual disabilities across the world live at home with their family, however, there is no reliable data to confirm exact numbers. In this chapter, we do not attempt tó analyse statistics; instead we adopt a human rights approach to thinking about how people with intellectual disabilities can find a place to live. Inevitably we cannot capture the experience of most people internationally. Moreover, the way human rights are formulated has a western-centric bias. That said, we still believe a human rights approach offers potential for progress in improving the conditions and life chances for the world's most vulnerable adult population including choices around where to live their lives.

We first consider the idea of *home* and then *rights*, focusing on Article 19 of the 2006 United Nations Convention on the Rights of Persons with Disabilities,

(CRPD) which is about living independently and being included in the community. We go on to explore the experience of people with intellectual disabilities in different accommodation settings, and critique the claim that institutions are in the past. In the final sections, we focus on practical application of Article 19 and draw on experience to explore how a rights-based approach may support people with intellectual disabilities to live happier, more fulfilling lives.

WHAT DOES 'HOME' MEAN FOR YOU?

Shelter is a fundamental requirement for health (World Health Organization, 1986), and a prerequisite for meeting all our other needs satisfactorily (McLeod, 2018). We need more than a place to stay, we need a *place to live*. When we think about what sort of place we want to live, we probably want a place to call home, on top of a checklist of features that are important. Many of us want a home that broadly corresponds with the society we live in, but we may also want our home to reflect our background or culture. A person with an intellectual disability is no different.

George lived with his Gypsy Traveller family on a large Gypsy and Traveller site. He has cerebral palsy and an intellectual disability. His parents had turned down offers of settled accommodation which had no space to keep a "wagon". With the help of a social worker and an occupational therapist, they were able to convert a large caravan into a home for George, with a wet room, wide doorways and ramps.

We like to think of home as a place of safety, privacy and comfort, even self-expression, but this is not always our experience. A person with an intellectual disability may be more likely to feel unsafe at home. In the UK around 1 in 7 adults with disabilities aged 16 to 59 years experienced domestic abuse in the year ending March 2019, compared with 1 in 20 adults without. Women with disabilities were more than twice as likely to have experienced domestic abuse than women without disabilities (Office of National Statistics, 2019a). As in other countries, people with intellectual disabilities in South Africa experience many rights violations, including abuse and involuntary confinement in family homes and care settings (Capri et al, 2018). Lack of support for carers increases the risk of home being a dangerous place (World Health Organization, 2012).

Perhaps we can understand home as how we experience the place we dwell. Whether we experience it as warm and secure is contingent on many factors, including how our body interacts with the environment. Poor housing design can reduce independence where it impedes self-management (Harrison and Davis, 2000), for example, when you are reliant on another person to move you from one room to another, and this will impact on how you feel about where you live (Imrie, 2004). Home should be a place that makes sense to us in terms of how we experience our existence in the world (Relph, 1976). One study (Lashewicz et al, 2020) used the idea of "existential insideness" to explore the contrasting experiences of two adults with intellectual disabilities in Canada. Sarah experiences her home as an "insider", confident that her preferences and privacy are respected, whereas Patrick experiences his high security residential home as an "outsider", the place he is taken to in handcuffs by the police after escaping.

We know a man who has his own home, but regards it as belonging to the people who are paid to support him. When the place you live is also a workplace for someone else, it may influence how you experience home (Dyck et al, 2005; Quinn et al, 2016), and we need to think carefully if care arrangements support a person to feel at home or alienate them from it. Another person, Agnes, is unequivocal about how she understands her home

"I was independent when I got my own front door key, because it's the first time I had a key in my life. I feel that I could have done what I like when I had my own key and nobody was bossing me about then – I was bossing myself about."

ARC Scotland, 2019

A Norwegian study of how people with intellectual disabilities in a shared housing complex felt about everyday life highlights the importance of a sense of home for well-being (Witsø and Hauger, 2020). One participant said: 'My home is important to me, it's a place where I can be myself and relax.' The study noted that it was important for participants to express the things they did for themselves, and the value they placed on having personal support to access things they wanted to do in the community. This contrasted with how participants described the complex where they lived, as "the shared accommodation" or "the base", and a tendency to describe themselves as "users" and support workers as "staff".

When helping to arrange housing for a person with an intellectual disability, you need to consider how that person might experience living in a particular place. What meanings might they derive from how the accommodation is structured and run? Are they likely to feel safe and at home there, or threatened, vulnerable and anxious? Is the accommodation and support malleable, so it can adapt to that person's preferred way of being; or is it rigid with the onus being on the person to adapt?

 READER ACTIVITY 24.1

What does the word 'home' mean to you and what aspects are most important?

Ask yourself this question and a sample of family members and colleagues.

Then, find out about housing allocation processes where you live. How well do you think they capture these aspects?

RIGHTS AND THE IDEA OF HOME

The Convention on the Rights of Persons with Disabilities (CRPD) came into force on 3 May 2008 and has been signed by most countries in the world (United Nations, 2020). The CRPD aims to ensure that people with disabilities enjoy the same human rights as everyone else and are afforded respect, non-discrimination and dignity. Article 19 – Living independently and being included in the community, says States parties must:

> "'recognize the equal right of all persons with disabilities to live in the community, with choices equal to others' and should take measures to promote 'full inclusion and participation in the community'.'"

There are three key elements to Article 19:

1   People with disabilities should have the same opportunity to choose where and with whom they live as is afforded to those without disabilities, and they should not have to live in any particular model of accommodation because of their disability.
2   They should have access to support, geared towards preventing isolation or segregation from the community, that enables them to live fully in the community.
3   Services and facilities used by everyone else should be accessible to them.

When helping someone with an intellectual disability to find a home we need to be thinking about all of these things, regardless of the person's diagnosis or circumstances. If at any time any of these elements are not available to a person, we should not give up, but continue to work towards achieving them all. Thinking about "home" (which implies something personal you need to create) and avoiding language like "placement" (which implies being put somewhere that already exists) may help cultivate a more creative and solution-focussed mindset.

The Committee on the Rights of Persons with Disabilities monitors implementation of the CRPD and provides clarification of the Articles to help put them into practice. The General Comment (GC) on Article 19 (Committee on the Rights of Persons with Disabilities, 2017), shows how failure to ensure the right to live independently and be included in the community impinges on other rights and responsibilities.

If people with intellectual disabilities are excluded from the community, they are denied full opportunity to develop and contribute, contravening Article 29 of the Universal Declaration of Human Rights (United Nations, 1948). Not allowing people to choose where they live is a breach of fundamental civil liberties, contravening Article 12 (1) of the International Covenant on Civil and Political Rights (United Nations, 1976a). Failure to provide adequate housing, or a home that most people in a given state would recognise as "adequate" for them, is a failure to treat people with intellectual disabilities as equal in dignity and worth, a fundamental human rights principle, and contravenes Article 11 of the International Covenant on Economic, Social and Cultural Rights (United Nations, 1976b). 'Adequate' housing means housing that offers legal security of tenure, affordability and accessibility.

Thus, the right to a home is more than a right to a roof over our heads. It is about the right to exist in equal worth to everybody else and be afforded dignity and respect, so we can develop, flourish and participate as full members of a society and as individuals.

> "Home is the foundation of our identity as individuals and members of a community, the dwelling-place of being. Home is not just the house you happen to live in, but an irreplaceable centre of significance."
>
> Relph, 2016, p. 1

READER ACTIVITY 24.2

Find out about your local and national government housing policies and plans for people with intellectual disabilities.

To what extent do these promote or hinder people's ability to choose their place of residence, access mainstream housing and access general community facilities and services on an equal basis with others?

FROM INSTITUTIONS TO COMMUNITY LIVING

This section of the chapter considers different models of accommodation currently provided to people with intellectual disabilities. Options for housing and support can be said to exist on a spectrum, from total institutions to supported living with reciprocal support. However, as this section will outline, this is not clear-cut. The story that is often told in the West, is that institutions are a thing of the past, but institutional structures, systems and practices can be present in a range of settings. It will be demonstrated that institutions continue to exist and professionals need to use their skills and creativity to avoid repeating or perpetuating mistakes of the past.

Institutions

When we think about institutions for people with intellectual disabilities, size and location are likely to spring to mind. An extreme example was the Leros Psychiatric Hospital, an institution based on a Greek island, where in the 1980s, people were accommodated on wards of 90–180 people and in one building alone there were 1,100 'inmates' (Karydaki, 2019). We need to understand other characteristics of institutions if we want to avoid perpetuating institutional accommodation for people with intellectual disabilities.

An institution can be understood as a place where, based on a certain attribute such as intellectual disability, people:

> "live together away from their families. Implicitly, a place in which people do not exercise full control over their lives and their day-to-day activities. An institution is not defined merely by its size."
> World Health Organization and World Bank, 2011, p. 305

An institution is also a place where

> "'residents are isolated from the broader community and/or compelled to live together' and where 'the requirements of the organisation itself tend to take precedence over the residents' individualised needs'."
> European Expert Group on the Transition from Institutional to Family Based Care, 2012, p. 25

We can think about institutions in terms of processes of institutionalisation. Following Goffman, in a "total institution" (Jones and Fowles, 1984), individuals are subjected to 'batch living', where everyday activities are undertaken as a group according to rules and schedules, and binary management, where managers (perhaps nurses or staff) organise and control. People may adopt the 'inmate role' (perhaps as patients or service users) where they not only learn their place but adopt their own strategies within that role, and sometimes behaviours that make sense in the context of the institution. The institution itself may then seek to validate itself by promulgating 'the institutional perspective',

where it pronounces the good work it does for people who can't live in the community, and creates an artificial sense of community by putting on social events, open days and such like.

Yet an "institution" can also have positive connotations, referring to social structures which have "normative and regulative elements that, together with associated activities and resources, provide stability and meaning to social life" (Scott, 1995, p. 48). If your home is institutional however, stability and meaning are imposed on you, and are resistant to change (Wiesel, 2020).

Thus institutions are incompatible with the concepts of independent and community living. Whilst a degree of choice and control may be possible in an institution, and people may have limited access to the community, the segregating character and imposition of key decisions means full realisation of human rights is not possible in institutionalised settings. The right to choose where to live requires realistic options of accessible housing to be available.

Institutions today

The end of the 20th century saw a wide commitment to shift from large-scale institutions to community care, and many countries developed legislation and policy to close institutions and develop community-based alternatives. However, institutions and institutionalised services persist, even in wealthy countries. In Austria, five out of nine provinces have institutions of over 100 persons (Kremsner et al., 2019); in 2016, it was reported that 5,385 French adults and 1,451 French children were placed in institutions in Belgium (Campion and Mouiller, 2016); in the USA only 14 States have closed their public institutions and in 2015, 3,541 people were living in State-run institutions in Texas (Lulinski and Shea Tanis, 2018). Spain has been criticised for spending public funds on building institutions and its lack of deinstitutionalisation strategy, and Turkey has yet to pass a legislation framework asserting the right of persons with disabilities to live independently and choose their place of residence (United Nations, 2019).

In Europe, there are particular issues with former Soviet Central Eastern European countries. For example, the Monitoring Committee on CRPD have condemned new EU Member States for using European

Structural and Investment Funds for maintaining insti-tutions (Bugarszki et al, 2017). They found the Czech Republic was investing more resources into institutions than community services, and in Slovakia, women with disabilities, in particular, continued to be institu-tionalised. In 2010 Human Rights Watch visited nine institutions in Croatia accommodating a total of 1,500 people where 70–100 percent of residents were admitted without their consent or the opportunity to challenge the decision (Human Rights Watch, 2010).

In the UK, people with intellectual disabilities can be detained in public or private hospitals for long periods, sometimes years, often on the grounds of having chal-lenging behaviour and there being no suitable accom-modation or support for them to be discharged to (MacDonald, 2018; Joint Committee on Human Rights, 2019). In 2019, a television programme exposed abuse in a private hospital for adults with intellectual dis-abilities in England (Panorama: Undercover Hospital Abuse Scandal, 2019) and the regulator rated six hos-pitals "inadequate". The Mental Welfare Commission in Scotland found that the environment in 12 of 18 state-run intellectual disability mental health units was not fit for purpose, and that people with intellectual disabilities were being detained twice as long as people without (Mental Welfare Commission for Scotland, 2016).

Large Care Homes

In the major period of deinstitutionalisation in the UK in the late 1980s/early 1990s, many people were dis-charged into residential care homes. In some instances, former workers from long-stay hospitals were able to acquire big old properties (often in post-industrial and ex-mining areas and seaside resorts) and literally take patients with them. These new private care homes were able to take advantage of welfare systems which allowed them to recruit new residents with minimal local authority involvement, advertising directly to families, often highlighting their lovely grounds. Later, many of these care homes targeted local authorities on the basis of being able to provide secure environments for high tariff clients. In more recent years, many of these have been taken over by large, sometimes multinational, corporations. A number of charitable organisations, established as alternatives to hospitals, also acquired buildings and in some cases developed significant campuses.

Intentional Communities

In a planned or intentional community, a shared (often religious) ideal is promoted through encouraging team-work and shared living. In intentional communities for people with intellectual disabilities, *assistants* (often vol-unteers who receive board and accommodation) choose to live and work alongside them, in theory as equal members of the community. A criticism is that whilst volunteers choose to join because of a shared belief or desire to live in a segregated project, people with intellectual disabilities are generally referred because of their disability, and admission can depend on will-ingness to work and how much support they will need (Montgomery, 2018).

Some suggest that a "sense of community" may be more important than being in *the* community. Some also suggest that people with intellectual disabilities are unlikely to find the dependable supportive relationships they need in the general community, but they may find this in groups of other people with intellectual disabili-ties (Cummins and Lau, 2003). However, some disabil-ity campaigners argue that such communities go against the anti-institution movement. One campaigner from Delaware ADAPT observed of an institution housing 600 people on a self-contained campus, that typically staff are the only neurotypical residents but "neurotyp-icals are always in charge" (Montgomery, 2018, p. 1).

Group Homes

Alongside these large-scale residential services, the group home model developed, where smaller groups of people were housed together like a family. In the USA numbers of group homes increased from approximately 40,000 in 1977 to 437,707 in 2007 (Alba et al., 2008) and in Australia, this was the main model of housing for people moving from institutions or from the fam-ily home (Clement and Bigby, 2010). The model of full board plus 24-hour care is often expensive, whilst generally leaving residents with only a small amount of pocket money to spend and no right to choose who they live with. However, many group homes worked hard on ordinary living principles and supported residents to make choices, sometimes for the first time.

Hostels

In the UK there was a period when housing related support was attached to housing welfare benefit. This created an incentive for authorities to develop hostel accommodation as an alternative to hospital, where 20 or more people lived in a block of bed-sit style accommodation with shared facilities. There is little research concerning these establishments which were built around the period 1960s-1980s, however one project, concerned with implementing the Supporting People programme on housing and support, records some of the tenants' experiences (Fyson et al, 2007). Premises were described as "too old and scruffy; "they didn't clean the toilet properly"; it was "a filthy, dreadful place; the bathroom and toilet stinked". Tenants complained about living in large groups, they "didn't like living on top of each other"; "there were people fighting with each other and people downstairs smoking"; "I was sick of living there with old people and people who had nowhere to go" (Fyson et al, 2007, p. 7).

Supported Living

The policy of closing long-stay hospitals in many Western countries attached funding for care to individuals which brought about the possibility of greater flexibilities. Why place people in expensive institutions or group homes, when individuals should have access to the same housing as everybody else, which could be cheaper social housing? Support could be offered to people based on assessed need, and whilst some might require constant supervision and high levels of personal care, others might require minimal help to maintain a tenancy. This might allow resources to be allocated more appropriately.

There is a lack of conclusive evidence in relation to the cost of institutions versus individual care, however, the inherent flexibility of individualised support allows for much greater scope to reduce costs. Institutions have a variety of fixed costs in relation to buildings and staffing, which are always the major factors in making this an expensive form of provision. Individuals supported in their own home may go through ups and downs in life, and support and cost can be adjusted accordingly. Once costs are invested in institutional services, there is a perverse incentive to fill all available places. Thus, people can be placed in inappropriate services with higher levels of support than they require in order to fill the voids of block commissioned services.

A fundamental idea of supported living was separating housing from support, so that in theory, it should be possible to help a person obtain housing through the normal routes (usually renting), giving them the rights and responsibilities of other householders, and giving them more say over how they get support. Support could be adjusted as their lives change but they would not have to move unless their accommodation became unsuitable. The development of person-centred planning allowed professionals to work creatively with families to design bespoke support, even for people with complex needs.

Studies in the US, the UK and Australia, all found that supported living offers greater choice and control and potentially, greater inclusion in the community, and is generally cheaper than a group home (Bigby et al, 2017). Yet it was also suggested that the absence of 24-hour support may negatively impact health, daily routines and personal safety. This is likely to be due to inadequate levels of support rather than the model itself. There are also concerns about loneliness particularly for people with mild or moderate disability (Sheppard-Jones et al, 2005). One study found that people with intellectual disabilities in England are seven times more likely to be lonely than the general population (Office of National Statistics, 2019b), however it is not clear that this is related to living in small settings or alone. One study suggested that loneliness is more of an issue for people living in larger settings of 7+ (Stancliffe et al, 2007) and another indicated that people who moved from congregated settings to their own home with personalised support express higher levels of personal wellbeing (McConkey et al, 2018). People living alone do express concerns about their vulnerability, and this is related to their experiences of abuse (Bond and Hurst, 2010).

There is often a presumption that supported living means living alone, and many supported living schemes offer only singleton accommodation. Some UK local authorities have had a policy to only fund single-person flats to promote ordinary living (Jackson and Irvine, 2013) and partly in response to a government policy that tied housing benefit to assessment of bedroom requirement. However, there is no reason to assume that a person with an intellectual disability wants to live alone any more than to assume they should live in a specialised facility.

Supported Living Schemes

This idea that supported living means having one's own front door has perhaps allowed schemes to be developed in obvious institutional settings, including on campuses that incorporate residential, respite and day services. The 'core and cluster' model, which might describe an arrangement where people live in their homes and access outreach support from a central site, is frequently construed as a congregated scheme, where people have individual tenancies often with communal areas and onsite support. Whilst these are an improvement on hostels, in that people generally have self-contained accommodation, residence may be dependent on accepting support from a provider chosen by a commissioner who doesn't know you.

Guidance in England says including six flats for people with intellectual disabilities in a block of twenty is acceptable, however, developing a block of twenty flats for people with intellectual disabilities could be considered an institution (Transforming Care Programme, 2016). Clustered accommodation aims to deliver economies of scale, but more dispersed housing is associated with better quality of life (Mansell and Beadle-Brown, 2009) as well as being more aligned with human rights.

Supported living is not a model of housing, but an approach which aims to make it easier for someone to live the way they want. The REACH standards (Paradigm, 2019) are a helpful guide to help you check how well housing and support arrangements protect rights (see Box 24.1).

Specialised Residential Services

Article 19 indicates that people with disabilities may require specialised services to enable them to be included in the community, however, some specialised residential services suggest they exist for people whose needs preclude them from living in the community. The GC says that specialised services should be provided to enable people to be "fully included and to participate in social life" (Committee on the Rights of Persons with Disabilities, 2017, p. 4), but often the main features in specialised services are size, remote location and high staffing levels, with care plans overseen by a clinical professional. Should access to specialised interventions or healthcare override the right for support to live in the community? It is possible for a service to support both the right to inclusion and the right to healthcare. For example, a person with epilepsy could be provided with a support worker trained in administering medication and seizure first aid, thus enabling them to live in their own home and participate in the community.

In the UK there is pressure to end 'out of authority placements' where people are accommodated away from the area they would normally live, often in hospitals, and one response has been to develop more local special accommodation services. Commissioners and town planners need to be careful they are not endorsing relocating institutions to local communities whenever there is a proposal to develop special accommodation. Specialist residential services are expensive and developing a bespoke service may be cheaper, as well as producing better outcomes.

Special accommodation may be sought when paid or unpaid caregivers find they cannot cope with difficult behaviour. Whilst there are emergency situations where a person can no longer reside in their current accommodation, and may need to move somewhere secure with support, this should not be seen as the end of a story, but a temporary response to crisis. In reality, people with intellectual disabilities, and other issues like challenging behaviour, can wait many years for a "specialised placement" to come up. A project set up to find housing and develop bespoke support for 13 people in hospital found that the shortest admission was 5 years and the longest was 15 years, compared to a national average prison sentence of 24.7 months (Sly, 2013). As social workers, the authors of this chapter found that throughout the years a person had been in hospital, there was rarely a conversation about housing or about what good support for that person might look like. Instead, reviews concluded that they couldn't be discharged until a specialised placement with high staffing was available. Consequently, professionals were waiting

---

📄 **BOX 24.1   The REACH Standards**

I choose who I live with

I choose where I live

I have my own home

I choose who supports me and how I am supported

I choose my friends and relationships

I get help to make changes in my life

I choose how to be healthy and safe

I choose how I am part of the community

I have the same rights and responsibilities as other citizens

for either someone to move out of a placement that could be hundreds of miles away, or for a new service to be built.

Reciprocity

When we think of human relations, we usually have an idea of reciprocity, of a two-way exchange that can potentially benefit all parties involved. Traditional models of housing and care tend towards a one-way relationship, with the person with a disability a passive recipient of resources and care. This risks turning people into commodities, such that their value is based on the employment and income generated from providing accommodation and support to them. Some models recognise people with intellectual disabilities as having something of worth to contribute as full human beings and build this into the approach.

Whereas most supported living schemes entail congregated living on a single site, a community living network links people who live near each other. A link worker lives in the network and offers low-level flexible support. If people require additional support, this can be arranged separately through the usual means. Members agree to meet up and help each other with the support of the link worker. In some schemes, people mutually choose to share their life together. Sometimes known as Family Placement, Adult Placement or Shared Lives, these schemes offer support and accommodation in the homes of individuals or families, often as a break from the family home, but sometimes providing a permanent residence, with the person with disabilities becoming an integral part of the family. Reciprocity may be a feature of intentional communities. Some may argue that in such communities, people with disabilities generate income for non-disabled people to follow a desired lifestyle, however, others would argue that the model is based on mutual support, with people with disabilities expected to contribute to, not just use the service.

 READER ACTIVITY 24.3

Fred's story in the online resource details his lengthy journey to his best home.

As you read it, make a note of your feelings at each move he experiences.

In particular, can you imagine how it must have felt for Fred?

BEING AT HOME IN THE COMMUNITY

This section draws on recommendations from the UN Committee on the Rights of Persons with Disabilities as to how Article 19 should be understood and implemented. The CRPD came in after the major deinstitutionalisation programmes and was intended to address continued failure in achieving human rights of people with disabilities. It became apparent that institutional practices persisted and that better community provision was necessary. This includes support for independent living, personal assistance and supported decision-making, as fundamental ingredients to enable a person with a disability to exercise their human rights.

When CRPD refers to community, it means *the* community, where people go about their daily lives. The GC makes clear that the right to be "included in the community" is not just about not living in an institution, it means "full and effective inclusion and participation in society", "being social" and "having access to all services offered by the community to its members" (Committee on the Rights of Persons with Disabilities, 2017, p. 4).

One reason for segregation may be ambivalence about the capacity of *community* to accommodate people perceived as vulnerable. Harassment, bullying and assault, coupled with inaccessible buildings and transport, are common experiences for many people with disabilities, and creating segregated communities may be a pragmatic response. One person described their experience to the authors of this chapter of being regularly bullied in the community, for example, when getting a bus, and how they had walked three miles home in the rain because they were too scared to get on a bus with schoolchildren. People with intellectual disabilities and their families are more likely to live in economically deprived areas (Allcock, 2019), which is a challenge for inclusion, thereby highlighting the need to look at deinstitutionalisation from both sides, i.e. at community development and community services.

Community living thus means being included and being able to participate in society like everybody else. People must have access to all aspects of political and cultural life and the same access to housing as everyone else.

INDEPENDENT LIVING

The concept of Independent Living (IL) predates the CRPD and is a key idea that informed its formulation, particularly Article 19 which sets out how fundamental human rights can be realised for people with disabilities. Article 19 can be understood as an attempt to codify IL within a human rights context. IL is a multi-faceted concept that combines self-determination, access and opportunity, including "the opportunity to make real choices and decisions regarding where to live, with whom to live and how to live" (European Network on Independent Living (ENIL), 2016). According to the GC, IL is essential for individual autonomy and freedom, upon which basis all human rights operate. A person with disabilities cannot realise their human rights if they are unable to live independently like non-disabled people.

Whilst it might be easy to see how IL might benefit someone with a mild intellectual disability, it is perhaps more difficult to make it a reality for someone with a more severe disability and communication difficulties. A study by the University of Girona's Research Group on Diversity (Fullana et al, 2019) found that families and professionals had low expectations about IL working for people with intellectual disabilities. This may be due to a lack of understanding of what IL means, for example, it does not mean living alone or having no support.

Those working with people with intellectual disabilities need to focus on participatory competence and self-determination. One approach to this is to simply start treating people as individuals with capacity to learn and develop. In the 1960s, Nirje adopted the term "normalization", to unite ordinary people behind the claim that institutions were incompatible with the human rights of people with intellectual disabilities (Goode, 1993). The "principle of normalization" was not about coercing people to appear more socially acceptable but about recognising that if people are denied "normal" lives, they are denied the possibility of functioning like everyone else. Helping people with intellectual disabilities achieve their rights had to be worked on. Normalization was superseded by Social Role Valorisation (Wolfensberger, 1998), however both became unfashionable, in part because of the language, and in part because of overly prescriptive application. People came to speak instead of 'ordinary living' and through the 1990s, drew on Connie and John O'Brien's 'five accomplishments' (O'Brien, 1997), which still offers a useful framework for making independent living a real possibility for people with all levels of intellectual disability (see Box 24.2).

BOX 24.2 O'Brien's Five accomplishments

- Sharing ordinary places
- Making choices
- Developing abilities
- Being treated with respect and having a valued social role
- Growing in relationships

Thus, independent living is an essential component of being able to exercise freedom. It means having control and making decisions about your own life, including about where you live and with whom.

Personal Assistance

Personal Assistance (PA) is a tool for independent living. The GC says that people who need PA should be able to "freely choose their preferred degree of personal control over service delivery according to their requirements, capabilities, life circumstances and preferences" (Committee on the Rights of Persons with Disabilities, 2017, p. 5). The PA model requires people with disabilities to receive payments so they can directly employ workers to undertake tasks they need help with, therefore governments need to adjust their welfare regimes accordingly. However, where a person doesn't choose or have the ability or support to manage a direct payment, they should still be involved in choosing who supports them.

There are various ways one might go about this, depending on the situation and the people concerned. One way might be helping people to think through the tasks they would want a Personal Assistant to perform and the characteristics they would want this person to have. From this, people can be supported to develop a person specification which they can use to help write a job advert, develop questions to ask at interview, and criteria they can use. Another way might be to draw up a profile of the person requiring support with family, friends and others who know them well. From this, you might start to develop a personalised profile for PA. People living in supported living schemes often don't get a say in what organisation provides the support, but they could and should be involved in drawing up criteria and selecting from potential applicants. We should also be looking critically at schemes which require tenants to receive support from the same organisation as everyone else. If the accommodation suits a person, they might still prefer to employ PA, and we need to look at ways to increase flexibilities.

Organisations founded on the principles of ordinary living and inclusion pioneered approaches that came to be broadly termed Person Centred Planning (PCP). PCP offers an alternative to service centred approaches, based on a simplistic understanding of 'community' as a place, which grew with the closure of institutions. Many services replacing hospitals came to replicate many of the traits of institutions, where people were typically segregated into group living situations on the basis of how their needs were assessed. Few people had access to PA, but were instead supported by a pool of staff who worked for the establishment they were 'placed' in.

By contrast, the organisations that grew out of the 'ordinary life' movement sought to recruit people who shared the values of inclusion and, crucially, who could help the person achieve the life they wanted. These organisations worked closely with families, and in partnership with the person being supported to maximise their control. PCP tools were developed which focussed on finding out what mattered to the person and what made them tick (O'Brien and Lyle O'Brien, 1988). Utilising direct payments and any other funds available, these organisations are able to pool the money that would have gone directly to a care establishment into an Individual Service Fund, enabling people to access PA. These individualised services enable people, regardless of level of disability, to live in mainstream housing, adapted to suit their particular requirements. The Vermont Self-Determination Project promoted system-wide change to encourage self-determination of people with intellectual disabilities as well as self-advocacy and circles of support (Aichroth et al, 2002).

A key idea behind this approach is that planning for where a person should live, and what support they need to do it, should follow what happens in everyday life. Normally, people think about they want, see what budget they have, then figure out what is really important, and it seemed to follow that people who are going to need PA to live their lives should know up-front what financial assistance they can get.

In summary, for people with intellectual disabilities to achieve independent and community living, personal assistance led by the person will probably be required. The easiest way to achieve this is to allocate funding for the assistance required to the person and

give them control over it. Where people don't want to have control over funding they should be able to decide how much control they want to have over service delivery.

Supported decision-making

The GC says that neither legal capacity or the level of support required can be grounds to deny the right to independent and community living. It says that control of PA, and considerations about where to live, can be through Supported Decision-Making (SDM). This means that professionals should not automatically assume decision-making powers, even when working as a multi-disciplinary team.

SDM broadly entails making adjustments and using tools and supports to help someone understand, make, and communicate their opinions and choices. One simple adjustment might be to provide better information in an appropriate form. Thus, whilst one person might appreciate easy-read information another person might prefer to have someone tell them the options, and another might prefer information to be conveyed using augmentative and alternative communication. A tool to help SDM could be a simple PCP tool such as *People, Places, and Activities*, where you help someone to think about these things by listing what they like/dislike, perhaps as part of Essential Lifestyle Planning (Smull and Sanderson, 2005). A more sophisticated tool might be an SDM Inventory (Shogren et al, 2017). Support might come from family, friends, existing support staff, amongst others, who might help a person understand and communicate, or who might be able to help understand a person's preferences.

The Everyday Decisions project classified decisions into three types – *everyday preferences*, *life choices*, and *difficult decisions* (Harding and Ezgi, 2018). They used this framework to explore the experiences people had of moving to a new accommodation service. The first tenants were just told they were moving and there was a suspicion that this was influenced by a strategic plan for re-provisioning services they had no involvement in. Later, prospective tenants received more information about where it was, who they'd be living with, etc. and were given the option of visiting and an overnight stay. This research found that people sought direct support from others to make decisions, more than they sought communication tools to help with decision-making. This wasn't just a matter of having someone who could interpret jargon, or give them more time, but the presence of someone they trusted alongside them.

In summary, supported decision-making is a way of keeping a person's will and preferences central to decision making, where impairment of intellectual and adaptive functioning affects ability to process information and communicate. Supported decision-making can help a person make a decision for themselves about where they live or how personal assistance is delivered. Supported decision-making can also help ensure that substitute decision-making reflects a person's will and preferences.

OTHER KEY INGREDIENTS

The previous section focussed on putting principles behind Article 19 into practice. This section offers practical advice for helping someone with an intellectual disability, regardless of condition or degree of impairment, to obtain a place to live.

A home that suits you

If the starting point for seeking accommodation is special provision, a person's options and their future prospects are blunted from the outset. When helping a person with an intellectual disability find a home, you should anticipate having to work at it, perhaps as you would if you are looking for your own ideal home. There are people who put years into finding (or even building) a place that suits them, and then spend the rest of their lives making it into "home". For people with intellectual disabilities, it can be a matter of being slotted into a vacancy, sometimes at short notice, or put on a list until one becomes available. In reality, where we live is often the result of a combination of economic necessity, social ties, personal preference, public policy and accident, but most of us would not want an outside agency to place us somewhere, except perhaps in an emergency, and then only for a short period of time. If we do have to live somewhere we wouldn't choose, it is expected that we, and perhaps our family, will seek out ways to change the situation. Choosing a place to live can be, but is often not, a once in a lifetime event. Many of us want to move house, maybe because of employment or support needs, or maybe because we discover on living somewhere that our home does not suit our lifestyle. If we reflect on how important it is for us to find the right home, and how much time and effort we put into it, we should expect to have to put at least as much work into developing accommodation and support for someone with unique and multiple needs.

The first consideration should be ordinary housing options that most people without disabilities would consider. Options might be a house or a flat, renting or buying, living with family, alone or with others, or whatever is a normal way to go about finding a home. As this book has an international focus, we do not go into detail about national housing policy or localised housing options as this will vary, depending on where you live, but we have included some links, in the online Useful resources section, to organisations that may help. However, if you are helping someone with an intellectual disability to find a home it is essential that you find out about mainstream housing rights and opportunities or seek out a housing rights professional. Help the person and their family understand their rights and if possible, involve an advocate if they are unable to understand what these are.

Housing location and design is important. In the UK, much social housing is spatially concentrated and not designed with disability in mind, but shouldn't be ruled out. A flat on a housing estate or scheme, might suit someone who wants to live around the corner from family, near their place of worship, or where there is an existing support network. On the other hand, social housing can be located in neighbourhoods with problems like high levels of anti-social behaviour, where a person with an intellectual disability would be vulnerable. Some people will need more bespoke housing, perhaps with thicker walls, or set back from the street. The authors recall two men who had been housed together in a terraced property but did not get on with each other, so one or the other was often in the garden making a lot of noise. There were frequent complaints from neighbours to the social work department.

A local housing office might be your first stop. Some projects that have supported people to leave institutions so they can live in the community have found organisations that can offer shared ownership. There are also housing associations which have a range of housing stock that may be more appropriate, and in some instances, have been able to invest in purpose-built housing. Private landlords may also be interested in renting to people with specific housing needs, who can be very reliable tenants.

Equipment, adaptations and technology can help people live independently and improve their quality of life. These can range from minor adaptations such as fitting grab rails, installation of tracking hoists, to remodelling a home to make it easier to move around. An Occupational Therapist (OT) is likely to have knowledge of equipment available, rights to funds and how to access these. Telecare services use technology to monitor people's movement, medication and home environment at a distance. Cost considerations have informed much of their development and utilisation in housing for people with intellectual disabilities, but it may also support independent living. However, we have to be careful that we are not falling into thinking that independent living means living without, or with less support. Telecare can reduce the need for intrusive checks, and allow help to be alerted, but it cannot enable participation in the community or promote freedom and choice. There is a risk that if used thoughtlessly, it could leave people trapped at home. Another concern is around surveillance, particularly where telecare is not an option but an integral part of housing.

Whilst mainstream housing should be the first consideration, options such as an existing Community Living Network or Supported Living Scheme may meet a person's housing and support plan or specification. When looking at existing schemes designed for people with intellectual disabilities, use the three key elements of Article 19 (section 3) to evaluate how well their rights will be protected there. The checklist on institutional characteristics outlined in Box 24.3 may help assess how well the scheme supports rights. If any of these apply can they be challenged or changed?

In the discussion on Specialised Residential Services, we considered situations where special provision is sometimes assessed as the "housing need" a person has, on the basis of certain characteristics, support needs, and very often "challenging behaviour", perhaps presented by a person with an intellectual disability and autism. However, like any other category we can put someone in, people on the autism spectrum do not form a homogenous group. If issues like lighting, non-intrusive appliances and clear delineation of spaces are present, they may be addressed in most types of housing. Likewise, if secure outdoor space is required, this is not inevitably only addressed by an institutional response. For example, a large garden with room for a trampoline addressed this issue for one person. If you experience

---

BOX 24.3   Checklist for institutional characteristics

- isolated / remote location
- segregated for people with intellectual disabilities
- large group of non-family members living together
- more than 6 individual living units for people with intellectual disabilities congregated on one site
- on a campus with other services for people with intellectual disabilities
- people are compelled to live together
- people have lived there for years with no review
- shared personal spaces
- can't have own possessions
- separate from wider community
- lack of privacy
- lack of liberty or freedom of movement
- strict schedule of activities / regime of acceptable behaviour
- division of power between staff and users with no balances (e.g. advocacy)
- work as well as live there
- no choice of support staff
- residence is contingent on support provision
- away from family and friends
- no control over when support is provided
- institutional language used e.g. "service users", "staff"
- do things as a group
- promotes an artificial community in place of the real community

---

the world differently it is all the more important that you have a home that can help you make sense of the space you are in. Inevitably, a specialist service (or an institution) caters for a group which means more variables and less ability for an individual to self-orientate, self-regulate and shape their environment.

Occasion may arise where some form of specialised residential service is the only option, but this must be for a specific purpose, and for a limited period of time. Many people with intellectual disabilities remain in hospital for long periods as informal patients, without them or their family being aware of their rights. Any person with an intellectual disability detained in hospital should have access to high quality advocacy, but any professional involved should ensure that they understand the rights of a person in hospital and are contributing to a discharge plan.

Planning

Planning ahead is a good idea for anyone who knows their living circumstances will change. Even if you are living with family, and will inherit the property or have succession rights to the tenancy, it is better to have information about the legal situation readily available, and a plan in place for if your support changes rather than wait for a crisis. One woman who lived with her elderly mother in what had become a mutual caring relationship, planned to stay in her home which she would inherit on her mother's death. Despite this, the local Community Learning Disability Team had her on a list of people for supported living schemes. It was critical that a plan was drawn up for if her mother went into hospital or died, as there was a real risk that she could be moved from her home into a scheme and would not have the ability to express an opposing view. David's story 24.1 in the accompanying online resource illustrates how continuity may be achieved.

Having a plan for where you will live, and how you will be supported next, is also important for young people in residential schools. The intention may be to return to the parents' house, but even here, thought needs to be given as to how this will work. Young adults can find it difficult to reintegrate into their childhood bedroom and role in the family household when they have been away, and this is particularly challenging for a young person who has been living in a residential school or intentional community for some years, in a highly structured and often spacious/rural environment. This can be a trigger point for problems at home, as families discover that what is available to their young child may be very different to what their adult child is able to access.

If you are living somewhere like a hostel, specialised residential service or a hospital, you should always have some sort of future housing and support plan, without which you might not be able to leave for years (or ever), or risk transferring to equally unsatisfactory living arrangements. Many people with intellectual disabilities have a long history of shifting from placement to placement, and of the "revolving door" where they are in and out of hospital, special units, prison, hostels, and

the only way to break this cycle is good planning. The long-term aim has to be achieving security of tenure/residence, with responsive support and meaningful relationships/connections that help a person to live the life that suits them.

How people are in hospitals may be very different to how they are when they move into the community. The hospital environment, and the way issues are managed (such as restraint, medication and seclusion), are not transferable to the community, therefore, information about how a person has presented in hospital will only give a partial picture of the person.

Individual Service Design

Even if you are not directly involved in arranging housing, you may be able to use your professional skills and knowledge of a person to contribute to a housing plan/specification and a support plan, which will be key components for *Individual Service Design*. The Service Design sets out what is needed and what is likely to make sense for the person. The following issues (and more) are likely to come up:

1 Housing - Location (both the geographical location and the sort of neighbourhood); who or what sort of person they might want to live with; what would they need to be able to do there; would it need a garden or outdoor space; type of building (flat/house etc.); rooms/space requirements; mobility requirements; any specific health needs that may be relevant.

2 Support - What sort of people could provide support (skills, attributes, availability, etc.); what would they need to do (supporting the person to participate in the community, help with shopping and budgeting, support with meal preparation, etc.); how to keep the person safe and well (e.g. how to support the person to mobilise safely); specific times support is required; any specific health needs that may be relevant (e.g. medication).

It is important to get as much fine detail in these specifications as possible, drawing on your professional expertise, knowledge of the person, and incorporating assessments from other professionals. Box 24.4 includes tips for planning for individual service design

Resilience is crucial. If this were easy it is unlikely that the person would have been stuck in an inappropriate setting. Detailed planning, based on the perspective of the person and those closest to them, reduces the chances of things going wrong, but even the best of

---

📄 BOX 24.4   Tips for planning for individual Service Design

- The person and those closest to them have the clearest experience of what works.
- Gather as much information as possible about the person's life from birth, schooling and onwards from the point of view of the person and their family. You will get a different perspective from case records.
- Give time to explore the person's early life with them and/or those who know them. Sometimes there are clues that have got lost in years of reports in different services.
- Try to record in meetings in an accessible way (perhaps using graphics), so everyone can see, challenge and think about what is being written down.
- Allocate plenty of time for any planning meeting and think about how to help it make sense for the person, e.g. having space to walk around or to come and go.
- Be creative. E.g. one planning meeting was held in the Director's box of the football club that a person was a big fan of; it helped make him feel that it really was his meeting.

- The aim of a planning meeting is to get into the detail of what's needed and what matters for the person, based on their experience. Detail is critical in determining features/location of housing, characteristics required of support workers and how the person will choose them.
- Once a Service Design has been developed, those involved need to 'sign up' to a plan of action as to how it might be achieved.
- Accommodation is unlikely to be available immediately, but someone needs to get the ball rolling by making relevant enquiries and applications.
- The process of recruitment should start as early as possible to give supporters and the person time get to know each other before the move.
- During the 'getting to know you' phase, develop a Working Policy. This is a practical 'how to' guide, which may include details of how to provide intimate personal care (we all brush our teeth in our own way) as well as detailed scenario planning – 'what if' … and actions/words the support worker should take/use. The Working Policy is a live document that is amended based on the experience of the person.

---

plans can. This is usually because insufficient or inaccurate detail was gathered at the planning stage, or those involved in providing support have not followed the Working Policy (see Box 24.4). 'Stickability' – not giving up on a person when things don't go to plan, characterises successful work with people with difficult histories. The problem is probably located in the response; for example, one man moved out of a long-stay hospital to his own home too quickly, before there was a good team in place. Too many irregular staff resulted in violent incidents and a return to hospital. The man moved back into his house when this was resolved, and he leads a good life there several years later.

Transitions

In the UK 'transition' is often used to describe the period when young people move from children's to adult services, but transitions occur other times in our lives, such as in bereavement and relationship breakdown, and are often accompanied with high emotional stress. You may have heard that moving home is one of the most stressful times in your life, though presumably that will depend on a number of factors. How we cope with stress is influenced by a multitude of factors which determine how resilient we are to change, and if our past experience has been lack of control, our coping strategies in the face of change will be fuelled by anxiety. Change can be difficult for us all, but if one has difficulty understanding the world beyond one's immediate experience, change may be even more challenging and possibly risk having ill effects for the rest of one's life.

The Summer Foundation identifies three key factors for a successful transition from an institutional setting to the community (Reynolds, 2017)

1   Individually tailored support and assistance - having adequate support that is tailored to the person, before, during and after the move, based on a good

understanding of what they want for life and in their new home. This will increase the likelihood that the right choices and priorities will be made as they go along.

2 Continuity of personnel - allows the person to have a sense of stability and also makes it easier for everyone to know where things are up to and how the person is doing. Having familiar people on the journey, supporting the person to adjust to a new environment and new routines are important considerations.

3 Trusted relationships - help the person maintain confidence in their capability to establish a successful life in their new home, air anxieties and make adjustments in response to new insights.

To this we would add

4 Having choice and control - the feeling that the move is happening because it has been chosen and is wanted by the person, not being done to them. Even where choice is limited, e.g. if a care home is closing or there are limited housing options, it is possible to maximise choice and give the person as much control as possible.

5 Quality of housing - moving to housing that is fit for purpose, meaning as well-adapted and suited to the person as possible, and a location that is safe and near to places and people that matter should clearly be the aim. Personalising the environment and crucially supporting the person to arrange things in a way that suits them.

Pace is important. Sometimes transitions happen too quickly, with people not having a chance to rationalise what is happening or get involved in the practical arrangements. If new objects/places/people just appear, there is no way of telling what else will happen. If the person has been fully involved throughout, they will have visited the accommodation, and the area, and will have seen it all come together. Sometimes, transitions can drag on for years, which can itself be confusing and demotivating (Wiesel et al, 2015).

A study in Ireland (Salmon et al, 2019) reinforces all these issues, including the importance of having trusted supporters throughout, being connected with the new locality, and also maintaining connections with the people and places one is moving away from. It also highlights how important it is for people with intellectual disabilities to feel safe where they live, and that one should not assume a person will feel safe in a congregated setting.

READER ACTIVITY 24.4

In Simon's story in the online resource, his reputation to challenge influenced the reluctance of the professionals involved to seek a better living situation for him, despite the cost of the service and a shared acknowledgement that it was unsatisfactory.

Having read Simon's story, and using the chapter content, how might you contribute to finding a solution for someone stuck in inappropriate accommodation?

The importance of relationships: a personal perspective

Those of us who become involved with people and their support through our jobs, will be familiar with the term 'keeping professional boundaries'. This is in recognition of the power imbalance that inevitably exists, and sadly reflecting occasions around the world, where the professional/support worker has exploited that relationship. However, sometimes this professional boundary can result in cold, compassionless interactions.

In our experience of providing support directly or organising support and housing, relationships are a critical factor, be it as a support worker, social worker, nurse or advocate. Establishing and maintaining an open dialogue is part of providing good support and learning to listen to an individual and understand what works for them. This has helped our service prove resilient in the face of COVID-19. Having a skilled team based round an individual fosters humane relationships which go beyond the traditional professional/client or service-user dynamic. This has helped teams maintain motivation and demonstrate high levels of commitment and problem solving at an individual level, whilst keeping all safe in this troubled time. It also helps to keep decision-making as close as possible to the person and their family and offers workers the opportunity for a wide range of career and skills development.

Positive and open relationships cannot be imposed. There are organisations which place great emphasis on matching a person providing direct support, by involving the supported person and those closest to them, in recruiting support workers. This does not mean recruiting 'friends', but taking account of factors beyond skills and knowledge, such as personality and interests. As well as increasing the likelihood of a "good match", this is more likely to foster a commitment or mutual stake between the supported person and the supporter. A relationship which includes mutual trust and respect, a relationship which does not see the person with an intellectual disability as a means to an end (e.g. career development or salary), but which sees the person with an intellectual disability as an end in themself (as we all see ourselves) is vital.

These relationships are not static. We all recognise the complexities of relationships and the necessary adjustments we make with our family, neighbours, colleagues or friends depending on time and context. Some organisations include a 'third party agreement' in the direct support worker's contract. This means where the worker is recruited to support an individual, employment with that individual is dependent on maintaining a positive working relationship. It gives the supported person, and those closest to them, the option of terminating the employment if the relationship breaks down. Because emphasis is placed on matching and involvement from the outset, the third party option is rarely used, but is seen as important in maintaining a healthy power balance. After all, who amongst us would want someone regularly coming into our home, sometimes providing intimate care, who we don't want to be there?

CONCLUSION

Whilst in this chapter we had the challenge of taking an international perspective on different living environments for people with intellectual disabilities, there is much scope for exploring this rich topic further. For example, there is overrepresentation of people with intellectual disabilities in prison across the world (García-Largo et al, 2020; Hellenbach, 2016) and levels of homelessness (Beer et al, 2019) which we think may be partly due to having inadequate housing and support at an earlier stage.

By taking a human rights perspective, we aim to allow the chapter to be relevant, wherever you are in the world. Along with the focus on rights, we have challenged dehumanising attitudes that perpetuate institutional practice, by encouraging the reader to relate the difficulties faced by people with intellectual disabilities in achieving a home, to their own experience. We encourage the reader to be ambitious for the people they encounter and get to know, and to see good housing and

support as not just meeting a need, but as allowing a person to lead a life. Finally, regardless of the model of housing and support, mutually respectful relationships are a crucial but sometimes overlooked factor, as important as the physical environment, in one really having a home of one's own.

REFERENCES

Aichroth, S., Carpenter, J., Daniels, K., et al. (2002). Creating a new system of supports: The Vermont Self-Determination Project. *Rural Special Education Quarterly*, 21(2), 16–28.

Alba, P., Prouty, R., Scott, N., et al. (2008). Changes in populations of residential settings for persons with intellectual and developmental disabilities over a 30–year period, 1977–2007. *Intellectual and Developmental Disabilities*, 46, 257–260.

Allcock, A. (2019). ESSS outline: disability, poverty and transitional support. *Iriss*. https://doi.org/10.31583/esss.20190121. [Accessed 27 October 2020].

ARC Scotland. (2019). *Independence* [film]. Edinburgh, Scotland: ARC Scotland.

Beer, A., Baker, E., Lester, L., et al. (2019). The relative risk of homelessness among persons with a disability: new methods and policy insights. *International Journal of Environmental Research and Public Health*, 16.

Bigby, C., Bould, E., & Beadle-Brown, J. (2017). Conundrums of supported living: the experiences of people with intellectual disability. *Journal of Intellectual & Developmental Disability*, 42(4), 309–319.

Bond, R., & Hurst, J. (2010). How adults with learning disabilities view living independently. *British Journal of Learning Disabilities*, 38(4), 286–292.

Bugarszki, Z., van Ewijk, H., Wilken, J., et al. (2017). *Comparative analysis of the implement of Article 19 of the United Nations Convention of the Rights of People with Disabilities in eight European countries*. Estonia: Estonian Ministry of Social Affairs.

Campion, C., & Mouiller, P. (2016). *Rapport D´Information Fait au nom de la commission des affaires sociales (1) sur la prise en charge de personnes handicapées en dehors du territoire français*. Available at: https://www.senat.fr/rap/r16-218/r16-2181.pdf. [Accessed 21 October 2020].

Capri, C., Abrahams, L., McKenzie, J., et al. (2018). Intellectual disability rights and inclusive citizenship in South Africa: what can a scoping review tell us? https://doi.org/10.4102/ajod.v7i0.396.

Clement, T., & Bigby, C. (2010). *Group homes for people with intellectual disabilities: encouraging inclusion and participation*. London: Kingsley.

Committee on the Rights of Persons with Disabilities. (2017). *General comment on Article 19: living independently and being included in the community*. United Nations.

Cummins, R., & Lau, A. (2003). Community integration or community exposure? A review and discussion in relation to people with an intellectual disability. *Journal of Applied Research in Intellectual Disabilities, 16*, 145–157.

Dyck, I., Kontos, P., Angus, J., et al. (2005). The home as a site for long-term care: meanings and management of bodies and spaces. *Health & Place, 11*, 173–185.

European Expert Group on the Transition from Institutional to Family Based Care. (2012). *Common European guidelines on the transition from institutional to community-based care*. Brussels: European Union.

European Network on Independent Living (ENIL). (2016). *Definitions*. Available at: http://enil.eu/independent-living/definitions/. [Accessed 20 October 2020].

Fullana, J., Pallisera, M., Vila, M., et al. (2019). Intellectual disability and independent living: professionals' views via a Delphi study. *Journal of Intellectual Disabilities, 24*(4), 433–447.

Fyson, R., Tarleton, B., & Ward, L. (2007). *Support for living? The impact of the Supporting People programme on housing and support for adults with learning disabilities*. Bristol: The Policy Press.

García-Largo, L., Gabriel Martí-Agustí, G., Martin-Fumadó, C., et al. (2020). Intellectual disability rates among male prison inmates. *International Journal of Law and Psychiatry, 70*.

Goode, P. B. (Director). (1993). *Ethics: the foundation of the principles of normalization* [Motion picture]. Available at: https://mn.gov/mnddc/bengtNirje/bengt_nirje02.html.

Harding, R., & Ezgi, T. (2018). Supported decision-making from theory to practice: implementing the right to enjoy legal capacity. *Societies, 8*(2), 25.

Harrison, M., & Davis, C. (2000). *Housing, social policy and difference: disability, ethnicity, gender and housing*. Bristol: The Policy Press.

Hellenbach, M. K. (2016). Intellectual disabilities among prisoners: prevalence and mental and physical health comorbidities. *Journal of Applied Research in Intellectual Disabilities, 30*(2), 230–241.

Human Rights Watch. (2010). *'Once you enter, you never leave'. Deinstitutionalization of persons with intellectual or mental disabilities in Croatia*. Available at: https://www.hrw.org/report/2010/09/23/once-you-enter-you-never-leave/deinstitutionalization-persons-intellectual-or. [Accessed 21 October 2020].

Imrie, R. (2004). Disability, embodiment and the meaning of the home. *Housing Studies, 19*(5), 745–763.

Jackson, R., & Irvine, H. (2013). The impact of ideology on provision of services for people with an intellectual disability. *International Journal of Developmental Disabilities, 59*(1), 20–34.

Joint Committee on Human Rights. (2019). *The detention of young people with learning disabilities and/or autism*. London: House of Commons and House of Lords. Available at: https://www.parliament.uk/business/committees/committees-a-z/joint-select/hum. [Accessed December 2020].

Jones, K., & Fowles, A. (1984). Goffman the radical. In K. Jones & A. Fowles (Eds.), *Ideas on institutions: analysing the literature on long-term care and custody* (pp. 12–16). London: Routledge & Kegan Paul.

Karydaki, D. (2019). A Greek neverland: the history of the Leros asylums' inmates with intellectual disability (1958–95). In J. Walmsley & S. Jarrett (Eds.), *Intellectual disability in the twentieth century: transnational perspectives on people, policy and practice* (pp. 79–98). Bristol: Policy Press.

Kremsner, G., Koenig, O., & Buchner, T. (2019). Tracing the historical and ideological roots of services for people with intellectual disabilities in Austria. In J. Walmsley & S. Jarrett (Ed.), *Intellectual disability in the twentieth century: transnational perspectives on people, policy and practice* (pp. 35–52). Bristol: Policy Press.

Lashewicz, B., Noshin, R., Boettcher, N., et al. (2020). Meanings of home: an illustration of insideness and outsideness for two adults with developmental disabilities. *Housing Studies*. https://doi.org/10.1080/02673037.2020.1796928.

Lulinski, A., & Shea Tanis, E. (2018). *The state of the states in intellectual and developmental disabilities*. Available at: https://www.colemaninstitute.org/wp-content/uploads/2018/04/SOS_SABE_brief_final.pdf. [Accessed 21 October 2020].

MacDonald, A. (2018). *Coming home: a report on out-of-area placements and delayed discharge for people with learning disabilities and complex needs*. Edinburgh: Scottish Government.

Mansell, J., & Beadle-Brown, J. (2009). Dispersed or clustered housing for adults with intellectual disability: a systematic review. *Journal of Intellectual & Developmental Disability, 34*(4), 313–323.

McConkey, R., Keogh, F., Bunting, B., et al. (2018). Changes in the self-rated well-being of people who move from congregated settings to personalized arrangements and group home placements. *Journal of Intellectual Disabilities, 22*(1), 49–60.

McLeod, S. A. (2018) Maslow's hierarchy of needs. Available at: https://www.simplypsychology.org/maslow.html. [Accessed 21 October 2020].

Mental Welfare Commission for Scotland. (2016). *No through road: people with learning disabilities in hospital*. Edinburgh: Mental Welfare Commission for Scotland.

Montgomery C. (2018). *Developmental disability community faces a housing crisis*. Available at: http://nosmag.org/disability-community-faces-a-housing-crisis-modern-asylums-not-a-solution-hcbs/. [Accessed 30 October 2020].

O'Brien, J. (1997). A framework for accomplishment. In H. K. Sanderson (Ed.), *People, plans and possibilities: exploring person centred planning*. Edinburgh: Scottish Human Services Trust.

O'Brien, J., & Lyle O'Brien, C. (1988). *A little book about person centred planning*. Toronto: Inclusion Press.

Office of National Statistics. (2019a). *Disability and crime*. Available at: https://www.ons.gov.uk/peoplepopulationandcommunity/healthandsocialcare/disability/bulletins/disabilityandcrimeuk/2019. [Accessed 20 October 2020].

Office of National Statistics. (2019b). *Disability, well-being and loneliness, UK: 2019 personal well-being (UK) and loneliness (England) outcomes for disabled adults, with analysis by age, sex, impairment type, impairment severity and country*. Available at: https://www.ons.gov.uk/peoplepopulationandcommunity/healthandsocialcare/disability/bulletins/disabilitywellbeingandlonelinessuk/2019#loneliness-by-disability-england. [Accessed 30 October 2020].

Panorama: Undercover Hospital Abuse Scandal. (2019). [Motion picture]. UK: BBC.

Paradigm. (2019). # *The reach standards practical guide*. Available at: https://paradigm-uk.org/what-we-do/reach-support-for-living/. [Accessed 27 October 2020].

Quinn, H. D., Zeeman, H., & Kendall, E. (2016). A place to call my own: young people with complex disabilities living in long-term care. *Journal of Prevention & Intervention in the Community*, 44, 258–271.

Relph, E. (1976). *Place and placelessness*. London: Pion.

Relph, E. (2016). *Placeness, place, placenessness*. Available at: https://www.placeness.com/529-2/. [Accessed 21 October 2020].

Reynolds, A. (2017). *A successful transition to more independent living*. Melbourne: Summer Foundation Ltd. Available at: https://www.summerfoundation.org.au/wp-content/uploads/2018/02/a-successful-transition-to-more-independent-living.pdf. [Accessed 10 November 2020].

Salmon, N., Garcia, E., Donohoe, B., et al. (2019). Our homes: an inclusive study about what moving house is like for people with intellectual disabilities in Ireland. *British Journal of Learning Disabilities*, 47, 19–28.

Scott, W. (1995). *Institutions and organizations*. Thousand Oaks, CA: Sage.

Sheppard-Jones, K., Thompson Prout, H., & Kleinert, H. (2005). Quality of life dimensions for adults with developmental disabilities: a comparative study. *Mental Retardation*, 43, 281–291.

Shogren, K. W. M., Uyanik, H., & Heidrich, M. (2017). Development of the supported decision making inventory system. *Intellectual and Developmental Disabilities*, 55(6), 432–439.

Sly, S. (2013). *Housing to end the prison of hospital*. Available at: https://www.centreforwelfarereform.org/library/housing-to-end-the-prison-of-hospital.html. [Accessed 20 October 2020].

Smull, M., & Sanderson, H. (2005). *Essential lifestyle planning for everyone*. Annapolis, MD: The Learning Community – Essential Lifestyle Planning.

Stancliffe, R., Lakin, C., Doljanac, R., et al. (2007). Loneliness and living arrangements. *Intellectual and Developmental Disabilities*, 45(6), 380–390.

Transforming Care Programme. (2016). *Building the right home: guidance for commissioners of health and care services for children, young people and adults with learning disabilities and/or autism who display behaviour that challenges*. London: NHS England, LGA and ADASS.

United Nations. (1948). *Universal Declaration of Human Rights*. Available at: https://www.un.org/en/universal-declaration-human-rights/. [Accessed 10 December 2019].

United Nations. (1976a). *International Covenant on Civil and Political Rights*. Available at: https://www.ohchr.org/en/professionalinterest/pages/ccpr.aspx. [Accessed 12 November 2019].

United Nations. (1976b). *International Covenant on Economic, Social and Cultural Rights*. Available at: https://www.ohchr.org/en/professionalinterest/pages/cescr.aspx. [Accessed 12 December 2019].

United Nations. (2019). CRPD - Convention on the Rights of Persons with Disabilities 21 Session (11/3/2019 – 5/4/2019). Available at: https://tbinternet.ohchr.org/_layouts/15/treatybodyexternal/SessionDetails1.aspx?SessionID=1304&Lang=en. [Accessed 5 November 2020].

United Nations. (2020). *Convention on the Rights of Persons with Disabilities (CRPD)*. https://www.un.org/development/desa/disabilities/convention-on-the-rights-of-persons-with-disabilities.html. [Accessed 20 October 2020].

Wiesel, I. (2020). Mainstream participation as an institution: commentary on "Legitimacy and ambiguity: institutional logics and their outcome for people with intellectual disabilities" (Ineland, 2020). *Research and Practice in Intellectual and Developmental Disabilities*, 7(1), 64–68.

Wiesel, I., Laragy, C., Gendera, S., et al. (2015). *Moving to my home: housing aspirations, transitions and outcomes of people with disability*. Sydney: Australian Housing and Urban Research Institute.

Witsø, E., & Hauger, B. (2020). 'It's our everyday life' – the perspectives of persons with intellectual disabilities in Norway. *Journal of Intellectual Disabilities*, 24(2), 143–157.

Wolfensberger, W. (1998). *A brief introduction to social role valorization: a high-order concept for addressing the plight of societally devalued people, and for structuring human services* (3rd ed.). Syracuse: NY: Training Institute for Human Services.

World Health Organization. (1986). *The Ottawa Charter for Health Promotion*. Available at: https://www.who.int/healthpromotion/conferences/previous/ottawa/en/. [Accessed 20 October 2020].

World Health Organization. (2012). *Prevalence and risk of violence against adults with disabilities: a systematic review and meta-analysis of observational studies*. Available at: https://www.who.int/disabilities/violence/en/. [Accessed 20 October 2020].

World Health Organization and World Bank. (2011). *World report on disability*. Geneva: World Health Organization.

25

Sexuality and relationships

Rebecca Fish and Kristín Björnsdóttir

KEY ISSUES

- People with intellectual disabilities have the same desires for intimate relationships as everyone else.
- They experience multiple barriers to establishing and maintaining relationships. Some of these barriers relate to paternalistic attitudes on behalf of health and social care professionals, parents and carers.
- People with intellectual disabilities have rights to be provided with accessible education and information about relationships, as well as practical support to meet people, access to transport, and privacy to maintain relationships. It is important that support

staff are trained in sexual rights and consent, as well as providing safeguarding support in a non-judgmental way.
- Policymakers should take into account the experiences and advice of people with intellectual disabilities when composing guidance.
- Some good practice examples are specialist dating agencies and clubs, websites with accessible multimedia resources that include guidance on legal aspects, and online toolkits for support staff and other professionals.

CHAPTER OUTLINE

INTRODUCTION

"It is important not to let the bureaucracy involved mean that we don't support people in a more positive way to have relationships. In our view, allowing people with learning [intellectual] disabilities to take acceptable risks, and helping them to assess risk, should help significantly to protect them from exploitation anyway."
Hall and Yacoub, 2008, p. 20

Sexuality and the intimate relationships of people with intellectual disabilities are increasingly being

recognised as social justice issues (Bahner, 2012; Turner and Crane, 2016). People with intellectual disabilities have the same desires and rights to express their sexuality as everyone else, although they experience many challenges along the way (National Development Team for Inclusion (NDTi), 2019; Rushbrooke et al, 2014). They face discriminatory attitudes and significant disadvantages in their desire to explore and maintain sexual and intimate relationships–indeed they may be actively discouraged from embarking on relationships by family and health, educational and support staff (Grieve et al,

451

2009; Lam et al, 2019; Rushbrooke et al, 2014). In this chapter we will explore some of these barriers in more detail, looking at how they are shaped by concepts of disability and gender and we suggest ways to address them.

WHAT INFLUENCES SEXUAL WELLBEING?

According to the World Health Organization (WHO), sexual wellbeing cannot be defined, understood, or made operational without a broad consideration of sexuality, which underlies important behaviours and outcomes related to sexual health. Their working definition of sexuality is:

> "… *a central aspect of being human throughout life [encompassing] sex, gender identities and roles, sexual orientation, eroticism, pleasure, intimacy and reproduction. Sexuality is experienced and expressed in thoughts, fantasies, desires, beliefs, attitudes, values, behaviours, practices, roles and relationships. While sexuality can include all of these dimensions, not all of them are always experienced or expressed. Sexuality is influenced by the interaction of biological, psychological, social, economic, political, cultural, legal, historical, religious and spiritual factors.*"
>
> *WHO, 2006, p. 5*

People with intellectual disabilities are able to experience sexuality – they value sensuality and intimacy (Turner and Crane, 2016), and also care and love in relationships (Yacoub and Hall, 2009). When asked, people with intellectual disabilities describe their intimate relationships as very important, allowing opportunities for increased self-esteem and independence whilst providing comfort and support, and for some, reparation for previous abuse (Bates et al, 2017b; Lafferty et al, 2013; O'Shea and Frawley, 2020; Webster, 2020).

Sexual wellbeing is therefore related to life satisfaction, but parents and service providers can place restrictions on privacy (personal time) and space for masturbation and sexual exploration. This may include placing limitations on bodily autonomy, resulting in people resorting to sex in places where they are not comfortable and less likely to practise safe sex (Fish, 2016; McLelland et al, 2012). Discussion around sexual desire and pleasure is generally missing in research with people with intellectual disabilities (Black and Kammes, 2019). Policies, parents and health and social care practitioners often refer to autonomy, empowerment and self-determination, but they may fail to address the underlying need for intimate

> ### BOX 25.1   Barriers to sexual and intimate relationships
>
> - Lack of knowledge about mental capacity and ability to consent to sexual relationships
> - Lack of awareness on behalf of support staff, carers and family members about how to support intimate relationships in practice
> - Concepts of 'vulnerability' contributing to feelings of over-protection by staff and families
> - People experiencing frequent placement moves throughout life
> - Congregate placements with insufficient private spaces
> - People having limited opportunities and limited resources to meet potential partners
> - People with intellectual disabilities not receiving sex education, or receiving overwhelmingly negative or inaccessible information about sex

relationships due to the focus on protection from risk (Bates et al, 2020; Lam et al, 2019; Neuman, 2019). We summarise the barriers experienced by people in relation to sexual and intimate relationships in Box 25.1.

The legacy of eugenics and institutionalisation has propagated stereotyped assumptions about people with intellectual disabilities - that they become promiscuous and dangerous when their sexuality is awakened, and therefore must be kept 'innocent' and asexual by protecting them and shielding them from knowledge about sex (Walmsley and Jarrett, 2019). Paternalistic approaches to working with people with intellectual disabilities reflect the historical, distinctly gendered attitudes to their sexuality. Arguably, this type of protection can be harmful because it can lead to the belief that sexual expression should either be ignored or suppressed, resulting in people being excluded from support or education about sexuality (Hollomotz, 2011; Rogers, 2009). Sex education for young people with intellectual disabilities is often discretionary and tends to be superficial and limited to safe sex, contraception and sexually transmitted infections (STIs) rather than discussing enjoyment and offering practical information (Frawley and Wilson, 2016), as we will discuss later.

When asked about what they needed to help them meet their needs in the area of relationships and sexuality, most people with intellectual disabilities wanted to know how to meet other people and how to talk to the people they are interested in (Chivers and Mathieson,

2000). There is a need to normalise sexuality and relationships for people with intellectual disabilities, in order to balance the important components of protection and empowerment (Lam et al, 2019).

Living arrangements

For the past four decades, the question of where people with intellectual disabilities live has been at the centre of disability policy in the Global North. It is now more common that people with intellectual disabilities live in community settings with or without support. Deinstitutionalisation and community integration allow people with intellectual disabilities greater access to society and various community resources. However, the support and services they receive may still have institutional qualities (Björnsdóttir and Traustadóttir, 2010), and the freedom to choose where to live and with whom has to a large extent not been granted to those who require support in their daily lives (Björnsdóttir et al, 2015).

For people living in residential settings it is difficult to develop intimate relationships. Bedrooms are often small and rarely have double beds (Brown et al, 2000). Privacy is commonly not respected – carers may enter rooms without knocking, and bedroom doors are seldom closed (Björnsdóttir and Stefánsdóttir, 2020). The lack of material space and privacy can make it almost impossible for individuals to create opportunities for intimacy with others (Hollomotz and Speakup Committee, 2009). Furthermore, service providers seldom include sexual support when planning services for people with intellectual disabilities (Björnsdóttir and Stefánsdóttir, 2020). In this instance, sexuality therefore becomes an afterthought or a reaction to a "problem".

The lack of attention to the relationships of people with intellectual disabilities has consequences - people with intellectual disabilities can internalise hegemonic and heteronormative gender roles, such as men as bread winners, and women as mothers, which leads them to feelings of failure (Björnsdóttir et al, 2017; Turner and Crane, 2016). Michelle McCarthy's (1999) study found that women felt they had very little choice or control over their sexual experiences, and experienced little or no enjoyment. These themes are also apparent in Barron's research in Sweden where women with intellectual disabilities did not see themselves as sexual beings, largely because they considered themselves to be sexually 'unavailable' (Barron, 2002, p. 69). Barron explains this is a result of the women having internalised views of themselves from others (parents and professionals), because there was much 'time and effort spent on training women with intellectual disabilities to behave in ways defined by others as proper and right for them to behave' (Barron, 2002, p. 59).

Wanting to have sex or masturbate is frequently labelled negatively for women by agency providers yet is seen as a more acceptable expectation for men (Fish, 2016; Williams and Nind, 1999). The fear of unwanted or unplanned pregnancy and the perceived inability of women with intellectual disabilities to become good mothers has influenced how caregivers approach their sexuality (Björnsdóttir et al, 2017); women with intellectual disabilities are still more likely to experience pressured preventive measures such as institutionalisation and sterilisation than men (Stefánsdóttir and Hreinsdóttir, 2013).

Although caregivers seem to be more at ease when considering men with intellectual disabilities as sexually active, men too face various barriers in relation to their sexuality. They have historically been constructed as sexual predators who have an uncontrollable sex drive (Björnsdóttir et al, 2017). The masturbation of men with intellectual disabilities has been described as a problem behaviour which needs treatment through behavioural or pharmaceutical therapy while little attention has been given to their need for education, safety and privacy (Murphy et al, 2007; Thompson and Beail, 2002). Box 25.2 describes a real-life example of good practice in relation to privacy and masturbation.

Locked wards

For people in inpatient, mental health or secure units, the notion of vulnerability is mixed with conceptions of dangerousness. Online Reader activity 25.1, Jane's story, illustrates this and encourages reflection on her experiences and service responses. People may encounter negative and controlling attitudes towards their sexuality and any form of sexual expression, with services regarding sexuality as a challenge which needs to be managed (Fish, 2016).

Johnson's ethnographic study on a locked ward for women with intellectual disabilities showed that sexuality *as a woman* was talked about as problematic in relation to impairment. This then became a reason for exerting more control over the women residents. Their sexuality was constructed as 'a problem related to their impairment which could be dealt with by isolating them from contact with others, containing their dangerousness and establishing strict measures of control over their

BOX 25.2   Good practice: privacy and masturbation

A young man with an intellectual disability who communicated with non-spoken language, was usually dressed in overalls and had his wrists tied to his wheelchair so he could not move his hands. This was because he had masturbated in public on occasion. He was also given drugs to decrease his sex drive. When he moved to a new residential home, his life changed dramatically. The new support staff viewed sexuality as a natural and important aspect of being human and made an effort to help him make choices in his everyday life. It was their understanding that he had masturbated in public in part because he was bored and did not have meaningful options to choose from in his daily life. They also made efforts to provide him with privacy and respected his privacy by knocking on his bedroom door before entering and incorporating "me-time" into his communication system for him to choose to masturbate in private and safe in his own room. There was no need to keep his hands tied to his wheelchair; he no longer needed to wear restrictive clothes, and he no longer masturbated in public.

BOX 25.3   Practice recommendations for inpatient services

- Local policy goals encouraging independence and progression through services should not override people's desire for relationships
- Policies should be individualised, flexible over time, and made in consultation with residents
- People should be clear about service policy on intimate relationships
- Private time and space should be provided whilst making sure the person is kept safe
- Clear, accessible information about sex should be provided
- Services should foster trust and rapport with residents, in order to support them individually, and allow them to discuss sexuality

behaviour' (Johnson, 1998, p. 67). Two of the women in Johnson's study were confined to the locked ward in part *because* of their sexual activities with men in other services. In each instance, it was the woman's behaviour that was seen as unacceptable and each was removed from her previous residence to the locked ward. Johnson concludes that women on the unit were considered to be sexually 'dangerous' (Johnson, 1998, p. 66).

Fish's research found that all spaces on locked wards were considered to be 'public', with implications on opportunities for exploring sexuality (Fish, 2016, 2018). Further, women on locked wards were often confused or unaware about policies on sexual and intimate relationships. Managerial staff were concerned about the women mixing with men because of their index offences and previous experiences, yet support staff invoked the Mental Capacity Act 2005 – arguing that women have the right to make unwise decisions. Fish concluded that both staff and residents required clear and accessible information about local and individual guidelines.

The literature provides an overwhelming picture of how people with intellectual disabilities are not expected

to have sexual desires, and when they show signs of sexual awareness, they are not provided with the support or information to make choices. In other words, other people are regulating their sexuality. This phenomenon seems to be exacerbated by the closed institutional lifestyle on locked wards.

In terms of recommendations for change, Fish's (2016) research proposed that guidelines on sexual and close relationships should be personalised and made in consultation with residents and their families at the beginning of their stay in a locked unit. People need to be made aware that there may be residents who are perpetrators of violent or sexual offences on locked wards. All guidelines should be made with the agreement of the resident so that they know they are coming from a policy of safeguarding rather than control, and should be dynamic and flexible over time. The wider literature points to further recommendations which we have summarised in Box 25.3.

SEXUAL RIGHTS AND CONSENT

There is considerable evidence that sexual behaviour amongst people with intellectual disabilities is often regarded as problematic or harmful. Whilst there has been noticeable recent improvements in the attitudes of care staff towards sexual expression in this group (Kelly et al, 2009; Yacoub and Hall, 2009), research shows that support staff are not generally expected to assist service users with this area of their lives (Bahner, 2012; Hollomotz, 2011).

To be free to, and have opportunities to express one's sexuality without interventions, violence, or harassment, can be understood as sexual rights. The Human Rights Act 1998, sets out the right to marry and have children, and the right to respect for a family life. Further, the UN Convention on the Rights of Persons with Disabilities (CRPD) (United Nations, 2006) states clearly that people with disabilities should have the freedom to make their own choices, recognising their right to participate in society. There are however, no specific statements or articles on sexual rights in the CRPD or other human rights conventions. Nevertheless, the CRPD recognises various rights that are linked to sexual rights, which are: equality and non-discrimination (Article 5), equal recognition before the law (Article 12), and respect for privacy, home and family (Article 22 and 23). There is also a special section which recognises the multiple discrimination of women and girls with disabilities. The World Health Organization (WHO) has published a working definition of sexual rights which refers to the human rights already widely recognised in international legislation:

"The fulfilment of sexual health is tied to the extent to which human rights are respected, protected and fulfilled. Sexual rights embrace certain human rights that are already recognised in international and regional human rights documents."

WHO, 2020

By defining sexual rights as human rights, states commit to ensuring that every person enjoys their sexuality and sexual freedom through protection from sexual abuse, exploitation and violence (Miller et al, 2015).

Despite the inclusion of relationships within these internationally ratified policies, support staff and health and social care staff may invoke a lack of capacity to consent as a way to limit sexual rights. James and Mitchell (2020) recognise this and recommend a collaborative exploration of actual risks:

"In adult social care, sexual desire is often conflated with concepts of risk and danger. Being able to work positively with professional constructions of risk arising from sex and desire involves a sophisticated understanding and exploration of the notion of risk, seeking to clarify the views of those involved, exploring the actual risks. This includes understanding the need for support and interventions that do not compromise the person's right to a private and personal life through
unnecessary and disproportionate state interference and social control."

James and Mitchell, 2020, p. 99

In the UK, the Mental Capacity Act (MCA) 2005, as an example, states that a person must always be assumed to have capacity unless it is established they lack capacity. The definition of incapacity is outlined in Section 2 of the MCA:

"A person lacks capacity in relation to a matter if at the material time he is unable to make a decision for himself in relation to the matter because of an impairment of, or a disturbance in the functioning of, the mind or brain."

To consent to sexual activity, the person must be able to understand the following:

- that they have a choice about whether to have sex and can refuse
- that they can change their mind at any time leading up to, and during, the sexual act
- the mechanics of sex, contraception, and the associated health risks, particularly the risk of sexually transmitted infections, and that sex between a man and a woman may result in the woman becoming pregnant.

The guidance states that where it is difficult to determine a person's capacity to consent to sexual relations, professional advice must be sought, which may result in cases being referred to the Court of Protection for determination. Providers should take steps to prevent people in their care having sex if they are deemed not to have capacity to consent to sex, for example, by speaking with the local safeguarding authority. Best interest decisions cannot be made in relation to a person's ability to consent to sex. This guidance is not always easy to follow; in their chapter on sexuality from the perspectives of social workers in the UK, James and Mitchell (2020) highlight the guidance complexities when making decisions about safeguarding, acknowledging the implications for caring relationships and people's long-term happiness.

Sex education

Research from around the globe suggests that people with intellectual disabilities lack access to sex education (Björnsdóttir et al, 2017; Wos et al, 2020). There are several intersecting reasons why.

Firstly, as a group, people with intellectual disabilities have limited or no opportunities to participate academically in general education classrooms and are frequently unprepared for adulthood (Björnsdóttir et al, 2015; Wilson and Frawley, 2016); whether students with intellectual disabilities receive sex education tends to vary greatly between schools and cultures (Doherty et al, 2014; Frawley and O'Shea, 2020; Wos et al, 2020). When disabled students are placed in inclusive school settings, sometimes they do not participate in sex education because their language or numeracy skills are prioritised. Also, research has shown that some educators are not comfortable teaching sex education with disabled students present (Björnsdóttir et al, 2017). One consequence of the lack of sex education is that people with intellectual disabilities learn (uncritically) about sex from TV, friends and the internet (Wos et al, 2020). Further, since people with intellectual disabilities have restricted access to education it is important to consider that they might have limited knowledge regarding anatomy and biology which calls for appropriate accommodations to allow them to access sex education instructional materials (Hollomotz, 2011; Löfgren-Mårtenson, 2012; Schaafsma et al, 2015). The content of special education classes and programmes that have been developed for people with intellectual disabilities varies greatly, but biological topics seem to be most common with emphasis on pregnancy and sexually transmitted infection (STI) prevention (Schaafsma et al, 2017). Adapted sexual programmes for people with intellectual disabilities have therefore been criticised for providing limited and poor information (Ferrante and Oak, 2020; Johnson et al, 2002; Löfgren-Mårtenson, 2012). Chapter 22 provides further commentary on the issue of sex education in schools.

Secondly, caregivers and parents are often concerned about the high risk of sexual abuse meaning that some adults with intellectual disabilities have been prevented from participating in sex education classes that are on offer in their community (Grove et al, 2018). Sex education is seen by some as increasing the risk of people with intellectual disabilities finding themselves in situations that are uncomfortable or dangerous regarding sexual behaviour (Rohleder, 2010). This has also meant that even some programmes intended for people with intellectual disabilities approach sexuality as problematic (Rohleder, 2010; Rohleder and Swartz, 2012; Schaafsma et al, 2015) and focus, for example, on how to avoid sexual abuse (Björnsdóttir et al, 2017) instead of safe and pleasurable sexual experiences.

Finally, as we have seen in our section on locked wards, people with intellectual disabilities are still being institutionalised in some regions of the world which further limits their access to sex education and sexual experience (Musopero, 2019). These restricted opportunities result in lack of knowledge about sexual health and rights.

Attitudes towards sex education

We have so far shown that negative attitudes and the idea that people with intellectual disabilities are victims rather than active sexual beings, can have negative impacts on their sexual experience (Williams and Nind, 1999). Thus, participation in sex education programmes has limited purpose if people are being met with negative attitudes by caregivers and absence of self-determination regarding their bodies, behaviours and daily lives (Hollomotz, 2011).

Hollomotz (2009) interviewed people with intellectual disabilities living in the community and found that they were often described as 'vulnerable' by their support staff. She critiques the concept of vulnerability, because it focuses analysis on the origin of the perceived risk posed to the individual. Indeed, she argues individual vulnerability 'assumes that a certain set of personal attributes and low self-defence skills combined, create risk' (Hollomotz, 2009, pp. 109–110). We begin to see that although elements of risk should be taken into account when safeguarding is needed, it seems that the use of the concept of vulnerability as a categorisation can result in greater regulation and less positive risk taking (see also Rushbrooke et al, 2014). Hollomotz makes recommendations for education in light of this. She argues that people need to have accessible education about sex in order to make decisions about sexual approaches, and skills to resist unwanted ones. These skills include having knowledge about sex and sexuality, the vocabulary needed to report sexual violence, awareness of one's rights to resist sexual contact, and self-esteem needed to effectively resist an unwanted sexual approach (see Chapters 6 and 8 for more discussion about positive risk taking and safeguarding).

As a response to negative attitudes, people with intellectual disabilities often feel guilt and secrecy about sexuality and have limited opportunities to talk and learn about feelings and emotions (Black and Kammes, 2019). Alexander and Taylor-Gomez (2017) show how sex education programmes for people with intellectual disabilities have neglected issues of pleasure, sensuality and feeling good, despite these issues being described by the WHO as the foundations for good sexual health and wellbeing (WHO, 2020). In order to reduce feelings of shame, it is important that sex education includes these aspects, including information about other positive aspects of relationships such as romance.

Sex education should therefore include a broad range of topics and not exclusively focus on safe sex and prevention of STIs or unwanted pregnancy (Alexander and Taylor-Gomez, 2017; Löfgren-Mårtenson, 2012; Schaafsma et al, 2017). Unfortunately, most existing sex education programmes have failed to involve people with intellectual disabilities in their development (Löfgren-Mårtenson, 2012; O'Shea and Frawley, 2020; Schaafsma et al, 2017).

 READER ACTIVITY 25.2

A man in his forties had considerable sexual experience and multiple sexual partners. He had participated in several sex education programmes since he left compulsory education. Although he had multiple sexual partners, he did not always use a condom. If he knew that his partners were, for example, using hormonal contraceptives, he believed he did not need to use a condom: "no condoms, no babies". He did not use condoms to prevent STIs.

Reflect on the reasons why the man only associated condoms with pregnancy prevention.

Think about the type of sex education this man should be offered, and the way this education should be delivered.

Since many people with intellectual disabilities have limited access to sexual experience and sex education, the consequences can be gendered. For example, men with intellectual disabilities may experience a significant lack of sexual understanding related to their behaviour. They are also most likely to receive sex education within a heterosexual context (Ferrante and Oak, 2020). Therefore, inadequate sex education, negative attitudes and absence of opportunities to express the emotional and sexual self has contributed to a wide variety of unwanted sexual behaviours (Yacoub and Hall, 2009). Further, there is a risk of unintended and unwanted pregnancies among women with intellectual disabilities,

and instead of educating them the solution has generally been abortions and sterilisation (Björnsdóttir et al, 2017; Hollomotz, 2011; Stefánsdóttir and Hreinsdóttir, 2013) as we discuss next.

Sterilisation

All over the world, women with intellectual disabilities have undergone systematic sterilisation to prevent them from having children (Llewellyn et al, 2010; Stefánsdóttir and Hreinsdóttir, 2013; Tilley et al, 2012). These measures were often taken without their knowledge or consent and were common during the times of eugenics and institutionalisation. People with intellectual disabilities were not considered capable of becoming parents, and by having children they were perceived to be polluting the gene pool. In Iceland, for example, at the onset of deinstitutionalisation, systematic sterilisation increased; people who wanted to keep their fertility had to remain in the institutions but if they agreed to be sterilised they had the option to move into community settings (Stefánsdóttir and Hreinsdóttir, 2013).

In most Global North countries, systematic sterilisation of people with intellectual disabilities is no longer practised. The CRPD states clearly that people with disabilities should retain their fertility equal to others. However, there is evidence that women and girls with intellectual disabilities are still being medically sterilised; they are often pressured by family members and sometimes not given accessible information about the consequences of such operations (Björnsdóttir et al, 2017). Activist groups such as Women With Disabilities Australia (WWDA, 2018) are working towards ending this practice as they argue that forced sterilisation - including forced contraception and menstrual suppression - is widespread and government sanctioned.

Hormonal contraceptives are commonly used with women with intellectual disabilities both for contraceptive and non-contraceptive purposes and serve as medical sterilisation (Hollomotz, 2011).Women are not commonly involved in making decisions about taking these medications, are given limited information about side-effects and are often not sexually active or having sex with men (Björnsdóttir and Stefánsdóttir, 2020; Hollomotz, 2011). The (medical) sterilisation practices in Iceland have been justified as an anti-abuse method. Under this rationale, sterilised women are protected from the consequences of sexual abuse, when in reality, the procedure only prevents pregnancy and therefore has the potential to hide ongoing abuse (Björnsdóttir et al, 2017; Björnsdóttir and Stefánsdóttir, 2020).

Men with intellectual disabilities may also experience discussions around their sterilisation, as Barton-Hanson (2015, p. 59) shows in her analysis of an English Court of Protection decision:

"what this really amounts to is a statement by the court that he can continue to have a sexual relationship but only on certain terms – those terms including that he is sterilized. The danger here is that in granting people with intellectual disability a measure of conditional freedom, it reinforces the idea that they can enjoy sexual freedom but at a cost."

Barton-Hanson's excellent overview of the legality of sterilisation concludes that the requirement for sexual freedom should not come at the price of sterilisation, and the least restrictive choice should always be taken. Moreover the views, wishes and interests of people with intellectual disabilities must be genuinely respected, and there should be acknowledgment that psychoactive medication has implications on sex drive, and therefore sexuality.

During the times of institutionalisation, more women with intellectual disabilities than men were sterilised (Stefánsdóttir 2014; Tilley et al, 2012). However, institutionalised men who were perceived as demonstrating inappropriate sexual behaviour such as masturbation were in some countries forced to undergo bilateral orchiectomies–a form of castration (Carlson et al, 2000). Castrations and sterilisations are permanent and involve surgical intervention. The sterilisation procedure for men is called vasectomy and does not influence sexual behaviour; they are common procedures for men in the Global North and most are successful. However, Carlson et al (2000) reported on studies which had associated vasectomies with chronic pain in one or both testes. While sterilisation should be on offer for men and women with intellectual disabilities, there is a need for appropriate support to help facilitate their decision making. Research has shown that while people with intellectual disabilities have given their consent for the surgery they have not always received appropriate information about the permanent consequences and associated risks (Björnsdóttir et al, 2017).

Hormonal drugs are commonly used for both women and men to control their sexuality. For men, hormonal drugs are used to block male sexual hormones, reduce sexual drive and reduce sperm production (Carlson et al, 2000). These drugs are used, for example, to reduce sexual preoccupation and number of days masturbated and reached orgasm (Sloan and Brewster, 2017). However, there are limited studies which aim at unpacking what constitutes problematic sexual behaviour and who should make that decision. What is, for example, an appropriate number of days masturbating to orgasm? Therefore, it is of the utmost importance that carers first examine how they might support the men in performing their sexuality safely and equally to others before requesting anti-libidinal therapy on their behalf. In many instances, quality accessible sex education could be beneficial to these men.

While hormonal drugs have been used to control the sexuality of men with intellectual disabilities, there are also other drugs that have negative effects on sexual performance. A Dutch study revealed that the prevalence of antipsychotic drug use among people with intellectual disabilities was 32.2% (de Kuijper et al, 2010). In general, more men with intellectual disabilities than women are prescribed antipsychotic drugs. Common adverse effects also include sexual dysfunction such as reduced libido, anorgasmia and erectile dysfunction (Stroup and Gray, 2018). In the Dutch study mentioned above, behavioural problems were the main reason for prescription of antipsychotics for people with intellectual disabilities, but in 18.5% no indication or reason for the prescription was noted in the medical record (de Kuijper et al, 2010). With such a high prevalence of prescribed antipsychotic drugs, there is need for research into the decision making processes including how well people are informed of the side effects of the long-term use of these drugs.

LGBTQIA EXPERIENCES

Public opinion towards lesbian, gay, bisexual, transgender, queer or questioning, intersex or asexual (LGBTQIA) people is generally positive, with multiple manifestations of gender and sexual identities operating around the world. However, people with intellectual disabilities have limited access to information and support around exploring and embracing such identities (Dinwoodie et al, 2020).

As we have mentioned, sex education for people with intellectual disabilities is focused on heterosexuality and they are presented with few opportunities to talk about homosexuality or bisexuality with others (Hellett, 2020; Richards, 2017). Research has shown that many people with intellectual disabilities express positive attitudes towards homosexuality (Hellett, 2020; Schaafsma et al, 2017) while some are still confused whether people with intellectual disabilities could be gay or if this identity is solely available to non-disabled people (Björnsdóttir et al, 2017); in many instances, their only knowledge about homosexuality comes from the media (Hollomotz, 2011).

Staff have reportedly claimed that they lack training and confidence in supporting gay people with intellectual disabilities (Abbott, 2015; Fish, 2016), which adds to the taboo status of their sexualities (Schaafsma et al, 2017). Löfgren-Mårtenson (2013) further states that the emphasis on heterosexuality and normalisation in education, support and policy reifies their status as outsiders. People identifying within non-heteronormative orientations report being frightened about what might be said if they make their feelings known (Abbott et al, 2005). The term 'challenging behaviour' may be used to characterise the unconventional sexual behaviour of men in this group, with cross-dressing, in particular, generating considerable professional and management concern (Cambridge and Mellan, 2000). Furthermore, support for lesbians or bisexual women with intellectual disabilities is lacking (Abbott et al, 2005, Löfgren-Mårtenson, 2009; McCarthy, 1999).

GENDER-BASED VIOLENCE AND ABUSE

Women with intellectual disabilities face oppression at the intersection of gender and disability, and this oppression means they are more likely to experience sexual violence and exploitation (Brown, 2004; McCarthy, 2014; McCarthy et al, 2019). Early attempts to communicate abuse are often not believed, and even when abuse is disclosed in adulthood this can be ignored by services or used as a way to increase restrictions–because women become seen as relationally incompetent (Pollack, 2007). Frequently, when women are offered support it is not the right kind (Traustadóttir and Johnson, 2000), and when they are seen as being particularly vulnerable or at risk for sexual abuse, this perceived vulnerability can act as a mechanism to deny their sexual desire (Gill, 2010).

McCarthy (1999) notes the very high levels of gender-based violence experiences amongst women with intellectual disabilities, with 82% of her participants having experienced sexual violence, including sexual abuse as children. More than half of those interviewed in Fish's

(2016) study disclosed experiences of abuse as children, or sexual violence as adults, even though they were not questioned directly about this.

Sexual abuse and harassment rarely go through the legal system and perpetrators are seldom charged, let alone convicted of their crime (Björnsdóttir et al, 2017; Björnsdóttir and Stefánsdóttir, 2020; Hollomotz, 2011). In Iceland, within the supported housing system, there are reports of women with intellectual disabilities who have been sexually harassed and abused by their carers. It seems common to view these acts of violence as organisational or employee issues to be dealt with within the home, workplace, or institution, for example by terminating the employment of the person in question without any aftermath or consequences (Björnsdóttir et al, 2017). International research also demonstrates that women with intellectual disabilities who have been sexually harassed or abused seldom receive any support or counselling due to perceptions that they are incapable of experiencing trauma because of their impairment, or that they lack the aptitude to benefit from psychological counselling (Bates et al, 2017a). Further, disability stigma and the hierarchy of gender may contribute to the high levels of gender-based violence experienced by people with intellectual disabilities (McCarthy et al, 2017). It is essential that services recognise trauma experiences and work together with people to balance risk and protection.

READER ACTIVITY 25.3

A woman in her forties was raped by a support staff member at the sheltered workshop where she worked. She was devastated and the carers at her group-home helped her press charges. It took the legal system months to decide if the abuser should be taken to court and the carers decided that it would be best for the woman to stop all social activities such as participation in leisure and self-advocacy groups until the legal process would be resolved. They also told her not to talk about her experience to anyone. She kept going to her job at the sheltered workshop.

Reflect on the following:

The possible reasons that the carers decided it was best for the woman to stop all social participation.

The way this decision affected her.

Steps that should have been taken.

Pornography

The opportunities for sexual expression amongst people with intellectual disabilities can be restricted by the belief systems of their parents and carers, who may make decisions on their behalf based on how they think they should live their lives (Bahner, 2013). For example, carers and parents may try to restrict their access to pornography (Maguire et al, 2019; Wilson et al, 2011). This is particularly true in institutional type settings such as hospitals (Yacoub and Hall, 2009) and group-homes (Björnsdóttir et al, 2017).

Some carers may fear that pornography could be harmful for youth and adults with intellectual disabilities because they have limited sexual experience and understanding of sexuality (Löfgren-Mårtenson et al, 2015). Furthermore, if people with intellectual disabilities are easily persuaded by gender stereotyping and unrealistic images of men and women (Löfgren-Mårtenson, 2012) it could be argued that viewing pornography could be harmful to them. Nevertheless, recent research suggests that some people with intellectual disabilities who view pornography are not fooled by the illusion of what they are viewing and claim that pornography does not influence how they would treat their sexual partners (Frawley and Wilson, 2016).

Although pornography has been criticised over the years for the exploitation of women (Ashton et al, 2018), a large number of people use it as part of normative sexual development, including people with intellectual disabilities (Frawley and Wilson, 2016; Löfgren-Mårtenson, 2012; Wilson et al, 2011; Yacoub and Hall, 2009). Most research on pornography and intellectual disabilities is gendered–the focus has been primarily on men and boys (Löfgren-Mårtenson et al, 2015). This is in line with sexuality research in general, especially research which is focused on sexuality as problematic or a pathological issue which needs to be treated. For example, much has been written on masturbation and men with intellectual disabilities but the literature focusing on women with intellectual disabilities and masturbation is almost non-existent.

Some staff members might experience discomfort in assisting people with intellectual disabilities to find pornography on the internet, and increased need for assistance might blur the line between access to information (pornography) and sexual facilitation. Further, when it comes to people with intellectual disabilities who have been labelled with severe or profound disabilities the issue of access to pornography becomes a non-issue since they are generally not perceived as sexual beings (Björnsdóttir and Stefánsdóttir, 2020; Maguire et al, 2019).

Since people with intellectual disabilities lack access to sex education, pornography can become their only source of information about sex (Björnsdóttir et al, 2017; Frawley and Wilson, 2016). It is important for carers, parents and educators to realise the differences between pornography and education. If people with intellectual disabilities could have access to quality sex education there might be fewer concerns that pornography is harmful to them or would lead to inappropriate behaviour. Also, research suggests that friends and family potentially have more influence on the moral development of people with intellectual disabilities than pornographic material (Frawley and Wilson, 2016). Nevertheless, it is important that critical appraisal and legality of pornography is explored during discussions about sex, as well as within sex education programmes and accessible information provision.

Sexual facilitation and sex work

Staff are generally not comfortable assisting people with intellectual disabilities regarding sexual activities. For example, personal care activities are interpreted differently if they are labelled as sexual. While staff might have no problem putting on a uridome (male urine disposal, resembling a condom) or assisting with undressing for bed or bath, they could find it troubling putting on a condom or undressing someone who was going to masturbate since that might be viewed as sexual facilitation (Bahner, 2013; Björnsdóttir and Stefánsdóttir, 2020). Even though the task is similar, the meaning attributed to it changes based on the supporter's own sexual values.

Because sexual facilitation can be problematic for staff, the issue of consent is of essence. Legislation on consent differs between countries. For example, Irish legislation defines an individual with an intellectual disability who lacks the capacity to consent to a sexual act as a "protected person" and therefore it is consequently an offence to engage in sexual acts with them (Law Reform Commission, 2005). The legislation in Iceland is however rather vague and does not clearly define competency and autonomy to provide consent. Furthermore, the general penal code there states that it is a punishable act (rape) to engage in a sexual act with an individual with an intellectual disability if they are "not in a condition to be able to resist the action or to understand its significance" (Althingi, 1997). Justifiably, staff remain ambiguous or insecure when it comes to sexual facilitation because there is no protocol in place to secure that informed consent is granted.

Views on sex work are culturally shaped and informed by the legislation of individual countries. Since it is illegal to buy any type of sex or prostitution in Iceland the issue of whether people with intellectual disabilities should or should not be allowed to do so is never raised. In other countries, such as the Netherlands, sex work is more common. Disabled and non-disabled people alike can buy services from sex workers and there are sex workers who specialise in sex care or sexual services for disabled people (Bahner, 2019). Sex care is therefore based on the idea that disabled people might be uncomfortable or embarrassed due to their impairments to buy sexual services from regular sex workers. However, there may be concerns that if support staff are enabling people to purchase sex, they may assume there is no longer a need to support or encourage regular intimate relationships (Bahner, 2019). Furthermore, there is danger of overstating the importance of sex to the cost of supporting friendship and intimacy (Shakespeare, 2000).

Unless sexual wellbeing is part of reflexive professional education, carers could potentially contribute to oppressive practices by reflecting normative attitudes to sexuality, due to lack of knowledge or discomfort in advocating for sexual citizenship.

READER ACTIVITY 25.4

John, a man with intellectual disabilities who also has physical impairments, needs assistance to masturbate. He has no difficulties expressing his will and desire and asks the staff to find pornography on his computer. He also needs assistance to get a grip on his penis so he can masturbate. Staff members have commented that their assistance is not taking part in his sexual act, they put on protective gloves which makes the act clinical and when John establishes a grip on his penis they leave the room.

Reflect on the potential issues with this arrangement from the point of view of staff.

Reflect on the possible problems with this arrangement from John's perspective.

GOOD PRACTICE

There is growing international interest in supporting people to meet and build relationships, demonstrated by the number of initiatives such as dating agencies and meet-up groups. McCarthy et al (2020) provide an overview of 10 specialist dating agencies in the UK, paying particular attention to what works well when supporting people to form and maintain relationships. The agencies offer educational workshops on sex and relationships, as well as organising seasonal events and activities. In order to minimise risk and maintain safety, they obtain references from professionals known to the members and provide chaperone services. They offer support on a personal level before and during relationships, and their members report feeling accepted, respected and valued within the organisations.

Turning to individual examples, a noteworthy community-driven and collaboratively developed programme is the Australian *Sexual Lives & Respectful Relationships* (SLRR, 2020), which is peer-led and developed in collaboration with people with intellectual disabilities at Deakin University. Peer educators and co-facilitators are trained to work together to promote inclusion and sexual health of people with intellectual disabilities. The lived experiences and agency of people with intellectual disabilities is at the forefront of the programme which emphasises their sexual rights and health (see also Johnson et al, 2002; O'Shea and Frawley, 2020). The programme is set up in four sessions covering four main themes: 1) talking about relationships and sexuality, 2) having rights and being safe, 3) respectful relationships, and 4) sexual identity.

Riksförbundet för Sexuell Upplysning (RFSU, 2020) is the Swedish Association for Sexuality Education and was founded in 1933. The association leads numerous initiatives around Sweden which aim to provide support for people with intellectual disabilities and carers. For example, *Sex for All* (Sex för Alla) is a sex education programme offered by RFSU in Malmö for people with intellectual disabilities and carers. The programme provides participants with information about sex, emotions, relationships, consent and sexual rights. They have published various short films on the topic of sexuality on their web page, and an accessible handbook (see online Useful resources). The programme also offers café meetings for people with intellectual disabilities where they can meet other people and discuss sex and relationships.

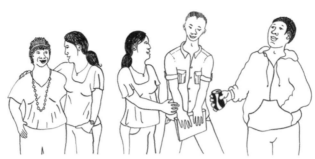

Figure 25.1 Example of accessible image to create easy-read information (Image copyright CHANGE at www.changepeople.org)

At the time of writing, Choice Support (2019) provides online guidance on specialist dating agencies throughout the UK (Bates, 2019). They provide a 'Supported Loving' web area with resources such as accessible information, toolkits and webinars for the use of people with intellectual disabilities and their supporters. Further, human rights organisation CHANGE (2020) offers easy-read leaflets about sexual wellbeing, as well as accessible resources and images for those who want to create their own easy-read information (see Figure 25.1).

Also in the UK, North-West based Meet 'N' Match provides a friendship and dating agency for adults with intellectual disabilities. They offer an exclusive matching service for members, to meet friends or potential partners. They also provide social activities and relationship advice and relationships training for staff members as well as organising meet-ups, and online information and support groups for LGBTQI members. Their website features useful videos of people talking about their experiences (Meet 'N' Match, 2020).

We feel encouraged by these examples, and the diverse and creative ways they are facilitating relationships. Turner and Crane (2016) categorise the ways people with intellectual disabilities can be supported into four areas: access to information, access to transportation, access to technology, and recognition of the systemic barriers that are put in place. Along with Harflett and Turner (2016), we recommend the following steps to sexual inclusion:

- Support plans at transition to adult services, and health care plans, should include arrangements to support relationships.

- Services should provide practical support, transport and living facilities for couples.
- Accessible information and sex education should include information about romance and pleasure, as well as sexual rights and risks.
- Support staff should receive training in sexual citizenship, including minority sexual identities and how to support these.
- Services should provide access to safeguarding, for example somewhere safe to go if things go wrong.

CONCLUSION

We have shown that people with intellectual disabilities can experience over-protection from care staff and families (who often have the best intentions towards the person but may find it easier to restrict than support sexual experiences). We argue that it is possible to support people to take balanced risks and make decisions about sexual relationships without over restriction. This can be achieved by: reducing barriers to finding accessible information about sexual rights, by facilitating access to potential partners, discussing sex in a positive way as well as informing people of the risks, and confronting systemic barriers when they present. Support staff, social workers and health professionals should have critical knowledge of the beliefs, values and myths about sexuality and people with intellectual disabilities, and be ready to both face and overcome barriers in supporting people to experience positive sexual and romantic relationships. We need to keep sexual citizenship on the agenda, but in a meaningful, caring and co-constructed way (Rogers, 2016; Rogers and Tuckwell, 2016).

REFERENCES

Abbott, D. (2015). Love in a cold climate: changes in the fortunes of LGBT men and women with learning disabilities? *British Journal of Learning Disabilities, 43*(2), 100–105.

Abbott, D., Howarth, J., & Glyde, K. (2005). *Secret loves, hidden lives? A summary of what people with learning difficulties said about being gay, lesbian or bisexual.* Bristol: Norah Fry Research Centre, University of Bristol.

Alexander, N., & Taylor Gomez, M. (2017). Pleasure, sex, prohibition, intellectual disability, and dangerous ideas. *Reproductive Health Matters, 25*(50), 114–120.

Althingi. (1997). *Act on legal competence.* No. 71/1997. Available at: https://www.althingi.is/lagas/nuna/1997071. html. [Accessed 11 May 2020].

Ashton, S., McDonald, K., & Kirkman, M. (2018). Women's experiences of pornography: a systematic review of research using qualitative methods. *The Journal of Sex Research, 55*(3), 334–347.

Bahner, J. (2012). Legal rights or simply wishes? The struggle for sexual recognition of people with physical disabilities using personal assistance in Sweden. *Sexuality and Disability, 30*(3), 337–356.

Bahner, J. (2013). The power of discretion and the discretion of power: personal assistants and sexual facilitation in disability services. *Vulnerable Groups & Inclusion, 4*(1), 20673.

Bahner, J. (2019). *Sexual citizenship and disability: understanding sexual support in policy, practice and theory.* Abington: Routledge.

Barron, K. (2002). Who am I? Women with learning difficulties (re) constructing their self-identity. *Scandinavian Journal of Disability Research, 4*(1), 58–79.

Barton-Hanson, R. (2015). Sterilization of men with intellectual disabilities: whose best interest is it anyway? *Medical Law International, 15*(1), 49–73.

Bates, C., Terry, L., & Popple, K. (2017a). Supporting people with learning disabilities to make and maintain intimate relationships. *Tizard Learning Disability Review, 22*(1), 16–23.

Bates, C. (2019). Supported loving–developing a national network to support positive intimate relationships for people with learning disabilities. *Tizard Learning Disability Review.*

Bates, C., Terry, L., & Popple, K. (2017b). The importance of romantic love to people with learning disabilities. *British Journal of Learning Disabilities, 45*(1), 64–72.

Bates, C., McCarthy, M., Milne Skillman, K., et al. (2020). 'Always trying to walk a bit of a tightrope': the role of social care staff in supporting adults with intellectual and developmental disabilities to develop and maintain loving relationships. *British Journal of Learning Disabilities, 48*(4), 261–268.

Björnsdóttir, K., Stefánsdóttir, Á., & Stefánsdóttir, G. V. (2017). People with intellectual disabilities negotiate autonomy, gender and sexuality. *Sexuality and Disability, 35*(3), 295–311.

Björnsdóttir, K., Stefánsdóttir, G. V., & Stefánsdóttir, Á. (2015). 'It's my life': autonomy and people with intellectual disabilities. *Journal of Intellectual Disabilities, 19*(1), 5–21.

Björnsdóttir, K., & Traustadóttir, R. (2010). Stuck in the land of disability? The intersection of learning difficulties, class, gender and religion. *Disability & Society, 25*(1), 49–62.

Björnsdóttir, K., & Stefánsdóttir, G. V. (2020). Double sexual standards: sexuality and people with intellectual disabilities who require intensive support. *Sexuality and Disability.* https://doi.org/10.1007/s11195-020-09643-2.

Black, R. S., & Kammes, R. R. (2019). Restrictions, power, companionship, and intimacy: a metasynthesis of people with intellectual disability speaking about sex and relationships. *Intellectual and Developmental Disabilities, 57*(3), 212–233.

Brown, H., Croft-White, C., Wilson, C., et al. (2000). *Taking the initiative: supporting the sexual rights of disabled people.* Brighton, UK: Pavilion.

Brown, H. (2004). A rights-based approach to abuse of women with learning disabilities. *Tizard Learning Disability Review, 9*(4), 41–44.

Cambridge, P., & Mellan, B. (2000). Reconstructing the sexuality of men with learning disabilities: empirical evidence and theoretical interpretations of need. *Disability & Society, 15*(2), 293–311.

Carlson, G., Taylor, M., & Wilson, J. (2000). Sterilisation, drugs which suppress sexual drive, and young men who have intellectual disability. *Journal of Intellectual & Developmental Disability, 25*(2), 91–104.

CHANGE. (2020). Our services. Available at: https://www.changepeople.org/. [Accessed 2 October 2020].

Chivers, J., & Mathieson, S. (2000). Training in sexuality and relationships: an Australian model. *Sexuality and Disability, 18*(1), 73–80.

Choice Support. (2019) Supported loving. Available at: https://www.choicesupport.org.uk/about-us/what-we-do/supported-loving/what-is-supported-loving. [Accessed 2 October 2020].

de Kuijper, G., Hoekstra, P., Visser, F., et al. (2010). Use of antipsychotic drugs in individuals with intellectual disability (ID) in the Netherlands: prevalence and reasons for prescription. *Journal of Intellectual Disability Research, 54*(7), 659–667.

Dinwoodie, R., Greenhill, B., & Cookson, A. (2020). 'Them two things are what collide together': understanding the sexual identity experiences of lesbian, gay, bisexual and trans people labelled with intellectual disability. *Journal of Applied Research in Intellectual Disabilities, 33*(1), 3–16.

Doherty, D., Ledger, S., Townson, L., et al. (2014). *Sexuality and relationships in the lives of people with intellectual disabilities: standing in my shoes.* London: Jessica Kingsley.

Ferrante, C. A., & Oak, E. (2020). 'No sex please!' We have been labelled intellectually disabled. *Sex Education, 1–15.*

Fish, R. (2016). 'They've said I'm vulnerable with men': doing sexuality on locked wards. *Sexualities, 19*(5–6), 641–658.

Fish, R. (2018). A feminist ethnography of secure wards for women with learning disabilities: locked away. *Routledge Interdisciplinary Disability Studies.*

Frawley, P., & O'Shea, A. (2020). 'Nothing about us without us': sex education by and for people with intellectual disability. *Sex Education, 20*(4), 413–424.

Frawley, P., & Wilson, N. J. (2016). Young people with intellectual disability talking about sexuality education and information. *Sexuality and Disability, 34*(4), 469–484.

Grieve, A., McLaren, S., Lindsay, W., et al. (2009). Staff attitudes towards the sexuality of people with learning disabilities: a comparison of different professional groups and residential facilities. *British Journal of Learning Disabilities, 37*(1), 76–84.

Grove, L., Morrison-Beedy, D., Kirby, R., et al. (2018). The birds, bees, and special needs: making evidence-based sex education accessible for adolescents with intellectual disabilities. *Sexuality and Disability, 36*(4), 313–329.

Gill, M. (2010). Rethinking sexual abuse, questions of consent, and intellectual disability. *Sexuality Research and Social, 7,* 201–213.

Hall, I., & Yacoub, E. (2008). Sex, relationships and the law for people with learning disability. *Advances in Mental Health and Learning Disabilities, 2*(2), 19–24.

Harflett, N., & Turner, S. (2016). *Supporting people with learning disabilities to develop sexual and romantic relationships.* Bath: National Development Team for Inclusion (NDTi).

Hellett, M. (2020). Sparkle and space. In S. Salman (Ed.), *Made possible: stories of Success by people with learning disabilities – in their own words* (pp. 161–182). London: Unbound.

Hollomotz, A., & Speakup Committee. (2009). 'May we please have sex tonight?'–people with learning difficulties pursuing privacy in residential group settings. *British Journal of Learning Disabilities, 37*(2), 91–97.

Hollomotz, A. (2009). Beyond 'vulnerability': an ecological model approach to conceptualizing risk of sexual violence against people with learning difficulties. *British Journal of Social Work, 39*(1), 99–112.

Hollomotz, A. (2011). *Learning difficulties and sexual vulnerability: a social approach.* London: Jessica Kingsley Publishers.

Human Rights Act (1998) Available at: https://www.legislation.gov.uk/ukpga/1998/42/contents [Accessed 30 September 2021].

James, E., & Mitchell, R. (2020). Love, hope and relationships. In E. James, R. Mitchell, & H. Morgan (Eds.), *Social work, cats and rocket science.* London: Jessica Kingsley.

Johnson, K. (1998). *Deinstitutionalising women: an ethnographic study of institutional closure.* Cambridge University Press.

Johnson, K., Frawley, P., Hillier, L., et al. (2002). Living safer sexual lives: research and action. *Tizard Learning Disability Review, 7*(3), 4–9.

Kelly, G., Crowley, H., & Hamilton, C. (2009). Rights, sexuality and relationships in Ireland: 'It'd be nice to be kind of trusted'. *British Journal of Learning Disabilities, 37*(4), 308–315.

Lafferty, A., McConkey, R., & Taggart, L. (2013). Beyond friendship: the nature and meaning of close personal relationships as perceived by people with learning disabilities. *Disability & Society, 28*(8), 1074–1088.

Lam, A., Yau, M., Franklin, R. C., et al. (2019). The unintended invisible hand: a conceptual framework for the analysis of the sexual lives of people with disabilities. *Sexuality and Disability, 37*(2), 203–226.

Law Reform Commission. (2005) Consultation paper on vulnerable adults and the law: capacity. Available at: https://www.lawreform.ie/_fileupload/consultation%20papers/Consultation%20Paper%20on%20Capacity.pdf. [Accessed 28 December 2020].

Llewellyn, G., Traustadóttir, R., McConnell, D., et al. (Eds.). (2010). *Parents with intellectual disabilities: past, present and futures.* Chichester: Wiley-Blackwell.

Löfgren-Mårtenson, L. (2009). The invisibility of young homosexual women and men with intellectual disabilities. *Sexuality and Disability, 27,* 21–26.

Löfgren-Mårtenson, L. (2013). 'Hip to be crip?' About crip theory, sexuality and people with intellectual disabilities. *Sexuality and Disability, 31,* 413–424.

Löfgren-Mårtenson, L. (2012). 'Hip to be crip?' About crip theory, sexuality and people with intellectual disabilities. *Sexuality and Disability, 30*(2), 209–225.

Löfgren-Mårtenson, L., Sorbring, E., & Molin, M. (2015). 'T@ngled up in blue': views of parents and professionals on Internet use for sexual purposes among young people with intellectual disabilities. *Sexuality and Disability, 33*(4), 533–544.

Maguire, K., Gleeson, K., & Holmes, N. (2019). Support workers' understanding of their role supporting the sexuality of people with learning disabilities. *British Journal of Learning Disabilities, 47*(1), 59–65.

McCarthy, M., Hunt, S., & Milne-Skillman, K. (2017). I know it was every week, but I can't be sure if it was every day: domestic violence and women with learning disabilities. *Journal of Applied Research in Intellectual Disabilities, 30*(2), 269–282.

McCarthy, M., Skillman, K. M., Elson, N., et al. (2020). Making connections and building confidence: a study of specialist dating agencies for people with intellectual disabilities. *Sexuality and Disability, 38*(1), 3–18.

McCarthy, M. (2014). Women with intellectual disability: their sexual lives in the 21st century. *Journal of Intellectual and Developmental Disability, 39*(2), 124–131.

McCarthy, M. (1999). *Sexuality and women with learning disabilities.* Jessica Kingsley Publishers.

McCarthy, M., Bates, C., Triantafyllopoulou, P., et al. (2019). 'Put bluntly, they are targeted by the worst creeps society has to offer': police and professionals' views and actions relating to domestic violence and women with intellectual disabilities. *Journal of Applied Research in Intellectual Disabilities, 32*(1), 71–81.

McClelland, A., Flicker, S., Nepveux, D., et al. (2012). Seeking safer sexual spaces: queer and trans young people labeled with intellectual disabilities and the paradoxical risks of restriction. *Journal of Homosexuality, 59*(6), 808–819.

Meet 'N' Match. (2020). Available at: http://www.meet-n-match.co.uk/. [Accessed 28 December 2020].

Mental Capacity Act (2005) Available at: https://www.legislation.gov.uk/ukpga/2005/9/contents [Accessed 30 September 2021].

Miller, A. M., Kismödi, E., Cottingham, J., et al. (2015). Sexual rights as human rights: a guide to authoritative sources and principles for applying human rights to sexuality and sexual health. *Reproductive Health Matters, 23*(46), 16–30.

Murphy, G., Powell, S., Guzman, A. M., et al. (2007). Cognitive-behavioural treatment for men with intellectual disabilities and sexually abusive behaviour: a pilot study. *Journal of Intellectual Disability Research, 51*(11), 902–912.

Musopero, O. (2019). Social integration: a pedagogical approach to disability generalisation of institutionalised children with mental challenges. *International Journal of Research in Social Sciences, 9*(1), 809–826.

NDTi. (2019). *The right to a relationship.* Bath: The National Development Team for Inclusion.

Neuman, R. (2019). Attitudes of direct support staff regarding couple relationships of adults with intellectual disability: implications for provision of support. *Journal of Social Service Research,* 1–13.

O'Shea, A., & Frawley, P. (2020). Gender, sexuality and relationships for young Australian women with intellectual disability. *Disability & Society, 35*(4), 654–675.

Pollack, S. (2007). 'I'm just not good in relationships'. Victimization discourses and the gendered regulation of criminalized women. *Feminist Criminology, 2*(2), 158–174.

RFSU. (2020) What is RFSU? Available at: https://www.rfsu.se/om-rfsu/om-oss/in-english/. [Accessed 2 September 2020].

Richards, M. (2017). 'Angry, when things don't go my own way': what it means to be gay with learning disabilities. *Disability & Society, 32*(8), 1165–1179.

Rogers, C., & Tuckwell, S. (2016). Co-constructed caring research and intellectual disability: an exploration of friendship and intimacy in being human. *Sexualities, 19*(5–6), 623–640.

Rogers, C. (2009). (S)excerpts from a life told: sex, gender and learning disability. *Sexualities, 12*(3), 270–288.

Rogers, C. (2016). Intellectual disability and sexuality: on the agenda? *Sexualities, 19*(5–6), 617–622.

Rohleder, P. (2010). Educators' ambivalence and managing anxiety in providing sex education for people with learning disabilities. *Psychodynamic Practice, 16*(2), 165–182.

Rohleder, P., & Swartz, L. (2012). Disability, sexuality and sexual health. *Understanding Global Sexualities: New Frontiers,* 138–152.

Rushbrooke, E., Murray, C., & Townsend, S. (2014). The experiences of intimate relationships by people with intellectual disabilities: a qualitative study. *Journal of Applied Research in Intellectual Disabilities, 27*(6), 531–541.

Schaafsma, D., Kok, G., Stoffelen, J. M. T., et al. (2017). People with intellectual disabilities talk about sexuality: implications for the development of sex education. *Sexuality and Disability, 35*(1), 21–38.

Schaafsma, D., Kok, G., Stoffelen, J. M., et al. (2015). Identifying effective methods for teaching sex education to individuals with intellectual disabilities: a systematic review. *Journal of Sex Research, 52*(4), 412–432.

Shakespeare, T. (2000) Disabled sexuality: toward rights and recognition. *Sexuality and Disability,* 18, 159–166. Available at: https://link.springer.com/article/10.1023/A:1026409613684. [Accessed 29 December 2020].

SLRR. (2020) Sexual lives & respectful relationships: rights and respect in sexuality and relationships. Available at: https://www.slrr.com.au/. [Accessed 2 September 2020].

Sloan, S., & Brewster, E. (2017). A review of the pharmacological management of sexually offending behaviour in learning disabled offenders. *Journal of Intellectual Disabilities and Offending Behaviour, 8*(4), 166–175.

Stefánsdóttir, G. V., & Hreinsdóttir, E. E. (2013). Sterilization, intellectual disability, and some ethical and methodological challenges: it shouldn't be a secret. *Ethics and Social Welfare, 7*(3), 302–308.

Stefánsdóttir, G. V. (2014) Sterilisation and women with intellectual disability in Iceland. *Journal of Intellectual & Developmental Disability, 39*(2), 188–197. https://doi.org/10.3109/13668250.2014.899327.

Stroup, T. S., & Gray, N. (2018). Management of common adverse effects of antipsychotic medications. *World Psychiatry, 17*(3), 341–356.

Thompson, A. R., & Beail, N. (2002). The treatment of auto-erotic asphyxiation in a man with severe intellectual disabilities: the effectiveness of a behavioural and educational programme. *Journal of Applied Research in Intellectual Disabilities*, 15(1), 36–47.

Tilley, E., Walmsley, J., Earle, S., et al. (2012). 'The silence is roaring': sterilization, reproductive rights and women with intellectual disabilities. *Disability & Society*, 27(3), 413–426.

Traustadottir, R., & Johnson, K. (2000). *Women with intellectual disabilities: finding a place in the world*. Jessica Kingsley.

Turner, G. W., & Crane, B. (2016). Sexually silenced no more, adults with learning disabilities speak up: a call to action for social work to frame sexual voice as a social justice issue. *The British Journal of Social Work*, 46, 2300–2317.

United Nations. (2006) General Assembly, Convention on the Rights of Persons with Disabilities: resolution. Available at: https://www.refworld.org/docid/45f973632.html. [Accessed 2 July 2020].

Walmsley, J., & Jarrett, S. (Eds.). (2019). *Intellectual disability in the twentieth century: transnational perspectives on people, policy, and practice*. Policy Press.

Webster, S. (2020). Father Shaun. In S. Salman (Ed.), *Made possible: stories of success by people with learning disabilities – in their own words* (pp. 161–182). London: Unbound.

Williams, L., & Nind, M. (1999). Insiders or outsiders: normalisation and women with learning difficulties. *Disability & Society*, 14(5), 659–672.

Wilson, N., Parmenter, T., Stancliffe, R., et al. (2011). Conditionally sexual: men and teenage boys with moderate to profound intellectual disability. *Sexuality and Disability*, 29(3), 275–289.

Wilson, N. J., & Frawley, P. (2016). Transition staff discuss sex education and support for young men and women with intellectual and developmental disability. *Journal of Intellectual & Developmental Disability*, 41(3), 209–221.

WWDA (Women with Disabilities Australia). (2018). End forced sterilization. Available at: https://wwda.org.au/2018/07/end-forced-sterilisation/. [Accessed 2 September 2020].

World Health Organisation. (2006). *Defining sexual health*. Geneva: WHO.

World Health Organisation. (2020) Sexual health. Available at https://www.who.int/health-topics/sexual-health#tab=tab_1. [Accessed 2 September 2020].

Wos, K., Kamecka-Antczak, C., & Szafrański, M. (2020). In search of solutions regarding the sex education of people with intellectual disabilities in Poland participatory action research. *European Journal of Special Needs Education*, 1–14.

Yacoub, E., & Hall, I. (2009). The sexual lives of men with mild learning disability: a qualitative study. *British Journal of Learning Disabilities*, 37(1), 5–11.

26

Growing older

Ruth Northway, Nathan Wilson and Stacey Rees

KEY ISSUES

- The number of older people with intellectual disabilities is increasing.
- Ageing can give rise to a range of physical and mental health problems.
- It is important to focus on the promotion of healthy ageing for people with intellectual disabilities and for this to begin from early adulthood.

- There are different models of support for older people with intellectual disabilities.
- A range of professionals have a key role to play in supporting healthy ageing, health monitoring and supporting older people with long term and often complex health problems.

CHAPTER OUTLINE

INTRODUCTION

Over recent years many reports have been published that highlight the health disparities experienced by people with intellectual disabilities (for example Rickard and Donkin, 2018) and the fact that they often suffer premature and avoidable deaths (for example Glover et al, 2017). However, it is also the case that, overall, the life expectancy of people with intellectual disabilities is increasing (Coppus, 2013). This means that many more people with intellectual disabilities are living into older age and facing the challenges that often accompany advanced years. This is a relatively new phenomenon and, as Bigby and Haveman (2010) observed, it was only in the 1980s that issues relating to ageing amongst

people with intellectual disabilities started to appear in the academic literature, at conferences and to inform service planning at a national level. In turn, this situation is presenting new challenges to families, carers and services that seek to provide support for this ageing population and, in particular, giving rise to a need to develop new knowledge and skills (Bigby and Haveman, 2010).

It is therefore important that we understand the ageing process and its particular implications for people with intellectual disabilities. We need to be aware of the impact on physical and mental health and, most importantly, how we can best promote healthy ageing whilst also effectively managing long term health conditions.

This means that we need to consider what models of support are likely to be most effective and the role of professionals in working within such services. These are therefore the areas that will be explored in this chapter before considering how best we can plan to meet future needs.

THE AGEING PROCESS

When we talk about ageing, and the ageing process, many people think about impacts on our health and well-being in later life. However, the ageing process starts from the moment we are born and continues throughout our lives. In the early years of life, we grow physically and psychologically, we then mature and often the later years of life are seen as a stage of decline. However, there is debate as to when this later stage of 'ageing' begins.

As we age, our bodies undergo a process of physiological change which places us at greater risk of a range of health problems, leads to a decline in capacity and ultimately to death (World Health Organisation (WHO), 2015). This might be referred to as biological ageing. However (as will be seen in this chapter), there are a range of factors that influence the speed at which this occurs, and it is not always a straightforward process of linear decline which is irreversible.

One approach to defining ageing is a chronological one in which individuals are considered to be 'older adults' when they reach a specified age. However, there are difficulties with such an approach since individuals who are the same chronological age can have very differing profiles in terms of their health and well-being. For example, we are all aware of some individuals in their seventies who appear very physically and/or mentally frail whilst others of the same age enjoy very fit, healthy and active lifestyles. WHO (2015) thus conclude that this diversity amongst older people often has little to do with chronological age, instead they note that these differences in health and well-being are influenced by personal characteristics (such as genetic makeup), lifestyle choices and also factors that may be outside the influence of individuals such as the physical and social environments that people live in. This is of particular relevance when we consider the situation of people with intellectual disabilities since they may have experienced a lifetime of health disparities which will impact on the ageing process and which (as will be discussed later in

this chapter) can lead to them experiencing age related health problems at a younger age when compared with their non-disabled peers.

It is also important to remember that the term 'people with intellectual disabilities' encompasses a diverse group of people and hence, within this group, experiences of ageing will vary greatly. Factors such as the level of disability and gender can have a significant difference on the ageing process and life expectancy. In addition, WHO (2000) note that most of the literature regarding ageing and intellectual disabilities originates from higher income countries meaning that the experiences of ageing amongst those in low and middle-income countries are largely hidden.

Another means that is often used in societies to determine who might be considered an 'older adult' is the retirement age within a country. However, as the number of older people within the population rises a number of countries have, for economic reasons, taken the decision to increase the retirement age thus confirming that the notion of retirement is a socially constructed one which can, and does, vary. In relation to people with intellectual disabilities, the use of the retirement age as a proxy for ageing can also be problematic since only a minority are likely to be in paid employment, and hence they do not retire in the commonly accepted understanding of the term.

Ageing is, therefore, a process rather than an event and there are many factors that can impact on how and when people with intellectual disabilities age. These factors will be explored further in the subsequent sections of this chapter.

PHYSICAL HEALTH

As we age we undergo many physiological changes affecting a range of bodily systems. For example, muscular-skeletal changes can lead to reduced strength and a slower gait, there can be a reduction in visual and auditory senses, immune function can be reduced, and skin can lose elasticity (WHO, 2015). Each of these changes can impact on quality of life but they can also impact on physical health. An increase in health problems as we age is therefore common.

Knowledge regarding the health needs of people with intellectual disabilities has increased significantly over recent years and with this our understanding of the specific needs of older people within this population. For example, a study undertaken by Haveman et al (2011) gathered data in relation to the health of 1253 people with intellectual disabilities aged 18 and over living in 14 different European Member States. Of these, 301 people were aged 55 or over. They found that an increase in age was positively linked to an increase in the presence of a number of health conditions including hearing disorders, cataracts, diabetes, hypertension, osteoarthritis and osteoporosis. Each of these conditions can have a significant impact on quality of life and also lead to further health problems – for example the presence of cataracts will impair vision which may lead to problems of mobility and potentially give rise to falls.

Such health conditions might, however, be considered by some as a common aspect of the ageing process and hence it is important to determine whether, and how, their prevalence amongst people with intellectual disabilities compares to the wider population. Morin et al (2012) compared data relating to 789 people with intellectual disabilities (43% of whom were aged 45 years or older) with data gathered regarding the wider Canadian population. Whilst low response rates amongst the sample of people with intellectual disabilities and the use of different approaches to collect data from the two populations might affect level of confidence in the findings of this study, higher rates of heart disease and thyroid problems were reported amongst the older population of people with intellectual disabilities compared with the wider population. Interestingly, lower reported rates of arthritis, migraine and skeletal pain amongst the population with intellectual disabilities were also found. Significantly, each of the conditions where a lower prevalence was noted are pain related conditions, therefore it may not be the case that they do not experience these conditions to the same extent but rather that they are not recognised, either by the person with an intellectual disability or their carers, and subsequently not treated; under-reporting and/or recognition of pain experienced by people with intellectual disabilities has been reported elsewhere (Findlay et al, 2014).

When considering the above studies it is, however, important to remember the caveat highlighted by WHO (2000) that much of our evidence regarding health and ageing comes from high income countries; the health of people with intellectual disabilities in low income countries may therefore differ given the different socio-economic circumstances and different healthcare systems within such countries. Nonetheless, it has been suggested that there is a level of consensus in the literature that regardless of country people with intellectual disabilities experience age related health problems at an earlier age than their non-disabled peers, and that often these occur during their 50s (Hermans and Evenhuis, 2014).

There are a number of issues that give rise to such a situation. Throughout their lives people with intellectual disabilities are at an increased risk of certain long-term health problems such as epilepsy (see Chapter 14). In addition, those with some specific syndromes experience an increased risk of related health problems. For example, those with Down syndrome are at increased risk of hypothyroidism and cardiac problems (Hermans and Evenhuis, 2014). Treatment for these (and other) conditions from an early age can mean that they are exposed over a long period to the side effects of essential medication. Hermans and Evenhuis thus argue that intellectual disability related physical health problems, unhealthy lifestyles and the metabolic effects of antipsychotic medication (prescribed for mental health problems or for behaviours that challenge) contribute to age related health problems occurring at a younger age and that they also place older people with intellectual disabilities at increased risk of multimorbidity.

Multimorbidity has been defined as having two or more chronic health problems (Hermans and Evenhuis, 2014) and this is generally viewed as a common feature of ageing (WHO, 2015). However, Hermans and Evenhuis (2014) studied 1047 adults with intellectual disabilities aged 50 or over and found that 79.9% were experiencing multimorbidity with increased age, the presence of severe or profound intellectual disability and Down syndrome all increasing the prevalence of such conditions. In 46.8% of those studied they found the presence of four or more health problems. They argue that there is a need to better understand the interaction between the different conditions and their treatments since treating conditions separately can lead to additional problems due to the conflicting effects of the different interventions. Whilst this study did not directly compare levels of multimorbidity amongst people with intellectual disabilities and the wider population, Hermans and Evenhuis (2014) assert that levels are higher amongst people with intellectual disabilities. Elsewhere a similar argument has been presented along with evidence that such multimorbidity amongst older people with intellectual disabilities gives rise to a greater risk of hospital readmissions (Axman et al, 2019).

It has also been suggested that multimorbidity can lead to frailty (Hermans and Evenhuis, 2014). The definition of frailty is contested (WHO, 2015) and many differing definitions can be found. However, Schoufour et al (2014, p. 2267) in their paper concerning frailty and people with intellectual disabilities, argue that it is 'a state of increased vulnerability to adverse health outcomes compared to others of the same age'. This suggests that it is important to consider not only the extent to which frailty is present amongst people with intellectual disabilities but also to consider how its prevalence amongst this population compares to their non-disabled peers. Indeed, Schoufour et al (2014) note levels of frailty amongst those with intellectual disabilities aged 50+ comparable to those amongst the general population aged 75+. Frailty is therefore linked with premature ageing amongst people with intellectual disabilities.

McKenzie et al (2017) studied 51,138 individuals with intellectual and developmental disabilities aged 18–99 living in Ontario, Canada and compared them with a 20% random sample of the Ontario population also aged 18–99 who did not have intellectual disabilities. They used the Frailty Marker (The Health Services Research and Development Center, the Johns Hopkins University, 2009) and routinely gathered data to determine and compare levels of frailty finding that the overall prevalence of frailty amongst those with intellectual and developmental disabilities was 8.9% compared with 3.1% amongst the general population. Being female, experiencing mental health problems and addictions also increased the risk of frailty amongst those with and without intellectual and developmental disabilities. Furthermore, they found that people with intellectual and developmental disabilities aged 18–24 had levels of frailty similar to those aged 60–64 who do not have intellectual and developmental disabilities.

It is, however, important to remember that targeted interventions can help to reverse, limit or slow the course of frailty. Schoufour et al (2014) therefore argue that it is important for those supporting older people with intellectual disabilities to recognise frailty so that interventions can be put in place to prevent further decline. The importance of seeking to promote healthy ageing is explored later in this chapter.

MENTAL HEALTH AND DEMENTIA

In Chapter 16, the specific issues of mental health were discussed. This chapter will focus on mental health in the older person with an intellectual disability, in particular dementia. People with intellectual disabilities experience the same mental health disorders as the wider population, but with greater prevalence (Sheerin et al, 2019). Previously published data from Ireland has found that 47.5% of adults with intellectual disabilities over 40 years had psychiatric disorders (McCarron et al, 2011). This replicates international findings (Cooper et al, 2007). Compared to the wider population, the prevalence of mental health disorders amongst people with intellectual disabilities increases with age. It is evidenced that rates of mental health disorders are higher among older age groups, women and those with severe or profound intellectual disabilities (McCarron et al, 2011).

Although few in number, those studies that have focused on psychiatric diagnoses among older people with intellectual disabilities report that ageing increases the risk of overall psychiatric morbidity, dementia, anxiety disorder and depression in this population (Deb et al, 2001). They may also be more vulnerable to developing mental health disorders due to factors such as heritable disorders (for example, the link between Down syndrome and Alzheimer's disease), poor coping skills and communication or language difficulties (Sheerin et al, 2019).

The prevalence of dementia in adults with intellectual disabilities aged 65 and older is up to five times higher than in the wider population (Strydom et al, 2013). The prevalence amongst people with Down syndrome is even higher (Strydom et al, 2013), with many such adults presenting with symptoms of early onset dementia in their late 40s or early 50s (McCarron et al, 2014).

It is reported that diagnosing dementia in people with intellectual disabilities is more complex than in the wider population due to fluctuating levels of pre-existing cognitive impairment, communication problems and a deficiency of knowledge among many health and social care professionals on how dementia presents in people with intellectual disabilities and the use of validated assessment tools specific to this population (Jokinen et al, 2013). Other factors which complicate recognition of advanced dementia in older people with intellectual disabilities are the differences in innate cognitive functioning and misunderstanding over whether these deficits relate to a person's intellectual disability or the development of dementia. This is known as diagnostic overshadowing; whereby, any presenting behavioural changes are attributed to the person's intellectual disability, rather than considering other causes (Kerr et al, 2011).

Further uncertainty in diagnosis of dementia in older people with intellectual disabilities (especially those with Down syndrome) arises due to an increased risk of other health conditions that often imitate dementia or confound diagnosis such as hypothyroidism, sensory impairments, B12 and folate deficiency and depression (Prasher, 2005). In addition, syndromes that are associated with advanced ageing (for example, Williams or Cockayne) may mean a quicker decline and shorter dementia duration (Janicki et al, 2005), however, there is a paucity of evidence on the prevalence of dementia in these syndromes.

FACILITATING HEALTHY AGEING

Given the global rise in life expectancy and the consequent increase in the number of older people within the population it is perhaps not surprising that international attention has focused on the need to promote and support healthy ageing (WHO, 2015). Healthy ageing has been defined as:

> "...the process of developing and maintaining the functional ability that enables well-being in older age."
>
> WHO, 2015, p. 28

For older individuals this has the potential to maintain independence and enhance quality of life whilst at a societal level reduce the burden of long-term illness and hence better contain economic costs. However, it has been suggested that at a policy and practice level the focus on healthy and active ageing has largely overlooked people with intellectual disabilities (Foster and Boxall, 2015; Buys et al, 2012). This is, in part, attributed to the fact that when active ageing is referred to in the wider population it is often linked with extending the economic contribution of individuals through longer working lives (Foster and Boxall, 2015). Since few people with intellectual disabilities are in employment they are not considered in this context.

WHO (2015, p. 8) argue that the diversity in the health and well-being of older people reflects the impact of 'cumulative inequities across the life-course'. As was mentioned earlier in this chapter, people with intellectual disabilities tend to experience age related health problems at an earlier age than their non-disabled peers and, whilst this can be attributed to very different life courses, strategies are available that could prevent or limit deterioration and the onset of frailty (Schepens et al, 2018).

WHO (2015) advocate a public health approach to the promotion of healthy ageing amongst the general population that offers a useful framework to guide the provision of support for people with intellectual disabilities. Within this approach three levels of 'capacity' are identified (see Box 26.1). As individuals age they

---

 BOX 26.1 Healthy Ageing and Levels of Capacity (WHO, 2015)

High and stable capacity
Declining capacity
Significant loss of capacity

 READER ACTIVITY 26.1

For each of the brief case studies below consider which of the levels of capacity suggested by WHO (2015) (Box 26.1) applies and what interventions might be used to support healthy ageing for the individual concerned.

Jenny is 75 years old. She has a mild intellectual disability and recently experienced a significant loss in mobility. She has had a couple of falls which have impacted on her confidence and this, in turn, has resulted in her becoming very withdrawn and depressed. She previously used to enjoy going out to bingo but now often says that she doesn't want to get out of bed.

David is 50 years old and has a severe intellectual disability. He enjoys going out for walks with his father but recently his father has experienced ill health and has been unable to accompany David on walks. David has started to put on weight and also greatly misses his walks.

Isobel is 63 years old and has a moderate intellectual disability. Recently she has started to become quite forgetful and at times seems very confused. Her behaviour has also started to change but the staff who support her in her supported living placement feel that this is just part of her intellectual disability and the fact that she is getting older.

are likely to move through these stages and experience increasing loss of capacity and the focus of support and intervention therefore needs to move from promoting behaviours that enhance capacity to removing barriers to participation and compensating for a loss of capacity. Each of these three stages warrants further consideration in relation to people with intellectual disabilities.

Where individuals have high and stable capacity then the WHO (2015) advocate a focus on the prevention of chronic conditions, early detection and effective control of such conditions. For example, Oppewal and Hilgenkamp (2019) found that physical fitness is predictive of a reduced mortality risk amongst people with intellectual disabilities and thus advocate that service systems should focus on improving physical fitness amongst those they support. However, given that age related health problems often occur at an earlier age in people with intellectual disabilities then it is also advocated that strategies to prevent frailty are also implemented at an earlier age (Schepens et al, 2018). For example, Finlayson (2018) suggests that people with intellectual disabilities often experience many lifelong risk factors for falls including epilepsy, medication and sedentary behaviours. Therefore, she advocates that falls prevention strategies should be targeted at people with intellectual disabilities from the age of 50 given that the consequences of falls can be a loss of confidence, injury and even death.

When individuals start to experience a decline in capacity then the focus of intervention and support should be on reversing or slowing this decline wherever possible. However, when individuals with intellectual disabilities experience health problems they are at risk of the aforementioned 'diagnostic overshadowing' meaning that such health problems are not identified and treated in a timely manner. Moreover, older people with intellectual disabilities appear to be at a risk of diagnostic overshadowing on two counts whereby changes in behaviour, health and well-being may be dismissed as either part of their intellectual disability or inappropriately dismissed as an inevitable consequence of ageing. Indeed, this tendency to interpret signs of illness as simply part of growing older has been noted amongst support staff who lack the knowledge and skills required to support older individuals who experience health problems (Roll and Bowers, 2017). However, if we consider the example of falls, Finlayson (2018) reminds us that falls are neither an inevitable consequence of ageing nor of having an intellectual disability.

Supporting older people with intellectual disabilities whose health is beginning to decline thus requires that health problems are recognised at an early stage, that effective pain relief is provided, that any required treatments are delivered in an effective and timely manner and that supports are increased as the ageing process advances (Schepens et al, 2018). In turn this requires that support staff are provided with the education required to recognise and address health issues in a proactive manner (Buys et al, 2012), that this is a formally recognised element of their role (Spassianu et al, 2019) and that service systems focus on the promotion of healthy ageing (Oppewal and Hilgenkamp, 2019). Unfortunately, such supports may not currently be in place (Spassianu et al, 2019).

Despite all efforts to promote and maintain capacity some older individuals with intellectual disabilities will experience a significant loss of capacity and here the WHO (2015) framework suggests that the focus of support needs to be on the management of advanced chronic health problems. In addition, barriers to participation in day to day activities need to be recognised and, where possible, removed through compensating for a lack of capacity. An example of an intervention at this stage might include ensuring that an individual who has experienced a loss of mobility and who becomes easily fatigued has access to a wheelchair and individual support to enable them to continue engagement in social activities thus promoting better mental health.

RETIREMENT

The most widely understood definition of retirement is the cessation, in later life, of one's main occupation and the transition into a new life stage. Oftentimes, people will start thinking about and planning for their retirement for some years before they actually do retire (Noone et al, 2013). This can include making financial plans, downsizing to a smaller house, reducing hours at work while increasing time spent pursuing leisure, and even joining a volunteer agency. Ideally, all members of society seek to participate in and enjoy the process of active ageing once they retire. However, as noted in the previous section, active ageing has not always been promoted for people with intellectual disabilities possibly due to the low numbers engaged in paid employment.

However, the absence of paid employment does not negate the right to experience healthy ageing, the desire to gradually change pace, and the right to pursue participation in other meaningful activities as one ages. Several research studies have reported that people with intellectual disabilities do want to be active and participate in inclusive retirement activities, but often need some support and/or don't know how to access such opportunities (Ellison and White, 2017). The most critical issue for all people who are nearing retirement age is the knowledge that whether retirement is voluntary, or not, being prepared for this new stage of life is positively associated with increased life satisfaction (Noone et al, 2013). Therefore, all people with intellectual disabilities should be supported to make person-centred plans for retirement as they start to age and/or experience age-related health issues regardless of chronological age. Critically, this support to people with intellectual disabilities should promote strategies to enable the person to be at the centre of choices and decision making about these plans.

Australian research on retirement for people with a lifelong disability offers some insights into how professionals might approach supporting people with intellectual disabilities who are facing voluntary or involuntary retirement (Stancliffe et al, 2013). The Transition To Retirement (TTR) project supported older adults with a lifelong disability to reduce their days at a sheltered workshop or day programme and start to 'practise' retirement one day a week by joining either a local community or volunteer group (Wilson et al, 2010). Examples of the types of groups joined were a local cat protection centre, a knitting group, an aviation museum, a community garden, and a Men's Shed. In Australia, Men's Sheds are community spaces where older men get together and work on projects, such as woodwork or metalwork, while they enjoy some social time together (Wilson et al, 2015). What was unique about this programme, was the use of existing members of the group to be mentors to the person with a lifelong disability rather than employing or using an outside 'disability expert'. Mentors were trained using a combination of disability awareness training and Active Support techniques that were underpinned by the principles of the co-worker model (Stancliffe et al, 2013).

Active Support acts as a support-worker led and targeted strategy to connect people with intellectual disabilities to participate in everyday activities (Stancliffe et al, 2008) (see also Heather's story 26.1). Outcomes for the older adults with intellectual disabilities from the programme included greater community participation, more social contacts, a reduction in hours at work, a significant increase in social satisfaction, and 10% of participants fully retired during the 3-year life of the programme (Stancliffe et al, 2015). Although no outcome measures were used with the mentors, qualitative insights highlighted many positive benefits to being a mentor and how getting to know people with intellectual disabilities enabled the mentors to see beyond the disability and that the person with intellectual disability was, in essence, no different to all group members (Wilson et al, 2013).

A separate 13-week Australian study, using the same techniques to train existing group members to be mentors, focussed on supporting older adults with intellectual disabilities to transition to retirement from their mainstream employment (Brotherton et al, 2016). These employees had been amongst the first in Australia to benefit from a change in government policy in 1986 that allowed people with intellectual disabilities to be employed in mainstream employment so they were employee pioneers in 1986 and retirement pioneers in 2019! This programme reported that support from the mentors significantly increased community participation of the people with intellectual disabilities and after the

HEATHER'S STORY 26.1

"Heather has an intellectual disability and has spent many years of her early life living in a secluded large residential complex. Heather was supported to join a local community kitchen. The community kitchen is a shared space where people with an interest in cooking meet each week to prepare and eat a meal together over several hours. Heather has a great love of cooking but had not had the chance to develop beyond her basic cooking skills. We taught the group the basics of person-centred active support – this means that the group members themselves learned how to teach Heather cooking skills in a way that she could understand. Heather now takes part in all the group activities, has learned a lot of new skills and has continued going to the community kitchen without any staff support for over a year" (Wilson et al, 2012, p. 6)

programme, 82% continued to attend their local community or volunteer group. What this, and the TTR project described above show, is that there are some retirement options that are fully inclusive and operate outside the disability 'system'. Moreover, that with the right kind of support and training to community mentors, that people with intellectual disabilities experience a range of positive outcomes such as more social contacts and a greater sense of social satisfaction. Likewise, as noted above, the older mentors also derived many reciprocal benefits from getting to know people with intellectual disabilities (Wilson et al, 2013).

DIFFERENT SERVICE MODELS TO SUPPORT OLDER PEOPLE WITH INTELLECTUAL DISABILITIES

There is unequivocal evidence of increased longevity of life in people with intellectual disabilities which is creating new challenges for contemporary models of service provision (Janicki, 2009). Previously, many people with intellectual disabilities may have lived in segregated long-stay residential complexes as they aged and until they died thus various residential and day units were able to accommodate changing levels and types of support needs (Jenkins, 2009). Contemporary service delivery models, however, no longer reflect these one-size-fits-all approaches and segregated options do not align with inclusive policy goals. The premature morbidity and mortality of people with intellectual disabilities has presented new issues as exemplified by the absence of any formal support and service models to support active ageing and retirement. Instead, disability services and families have been forced to develop ad-hoc support responses, often from a crisis such as health decline or the death of ageing family caregivers, to ensure that individual needs are met (McDermott et al, 2009). This will typically mean that the support services offered to the person are fragmented, lack choice and have limited specialisation on ageing issues (Hatzidimitriadou and Milne, 2005). These issues are also compounded by the reality that most generic ageing services have no capacity and/or lack the specialist skills to support older people with intellectual disabilities. In their previous chapter on growing older, Jenkins and Steff (2011) argued that, although lacking in policy clarity, literature on the topic pointed to there being three broad models

> **BOX 26.2   Models of care and support (adapted from Grant, 2001)**
>
> - Age- integrated models of care and support
> - Specialist models of care and support
> - Generic models of care and support

of support that are typically offered to older people with intellectual disabilities (see Box 26.2).

Age-integrated model

The basis of this model is the principle of 'ageing in place', where an older person with an intellectual disability is supported by intellectual disability services to stay in their home as they age, as safely and as independently as possible. What this means for disability services is the need to review the home context and modify this accordingly to support the person's changing needs. While a laudable goal within itself, there are some potentially significant costs and practicalities associated with making the necessary adjustments to the environmental context in addition to balancing the needs of everyone who may live in the home.

Indeed, where these adjustments are simply not feasible and the person's support needs can no longer be met by the service, the person with intellectual disability may have to move out of their own home (Jenkins, 2009). As was illustrated by the case example in Jenkins' UK-based study of an older person with intellectual disability being carried up and down stairs just to remain at home, unsafe working practices can result where the context is no longer suitable. In these instances, staying at home under an 'ageing in place' philosophy is not always feasible.

There are, however, practice examples where innovative modifications are possible and can make a positive difference. Mirza and Hammel's (2009) US study used a modified version of an intervention framework used in adults without intellectual disabilities who had dementia. In this study they co-produced, with older people with intellectual disabilities, an array of goals to modify aspects of their lives using a range of assistive technology and environmental modification. Using assistive technology includes interventions such as eliminating areas of pooled darkness in the home, changing the height of various surfaces, and changing default settings to water temperature. These might be viewed as further examples of compensating for a loss of capacity as identified by WHO (2015).

Importantly, working in partnership with people with intellectual disabilities who are ageing to identify problem areas in the home and develop solutions, is more effective than without their input. People with intellectual disabilities, when asked what they want from services as they age, expressed a desire to 'age in place', to have access to residential options that do not isolate them from existing social contacts and are not in small-scale dispersed housing, rather preferring proximity to more, rather than fewer, people (Shaw et al, 2011).

Specialist service model

This model is the result of intellectual disability services creating disability- and age-specific services for older people with intellectual disabilities. Although the possibilities for such models are likely to be quite wide-ranging, they are nonetheless segregated service models that may not promote other active ageing goals such as community participation and social inclusion. It has also been argued that such models are a default option in the absence of more inclusive options. For instance, Bigby et al (2011) reported that segregated disability-specific options were typically proposed by disability service providers.

One such model, a retirement programme created for the older workers of a sheltered workshop, has been developed and evaluated in Australia (Burke, 2006). Although segregated and intellectual disability-specific, this programme resembled a mainstream retirement day centre where, rather than going to work every day, older employees of the sheltered workshop attended the retirement programme one or two days a week and participated in centre-based or community activities. The critical issue here is that this service resulted from the absence of any alternatives and the moral need to offer something meaningful to employees who, in the case of many, had been working at the sheltered workshop for decades. Most importantly, this was a model that excluded the home where the person lived and so, although beneficial and enjoyable for many, it only solved one age-related service problem. For residential supports, other solutions are needed and there are very few examples of evidence-based residential services for older people with intellectual disabilities reported in the literature. Jenkins (2009) offered a positive description of an aged care facility in the UK specifically designed

for older people with intellectual disabilities who also had dementia, a particular feature for some people with Down syndrome.

Generic service model

This model is the utilisation of ageing services that are designed for and used by the general population. Bigby (2008) reported that where disability services are unable to adapt to the needs of people with intellectual disabilities who are ageing, they may in fact move into residential aged care settings prematurely. In fact, a national survey of aged care facilities conducted in Australia showed that people with intellectual disabilities were not only younger on average than other residents of aged care facilities, but also stayed there longer (Bigby et al, 2008). Critical issues were not fitting in with other residents and few meaningful relationships. This supports Jenkins and Steff's (2011) assertion that the model of mainstream aged care services requires the person to adapt to the service, rather than the service modifying models of care and tailoring supports to be individualised and person-centred.

 READER ACTIVITY 26.2

Consider the suitability of each of the service models identified by Grant (2001) in your area of practice. Identify strengths and weaknesses of each model. Are all three necessary or should a new model be developed?

THE ROLE OF PROFESSIONALS IN IDENTIFYING AND MEETING NEEDS

Older people with intellectual disabilities may have very complex care needs and these will imply that a variety of health and social care professionals will be involved in their care. In a multi-disciplinary team (MDT) context, this may include support staff, social workers, physiotherapists, dieticians, psychologists, speech and language therapists, occupational therapists, drama and music therapists as well as a range of specialist nurses, each with their different but complementary skill sets. However, there appears to be lack of guidance for professionals working with this vulnerable group (Jenkins, 2012).

The number of older people with unmet care and support needs is increasing substantially due to the challenges facing the formal and informal care system in many countries (Lin et al, 2016; Navas et al, 2019), with growing recognition of this as an urgent public health priority (Abdi et al, 2019). A study conducted in Ireland reports on the range of unmet service and support needs for older adults with intellectual disabilities (McCausland et al, 2010). They report on a paucity of basic education and budgeting information and a lack of transport to available services for older adults with intellectual disabilities. They argue for more lifelong learning to help individuals prepare and subsequently cope with the changes retirement will bring, as they transition from adult to older adult service provision.

Concerns have been raised in relation to the preparedness of staff within social care settings to meet the health needs of the growing number of older people with intellectual disabilities (McGhee and Dorsett, 2011). For example, in Wales there were particular concerns raised by local authorities, that people with intellectual disabilities over 50 can be placed in care homes for the elderly, and be labelled as 'elderly', resulting in becoming unknown to public services for their intellectual disability and not being able to access appropriate adjustments to meet their needs (Welsh Government, 2018). In addition, some people with intellectual disabilities may have been living with their parents for most of their life. As parents become older, they may experience ill health or die. Therefore, they may no longer be able to provide the care to their child they previously had. This can result in the person with intellectual disability moving into service-based accommodation, either in a setting for older adults or into supported living accommodation for people with intellectual disabilities (see previous section regarding models of care). Often these changes can be sudden or unexpected given that many older carers may have been unwilling or unable to make plans for the future (Dillenburger and McKerr, 2010). It is suggested that older carers need proactive support from professionals with planning for the future (Bowey and McGlaughlin, 2007).

However, there may also be a lack of information around housing options (Gilbert et al, 2008) and less than optimum support from professionals that add to poorly planned transitions in care (Llewellyn et al, 2010). Another challenge that has been raised in connection with older people is the need for greater palliative/end-of-life care planning for people with intellectual disabilities (Hunt et al, 2019). Although premature mortality has been highlighted as a concern for all adults with intellectual disabilities, the risk of death is higher for older parts of this population (Todd et al, 2019). Research conducted by McCarron et al, (2017) highlighted gaps in end-of-life care for the person with an intellectual disability. This included poor pain management, transitions, crisis-led decision making, health care professionals not understanding the needs of the person and not having the skills to engage in conversations about death.

Although the risk of death is higher for older people with intellectual disabilities, many of their deaths are not anticipated by support staff; this presents an additional difficulty in supporting people with intellectual disabilities in the last years of life (Todd et al, 2019). Death and dying further complicates the delivery of care to older adults and involves input from a range of different health professionals (Northway et al, 2018). Links between specialist intellectual disability services and palliative care services need to be made (Tuffrey-Wijne and Davidson, 2018). However, international literature suggests that some specialist intellectual disability professionals report a lack of knowledge and skill to deliver palliative/end-of-life care and therefore need specialised palliative care training and support (Wiese et al, 2014; Cross et al, 2012). It is essential that both palliative/end-of-life care and intellectual disability service providers work in collaboration, including involving families. It is also important that care is person-centred, and that there is a focus on staff training and the use of adapted or accessible tools (Tuffrey-Wijne and Davidson, 2018). End of life is covered extensively in Chapter 27.

In general, little research has been undertaken into the role of professionals in identifying and meeting the needs of older people with intellectual disabilities (Jenkins, 2009, 2012). However, they have a role to ensure that older people with intellectual disabilities have access to appropriate health services, whether it is an age-integrated, specialist service, or generic service model. One of the challenges as people with intellectual disabilities age is the increasing complexity of providing appropriate services and professionals for the individual and any carers. Heslop et al (2013) acknowledge the problem of poor coordination between and across services as a contributory factor for premature mortality in people with intellectual disabilities. Whilst that study focused on people with intellectual disabilities across the lifespan, it could be argued that these issues would be more likely to impact the ageing population owing to their greater reliance on paid care provided within social rather than healthcare.

In many countries, older people with intellectual disabilities live in supported living or group home settings which may mean that they will rely heavily on social care staff to support their health needs, to help manage chronic health conditions and to support them to access healthcare services when required (Northway et al, 2017). Therefore, professionals working with older people living in supported living settings will inevitably work across service and organisational boundaries; across health and social care, and across specialist intellectual disability services, generic health services and older adult services.

LOOKING TO THE FUTURE

As has been noted in previous sections of this chapter, the life expectancy of people with intellectual disabilities is increasing which means that looking to the future there is a pressing need to ensure that we have effective and appropriate systems of support in place to identify and meet their needs. This will require effective working across organisational, service and professional boundaries to ensure that such support is coordinated and delivered at an appropriate time. It also requires that we take a lifespan approach recognising that the foundations of health in older age are laid during our younger years and hence we should be seeking to ensure that these foundations are as strong as possible.

Central to such future systems of support therefore is the need to more effectively promote healthy ageing for people with intellectual disabilities and to ensure that a proactive approach is taken. The view that declining health is an inevitable consequence of both having an intellectual disability and getting older needs to be robustly challenged. Indeed, Oppewal and Hilgenkamp (2019) argue that service systems need to have a focus on keeping people with intellectual disabilities physically active and fit, that simply promoting physical activity is insufficient and that improving physical fitness should become a basic part of the support we provide for adults with intellectual disabilities.

To effect such change, however, requires more than simply stating that it should happen. Spassiani et al (2019) suggest that there needs to be a commitment of financial and other resources and also clarity regarding responsibilities. Indeed, they suggest that responsibilities need to be set out in agency policies and in job descriptions. Elsewhere, Roll and Bowers (2017) argue that staff training needs to be provided since many support staff lack the knowledge required to effectively support people with intellectual disabilities who develop age related health problems.

It is not only paid carers, however, that require support to fulfil their role in relation to the promotion of healthy ageing. Many older people with intellectual disabilities live with their families, who may themselves be very old and sometimes frail. Families therefore also need to understand the importance of active ageing and where they are unable to provide the support themselves to enable this to happen, additional supports may be required.

Finally, and most importantly, older people with intellectual disabilities themselves need to be supported to play a central role in shaping future provision to meet their needs and wishes. Unfortunately, however, a limited understanding of the ageing process (Buys et al, 2012) and how they can contribute to active ageing (Spassianu et al, 2019) has been noted amongst people with intellectual disabilities. There would thus appear to be a need to ensure that people with intellectual disabilities are supported to understand the ageing process and that they are enabled to express their views concerning what supports they need as they age.

CONCLUSION

This chapter has explored the ageing process in relation to people with intellectual disabilities and has argued that whilst their pattern of mental and physical health often differs from that of their non-disabled peers such differences may be amenable to change. An argument has therefore been presented for greater attention to be paid to the promotion of healthy ageing which includes not only a focus on physical health but also on positive mental well-being through, for example, supporting engagement in social activities. It is recognised, however, that whilst much can be done to promote more active and healthy ageing, the needs of individuals are likely to change as they age and hence there is the need for more effective and appropriate patterns of support to be developed to meet such changing needs.

REFERENCES

Abdi, S., Spann, A., Borilovic, J., et al. (2019). Understanding the care and support needs of older people: a scoping review and categorisation using the WHO international classification of functioning, disability and health framework (ICF). *BMC Geriatrics, 19*(195).

Axman, A., Bjorkman, M., & Ahlstrom, G. (2019). Hospital readmissions among older people with intellectual disabilities in comparison with the general population. *Journal of Intellectual Disability Research, 63*(6), 593–602.

Bigby, C. (2008). Beset by obstacles: a review of Australian policy development to support ageing in place for people with intellectual disability. *Journal of Intellectual and Developmental Disability, 33*(1), 76–86.

Bigby, C., & Haveman, M. (2010). Ageing: a continuing challenge. *Journal of Policy and Practice in Intellectual Disabilities, 7*(1), 1–2.

Bigby, C., Webber, R., Bowers, B., et al. (2008). A survey of people with intellectual disabilities living in residential aged care facilities in Victoria. *Journal of Intellectual Disability Research, 52*(5), 404–414.

Bigby, C., Wilson, N. J., Balandin, S., et al. (2011). Disconnected expectations: staff, family and supported employee perspectives about retirement. *Journal of Intellectual and Developmental Disability, 36*, 167–174.

Bowey, L., & McGlaughlin, A. (2007). Older carers of adults with a intellectual disability confront the future: issues and preferences in planning. *Journal of Social Work, 37*(1), 39–54.

Brotherton, M., Stancliffe, R. J., Wilson, N. J., et al. (2016). Supporting workers with intellectual disability in mainstream employment to transition to socially-inclusive retirement. *Journal of Intellectual and Developmental Disability, 41*(1), 75–80.

Burke, M. E. (2006). *Daily activities linking initiative (DALI): stage one report*. Wollongong, NSW, Australia: Greenacres Association.

Buys, L., Aird, R., & Miller, E. (2012). Service providers' perceptions of active ageing among older adults with lifelong intellectual disabilities. *Journal of Intellectual Disability Research, 56*(12), 1133–1147.

Coppus, A. M. W. (2013). People with intellectual disability: what do we know about adulthood and life expectancy? *Developmental Disabilities Reviews, 18*, 6–16.

Cooper, S. A., Smiley, E., Morrison, J., et al. (2007). Mental ill-health in adults with intellectual disabilities: prevalence and associated factors. *The British Journal of Psychiatry, 190*(1), 27–35.

Cross, H., Cameron, M., Marsh, S., et al. (2012). Practical approaches toward improving end-of-life care for people with intellectual disabilities: effectiveness and sustainability. *Journal Of Palliative Medicine, 15*(3), 322–326.

Deb, S., Thomas, M., & Bright, C. (2001). Mental disorder in adults with intellectual disability. I: prevalence of functional psychiatric illness among a community-based population aged between 16 and 64 years. *Journal of Intellectual Disability Research, 45*(6), 495–505.

Dillenburger, K., & McKerr, L. (2010). How long are we able to go on? Issues faced by older family caregivers of adults with disabilities. *British Journal of Intellectual Disabilities, 3*, 929–938.

Ellison, C. J., & White, A. L. (2017). Exploring leisure and retirement for people with intellectual disabilities. *Annals of Leisure Research, 20*(2), 188–205.

Findlay, L., Williams, A. C., & Scior, K. (2014). Exploring experiences and understandings of pain in adults with intellectual disabilities. *Journal of Intellectual Disability Research, 58*(4), 358–367.

Finlayson, J. (2018). Fall prevention for people with intellectual disabilities: key points and recommendations for practitioners and researchers. *Tizard Intellectual Disability Review, 23*(2), 91–99.

Foster, L., & Boxall, K. (2015). People with intellectual disabilities and 'active ageing'. *British Journal of Intellectual Disabilities, 43*, 270–276.

Gilbert, A., Lankshear, G., & Petersen, A. (2008). Older family-carers' views on the future accommodation needs of relatives who have an intellectual disability. *International Journal of Social Welfare, 17*, 54–64.

Glover, G., Williams, R., Heslop, P., et al. (2017). Mortality in people with intellectual disabilities in England. *Journal of Intellectual Disability Research, 61*(1), 62–74.

Grant, G. (2001). Older people with intellectual disabilities: Health, community inclusion and family caregiving. In M. Nolan, S. Davies, & S. Grant (Eds.), *Working with older people and their families: Key issues in policy and practice*. Buckingham: Open University Press.

Hatzidimitriadou, E., & Milne, A. (2005). Planning ahead: meeting the needs of older people with intellectual disabilities in the United Kingdom. *Dementia. The International Journal of Social Research and Practic,e, 4*(3), 341–359.

Haveman, M., Perry, J., Salvador-Canula, L., et al. (2011). Ageing and health status in adults with intellectual disabilities: results of the European POMONA II study. *Journal of Intellectual Disability Research, 36*(1), 49–60.

Hermans, H., & Evenhuis, H. M. (2014). Multimorbidity in older adults with intellectual disabilities. *Research in Developmental Disabilities, 35*, 776–783.

Heslop, P., Blair, P., Fleming, P., et al. (2013). *Confidential inquiry into premature deaths of people with learning disabilities*. Bristol: Norah Fry Research Centre, University of Bristol.

Hunt, K., Bernal, J., Worth, R., et al. (2019). End-of-life care in intellectual disability: a retrospective cross-sectional study. *BMJ Supportive and Palliative Care*. Available at: https://spcare.bmj.com/content/early/2019/10/16/bmjspcare-2019-001985.info.

Janicki, M. P. (2009). The aging dilemma: is increasing longevity among people with intellectual disabilities creating a new population challenge in the Asia-Pacific region? *Journal of Policy and Practice in Intellectual Disabilities, 6*(2), 73–76.

Janicki, M. P., Dalton, A. J., McCallion, P., et al. (2005). Group home care for adults with intellectual disabilities and Alzheimer's disease. *Dementia: The International Journal of Social Research and Practice, 4*(3), 361–385.

Jenkins, R. (2009). Nurses' views about services for older people with intellectual disabilities. *Nursing Older People, 21*(3), 23–27.

Jenkins, R., & Steff, M. (2011). Growing older: meeting the needs of people with intellectual disabilities. In H. L. Atherton & D. J. Crickmore (Eds.), *Learning disabilities: toward inclusion* (pp. 519–534). London: Churchill Livingstone.

Jenkins, R. (2012). Meeting the health needs of older people with intellectual disabilities. *British Journal of Nursing, 21*(8), 468–473.

Jokinen, M. P., Janicki, S. M., Keller, P., et al., & the National Task Group on Intellectual Disabilities and Dementia Practices. (2013). *Guidelines for structuring community care and supports for people with intellectual disabilities affected by dementia*. Washington, DC: AADMD. Available at: http://aadmd.org/sites/default/files/NTG_Guidelines-posting-version.pdf.

Kerr, D., Cunningham, C., & Wilkinson, H. (2011). Responding to the pain experiences of people with an intellectual difficulty and dementia. *International Medical Review on Down Syndrome, 15*, 2–7.

Lin, J., Lin, L., & Hsu, S. (2016). Ageing People with intellectual disabilities: current challenges and effective interventions. *Review Journal of Autism and Developmental Disorders, 3*(3), 266–272.

Llewellyn, G., McConnell, D., Gething, L., et al. (2010). Health status and coping strategies among older parent-carers of adults with intellectual disabilities in an Australian sample. *Research in Developmental Disabilities, 31*(6), 1176–1186.

McCarron, M., Swinburne, J., Burke, E., et al. (2011). *Growing older with an intellectual disability in Ireland 2011: first results from the Intellectual Disability Supplement to the Irish Longitudinal Study on Ageing (IDS-TILDA)*. Dublin: Trinity College Dublin.

McCarron, M., McCallion, P., Reilly, E., et al. (2014). Responding to the challenges of service development to address dementia needs for people with an intellectual disability and their caregivers. In K. Watchman (Ed.), *Intellectual disability and dementia: research into practice* (pp. 241–269). London: Jessica Kingsley.

McCarron, M., Burke, E. M., White, P. O., et al. (2017). *'He'd mind you, you mind him': experiences of end of life care for people with an intellectual disability as perceived by staff carers. Findings from the End of Life Interviews of the Intellectual Disability Supplement to the Irish Longitudinal Study on Ageing (IDS-TILDA)*. Dublin: Trinity College Dublin.

McCausland, D., Guerin, S., Tyrell, J., et al. (2010). *Research in Developmental Disabilities, 31*, 381–387.

McDermott, S., Edwards, R., Abello, D., et al. (2009). *Ageing and Australian disability enterprises: final report*. Sydney: Social Policy Research Centre, University of New South Wales.

McGhee, A., & Dorsett, P. (2011). Ageing of people with intellectual disability: effective training for frontline workers. *Journal of Social Inclusion, 2*(1), 65–81.

McKenzie, K., Ouellette-Kuntz, H., & Martin, L. (2017). Applying a general measure of frailty to assess the age related needs of adults with intellectual and developmental disabilities. *Journal of Policy and Practice in Intellectual Disabilities, 14*(2), 124–128.

Mirza, M., & Hammel, J. (2009). Consumer-directed goal planning in the delivery of assistive technology services for people who are ageing with intellectual disabilities. *Journal of Applied Research in Intellectual Disabilities, 22*, 445–457.

Morin, D., Merineau-Cote, J., Ouellette-Kuntz, H., et al. (2012). A comparison of the prevalence of chronic disease among people with and without intellectual disabilities. *American Journal of Intellectual and Developmental Disabilities, 117*(6), 455–463.

Navas, P., Llorente, E. S., Garcia, L., et al. (2019). Improving healthcare access for older adults with intellectual disability: what are the needs? *Journal of Applied Research in Intellectual Disabilities, 32*(6), 1453–1464.

Noone, J., O'Loughlin, K., & Kendig, H. (2013). Australian baby boomers retiring 'early': understanding the benefits of retirement preparation for involuntary and voluntary retirees. *Journal of Aging Studies, 27*(3), 207–217.

Northway, R., Holland-Hart, D., & Jenkins, R. (2017). Meeting the health needs of older people with intellectual disabilities: exploring the experiences of residential social care staff. *Health and Social Care in the Community, 25*(3), 923–931.

Northway, R., Todd, S., Hunt, K., et al. (2018). Nursing care at end of life: a UK-based survey of the deaths of people living in care settings for people with intellectual disability. *Journal of Research in Nursing, 24*(6), 366–382.

Oppewal, A., & Hilgenkamp, T. I. M. (2019). Physical fitness is predictive for 5-year survival in older adults with intellectual disabilities. *Journal of Applied Research in Intellectual Disabilities, 32*, 958–966.

Prasher, V. (2005). *Alzheimer's disease and dementia in down syndrome and intellectual disabilities.* Oxford: Radcliffe.

Roll, A. E., & Bowers, B. J. (2017). Promoting healthy aging of individuals with developmental disabilities: a qualitative case study. *Western Journal of Nursing Research, 39*(2), 234–251.

Rickard, W., & Donkin, A. (2018). *A fair, supportive society.* London: Institute of Health Equity.

Shaw, K., Cartwright, C., & Craig, J. (2011). The housing and support needs of people with an intellectual disability into older age. *Journal of Intellectual Disability Research, 55*(9), 895–903.

Sheerin, F., Fleming, S., Burke, E., et al. (2019). Exploring mental health issues in people with an intellectual disability. *Intellectual Disability Practice, 23*(1), 13–17.

Stancliffe, R. J., Bigby, C., Balandin, S., et al. (2015). Transition to retirement and participation in mainstream community groups using active mentoring: a feasibility and outcomes evaluation with a matched comparison group. *Journal of Intellectual Disability Research, 59*(8), 703–718.

Stancliffe, R. J., Jones, E., Mansell, J., et al. (2008). Active support: a critical review and commentary. *Journal of Intellectual & Developmental Disability, 33*, 196–214.

Stancliffe, R. J., Wilson, N. J., Gambin, N., et al. (2013). *Transition to retirement: a guide to inclusive practice.* Sydney, Australia: Sydney University Press.

Strydom, A., Chan, T., King, M., et al. (2013). Incidence of dementia in older adults with intellectual disabilities. *Research in Developmental Disabilities, 34*(6), 1881–1885.

Schepens, H. R. M. M., Van Puyenbroek, J., & Maes, B. (2018). How to improve the quality of life of elderly people with intellectual disability: a systematic literature review of support strategies. *Journal of Applied Research in Intellectual Disabilities, 32*, 483–521.

Schoufour, J. D., Mitniski, A., Rockwood, K., et al. (2014). Predicting disabilities in daily functioning in older people with intellectual disabilities using a frailty index. *Research in Developmental Disabilities, 35* 2267–2227.

Spassianu, N. A., Mesner, B. A., Abou Chacra, M. S., et al. (2019). What is and isn't working: factors involved in sustaining community-based health and participation initiatives for people ageing with intellectual disabilities. *Journal of Applied Research in Intellectual Disabilities, 32*, 1465–1477.

The Health Services Research and Development Center at the Johns Hopkins University. (2009). *ACG System: technical reference guide version 9.0.* Baltimore, MD.

Todd, S., Brandford, S., Worth, E., et al. (2019). Place of death of people with intellectual disabilities: an exploratory study of death and dying within community disability service settings. *Journal of Intellectual Disabilities.* Available at: https://journals.sagepub.com/doi/10.1177/1744629519886758.

The Learning Disabilities Mortality Review Programme (LeDeR). (2017). *Annual report.* Bristol: University of Bristol.

Tuffrey-Wijne, I., & Davidson, J. (2018). Excellence in palliative and end-of-life care provision for people with intellectual disability. *International Journal of Palliative Nursing, 24*(12), 598–610.

Welsh Government. (2018). *Intellectual disability: Improving Lives Programme.* Available at: https://gov.wales/topics/health/professionals/nursing/intellectual/?lang=en.

Wiese, M., Stancliffe, R. J., Dew, A., Balandin, S., & Howarth, G. (2014). What is talked about? Community living staff experiences of talking with older people with intellectual disabilities about dying and death. *Journal of Intellectual Disability Research, 58*(7), 679–690.

Wilson, N. J., Stancliffe, R. J., Bigby, C., et al. (2010). The potential for active mentoring to support a positive transition into retirement for older adults with a lifelong disability. *Journal of Intellectual & Developmental Disability.* 35(3), 211–214. Doi: 10.3109/13668250.2010.481784.

Wilson, N. J., Stancliffe, R. J., Bigby, C., et al. (2012). Creating opportunities for social inclusion: older adults with a lifelong disability in the transition to retirement phase of life. *VOICE, 1*(3), 4–6.

Wilson, N. J., Bigby, C., Stancliffe, R. J., et al. (2013). Mentors' experiences using the active mentoring model to support older adults with intellectual disability to participate in community groups. *Journal of Intellectual & Developmental Disability, 38*(4), 344–355.

Wilson, N. J., Stancliffe, R. J., Gambin, N., et al. (2015). A case study about the supported participation of older men with lifelong disabilities at Australian community-based Men's Sheds. *Journal of Intellectual and Developmental Disability*, *40*(4), 330–341.

World Health Organisation. (2000). *Ageing and intellectual disability*. Geneva: WHO.

World Health Organisation. (2015). *World report on ageing and health*. Geneva: WHO.

27

End of life: holistic approaches to loss, dying & death

Sue Read and Michele Wiese

KEY ISSUES

- Death is a universal experience.
- People with intellectual disabilities, their families, and professional carers experience a range of losses associated with the end of life.
- Carers need to consider the voices of people with intellectual disabilities; their experiences of loss, dying and death, and how such experiences can help shape effective care and support.
- It is important to recognise the range of losses associated with end-of-life care for individuals with intellectual disabilities, their families and professional carers.

- Identifying the inherent and persistent challenges to providing effective support at the end of life from a holistic perspective is crucial in order for them to be addressed.
- People with intellectual disabilities are likely to experience disenfranchised death and grief.
- Carers need to adopt a creative approach to the effective care and support of people with intellectual disabilities when they experience dying, death and loss.

CHAPTER OUTLINE

INTRODUCTION

The aim of this chapter is to consider the loss issues surrounding end of life and the persistent and inherent challenges of supporting, empowering and enabling individuals with intellectual disabilities to become actively involved in decision making processes. The chapter adopts an international perspective, incorporating current research on end-of-life support to this marginalised group. Death never occurs in a vacuum but within a social context (Read, 2008), significantly influencing how the person faces the end of their life and how survivors

accommodate the death of their friend/family member. This chapter considers such social contexts and how they ultimately affect individuals and the support provided.

As we steer towards the end of this book it reminds us that we are all travelling along the same path as we age and face the challenges inevitable at the end of life. This chapter explores the importance of living well until death, and how people with intellectual disabilities can be best supported as they move towards the dying phase. The chapter also explores the aftermath of death, as survivors cope with losing their loved one in a world that will be forever different. These are important journeys; journeys that cannot be rehearsed nor repeated. For some people who have cognitive impairments, it may seem like trying to make sense out of nonsense; trying to truly comprehend what is happening around them with a limited capacity to understand the complex realities of ill health, dying and death. For those people who cannot understand abstract concepts such as loss, dying or death, carers need to explore creative approaches of engagement. We owe it to all people travelling towards the end of life to get it right, and to celebrate the companionship along this difficult path. For people with intellectual disabilities, this journey may be the same as for anyone else, but the routes taken to get there may be different, as carers and people with intellectual disabilities themselves cope with all the challenges that having intellectual disabilities might bring.

This chapter will introduce death within a range of loss experiences: exploring the concept of loss particularly in relation to people with intellectual disabilities; exploring end-of-life and the care required at this intersection; and identifying the persistent and inherent challenges to effective and practical support.

DEATH AS LOSS

Life is characterised by movement and change and therefore, by its very nature, by transitions, losses and grief (Thompson, 2002); loss and death are omnipresent. Death is often perceived as the ultimate loss and, along with birth, one of two life's certainties. Death is sometimes a regular companion, for example those living for many years with life-threatening conditions. Death can be a sudden and unexpected visitor, arriving without warning or time to prepare. Death can be a welcomed friend, following extended, enduring pain with no expectation of release. Death can also be a stranger, shrouded in secrecy and not disclosed to individuals until absolutely necessary, if at all, unfortunately an all too common experience for those with intellectual disabilities (Wiese et al, 2013).

There are a range of responses to the loss of a loved one which can be influenced by many factors including the relationship to the deceased, the nature of the death, and existing coping styles – all of which may influence the full impact of loss. Whether anticipated, unexpected, welcomed or disguised, death can create a huge chasm in the lives of survivors as they learn to accommodate

> ### 📋 READER ACTIVITY 27.1
>
> For just one moment, imagine if you never got to say a final goodbye to your loved one; imagine if you had no pictures or other mementoes of that person; imagine if no one told you about the funeral; imagine if no one asked you if you wanted to go to the funeral, or take flowers. Imagine living in a world where other people make decisions for you around loss and death, as to whether, for example, you should visit the hospice to see a dying relative. Imagine not having the voice to articulate your feelings, concerns or questions, or not having anyone who asks you how you are feeling. Make a note of how this might make you feel.

their loss and relearn new life roles in the absence of companions (Attig, 1996), whilst remembering loved ones across the ensuing years (Klass et al, 1996).

How might you have felt?

Working through Reader activity 27.1, you might have noted that you felt confused, sad or angry but couldn't explain why. You might have felt frustrated because of the mixed emotions but not had the words to verbalise these feelings in a meaningful way. You might have felt lonely because you had no one to share the fears and anxieties with; believing that no one had the time or could possibly understand what you are going through as you tried to express your pain.

Sudden deaths are often hardest to accommodate, perhaps because survivors may be unprepared, have unfinished business, and because these deaths can be tragic and traumatic. Anticipated deaths are different; the dying person may have an incurable illness and there is time to prepare for its arrival. People with intellectual disabilities may be exposed to sudden deaths, but perhaps more often protected from knowing about anticipated deaths. Carers may be fearful of exposing the individual to the stark reality of loved ones dying; may lack the skills to provide support; feel uncomfortable talking about death themselves; or want to protect people from distress.

Despite clear evidence that talking about the end of life with people who have intellectual disabilities does not cause harm, the contrary may be so. Not approaching the topic openly and with compassion may in fact be causing harm (Stancliffe et al, 2021; Wiese et al, 2015). Some carers may feel that people with intellectual disabilities simply do not have the capacity to understand loss and grief (Lord et al, 2017). Loss can be disempowering for anyone, but for people with intellectual disabilities loss can be *totally* disempowering and overwhelming.

Although loss and death are embedded threads woven into the fabric of life, people with intellectual disabilities rarely get constructive opportunities to talk or learn about them. Subsequently, accommodating loss can be difficult for them, whether they are accommodating the loss or death of others, or facing their own impending death.

END-OF-LIFE CARE

The provision of care for dying people in contemporary society is described as end-of-life care, and "How we care for the dying is an indicator of how we care for all sick and vulnerable people" (Department of Health (DH), 2008).

Palliative care involves active total care, and is defined as:

"an approach that improves the quality of life of patients (adults and children) and their families who are facing problems associated with life-threatening illness. It prevents and relieves suffering through the early identification, correct assessment and treatment of pain and other problems, whether physical, psychosocial or spiritual."

World Health Organization (WHO), 2020

Palliative care aims to affirm life and regards dying as a normal process. It is a support system that:
- accompanies the patient and family throughout the illness course
- intends neither to hasten or postpone death; providing treatment where needed to achieve adequate comfort in line with the patient's values
- integrates with and complements prevention, early diagnosis and treatment of serious or life-limiting health problems
- provides an alternative to treatment of questionable value near the end of life, and assists decision-making about optimum use of life-sustaining treatment
- is applicable to those with long-term physical, psychological, social or spiritual sequelae of serious or life-threatening illnesses or of their treatment
- helps the family cope during the patient's illness and in their own bereavement

- should be applied by health care workers across all levels of health care systems, and accessible, including in patients' homes
- aims to enhance quality of life, promotes dignity and comfort, and may also positively influence the course of illness
- is applicable early in the course of illness, in conjunction with other therapies that are intended to prolong life
- encourages active involvement by communities and community members
- seeks to mitigate effects of poverty on patients and their family and protect them from financial hardship due to illness or disability
- improves continuity of care, thereby strengthening health systems

(World Health Organization, 2018)

Palliative care is delivered in various care settings (i.e. hospital, hospice, home), by a range of health and social care workers. The social context in which people live (and sometimes the labels which have been ascribed to them) may impact on the end-of-life care accessed (Oliviére and Monroe, 2004) and subsequent care received (Read and Thompson-Hill, 2009). Whilst a holistic approach is the perceived basis for high-quality palliative care and support (Department of Health (DH) 2008), some marginalised groups (e.g., people with low socioeconomic status; people with intellectual disabilities) may struggle to access appropriate palliative care and support. While it is argued that "... *people with a learning disability {sic} have poorer health, greater health needs and shorter lives*" (Mencap, 2004, p. 31), end-of-life care for this population remains inconsistent across the UK and across the globe (Tuffrey-Wijne et al, 2007). In Australia and China, for example, palliative care professionals report a number of challenges that mediate their ability to provide quality care to the dying person with an intellectual disability. These include (but are not limited to) referral timeliness to the palliative care team; managing symptoms when the person may have difficulties communicating pain; ethical dilemmas around understanding the illness and decision making; and navigating the complex and often siloed health and social care systems (Li et al, 2018; Foo et al, 2021).

In the UK, the majority of the general population still die in institutionalised care, whether a nursing

BOX 27.1   Where people die
(Public Health England, 2019)

452,859 people died in England in 2011 in the following places:

230,850 in hospital and communal establishments
98,645 at home
88,082 in care homes
1,381 in other communal establishments
24,495 in hospices.

home, hospital or hospice (see Box 27.1). Places where group dying takes place (i.e. hospices, hospitals) can be perceived as creating an 'atypical visibility' which serves to entrench the social devaluation of people who are dying (Sinclair, 2007) rather than supporting the individual to die in a familiar place where they have lived all their life.

Dying and death are often referred to as the 'last taboo' within society and only 34% of people are believed to have discussed or shared their end of life wishes with anyone else (National Council for Palliative Care (NCPC), 2009). For people with intellectual disabilities, this figure is likely to be *significantly* lower, with research from Europe, the USA and Australia suggesting that they are rarely consulted about their final wishes (Kirkendall et al, 2017; Stancliffe et al, 2016; Zaal-Schuller et al, 2018). Unless the discomfort about this topic is overcome, people with intellectual disabilities will remain disenfranchised from determining the course of their end-of-life care.

End-of-life care and people with intellectual disabilities

Loss experiences usually increase with age. One of the many features associated with ageing is that as the person draws nearer to death, perceptions of mortality and all this entails become more acute as those around them age and die too. While people with intellectual disabilities are enjoying increased longevity (Lauer and McCallion, 2015), many will come to have a dying phase in their lives as opposed to dying suddenly. The problems associated with ageing have been recognised for some time (Foundation for People with Learning Disabilities, 2002; Holland, 2018; National Institute for Clinical Excellence (NICE), 2018). For example, people with Down syndrome are living longer, yet the incidence of dementia increases significantly with age for this population (Prasher and Chung 1996; Prasher, 2005). Conversely, children with profound and multiple intellectual disabilities are surviving where previously they might not (Emerson, 2009), driving developments in children's palliative care (e.g., Together for short lives, 2020). Therefore, children, young people, and older populations with intellectual disabilities may present noteworthy groups that have not been fully considered by either the research or care communities.

Despite preferred wishes about care and death at home, in Australia, like the UK (see Box 27.1) most people die in hospital or hospice (Virdun et al, 2015). The picture is similar for people with intellectual disabilities, with research from New Zealand and Australia suggesting deaths in hospital are most common (Todd et al, 2019; Wiese et al, 2019b). Paradoxically, however, people with intellectual disabilities benefit from familiarity of place, people and routines; it is also clear from research across the world including the UK, Europe, the USA and Australia, that carers want to, within safe and practical means, provide end-of-life care in the familiarity of the dying person's home (Bekkema et al, 2014; Wiese et al, 2012). Yet the unfamiliar setting of hospital, with arguably inequitable access to care (Lauer and McCallion, 2015), remains the prevailing place of death for this group.

Recognising ill health

Chapter 9 discussed the range of inherent social problems (i.e. limited exercise; restricted social activities), poor diet and additional health problems, (i.e. epilepsy, dementia) that compound the health status of people with intellectual disabilities (Mencap, 2007; Emerson and Baines, 2011; Emerson et al, 2016).

While there is a developing evidence base driven by policy around general end-of-life principles for health care providers (DH, 2008), there is relatively little empirical evidence around applying such principles to marginalised groups (i.e. people with intellectual disabilities).

 READER ACTIVITY 27.2

Think about the last time you talked about death and dying, and under what circumstances.

Now think about the last time you talked with a person with an intellectual disability about loss, death or dying.

Compare the two experiences.

People with intellectual disabilities may not recognise symptoms or changes in their body that indicate ill health and disease, while some people may have had bad experiences of hospitals, doctors and nurses and are reluctant to voice any noticeable symptoms. Some may simply be too afraid to report any recognised symptoms for fear of a poor diagnosis (Read and Morris, 2009). John Davies, a man with an intellectual disability, knew that he was ill (he had penile cancer) but had ignored his illness for many months because of fear and urged everyone to visit the doctor as soon as they noticed something amiss (Tuffrey-Wijne and Davies, 2007). There is also evidence in Australia suggesting that carers may be referring to health and palliative care services too late, leading to delayed diagnosis, unnecessary pain, and fragmented palliative care to the dying person and caregivers (Foo et al, 2021). Carers and supporters of people with intellectual disabilities must remain vigilant in recognising signs of potential ill health that may require further investigations (see Box 27.2).

Symptom recognition and identification may be difficult with this population because of communication difficulties and diagnostic overshadowing (Brown et al, 2003). Pain and other symptoms may also be difficult to manage and assess, as the person struggles to indicate worsening symptoms and carers struggle to understand when to offer, administer or increase prescribed medication. Macmillan Cancer Support (2003) identified four key barriers restricting access to cancer care services in particular: physical, professional, emotional and social, cultural or religious/spiritual. For individuals with intellectual disabilities, knowledge and attitudinal beliefs around the disability itself are also important factors that influence equitable access to, and receipt of, quality care (Read and Morris, 2009). People with intellectual disabilities are often lost behind barriers that make access to end-of-life care and support difficult, further compounded for older people with intellectual disabilities (Jenkins, 2005), or dementia (Frey, 2006).

Whilst professional carers of this population are committed to providing good quality care and support, they may not have the appropriate knowledge and skills to provide end-of-life care (Wiese et al, 2012, 2019a). Many face 'role blurring', as they try to move seamlessly between various roles, such as carer, advocate or friend. Many may be unfamiliar with the concept of palliative care but have had to learn quickly in order to support the people they care for (Read and Morris, 2009). Carers may become experts relatively quickly as they learn to provide end-of-life care for the dying person, but afterwards, as life quickly reverts to a sense of normality, eventually lose this expertise and begin again to focus on the living well (as opposed to the dying well) aspects of their caring role.

> ### READER ACTIVITY 27.3
>
> Should a person with an intellectual disability that you support be diagnosed with a life-limiting condition, what might you do to include the person in the choices around their care?
>
> How might you prepare them as death approaches?

BOX 27.2   Simple things to look out for (Read and Morris, 2009)

- Swellings or lumps.
- Clothes not fitting properly.
- Weight loss or gain.
- Personality changes.
- Changes in eating habits.
- Changes in toilet habits.
- Generally feeling unwell.
- Tiredness or lethargy.
- Changes in behaviour.
- Asking for pain relief more often than usual.

Working through Reader activity 27.3, one could consider how able the person is and what they already understand about their condition. Even if they have not been told about the severity of the illness, many people often guess that something is wrong, perhaps because of the number of doctor and hospital appointments recently, or the deterioration in health over time, or the simple fact that people are perhaps more-than-usually kind. Breaking difficult news is never easy, but practical tips around difficult diagnosis can be found at this helpful website, "Talking End of Life...with people with intellectual disability (TEL)" which gives caregivers the knowledge, skills and confidence to approach discussing the end of life with people with intellectual disabilities (Talking End of Life, 2018). Importantly, whatever is happening, the person who is about to die remains the most important person within this care context, and everything that is done is done because it will help them in some way. You might think about the person's circle of support and who is important to that person. You should explore what the person's end-of-life preferences are (if possible) and whether they have specific ideas about their own funeral. Religious and spiritual beliefs remain important, and sometimes individuals who may not have been actively practicing any religious preferences, as the end of life draws increasingly closer, may turn to their religious leader for help, support and comfort. The amount of active involvement depends entirely on the needs of the person and their ability to understand what is happening to them (and those around them), and they have a choice to be involved if they are able, and indeed want, to be included in this part of their life. No one should be forced, for example, to make a Will, or to complete funeral plans, if they do not want to. Carers should help individuals to understand end-of-life information and to support them with honesty, empathy and compassion. A series of free, accessible leaflets and booklets specifically developed to help personal and professional carers and individuals with intellectual disabilities at the end of life can be found in the online Useful resources section for this chapter.

Hospice professionals need to be aware of the challenges that supporting people with intellectual disabilities may incur; should recognise the importance of being able to access specialist intellectual disability expertise; appreciate the importance of effective communicating; and understand what having an intellectual disability really means (Cartlidge and Read, 2010). How a person with an intellectual disability dies could be perceived as a barometer against which one can measure how the person lived, and the value placed on their lives.

From a pro-active perspective, carers need to ensure that people with intellectual disabilities access national screening programmes (e.g., bowel cancer screening) to promote healthier outcomes (Read and Latham, 2009) and address the issue of gatekeepers, who may govern access to patients and clients as in the hospice environment and who can facilitate this active involvement. An acronym (AWARE) developed to promote

 BOX 27.3   AWARE: promoting health for people with intellectual disabilities (Read and Morris, 2009)

A– Alert people to the potential for ill health.

W– Watchful and vigilant: regarding regular personal body checking; carers need to notice any changes in any aspect of the person that might be an indicator of ill health.

A– Attend regular screening programmes: encourage and support individuals to attend health checks such as mammograms, cervical screening and testicular checking. Identifying disease early can impact on treatment and outcomes.

R– Remember to encourage people to tell someone if they don't feel well or they notice any changes in their body. Talking about such sensitive issues may be difficult, and carers need to give people opportunities to explore how they feel in a way that the person feels most comfortable with (e.g. using pictures, drama, role play).

E– Encourage and enable people to attend appointments and to understand what might happen to them if they don't. Some people may need more time at clinics to help with communication issues; some may need to visit the clinic/hospital prior to the appointment to familiarise themselves with the venue; a familiar carer should accompany the person at appointments to promote consistency of support and minimise distress for the person.

health for people with intellectual disabilities is a useful framework for all carers supporting this population (see Box 27.3).

LIVING WITH LOSS

"Loss can be described as a sense of being deprived or being without, and as such can be expected or unexpected."

Read, 2014, p. 29

Some of the major losses related to death experiences are positively validated by society (such as the death of a parent) but some are not (such as abortion). The literature recognises that grief responses are not solely related to death explicitly but can relate to other forms of loss. For example loss associated with altered body image, disability or some aspect of self; loss related to divorce or separation; material losses (both tangible and intangible); maturational or developmental losses (Hess, 1980; Machin, 1998), invisible loss (Machin, 2010; McNutt and Yakushko, 2013), and non-finite loss (Bruce and Schultz, 2001), all embody feelings of grief reactions as the loss is accommodated into the life of the living (Worden, 2009). Life is a journey, a journey full of losses (Machin, 2014), and having an intellectual disability can imply numerous invisible losses inherent with the label itself: e.g., one's social role in society and how devaluing this can be. Each loss carries with it the threat of additional losses and the potential for future associated losses, hence losses are often multiple, complex and successive (Elliott, 2003; Parkes, 2014).

While bereavement is perceived as being the most common type of loss, having a child with an intellectual disability can mean confronting numerous losses, synchronous with hopes, wishes, ideals and expectations (Parkes, 2014). This is echoed poignantly in an article written by a parent of a daughter with Rett syndrome describing a lifetime of disappointment, loss, frustration, sadness and pain as she continually tried to access the appropriate support required for her daughter during more than 40 years of parenting (Babb, 2007). Babb related explicitly to the concept of shattered dreams (Bowman, 2001, 2004), where a loss (e.g. childlessness, the role of family and parenting) forces individuals to create new dreams in keeping with their current situations.

As previously stated, generally, as people age, their experiences of loss will increase. The older one gets, the more one is likely to experience death, as family and friends confront ill health, the associated complexities and subsequent impact. Loss and death are omnipresent, since "*death is inevitable and loss universal*" (Kellehear, 2005, p. 16), yet there is limited research around how people with intellectual disabilities are supported in death and dying and how death is managed from a professional caring perspective (Todd and Blackman, 2005). The losses across the life cycle may be entirely different for a person with an intellectual disability.

Loss and intellectual disability

People with intellectual disabilities are more likely to "*... function on a developmental level that is inconsistent with their chronological age*" (Lavin, 2002, p. 314), and carry a history of marginalisation, devaluation and stigma. In an evolving society where great esteem is placed on good health, intelligence, independence, wealth, youth and perfection (Blackman, 2003), being different is usually negatively perceived. Many people with intellectual disabilities still have limited choices and restricted lifestyles, often living with people they have no choice about being with, as illustrated in the classification of care by Nolan et al (1994) (Table 27.1).

Although much care is provided *in the community* and *by the community*, care *for the community*, where people with intellectual disabilities are identified as *contributing to* communities, is increasingly apparent but still remains the exception rather than the rule. A general pattern of life cycle for a person with an intellectual disability may involve moving to up to a dozen

TABLE 27.1 Classification of care (Nolan et al, 1994)	
Perceptions of care outside of hospital	**Perceptions of care inside of hospital**
Care outside the community.	In long-stay hospitals
Care in the community by professionals and paid unqualified people	All care provided in small community. Own homes.
Care by the community.	Care by unpaid family carers and volunteers in local communities. This care mirrors a commitment to ordinary or valued lifestyles.
Care for the community.	Care that is committed to the support of family carers. It also acknowledges that the person with an intellectual disability can contribute to the community.

different care facilities in a lifetime; meeting numerous carers and support staff; changing carers too numerous to mention; having the support of a range of other care professionals to meet various individual (and sometimes complex) needs; and having reams of paperwork and various assessments completed about them by numerous professionals and stored indefinitely. The losses associated with this lifestyle are rarely recognised; barely acknowledged; and are inconsistently supported.

Death never occurs in a vacuum, but from within a social context, and varied social contexts can often impact upon the nature and circumstances surrounding the death itself (Oliviére and Monroe, 2004), and the subsequent effects upon those survivors left behind. Loss can impact upon an individual in a physical, emotional, psychosocial and/or spiritual way (Worden, 2009). Considering the potential for pain associated with loss, some might think "... loss is hard to bear, but is it worse than having nothing to lose?" (Cordy, 2004, p. 258). Yet having a life without companionship, connections, bonds and ties would be perceived to be a barren and unfulfilled existence for many.

Death remains shrouded in mystery, and is often misunderstood (Kellehear, 2005), particularly if you are part of a marginalised group that has historically been viewed as 'different' from the rest of society. In this situation, people may lack the voice to be heard and are often overlooked when psychosocial/emotional support needs are concerned. They may be ignored when issues around loss, dying, death and grief arise, described as disenfranchised death (Read, 2006) and grief (Doka, 1989, 2002). Disenfranchised death (see Box 27.4) means that the autonomy of the dying person is not recognised; the pending death is not recognised or legitimised; and the person's 'rights to know' are overlooked (Read, 2006).

Similarly, marginalised groups (i.e. people with mental health challenges; people diagnosed with HIV and AIDS;

 **BOX 27.4   Disenfranchised death·
(Read, 2006, p. 96)**

... death that is not openly acknowledged with the dying person, where the dying person is socially excluded from the process of dying and deliberately excluded from the decision-making process surrounding the terminal illness.

 BOX 27.5   Disenfranchised grief

... the grief that persons experience when they incur a loss that cannot be openly acknowledged, publicly mourned, or socially supported ...
- The relationship is not recognised.
- The loss is not recognised.
- The griever is not recognised (Doka, 1989).
- The circumstances surrounding the death.
- The ways that individuals grieve (Doka, 2002).

READER ACTIVITY 27.4

Having reflected on the variety of losses experienced by people with intellectual disabilities in their lifetime, you might consider how loss is a focus in the lives of people you care for and how many of these losses are acknowledged or overlooked.

You might think about how you could pro-actively talk about loss to people with intellectual disabilities, by making use of naturally occurring events on the television or other media.

and people with intellectual disabilities), may struggle to have their grief needs acknowledged or responded to in a constructive way and experience disenfranchised grief (Box 27.5). Addressing disenfranchised grief involves acknowledging the loss and legitimising the emotional pain associated with that loss; active listening; empathy; and exploring meaning making (finding benefits or giving purpose) throughout the lived experiences of grief (Doka, 2002). Loss is universal and can have a profound impact on individuals throughout life.

BEREAVEMENT AND PEOPLE WITH INTELLECTUAL DISABILITIES

People with intellectual disabilities do experience grief (Hollins and Esterhuyzen, 1997; Oswin, 2000), but the impact of grief is varied and often complex (Conboy-Hill, 1992; MacHale and Carey, 2002). While "*response to bereavement by adults with learning disabilities [sic] is similar in type, though not in expression, to that of the general population*" (Bonell-Pascual et al, 1999, p. 348), they are often neither encouraged nor expected to grieve or express their grief in any way. Subsequently, grief work may be delayed, sometimes indefinitely, as the person is exposed to other successive losses. For the person with an intellectual disability, as time passes, the likelihood of their loss being remembered by carers is reduced, and in some cases not recorded at all. Some bereaved individuals with an intellectual disability may struggle to accept the reality of the loss and accepting the finality and irreversibility of loss may take many months or years, particularly if the person does not receive appropriate support around the time of the death.

Challenges to effective support

The emotional needs of people with intellectual disabilities are often neglected (Arthur, 2003), perhaps because of varied perceptions of their ability to grieve (Elliott, 1995; McLoughlin, 1986; Read, 2007), overprotectiveness by carers (Deutsch, 1985), or carers' feelings of fear, inadequacy and uncertainty (Emerson, 1976; Thurm, 1989). Conboy-Hill recognised the role of carers as she argued that:

> "…failure to recognise the impact of loss on people with learning {sic} disabilities arises from our need to see such people as lacking in effective emotional apparatus … this conveniently feeds our own need to avoid discussion of pain and grief and so the cycle of ignorance and inaction has been perpetuated."
>
> ### Conboy-Hill, 1992, p. 151

People with intellectual disabilities are vulnerable as many have an external locus of control, remaining reliant on so many people (often professional carers) for so much, and they are actively excluded from responding to death and dying (Read and Elliott, 2003). There appears to be an increasing factorial effect with people with intellectual disabilities that precludes active involvement in the sad business of death, where the more complex the needs, such as having communication impairment or behaviours that may challenge services, the less likelihood they have of being involved (Read and Elliott, 2003).

Such issues potentially make grief support complicated or hard to access, and many people with intellectual disabilities may not receive the support they need following bereavement, and consequently many experience disenfranchised grief (Doka, 1989, 2002) (see Box 27.5). Those experiencing disenfranchised grief may have intensified emotional responses to loss (feelings of anger, guilt or powerlessness); they may experience ambivalent relationships and concurrent life crises, which can complicate grief, or the factors that facilitate mourning may be missing (e.g. grief rituals). Ultimately, the very nature of disenfranchised

grief precludes social support, at the time when such support is seen as crucial (Doka, 2002).

READER ACTIVITY 27.5

Case study 27.1 in the online resource (Jacky's story of loss: part one) describes the personal experiences of a woman with an intellectual disability who, following the loss of her son due to a termination, experienced multiple losses.

Read through the case study and consider the losses that Jacky experienced as a result of having her termination.

Responding to loss and grief

A continuum of bereavement support is a useful framework to provide holistic support and to minimise disenfranchised grief (Read, 2005; Read and Elliott, 2007). This involves a broad range of support strategies that are available at many different levels and subsequently provided by a range of different people (see Figure 27.1). These strategies range from general preparation *before* loss or death has occurred (education) to portraying loss and death as *natural life events* (participation) or providing consistent support *after* the death has occurred (facilitation) and identifying the need for *specific help* (therapeutic interventions). Using every day, natural opportunities to talk, explore and express feelings in a broader context, rather than relying on a reactive approach, involves developing and using a range of resources (e.g. Hollins and Sireling, 2004a,b) and utilising a variety of media to communicate effectively, including pictures, books, videos and DVDs, television and radio. While such resources can help in various constructive ways, there is no empirical evidence of what works and why, with respect to bereaved people with intellectual disabilities.

Read Case study 27.2 (Jacky's story of loss: part 2) in the online resource to see how Jacky was helped to deal with her loss.

Story telling

Jennings (2005) reminds us of the importance of storytelling highlighting their healing nature (through listening); explaining how different spaces (as in different places) are conducive to different story telling opportunities. Consequently, the stories that you hear in a doctor's waiting room may be significantly different from the stories in a maternity waiting room, or while waiting at a train station or being stranded in an airport lounge. Stories are concrete and can be permanent when written down using paper or on a computer. Recounting stories in grief work can be particularly helpful with people with intellectual disabilities, and whether as life story or memory work, can be cathartic in the bereavement context (Read and Bowler, 2007). Many people with intellectual disabilities lack personal heritage and history, and stories of life (and death) can help to construct a meaningful, visible and valued identity for the person once well-constructed (see also Chapter 2). Such stories can also be shared, with consent, by others and help to accentuate the uniqueness of the individual and their life experiences.

READER ACTIVITY 27.6

Think about how you might help a person with an intellectual disability to attend the funeral of a loved one.

What might you do to prepare them for this event?
How might you involve them in the funeral rituals?

No one prescription fits all bereaved people, so in answer to the questions in Reader activity 27.6, there are a range of helpful activities that can be very useful to some people, but unhelpful to others. However, you might have considered finding out what previous experience the person had had of death, dying and funerals. You need to establish what the person understands about death. This might be done with simple questions or using books from the *Books Beyond Words* series or seeking the available strategies from the *Talking End of Life…with People with Intellectual Disability (TEL)* website resource (Talking End, of Life, 2018). Checking previous case notes and life story books might be a way of ascertaining this involvement. Exploring if the person wants to attend the funeral is crucial to this work and no one should ever be forced to attend if they choose not to, despite what other people believe is the right and proper thing to do. You might use a video to explain the difference between burial and cremation. Taking the person to where the service will take place before the day of the funeral might help to allay fears and anxieties. With regards to active involvement, the bereaved person could be encouraged to select special clothes to go to the funeral and perhaps personally selecting flowers to send.

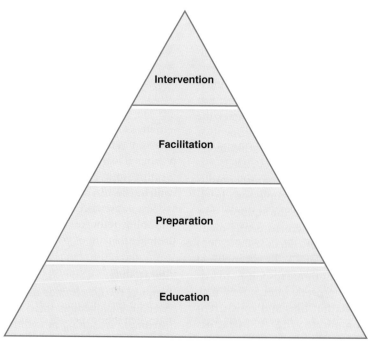

Figure 27.1 A continuum of bereavement support

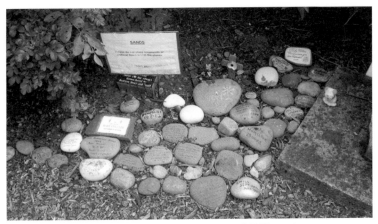

Figure 27.2 Decorated pebbles in SAND garden

The person might want to write or draw something that could be put with the flowers. They could choose who they would like to go with them (e.g. a special staff member or friend). They might even want to say a few words themselves at the ceremony, and you can help them to prepare for this in advance. Taking pictures after the ceremony of the flowers or place of rest might help to affirm the death to the bereaved person and can be really useful afterwards when constructing life story or memory books with the bereaved person.

Endings are really important in loss work. As Jacky recalled: "When I had the abortion I never had a chance to say goodbye to my baby". Her counsellor explored with her what sort of ending might help her so long after the loss. Jacky said that she wanted somewhere that she could visit and take flowers when she felt like it (see Case study 27.3 Jacky's story of loss: Part 3 in the online resource).

Rituals that recognise and commemorate loved ones are an important part of grief work as they can act as strong therapeutic tools. They can involve funerals; rituals of continuity, transition, reconciliation and rituals of affirmation (Doka, 2002). Rituals play an important role in the lives of people with intellectual disabilities too, as Jacky described in her story (see Case study 27.3 Jacky's story of loss: Part 3 in the online resource).

The National Memorial Arboretum at Alrewas, Staffordshire, UK, remains a poignant reminder of the number of people who have died (and continue to die) in the armed forces and other professional groups. There are many pebbles in the SANDS garden, all decorated differently and personally, in memory of lost children (see Figure 27.2). Jacky recognised the need to

say goodbye so that she could move on, and she chose a memorial that she could visit in the future and would always know where her pebble would be. The memory of her son would live on forever. However, she would never have independently selected this ending if someone hadn't known about the memorial and was able to offer the suggestion as one of several potential endings in this case.

Case studies provide a rich source of data that can illustrate phenomena within their own particular contexts. Yin (2009) defines them as

> "...an empirical study that investigates a contemporary phenomenon in depth and within its real-life context, specifically when the boundaries between phenomenon and context are not clearly evident.
>
> **Yin, 2009, p. 18**

The case study within this chapter, Jacky's story of loss, has been used to illustrate the complexities of peri-natal loss within an intellectual disability context, resulting in disenfranchised grief (Doka, 2002). While counselling and support can never undo the pain and sadness experienced, it can help individuals to accept the reality of the loss; explore the feelings surrounding the loss and pain of grief; to reflect on, and adjust to, a world that is different; and to emotionally relocate the dead person, integrating their memory into the world of the living (Worden, 2009). Such approaches can also help the person to learn how to cope with loss so that when they experience loss again in the future, they are better placed to deal with it. The case study illustrates well the importance of ritual when facilitating grief work with people with intellectual disabilities; demonstrating the reality of practice and constructively informing the link between theory and meaningful practice.

CONCLUSION AND RECOMMENDATIONS

This chapter has explored and addressed issues around end of life, loss and bereavement for one particular marginalised population. The authors have deliberately woven the issues inherent to effective support for people with intellectual disabilities within the general grief literature, since people with intellectual disabilities have more similarities *to us* than differences *from us* (Read, 2006), particularly in relation to death and dying.

It is critical to recognise that for carers, engaging with people with intellectual disabilities about the end of life is undeniably difficult and complex. This, however, does not abrogate any responsibility to do so. People with intellectual disabilities have a human right to learn about death, plan for it if they wish to, care for their dying loved ones, and engage with their own, and others, death.

More research is needed around where and how people with intellectual disabilities die, and whether professional carers are fully prepared with the holistic nature of end-of-life care and the type of skills and support needed. Practical issues surrounding accessibility (e.g. to hospice care) needs critically exploring, to ensure the key factors to fully accessible services are recognised. The Palliative Care for People with a Learning Disability network is a useful resource for carers and has a website incorporating resources and research around end-of-life care (PCPLD, 2020).

Similarly, many research questions remain unanswered in the loss and bereavement arena involving people with intellectual disabilities. While there are a variety of bereavement resources available, we have no evidence as to which are useful and which bereavement interventions work better than others. Sensitively supporting people with more severe, complex needs remains challenging. Collaborative education across generic and specialist palliative services (involving both intellectual disability and palliative care professionals) is the key to effective palliative care and support (Read, 2006) and should include focused discussions around topics such as communication; management of conditions; and knowledge of intellectual disability itself (Cartlidge and Read, 2010). Many of the skills required

 BOX 27.6 Learning from experiences of people with intellectual disabilities

If palliative care services get it right for people with an intellectual disability, then they are highly likely to get it right for all of their patients (Cartlidge and Read, 2010, p. 98).

to support a person with an intellectual disability can be translated across and generalised to other vulnerable groups (see Box 27.6). Subsequently, there is much learning still to be done.

Acknowledgement

We would like to thank Jacky for sharing her story and giving permission for it to be used within this chapter and the accompanying online resource.

REFERENCES

Arthur, A. R. (2003). The emotional lives of people with learning disability. *British Journal of Learning Disabilities*, *31*, 25–30.

Attig, T. (1996). *How we grieve: relearning the world*. New York: Oxford University Press.

Babb, C. (2007). Living with shattered dreams: a parent's perspective of living with learning disability. *Learning Disability Practice*, *10*(5), 14–18.

Bekkema, N., de Veer, A. J. E., Wagemans, A. M. A., et al. (2014). Decision making about medical interventions in the end-of- life care of people with intellectual disabilities: A national survey of the considerations and beliefs of GPs, ID physicians and care staff. *Patient Education and Counseling*, *96*, 204–209.

Blackman, N. (2003). *Loss and learning disability*. London: Worth.

Bonell-Pascual, E., Huline-Dickens, S., Hollins, S., et al. (1999). Bereavement and grief in adults with learning disabilities. *British Journal of Psychiatry*, *175*, 348–350.

Bowman, T. (2001). *Finding hope when dreams have shattered*. Minneapolis: Bowman.

Bowman, T. (2004). *Loss of dreams: a special kind of grief* (8th ed.). Minneapolis: Bowman.

Brown, H., Burns, S., & Flynn, M. (2003). Please don't let it happen on my shift! Supporting staff who are caring for people with learning disabilities who are dying. *Tizard Learning Disability Review*, *8*(2), 32–41.

Bruce, E. J., & Schultz, C. L. (2001). *Nonfinite loss and grief: a psychoeducational approach*. London: Jessica Kingsley.

Cartlidge, D., & Read, S. (2010). Exploring the needs of hospice staff supporting people with an intellectual disability: a UK perspective. *International Journal of Palliative Nursing*, 16(2), 93–98.

Conboy-Hill, S. (1992). Grief, loss and people with learning disabilities. In A. Waitman & S. Conboy-Hill (Eds.), *Psychotherapy and mental handicap* (pp. 150–170). London: Sage.

Cordy, M. (2004). *The venus conspiracy*. London: Corgi.

Department of Health. (2008). *End of life care strategy: promoting high quality care for all adults at the end of life*. London: HMSO. Available at: https://www.gov.uk/ government/publications/end-of-life-care-strategy-promoting-high-quality-carefor-adults-at-the-end-of-their-life. [Accessed 28 December 2020].

Doka, K. J. (1989). *Disenfranchised grief: recognising hidden sorrow*. Toronto: Lexington Books.

Doka, K. J. (2002). In K. J. Doka (Ed.), *Disenfranchised grief: new directions, challenges and strategies for practice 2002*. IL: Research Press.

Deutsch, H. (1985). Grief counselling with mentally retarded clients. *Psychiatric Aspects of Mental Retardation Reviews*, 4(5), 17–20.

Emerson, E. (2009). *Estimating future numbers of adults with profound multiple learning disabilities in England*. Lancaster: CeDR.

Emerson, P. (1976). Covert grief reactions in mentally retarded clients. *Mental Retardation*, 15(6), 27–29.

Elliott, D. (1995). Helping people with learning disabilities to handle grief. *Nursing Times*, 91(43), 27–29.

Elliott, D. (2003). Loss and bereavement. In M. Jukes & M. Bollard (Eds.), *Contemporary learning disability practice*. Wiltshire: Quay Books.

Emerson, E. B., & Baines, S. (2011). Health inequalities and people with learning disabilities in the UK. *Tizard Learning Disability Review*, 16(1), 42–48.

Emerson, E. B., Hatton, C. R., Baines, S. M. J., et al. (2016). The physical health of British adults with intellectual disability: cross sectional study. *International Journal for Equity in Health*, 15(9), 11.

Frey, M. (2006). Special needs require special measures. *Community Living*, 20(2), 22–23.

Foo, B., Wiese, M. Y., Curryer, B., et al. (2021). Australian specialist palliative care staff's experiences of talking to people with intellectual disability about their dying and death. *A thematic analysis of in-depth interviews Palliative Medicine*, 35(4), 738–749.

Foundation for People with Learning Disabilities. (2002). *Today and tomorrow – the report of the Growing Older with Learning Disabilities programme*. London: Foundation for People with Learning Disabilities.

Hess, P. (1980). *Nursing and the concept of loss*. London: John Wiley & Sons.

Holland, A. J. (2018). Ageing and learning disability. *British Journal of Psychiatry*, 176(1), 26–31.

Hollins, S., & Esterhuyzen, A. (1997). Bereavement and grief in adults with learning disabilities. *British Journal of Psychiatry*, 170, 497–501.

Hollins, S., & Sireling, L. (2004a). *When dad died*. London: St George's Hospital Medical School.

Hollins, S., & Sireling, L. (2004b). *When mum died*. London: St George's Hospital Medical School.

Jenkins, R. (2005). Older people with learning disabilities: part 2. Accessing care and the implications for nursing practice. *Nursing Older People*, 17(1), 32–35.

Jennings, S. (2005). *Creative storytelling with adults at risk*. Bicester: Speechmark.

Kellehear, A. (2005). *Compassionate cities: public health and end of life care*. London: Routledge.

Kirkendall, A., Linton, K., & Farris, S. (2017). Intellectual disabilities and decision making at the end of life: a literature review. *Journal of Applied Research in Intellectual Disabilities*, 30(6), 982–994.

Klass, D., et al. (1996). In D. Klass, P. R. Silverman, & S. L. Nickman (Eds.), *Continuing bonds: new understandings of grief*. Washington, DC: Taylor & Francis.

Lavin, C. (2002). Disenfranchised grief and individuals with developmental disabilities. In K. J. Doka (Ed.), *Disenfranchised grief: new directions, challenges and strategies for practice* (pp. 307–322). IL: Research Press.

Lauer, E., & McCallion, P. (2015). Mortality of people with intellectual and developmental disabilities from select US state disability service systems and medical claims data. *Journal of Applied Research in Intellectual Disabilities*, 28(5), 394–405.

Li, C. W., Wong, Y. C., Lo, Y. M., et al. (2018). Embracing the setting sun: provision of palliative care via a collaborative model between hospital and community for patients with intellectual disabilities. *Annals of Palliative Medicine*, 7(3), 365–367.

Lord, A. J., Field, S., & Smith, I. C. (2017). The experiences of staff who support people with intellectual disability on issues about death, dying and bereavement: a metasynthesis. *Journal of Applied Research in Intellectual Disabilities*, 30(6), 1007–1021.

MacHale, R., & Carey, S. (2002). An investigation into the effects of bereavement on mental health and challenging behaviour in adults with learning disability. *British Journal of Learning Disabilities*, 30, 113–117.

Machin, L. (1998). *Looking at loss: bereavement counselling pack* (2nd ed.). Brighton: Pavilion.

Machin, L. (2010). *Working with loss and grief: a new model for practitioners.* London: Sage.

Machin, L. (2014). Loss and resilience. In S. Read (Ed.), *Supporting people with intellectual disabilities experiencing loss and bereavement: theory and compassionate practice.* London: Jessica Kingsley.

Macmillan Cancer Support. (2003). *Barriers to accessing cancer services. The report of the Barriers to Access Project Steering Group (Nov. 2002–2003).* London: Macmillan Cancer Support.

McLoughlin, I. J. (1986). Care of the dying: bereavement in the mentally handicapped. *British Journal of Hospital Medicine,* 256–260.

McNutt, B., & Yakushko, O. (2013). Disenfranchised grief among lesbian and gay bereaved individuals. *Journal of LBGT Issues in Counselling,* 7(1), 87–116.

Mencap. (2004). *Treat me right!* London: Mencap.

Mencap. (2007). *Death by indifference.* London: Mencap.

National Council for Palliative Care. (2009). *End of life care manifesto for 2010.* London: The National Council for Palliative Care.

National Institute for health and Care Excellence (NICE). (2018). *Care and support of people growing older with learning disabilities.* London: NICE.

Nolan, M., Grant, G., Caldock, K., et al. (1994). *A framework for assessing the needs of family carers: a multidisciplinary guide.* Bangor: University of Wales.

Oliviére, D., & Monroe, B. (2004). *Death, dying and social differences.* Oxford: Oxford University Press.

Oswin, M. (2000). *Am I allowed to cry?* (2nd ed.). London: Souvenir Press.

Palliative Care for People with Learning Disabilities. (2020). Available at: www.pcpld.org. [Accessed 17 August 2020].

Parkes, M. (2014). Living with shattered dreams: a parent's perspective. In S. Read (Ed.), *2014 Supporting people with intellectual disabilities experiencing loss and bereavement: theory and compassionate practice.* London: Jessica Kingsley.

Prasher, V. P., & Chung, M. C. (1996). Causes of age-related decline in adaptive behavior of adults with Down syndrome: differential diagnoses of dementia. *American Journal of Mental Retardation,* 101, 175–183.

Public Health England. (2019). *Classification of place of death: a technical bulletin from the National End of Life Care Intelligence Network.* London: Public Health England. Available at: https://fingertips.phe.org.uk/profile/end-of-life. [Accessed 27 December 2020].

Prasher, V. P. (2005). *Alzheimer's disease and dementia in Down syndrome and intellectual disabilities.* Oxford: Radcliffe.

Read, S. (2005). Loss, bereavement and learning disability: providing a continuum of support. *Learning Disability Practice,* 8(1), 31–37.

Read, S. (2007). *Bereavement counselling for people with learning disabilities.* London: Quay Books.

Read, S. (2006). *Palliative care for people with learning disabilities.* London: Quay Books.

Read, S. (2008). Loss, bereavement, counselling and support: an intellectual disability perspective. *Grief Matters: The Australian Journal of Grief and Bereavement,* 11(2), 54–59.

Read, S., & Bowler, C. (2007). Life story work and bereavement: shared reflections on its usefulness. *Learning Disability Practice,* 10(4), 10–15.

Read, S., & Elliot, D. (2003). Death and learning disability: a vulnerability perspective. *Journal of Adult Protection,* 5(1), 5–14.

Read, S., & Elliott, D. (2007). Exploring a continuum of support for bereaved people with intellectual disabilities. *Journal of Intellectual Disabilities,* 11(2), 167–182.

Read, S., & Latham, D. (2009). Bowel cancer screening: involving people with learning disabilities. *Journal of Gastrointestinal Nursing,* 7(7), 10–16.

Read, S., & Morris, H. (2009). *Living and dying with dignity: the best practice guide for end of life care for people with learning disability.* London: Mencap.

Read, S., & Thompson-Hill, J. (2009). Palliative care nursing in relation to people with intellectual disabilities. *International Journal of Palliative Nursing,* 15(5), 226–232.

Read, S. (2014). Loss in the caring context. In S. Read (Ed.), *2014 Supporting people with intellectual disabilities experiencing loss and bereavement: theory and compassionate practice.* London: Jessica Kingsley.

Sinclair, P. (2007). *Rethinking palliative care: a social role valorisation approach.* Bristol: Policy Press.

Stancliffe, R. J., Wiese, M. Y., Read, S., et al. (2016). Knowing, planning for and fearing death: Do adults with intellectual disability and disability staff differ? *Research in Developmental Disabilities,* 49(50), 47–59.

Stancliffe, R. J., Wiese, M. Y., Read, S., et al. (2021). Does talking about the end of life with adults with intellectual disability cause emotional discomfort or psychological harm? *Journal of Applied Research in Intellectual Disabilities,* 34(2), 649–669.

Talking end of life…with people with intellectual disability (TEL). (2018). *A toolkit for disability support professionals to assist them to help people with intellectual disability understand dying and death.* Available at: https://www.caresearch.com.au/TEL/. [Accessed 27 December 2020].

Thurm, A. (1989). I've lost a good friend. *Nursing Times,* 85(32), 66–68.

Thompson, N. (2002). *Loss and grief: a guide for human services practitioners.* London: Palgrave Macmillan.

Todd, S., & Blackman, N. (2005). Reconnecting death and intellectual disability. *European Journal of Palliative Care*, *12*(1), 32–34.

Todd, S., Brandford, S. W. R., & Shear, J. B. J. (2019). Place of death of people with intellectual disabilities: an exploratory study of death and dying within community disability service settings. *Journal of Intellectual Disabilities*. https://doi.org/10.1177/1744629519886758.

Together for short lives. (2020). Available at: https://www. togetherforshortlives.org.uk. [Accessed 27 December 2020].

Tuffrey-Wijne, I., & Davies, J. (2007). This is my story: I've got cancer. 'The Veronica Project': an ethnographic study of experiences of people with learning disabilities who have cancer. *British Journal of Learning Disabilities*, *35*, 7–11.

Tuffrey-Wijne, I., Hogg, J., & Curfs, L. (2007). End of life and palliative care for people with intellectual disabilities who have cancer or other life-limiting illness: a review of the literature and available resources. *Journal of Applied Research in Intellectual Disabilities*, *20*(4), 331–344.

Virdun, C., Luckett, T., Davidson, P. M., et al. (2015). Dying in the hospital setting: a systematic review of quantitative studies identifying the elements of end-of-life care that patients and their families rank as being most important. *Palliative Medicine* (9), 774–796.

Wiese, M., Stancliffe, R. J., Balandin, S., et al. (2012). End-of-life care and dying: issues raised by staff supporting older people with intellectual disability in community living services. *Journal of Applied Research in Intellectual Disabilities*, *25*(6), 571–583.

Wiese, M., Dew, A., Stancliffe, R. J., et al. (2013). 'If and when?': experiences of community living staff engaging older people with intellectual disability to know about dying. *Journal of Intellectual Disability Research*, *57*(10), 980–992.

Wiese, M., Stancliffe, R. J., Read, S., et al. (2015). Learning about dying, death and end-of-life planning: current issues informing future actions. *Journal of Intellectual & Developmental Disability*, *40*(2), 230–235.

Wiese, M. Y., Stancliffe, R. J., Wilson, N. J., et al. (2019a). Multidisciplinary palliative care team experiences when caring for people with intellectual disability who are dying [Abstract]. *Journal of Intellectual Disability Research*, *63*(7), 648.

Wiese, M. Y., Stancliffe, R., Durvasula, S., et al. (2019b). The place of death and associated variables for clients in out-of-home care in New South Wales Australia [Abstract]. *Journal of Intellectual Disability Research*, *63*(7), 648.

Worden, J. W. (2009). *Grief and grief therapy: a handbook for mental health practitioners* (4th ed.). London: Routledge.

World Health Organization. (2018). *Integrating palliative care and symptom relief into primary health care: a WHO guide for planners, implementers and managers.* Available at: https://apps.who.int/iris/bitstream/han dle/10665/274559/9789241514477-eng.pdf?ua=1. [Accessed 29 December 2020].

World Health Organization. (2020). *Palliative care. Available at:* https://www.who.int/news-room/fact-sheets/detail/ palliative-care. [Accessed 28 December 2020].

Yin, R. K. (2009). *Case study research: design and methods* (4th ed.). London: Sage.

Zaal-Schuller, I. H., Willems, D. L., Ewals, F. V. P. M., et al. (2018). Considering quality of life in end-of-life decisions for severely disabled children. *Research in Developmental Disabilities*, *73*, 67–75.

Note: Page numbers followed by 'f' indicate figures, those followed by 't' indicate tables, those followed by 'b' indicate boxes and those followed by 'elt' indicate electronic resource table.